# Essential Concepts for
# Healthy Living

### Sixth Edition

**Sandra Alters, PhD**
**Wendy Schiff, MS, RD**

JONES & BARTLETT
LEARNING

*World Headquarters*
Jones & Bartlett Learning
5 Wall Street
Burlington, MA 01803
978-443-5000
info@jblearning.com
www.jblearning.com

Jones & Bartlett Learning books and products are available through most bookstores and online booksellers. To contact Jones & Bartlett Learning directly, call 800-832-0034, fax 978-443-8000, or visit our website, www.jblearning.com.

Copyright © 2013 by Jones & Bartlett Learning, LLC, an Ascend Learning Company

**Production Credits**

Chief Executive Officer: Ty Field
President: James Homer
SVP, Editor-in-Chief: Michael Johnson
SVP, Chief Technology Officer: Dean Fossella
SVP, Chief Marketing Officer: Alison M. Pendergast
Publisher: Cathleen Sether
Executive Editor: Shoshanna Goldberg
Editorial Assistant: Agnes Burt
Editorial Assistant: Sean Coombs
Production Manager: Julie Champagne Bolduc
Senior Production Editor: Renée Sekerak

Production Editor: Angela Dooley
Marketing Manager: Jody Yeskey
V.P., Manufacturing and Inventory Control: Therese Connell
Composition: Publishers' Design and Production Services, Inc.
Cover Design: Kristin E. Parker
Photo Researcher: Sarah Cebulski
Cover Image: © iStockphoto/Thinkstock
Printing and Binding: Courier Companies
Cover Printing: Courier Companies

**To order this product, use ISBN: 978-1-4496-5193-0.**

Some images in this book feature models. These models do not necessarily endorse, represent, or participate in the activities represented in the images.

**Library of Congress Cataloging-in-Publication Data**
Alters, Sandra.
  Essential concepts for healthy living / Sandra Alters, Wendy Schiff. -- 6th ed.
      p. cm.
  Includes bibliographical references and index.
  ISBN 978-1-4496-3062-1 (alk. paper)
1.   Health.   I. Schiff, Wendy. II. Title.
  RA776.5.A596 2013
  613--dc23
        2011043128
6048

Printed in the United States of America
16  15  14  13     10  9  8  7  6  5  4

# Brief Contents

# Contents

## CHAPTER 8
## Alcohol and Tobacco 231

## CHAPTER 9
## Nutrition 271

## CHAPTER 10
## Body Weight and Its Management 311

# Features

## Across the Life Span

# *Essential Concepts for Healthy Living, Sixth Edition,*

## challenges students to think seriously about health-related information by using critical-thinking strategies.

What is critical thinking? What does a critical-thinking textbook do?

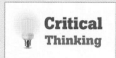

Critical thinking encompasses a variety of cognitive skills such as

- Synthesizing
- Analyzing
- Applying
- Evaluating

Throughout the textbook, a critical-thinking icon identifies features that focus specifically on these skills.

In the health sciences, critical-thinking skills are necessary to understand and evaluate health information as well as apply it to daily life. This book *teaches* critical-thinking skills that help students develop expertise in important cognitive functions:

- Differentiating between verifiable facts and value statements
- Distinguishing relevant information from irrelevant information
- Determining the factual accuracy of health claims
- Making responsible health-related decisions

To think critically, students need a solid foundation of personal health information. *Essential Concepts for Healthy Living* has been developed from the latest scientific and medical research, relying heavily on primary sources, which are cited in the text. Because understanding health involves understanding science, this text includes basic scientific information that relates to health and presents it in an easy-to-understand manner.

## New to the *Sixth Edition*

*Essential Concepts for Healthy Living, Sixth Edition*, continues to discuss major health topics, including the following:

- Genomics
- The 2010 Dietary Guidelines and the MyPlate food guide

- *Healthy People 2020*
- Updated discussion of extended cycle oral contraceptives
- Updated discussion of postmenopausal hormone therapy
- New information on antidrug vaccines, alcohol-related injury deaths in college students, and the rise in the incidence of stroke in young people
- Updated discussion on targeted cancer therapies
- New Analyzing Health-Related Information boxes about strategies to reduce college drinking, the link between tanning beds and an increased risk of melanoma, trans fat labeling, and Gardasil (the human papillomavirus vaccine) and anal cancer

The *Sixth Edition* also provides the most current statistical data on a comprehensive array of health and wellness topics and issues, including the latest information on:

- Healthcare costs
- Binge drinking
- Alternative medical therapies
- Mental illness and depression
- Sexually transmitted infections
- Physical activity and health
- Eating disorders
- Cervical and prostate cancer
- Drug use and abuse

In addition, the *Sixth Edition* contains a built-in critical-thinking workbook that allows students to assess and improve their health-related behaviors and attitudes. (See the Student Workbook at the end of this text for more information.)

*Essential Concepts for Healthy Living* focuses on teaching behavior change, personal decision making, and up-to-date personal health concepts. The critical-thinking approach encourages students to consider their own behaviors in light of the knowledge they are gaining. The pedagogical aids that appear in the chapters are described in the following pages.

The organization of ideas is an integral part of learning comprehension. The chapters are structured with a consistent format throughout the text. Each chapter begins and ends with a section that points out the key concepts and ties the information together.

# Chapter-Opening Pedagogy

Each chapter-opening spread shows students the organization of the chapter using a chapter overview and a list of the special boxed features. It also lists activities in the companion Student Workbook (included at the back of this text) and topics explored on the companion website, **go.jblearning.com/alters6e.**

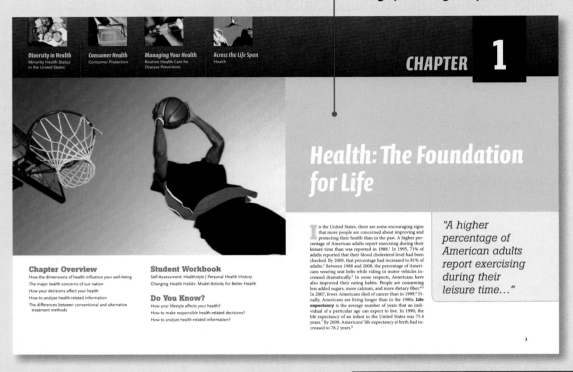

**Diversity in Health**
Minority Health Status in the United States

**Consumer Health**
Consumer Protection

**Managing Your Health**
Routine Health Care for Disease Prevention

**Across the Life Span**
Health

**CHAPTER 1**

## Health: The Foundation for Life

In the United States, there are some encouraging signs that more people are concerned about improving and protecting their health than in the past. A higher percentage of American adults report exercising during their leisure time than was reported in 1988.[1] In 1995, 71% of adults reported that their blood cholesterol level had been checked. By 2009, that percentage had increased to 81% of adults.[2] Between 1988 and 2008, the percentage of Americans wearing seat belts while riding in motor vehicles increased dramatically.[3] In some respects, Americans have also improved their eating habits. People are consuming less added sugars, more calcium, and more dietary fiber.[4,5] In 2007, fewer Americans died of cancer than in 1999.[6] Finally, Americans are living longer than in the 1980s. **Life expectancy** is the average number of years that an individual of a particular age can expect to live. In 1990, the life expectancy of an infant in the United States was 75.4 years.[7] By 2009, Americans' life expectancy at birth had increased to 78.2 years.[8]

*"A higher percentage of American adults report exercising during their leisure time..."*

**Chapter Overview**
How the dimensions of health influence your well-being
The major health concerns of our nation
How your decisions affect your health
How to analyze health-related information
The differences between conventional and alternative treatment methods

**Student Workbook**
Self-Assessment: Healthstyle | Personal Health History
Changing Health Habits: Model Activity for Better Health

**Do You Know?**
How your lifestyle affects your health?
How to make responsible health-related decisions?
How to analyze health-related information?

3

# Chapter Summaries

Research says that students learn how to identify the key ideas of stories in elementary school, but that they often have difficulty identifying key ideas in textbooks in their later schooling. Chapter summaries help students with this task. The chapter summaries follow the organization of the chapter.

## CHAPTER REVIEW

### Summary

Drugs are nonfood chemicals that alter the way a person thinks, feels, functions, or behaves. Many drugs have beneficial uses as medicines, but these substances can have serious negative effects on the health and well-being of people who use them improperly. People often abuse psychoactive, or mood-altering, drugs. Drug abuse contributes to numerous social problems that plague our society, such as crime, unemployment, and family violence and dissolution.

By interacting with nerve cells in the brain, psychoactive drugs influence perceptions, thought processes, feelings, and behaviors. Additionally, environmental factors can affect how people act and feel while under the influence of psychoactive drugs.

In most instances, the liver converts drugs into less dangerous compounds that can be eliminated in urine, feces, or exhaled breath. When the body is unable to detoxify and eliminate excessive amounts of a drug rapidly, the characteristic signs and symptoms of intoxication occur. Drug overdoses and polyabuse may produce serious, even deadly, effects.

In 2009, an estimated 21.8 million Americans older than 12 years of age were current illicit drug users. Rates of illicit drug use are especially high among teenagers and young adults. Initially, these individuals typically use alcohol, nicotine, or inhalants; they then may move on to marijuana. Some persons experiment with or use other illicit drugs after marijuana. In general, illicit drug use declines after age 20 years.

Dependency and addiction describe any habitual behavior that interferes with a person's health, work, and relationships. Drug dependence or addiction occurs when users develop a pattern of taking drugs that usually produces a compulsive need to use these substances, a tolerance for them, and withdrawal when they are discontinued. The type of substance taken, the social environment of the person, his or her personality, and genetics influence an individual's chances of developing a drug dependency.

Depressants such as alcohol and barbiturates slow the activity of the cerebral cortex, producing seda-

tive and hypnotic effects as well as drowsiness. Thus, people should not drive or operate machinery while under the influence of depressants. Misusing depressants can be deadly.

Stimulants enhance chemical activity in parts of the brain that influence emotions, sleep, attention, and learning. Caffeine is the most commonly consumed legal stimulant in this country. Stimulants such as Ritalin and cocaine have few medical uses. Cocaine is addictive and frequently abused. Methamphetamine use in U.S. college students has declined since 1999, from 3.3% in that year to 0.3% in 2009.

Opiates have important medical uses as sedatives, analgesics, and narcotics. When misused, opiates are highly addictive and extremely dangerous.

Marijuana, which contains THC as its major psychoactive compound, is the most widely used illicit drug in the United States. Although marijuana does not produce physiologic dependence, some people become compulsive users. Marijuana smoke contains numerous irritants that can damage the bronchial tubes and lungs.

Hallucinogens alter the brain's ability to perceive sensory information, producing abnormal and unreal sensations. In the United States, the most potent and commonly abused hallucinogens are mescaline, psilocybin, LSD, ketamine, and PCP. High doses of PCP and ketamine can be deadly.

Many common household products release toxic fumes that can produce psychoactive effects when inhaled. Teenagers may use inhalants before they move on to other psychoactive drugs. Inhalants can depress respiration, resulting in coma or death.

Designer drugs are made by altering the chemical structures of controlled substances. In some cases, these drug analogs are more toxic than the compounds from which they were derived.

The FDA regulates the production and marketing of all medications in the United States. Some health food and OTC products contain substances that are harmful or that produce psychoactive effects, especially when they are misused or abused.

**go.jblearning.com/alters6e**

226    **Chapter 7** Drug Use and Abuse

*Essential Concepts for Healthy Living, Sixth Edition,* encourages students to adopt healthier lifestyles, and the boxed features throughout the text recommend practical ways to do so.

## Healthy Living Practices

Unique to this text, these short lists of bulleted statements throughout the chapters summarize key points and concisely state concrete yet simple actions students can take to improve their own health.

## Managing Your Health

This feature contains short essays or lists of tips that focus on ways to live a healthier life.

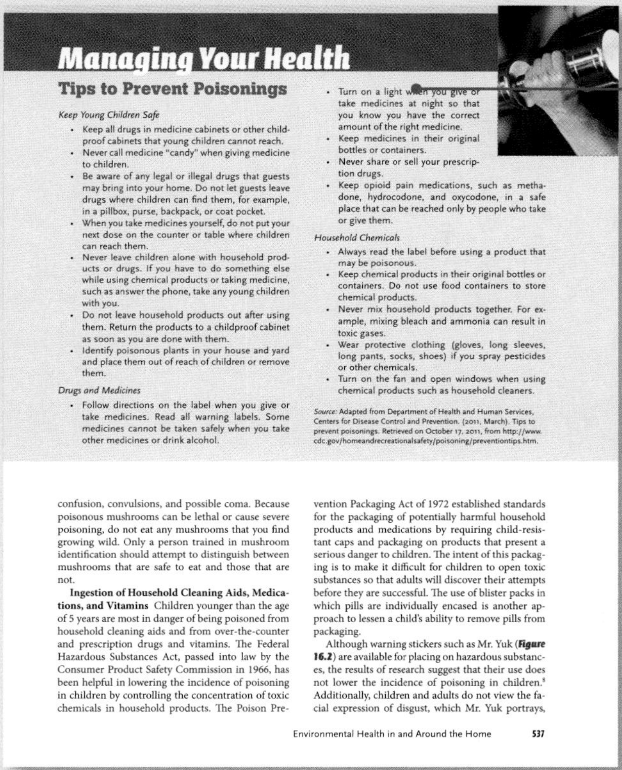

## Managing Your Health

### Tips to Prevent Poisonings

*Keep Young Children Safe*

- Keep all drugs in medicine cabinets or other childproof cabinets that young children cannot reach.
- Never call medicine "candy" when giving medicine to children.
- Be aware of any legal or illegal drugs that guests may bring into your home. Do not let guests leave drugs where children can find them, for example, in a pillbox, purse, backpack, or coat pocket.
- When you take medicines yourself, do not put your next dose on the counter or table where children can reach them.
- Never leave children alone with household products or drugs. If you have to do something else while using chemical products or taking medicine, such as answer the phone, take any young children with you.
- Do not leave household products out after using them. Return the products to a childproof cabinet as soon as you are done with them.
- Identify poisonous plants in your house and yard and place them out of reach of children or remove them.

*Drugs and Medicines*

- Follow directions on the label when you give or take medicines. Read all warning labels. Some medicines cannot be taken safely when you take other medicines or drink alcohol.
- Turn on a light when you give or take medicines at night so that you know you have the correct amount of the right medicine.
- Keep medicines in their original bottles or containers.
- Never share or sell your prescription drugs.
- Keep opioid pain medications, such as methadone, hydrocodone, and oxycodone, in a safe place that can be reached only by people who take or give them.

*Household Chemicals*

- Always read the label before using a product that may be poisonous.
- Keep chemical products in their original bottles or containers. Do not use food containers to store chemical products.
- Never mix household products together. For example, mixing bleach and ammonia can result in toxic gases.
- Wear protective clothing (gloves, long sleeves, long pants, socks, shoes) if you spray pesticides or other chemicals.
- Turn on the fan and open windows when using chemical products such as household cleaners.

*Source:* Adapted from Department of Health and Human Services, Centers for Disease Control and Prevention. (2011, March). Tips to prevent poisonings. Retrieved on October 17, 2011, from http://www.cdc.gov/homeandrecreationalsafety/poisoning/preventiontips.htm.

confusion, convulsions, and possible coma. Because poisonous mushrooms can be lethal or cause severe poisoning, do not eat any mushrooms that you find growing wild. Only a person trained in mushroom identification should attempt to distinguish between mushrooms that are safe to eat and those that are not.

**Ingestion of Household Cleaning Aids, Medications, and Vitamins** Children younger than the age of 5 years are most in danger of being poisoned from household cleaning aids and from over-the-counter and prescription drugs and vitamins. The Federal Hazardous Substances Act, passed into law by the Consumer Product Safety Commission in 1966, has been helpful in lowering the incidence of poisoning in children by controlling the concentration of toxic chemicals in household products. The Poison Prevention Packaging Act of 1972 established standards for the packaging of potentially harmful household products and medications by requiring child-resistant caps and packaging on products that present a serious danger to children. The intent of this packaging is to make it difficult for children to open toxic substances so that adults will discover their attempts before they are successful. The use of blister packs in which pills are individually encased is another approach to lessen a child's ability to remove pills from packaging.

Although warning stickers such as Mr. Yuk (**Figure 16.2**) are available for placing on hazardous substances, the results of research suggest that their use does not lower the incidence of poisoning in children.[8] Additionally, children and adults do not view the facial expression of disgust, which Mr. Yuk portrays,

Environmental Health in and Around the Home 537

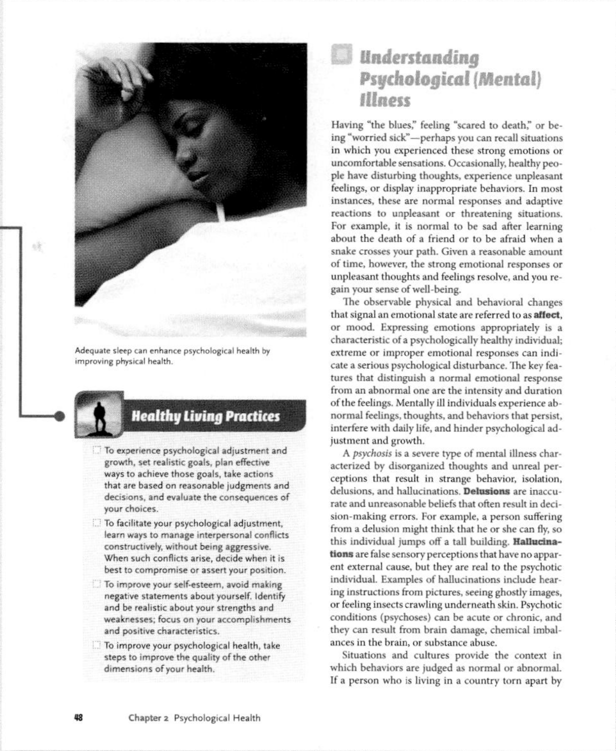

Adequate sleep can enhance psychological health by improving physical health.

### Healthy Living Practices

- To experience psychological adjustment and growth, set realistic goals, plan effective ways to achieve those goals, take actions that are based on reasonable judgments and decisions, and evaluate the consequences of your choices.
- To facilitate your psychological adjustment, learn ways to manage interpersonal conflicts constructively, without being aggressive. When such conflicts arise, decide when it is best to compromise or assert your position.
- To improve your self-esteem, avoid making negative statements about yourself. Identify and be realistic about your strengths and weaknesses; focus on your accomplishments and positive characteristics.
- To improve your psychological health, take steps to improve the quality of the other dimensions of your health.

### Understanding Psychological (Mental) Illness

Having "the blues," feeling "scared to death," or being "worried sick"—perhaps you can recall situations in which you experienced these strong emotions or uncomfortable sensations. Occasionally, healthy people have disturbing thoughts, experience unpleasant feelings, or display inappropriate behaviors. In most instances, these are normal responses and adaptive reactions to unpleasant or threatening situations. For example, it is normal to be sad after learning about the death of a friend or to be afraid when a snake crosses your path. Given a reasonable amount of time, however, the strong emotional responses or unpleasant thoughts and feelings resolve, and you regain your sense of well-being.

The observable physical and behavioral changes that signal an emotional state are referred to as **affect**, or mood. Expressing emotions appropriately is a characteristic of a psychologically healthy individual; extreme or improper emotional responses can indicate a serious psychological disturbance. The key features that distinguish a normal emotional response from an abnormal one are the intensity and duration of the feelings. Mentally ill individuals experience abnormal feelings, thoughts, and behaviors that persist, interfere with daily life, and hinder psychological adjustment and growth.

A *psychosis* is a severe type of mental illness characterized by disorganized thoughts and unreal perceptions that result in strange behavior, isolation, delusions, and hallucinations. **Delusions** are inaccurate and unreasonable beliefs that often result in decision-making errors. For example, a person suffering from a delusion might think that he or she can fly, so this individual jumps off a tall building. **Hallucinations** are false sensory perceptions that have no apparent external cause, but they are real to the psychotic individual. Examples of hallucinations include hearing instructions from pictures, seeing ghostly images, or feeling insects crawling underneath skin. Psychotic conditions (psychoses) can be acute or chronic, and they can result from brain damage, chemical imbalances in the brain, or substance abuse.

Situations and cultures provide the context in which behaviors are judged as normal or abnormal. If a person who is living in a country torn apart by

48 Chapter 2 Psychological Health

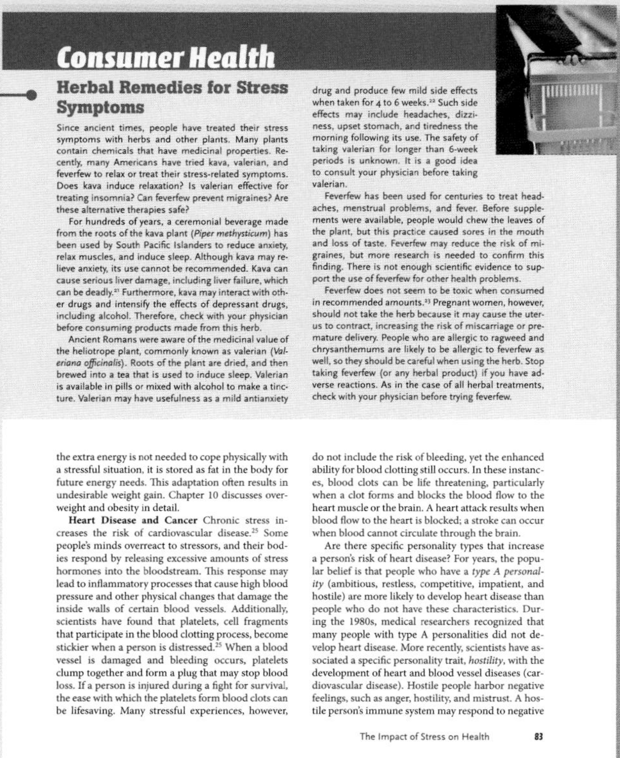

## Consumer Health

### Herbal Remedies for Stress Symptoms

Since ancient times, people have treated their stress symptoms with herbs and other plants. Many plants contain chemicals that have medicinal properties. Recently, many Americans have tried kava, valerian, and feverfew to relax or treat their stress-related symptoms. Does kava induce relaxation? Is valerian effective for treating insomnia? Can feverfew prevent migraines? Are these alternative therapies safe?

For hundreds of years, a ceremonial beverage made from the roots of the kava plant (*Piper methysticum*) has been used by South Pacific Islanders to reduce anxiety, relax muscles, and induce sleep. Although kava may relieve anxiety, its use cannot be recommended. Kava can cause serious liver damage, including liver failure, which can be deadly.[21] Furthermore, kava may interact with other drugs and intensify the effects of depressant drugs, including alcohol. Therefore, check with your physician before consuming products made from this herb.

Ancient Romans were aware of the medicinal value of the heliotrope plant, commonly known as valerian (*Valeriana officinalis*). Roots of the plant are dried, and then brewed into a tea that is used to induce sleep. Valerian is available in pills or mixed with alcohol to make a tincture. Valerian may have usefulness as a mild antianxiety drug and produce few mild side effects when taken for 4 to 6 weeks.[22] Such side effects may include headaches, dizziness, upset stomach, and tiredness the morning following its use. The safety of taking valerian for longer than 6-week periods is unknown. It is a good idea to consult your physician before taking valerian.

Feverfew has been used for centuries to treat headaches, menstrual problems, and fever. Before supplements were available, people would chew the leaves of the plant, but this practice caused sores in the mouth and loss of taste. Feverfew may reduce the risk of migraines, but more research is needed to confirm this finding. There is not enough scientific evidence to support the use of feverfew for other health problems.

Feverfew does not seem to be toxic when consumed in recommended amounts.[23] Pregnant women, however, should not take the herb because it may cause the uterus to contract, increasing the risk of miscarriage or premature delivery. People who are allergic to ragweed and chrysanthemums are likely to be allergic to feverfew as well, so they should be careful when using the herb. Stop taking feverfew (or any herbal product) if you have adverse reactions. As in the case of all herbal treatments, check with your physician before trying feverfew.

the extra energy is not needed to cope physically with a stressful situation, it is stored as fat in the body for future energy needs. This adaptation often results in undesirable weight gain. Chapter 10 discusses overweight and obesity in detail.

**Heart Disease and Cancer** Chronic stress increases the risk of cardiovascular disease.[25] Some people's minds overreact to stressors, and their bodies respond by releasing excessive amounts of stress hormones into the bloodstream. This response may lead to inflammatory processes that cause high blood pressure and other physical changes that damage the inside walls of certain blood vessels. Additionally, scientists have found that platelets, cell fragments that participate in the blood clotting process, become stickier when a person is distressed.[25] When a blood vessel is damaged and bleeding occurs, platelets clump together and form a plug that may stop blood loss. If a person is injured during a fight for survival, the ease with which the platelets form blood clots can be lifesaving. Many stressful experiences, however, do not include the risk of bleeding, yet the enhanced ability for blood clotting still occurs. In these instances, blood clots can be life threatening, particularly when a clot forms and blocks the blood flow to the heart muscle or the brain. A heart attack results when blood flow to the heart is blocked; a stroke can occur when blood cannot circulate through the brain.

Are there specific personality types that increase a person's risk of heart disease? For years, the popular belief is that people who have a *type A personality* (ambitious, restless, competitive, impatient, and hostile) are more likely to develop heart disease than people who do not have these characteristics. During the 1980s, medical researchers recognized that many people with type A personalities did not develop heart disease. More recently, scientists have associated a specific personality trait, *hostility*, with the development of heart and blood vessel diseases (cardiovascular disease). Hostile people harbor negative feelings, such as anger, hostility, and mistrust. A hostile person's immune system may respond to negative

The Impact of Stress on Health 83

## Consumer Health

These commentaries and tips provide practical information and suggestions to help students become more careful consumers of health-related goods and services. In addition to being highlighted in this feature, consumer topics are integrated throughout the book and are the subject of scrutiny in the Analyzing Health-Related Information activities.

The focus of education today is not simply to give students information, but to teach them how to acquire and evaluate information. Unlike other personal health textbooks, the critical-thinking features in this text teach students higher-order thinking skills and give them ways to practice these skills in every chapter.

## Diversity in Health

This feature cultivates an interest in and an appreciation for the health status and practices of various ethnic, cultural, and racial groups in the United States, as well as people around the world. Although the diversity essays focus specifically on multiculturalism, additional multicultural information is woven throughout the book.

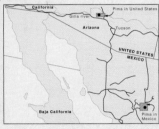

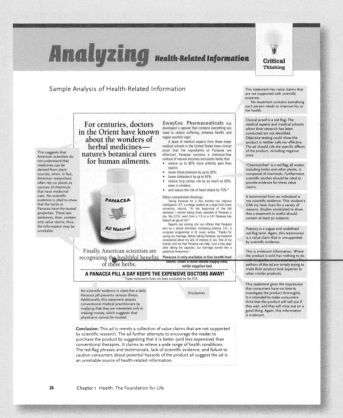

## Analyzing Health-Related Information

This innovative feature teaches students the critical-thinking skill of analysis. Students use this skill and the model provided to determine the reliability of health-related information in articles, advertisements, websites, and other sources. Learning such a skill and practicing it helps students become knowledgeable consumers of health-related information and products.

## Applying What You Have Learned

This unique end-of-chapter feature is a series of questions and activities that require critical thinking—application, analysis, synthesis, and evaluation. Each question is labeled with what type of critical thinking is required, and a key provides a brief explanation of the process students need to follow to complete the question or activity.

## Reflecting on Your Health

This end-of-chapter journal-writing activity stimulates students to consider what they have learned and to understand how their thoughts and feelings about health might have changed as a result of their new knowledge. Compiling these activities and reviewing them from time to time, especially at the end of the semester, can offer tangible evidence of changes and psychological and intellectual growth.

## The Integrated Teaching and Learning Package

Integrating the text and ancillaries is crucial to deriving their full benefit. Based on feedback from instructors and students, the following supplements are offered with *Essential Concepts for Healthy Living, Sixth Edition.*

## *Applying Concepts for Healthy Living: A Critical-Thinking Workbook*

*Applying Concepts for Healthy Living: A Critical-Thinking Workbook,* included at the back of the textbook, contains two types of activities that address self-assessment and changing health habits. Together, these features help students assess their behaviors and attitudes and provide a mechanism that will help students change health-related behaviors if they choose. The authors do not tell students which decisions are most valuable; instead, they provide background information and guidance through the use of thought-provoking techniques to make responsible decisions.

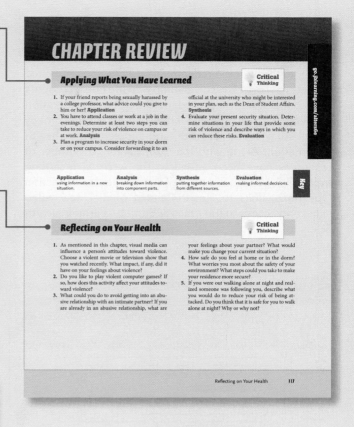

## Companion Website

**go.jblearning.com/alters6e**

This interactive and informative website is accessible to students through the redeemable access code provided in every new text. The companion website offers students and educators an unprecedented degree of integration between the text and the online world through many useful study tools, activities, and supplementary health information. Along with the *Sixth Edition*, a number of resources have been added to the website, including expanded Web links and Self-Assessments, Reflection Questions, links to Health-Related Media, new video clips, and access to the Jones & Bartlett Learning Health Statistics website.

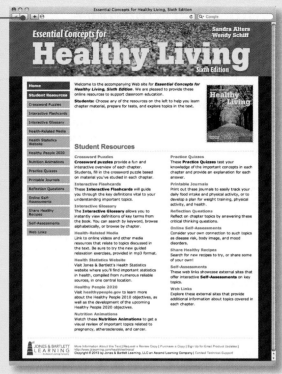

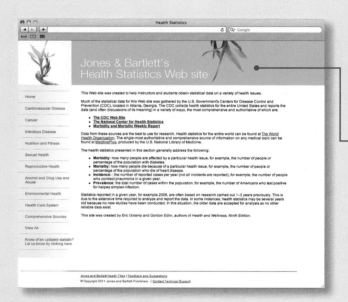

## Health Statistics Website

**go.jblearning.com/healthstats**

Jones & Bartlett's Health Statistics website provides current statistics on a variety of health topics in one central location. Data are compiled from numerous reliable sources, such as the Centers for Disease Control and Prevention (CDC), the World Health Organization (WHO), and MedLine Plus, a comprehensive website of medical topics produced by the U.S. National Library of Medicine.

## Instructor's Media CD

The Instructor's Media CD includes Lecture Outlines, PowerPoint Presentations, Warm-Up Exercises, and an Image Bank. A computerized Test Bank is also available as a free, secure download. All materials are formatted for online course management systems.

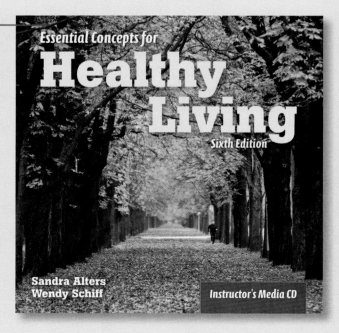

# Acknowledgments

The authors' writing is only one small portion of the work that goes into the development and production of a textbook. Many people work long hours with a shared goal: to produce a visually appealing, error-free, up-to-date, high-quality textbook for students. We would like to acknowledge the dedication and hard work of these individuals, for without them this project never would have been realized.

Our thanks to Shoshanna Goldberg, executive editor; Agnes Burt, editorial assistant; and Jody Yeskey, marketing manager, for their contributions to the project. These members have helped all involved in the book's development to remain focused on the needs of our audience. Renée Sekerak, Angela Dooley, and Sarah Cebluski managed the production of *Essential Concepts for Healthy Living*, doing an amazing job to keep an incredibly complex process running smoothly. A heartfelt thanks to you all. Thank you also to Virginia Thomas for updating the PowerPoints, lecture outlines, warm-up exercises, and Web content.

Jones & Bartlett is a company on the cutting edge of integrating technology with print materials for learning. The superb Web-based materials that are a part of the *Essential Concepts for Healthy Living* program could not have been developed without help from the Jones & Bartlett technology group.

Sandra Alters
Wendy Schiff

# Reviewers

Many health teachers and researchers have made significant contributions to the development of this book. Our gratitude goes to the following reviewers whose expertise gave invaluable direction to the development of the sixth edition of *Essential Concepts for Healthy Living*:

Carol Allen, *Lane Community College*

Robert E. Alman II, *Indiana University of Pennsylvania*

H. Giovanni Antunez, *St. Cloud State University*

Debra Atkinson, *Iowa State University*

Linda G. Beatty, *Mclennan Community College*

Carol M. Biddington, *California University of Pennsylvania*

Elaine D. Bryan, *Georgia Perimeter College*

Elizabeth G. Calamidas, *The Richard Stockton College of New Jersey*

Gordon Chalmers, *Western Washington University*

Elisabeth K. Constandy, *UNC Wilmington*

William E. Dunscombe, *Union County College*

Karen Edwards, *University of Delaware*

Jennifer Rogers Fagenbaum, *Davenport University*

Maqsood Faquir, *Palm Beach Community College*

Brian W. Findley, *Palm Beach Community College*

James W. Forkum, *Sierra College*

Deborah Galanski-Maciak, *Davenport University (Online)*

Marilyn M. Gardner, *Western Kentucky University*

Deborah J. Gibson, *University of Tennessee at Martin*

Ellen L. Glascock, *St. Francis College*

Valerie Greenberg, *Ventura College*

Jennifer L. Han, *University of Oklahoma*

David W. Hey, *California Polytechnic State University*

Marlene Hollick, *Monroe College*

Linda Hoogendijk, *Evergreen Valley College*

Younghee Kim, *Bowling Green State University*

Jerrilee LaMar, *University of Evansville*

Pat Lefler, *Bluegrass Community and Technical College*

Raymond A. Lomax, *Kean University*

Donna McGill-Cameron, *Woodland Community College*

Cynthia K. Miller, *Ball State University*

Paula Myslivecek, *Palm Beach Community College*

Shelley M. Patterson, *Davenport University*

Pamela Rost, *Buffalo State College*

Carole A. Sloan, *Henry Ford Community College*

Kimberli A. Stassen, *Ball State University*

Ruth A. Taylor, *Davenport University*

Debra Tavasso, *East Carolina University*

Blonnie Y. Thompson, *Eastern University*

Amy Townsend, *Emporia State University*

Sol M. Velazquez, *Monroe College*

# About the Authors

*Essential Concepts for Healthy Living, Sixth Edition*, was written by an author team with extensive credentials and backgrounds in biology, health, nutrition, and education. Sandra Alters holds a doctorate degree in science education and a master's degree in biology. Formerly a tenured professor in biology and education, Dr. Alters now writes full time in the areas of biology, personal health, and education. She has authored several textbooks and other books in addition to *Essential Concepts for Healthy Living*, including a variety of science, health, and education-related titles for the Information Plus reference book series; children's science books; many articles in the professional literature; and more than 60 chapters and features in books. Additionally, she has written the instructional design for a variety of science-related software products for students. With 25 years of teaching experience, Dr. Alters brings her education expertise, background in biology and human biology, and extensive writing experience to this author team.

Wendy Schiff holds a master's degree in human nutrition. She is a registered dietitian and a former adjunct instructor in the Department of Physical Education at St. Louis Community College–Meramec. Ms. Schiff has authored a college-level nutrition textbook, two health education manuals, and a low-calorie cookbook, and has published articles in professional journals. She has served as a consulting nutritionist, reviewer of health education and nutrition materials, and freelance health and nutrition essayist. With her educational background in health and her experience teaching college health, nutrition, stress management, and sexuality classes, Ms. Schiff complements Dr. Alters' expertise in biological sciences and science education.

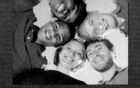

**Diversity in Health**
Minority Health Status
in the United States

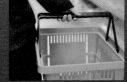

**Consumer Health**
Consumer Protection

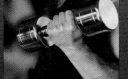

**Managing Your Health**
Routine Health Care for
Disease Prevention

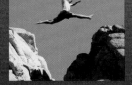

**Across the Life Span**
Health

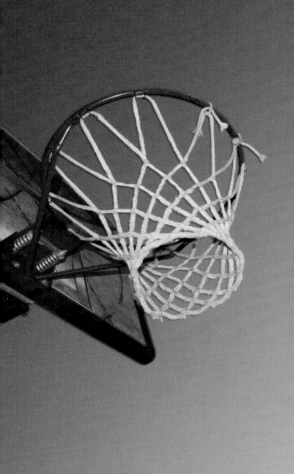

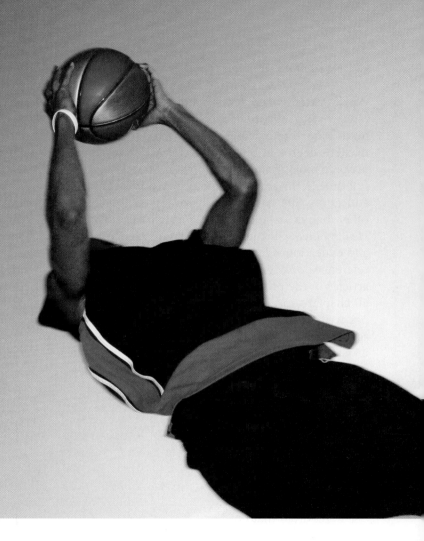

# Chapter Overview

How the dimensions of health influence your well-being

The major health concerns of our nation

How your decisions affect your health

How to analyze health-related information

The differences between conventional and alternative
treatment methods

# Student Workbook

Self-Assessment: Healthstyle | Personal Health History
Changing Health Habits: Model Activity for Better Health

# Do You Know?

How your lifestyle affects your health?

How to make responsible health-related decisions?

How to analyze health-related information?

# Health: The Foundation for Life

In the United States, there are some encouraging signs that more people are concerned about improving and protecting their health than in the past. A higher percentage of American adults report exercising during their leisure time than was reported in 1988.[1] In 1995, 71% of adults reported that their blood cholesterol level had been checked. By 2009, that percentage had increased to 81% of adults.[2] Between 1988 and 2008, the percentage of Americans wearing seat belts while riding in motor vehicles increased dramatically.[3] In some respects, Americans have also improved their eating habits. People are consuming less added sugars, more calcium, and more dietary fiber.[4,5] In 2007, fewer Americans died of cancer than in 1999.[6] Finally, Americans are living longer than in the 1980s. **Life expectancy** is the average number of years that an individual of a particular age can expect to live. In 1990, the life expectancy of an infant in the United States was 75.4 years.[7] By 2009, Americans' life expectancy at birth had increased to 78.2 years.[8]

*"A higher percentage of American adults report exercising during their leisure time..."*

**life expectancy** The average number of years that an individual of a particular age can expect to live.

**lifestyle** A way of living including behaviors that promote or impair good health and longevity.

**risk factor** A characteristic that increases an individual's chances of developing a health problem.

Other findings about Americans' current health status and health-related behaviors, however, are less encouraging. Cigarette smoking and alcohol abuse are widespread behaviors, particularly among young people. Tobacco use is the leading cause of preventable illness and death in the United States.[9] In 2009, adults smoked fewer cigarettes than in 1985, but about one in five Americans who were 18 years of age and older smoked cigarettes.[10] U.S. public health officials are also concerned about Americans who use alcohol irresponsibly. In 2008, excessive alcohol consumption was the third leading cause of preventable deaths in the United States, including traffic-related fatalities.[11] Fifteen percent of adult Americans and 25% of high school students reported that they engaged in *binge drinking* in 2009.[12] Binge drinking is defined as consuming five or more alcoholic drinks per occasion (males) and four or more drinks per occasion (females). Americans who are 18 to 24 years of age are more likely to binge drink than other members of the population. According to results of one study, about one in four college students indicated that their drinking behaviors contributed to serious academic problems, including missing classes, performing poorly on exams, and lowering their grade point averages.[13] The typical American does not meet the federal government's recommendations concerning healthy food choices. The majority of the U.S. population does not eat enough vegetables, whole grains, fruits, milk, and oils ("healthy" fats).[14] An important sign of Americans' poor nutritional practices is the high prevalence of *obesity* in the United States. Between 1988 and 1994, 10% of children[15] and almost 23% of adults[16] were obese. By 2008, 17% of American children and more than 33% of American adults were obese.[17] Between 1994 and 2008, the prevalence of obesity increased dramatically among all groups of Americans regardless of their age, sex, race, ethnicity, socioeconomic status, region of the country, and educational level. Excess body fat is associated with the development of many serious diseases, including high blood pressure, heart disease, certain cancers, and *type 2 diabetes*, a serious disorder char-

acterized by the body's inability to regulate its blood sugar normally.

Although Americans are living longer than in the past, living longer is not always a sign that people are living *better*. Many older adults suffer from conditions that reduce their ability to enjoy life and perform important daily activities such as bathing and dressing. Heart disease, stroke, cancer, Alzheimer's disease, impaired vision, hearing loss, osteoporosis, and depression not only create much misery for millions of older adults but also for the family members who struggle to care for their disabled relatives.

The results of many studies show that exercising regularly, eating a more nutritious diet, and avoiding smoking and excess alcohol consumption promote good health. Incorporating these and other healthy habits into your *lifestyle*, while you are still young, can improve your health and well-being and increase your chances of living a longer and healthier life than your parents and grandparents.

**Lifestyle** is a way of living. As a college student, your lifestyle includes a variety of behaviors that promote or impair good health and longevity. Although you may be unable to prevent severe birth defects or inherited disorders from affecting your health, you can modify many health *risk factors*, reducing the likelihood that you will develop serious medical problems. A **risk factor** is a characteristic that increases an individual's chances of developing a health problem. For example, physical inactivity, tobacco use, emotional stress, and obesity are risk factors for heart disease, *hypertension* (persistent high blood pressure), and certain types of cancers. You can dramatically lower your chances of developing these conditions by incorporating exercise into your daily schedule, choosing not to use tobacco products, practicing relaxation techniques, and eating a more nutritious diet. Of course, the decision to adopt a healthier lifestyle is up to you.

To evaluate the impact of your lifestyle on your health, answer the questions in the "Healthstyle" assessment in the Student Workbook at the end of the book. You can use the results of this assessment to determine which health-related behaviors need to be changed to reduce your risk of certain diseases.

Are you concerned about your health? What are you doing to protect it? What steps can you take to enhance your state of health so that you can enjoy life more fully? Where can you find reliable information concerning health? This textbook presents findings from current scientific research for you to use in making choices that will improve your health.

# The Dimensions of Health

## What Is Health?

Most people can describe how it feels to be healthy or ill, but trying to define *health* is not an easy task. In 1948, the World Health Organization (WHO) constitution defined health as "a state of complete physical, mental, and social well-being and not merely the absence of disease or infirmity."[18] This definition, however, is too limited. Consider the people in **Figure 1.1**. Although they are in wheelchairs, they are able to compete as athletes. If you judged their state of health using WHO's 1948 definition, you might conclude that they are unhealthy. Many physically disabled people are able to function adequately in society and do not consider themselves ill or infirm.

The Ottawa Charter for Health Promotion defines *health* as "a resource for everyday life . . . a positive concept emphasizing social and personal resources, as well as physical capabilities."[19] According to this charter, health requires "peace, shelter, education, food, income, a stable ecosystem, sustainable resources, social justice and equity." In addition to these conditions, most healthy adults want to function independently; enjoy eating, sexual, and physical activities; feel good about themselves; and enjoy being with family and friends.

Behavioral scientist Godfrey Hochbaum proposed a simple definition for health: "Health is what helps me be what I want to be . . . do what I want to do

**good health** The ability to function adequately and independently in a constantly changing environment.

**optimal wellness** A sense that one is functioning at his or her best level.

. . . [and] live the way I would like to live."[20] Using Hochbaum's definition, you might conclude that the wheelchair-bound athletes in Figure 1.1 are as healthy as people who are capable of running.

## Health and Wellness

Health and wellness are related concepts. **Good health** enables one to function adequately and independently in a constantly changing environment; **optimal wellness** is a sense that one is functioning at one's best level. **Figure 1.2** illustrates the concept of health as a continuum; there are degrees of health. The absence of functioning (premature death) is at one end of this continuum, and the highest level of functioning (optimal well-being) is at the other end. Many people accept responsibility for the quality of their health and well-being. These people are willing to take various steps to improve their health, achieving a higher degree of wellness in the process.

Most health educators agree that health and wellness are **holistic**; that is, they involve all aspects of the individual. Thus, the holistic concept of health encompasses not only the physical, psychological, and social aspects, but also the intellectual, spiritual, and environmental dimensions of a person. Each dimension is an integral part of a person's health, and

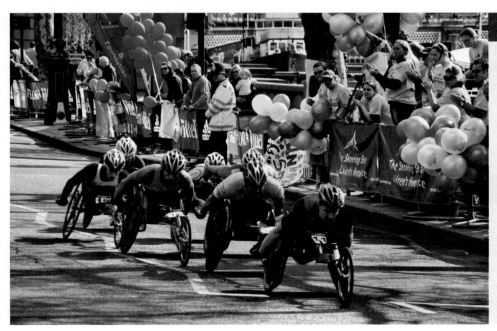

### Figure 1.1

**Wheelchair Athletes.** Many physically disabled people do not consider themselves ill or infirm because they can function well in society. According to Hochbaum's definition of health, individuals with physical disabilities can be healthy and enjoy life.

**holistic** (hole-IS-tic) A characteristic involving all aspects of the person.

**signs** Observable and measurable features of an illness.

**symptoms** Subjective complaints of illness.

**acute** A condition or illness that tends to develop quickly and resolve within a few days or weeks.

**chronic** A condition or disease that often takes months or years to develop, progresses in severity, and can affect a person over a long period.

any change in the quality of one component of health affects the others. For example, individuals who exercise with others to increase their level of physical health often report a sense of improved psychological and social health.

## The Components of Health

**Physical Health** *Physical health* refers to the overall condition of the organ systems, such as the cardiovascular system (heart and blood vessels), respiratory system (lungs), reproductive system, and nervous system. A healthy person's systems function properly; the individual feels well and is free of disease. When organs do not function adequately, a person has various signs and symptoms of illness. **Signs** are the observable and measurable features of an illness, such as fever, rash, and abnormal behavior. **Symptoms** are the subjective complaints of an illness, such as reports of fatigue, headaches, and numbness. An **acute** condition or illness, such as the common cold or a food-borne infection, tends to develop quickly and resolve within a few days or weeks. A **chronic** condition or disease often takes months or years to develop, progresses in severity, and can affect a person over a longer period, in some cases, throughout his or her lifetime.

**Psychological Health** Psychological (mental) health involves the ability to deal effectively with the psychological challenges of life. Psychologically healthy people accept responsibility for their behavior, feel good about themselves and others, are comfortable with their emotions (feelings), and have positive, realistic outlooks on life. Although experiences such as losing a job or a family member cause stress or grief, psychologically healthy people are able to limit the extent to which crises affect their lives. Chapter 2 focuses on the topic of psychological health.

**Social Health** Social health is the sense of well-being that an individual achieves by forming emotionally supportive and intellectually stimulating relationships with family members, friends, and associates. Living in communities rather than in isolation, identifying with social groups, and belonging to organizations strengthen the social dimension of health. When social networks break down, health declines.

**Intellectual Health** Intellectual health is the ability to use problem solving and other higher-order thinking skills to deal effectively with life's challenges. Healthy people analyze situations, determine alternative courses of action, and make decisions. After making decisions, intellectually healthy individuals are able to judge the effectiveness of their choices and learn from their experiences. Effective intellectual skills enable people to feel in control of their lives.

**Spiritual Health** Spiritual health is the belief that one is a part of a larger scheme of life and that one's life has purpose. Identifying with a religion and having religious beliefs influence the spiritual health of many people. However, spirituality is not confined to those who belong to organized religious groups or have religious beliefs. People can develop spirituality without practicing a particular religion or believing in the power of a supreme being. Whatever the nature of their spirituality, many individuals achieve a sense

### Figure 1.2

**A Health Continuum.** Some people view health as a continuum; that is, there are degrees of health. Premature death is at one end of this continuum, and optimal well-being is at the other end.
*Source:* Modified from Ebersole, P., & Hess, P. (1994). *Toward healthy aging* (4th ed.). St. Louis, MO: Mosby. Copyright © 1994 with permission from Elsevier.

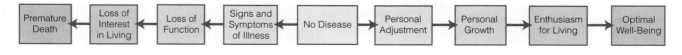

Premature Death ← Loss of Interest in Living ← Loss of Function ← Signs and Symptoms of Illness ← No Disease → Personal Adjustment → Personal Growth → Enthusiasm for Living → Optimal Well-Being

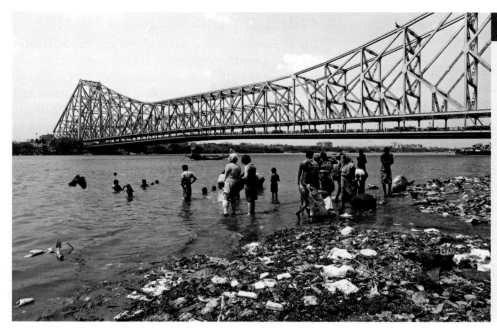

**Figure 1.3**

**Environmental Health.** The state of the environment in which people live, work, and play affects the quality of their health. People cannot achieve a high degree of wellness if their environment is polluted or unsafe.

of inner peace and harmony as well as emotional ful-fillment by believing that their lives have a purpose. As in the other wellness dimensions, a breakdown in spiritual health can have a negative impact on one's well-being.

**Figure 1.4**

**The Components of Health.** The components of health are interrelated. According to this model, the social, intellectual, and spiritual components of health are in the larger spheres of physical and psychological health, which are in the largest sphere of environmental health.

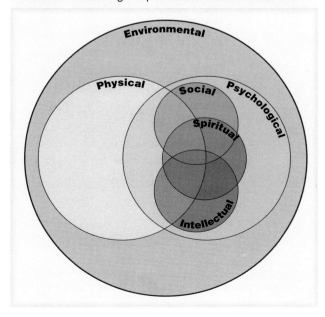

**Environmental Health** Nothing affects the qual-ity of wellness components as much as the state of the environment—the conditions where people live, work, and play. Environmental concerns that influ-ence wellness include the provision of clean water and air, the management of wastes, and the control of distressing social problems such as crime and fam-ily violence. Humans cannot achieve a high degree of wellness if their environment is polluted or unsafe (**Figure 1.3**). Chapter 16 discusses environmental health concerns.

**Figure 1.4** is a model that illustrates how these six components of wellness are related and inte-grated into a holistic approach to understanding health. This model has the physical and psychologi-cal health components at the core of the larger en-vironmental component. The social, intellectual, and spiritual components involve thought processes; therefore, they are found in the psychological health dimension. Note how the physical and psychologi-cal spheres overlap to illustrate how the body and mind are closely integrated. When the components of health function well together, the individual has a sense of well-being.

## The Nation's Health

Health involves more than just personal health—health is a national concern, too. Many of the cru-cial social, political, and economic issues facing this country are health related, such as domestic violence, terrorism, care of the aged, and access to health care and insurance.

Lack of health insurance and the high cost of health care are major barriers to obtaining routine preventive medical care and proper treatment. The United States spends more on health-related care per person than any other country.[7] According to the U.S. Department of Health and Human Services, total healthcare costs reached $2.3 *trillion* in 2008 and were projected to reach $2.8 trillion in 2012.[21] Americans generally rely on themselves and their employers, as well as private and public health insurance programs, to pay for some of their health care. Millions of Americans, however, do not have health insurance or they have inadequate insurance coverage. In 2009, an estimated 17.5% of Americans younger than 65 years of age were not covered by health insurance.[22] A major illness, serious accident, or hospitalization can quickly exhaust a person's financial resources and create enormous personal debt; therefore, it is important to have adequate health insurance to cover such expenses.

# Tracking the Nation's Health

The U.S. government, particularly the Public Health Service of the Department of Health and Human Services, monitors the nation's health in a variety of ways. One way is by recording cases of certain diseases and causes of death. **Table 1.1** shows preliminary data for the 10 leading causes of death for all Americans in 2009. In the United States, heart disease was the leading cause of death, followed by cancer, chronic lower respiratory diseases, and strokes.[8]

The major causes of death differ for members of various age groups. **Table 1.2** shows preliminary data concerning the leading causes of death in two age categories: 15 to 24 years and 25 to 44 years. In 2009, unintentional injuries (accidents), homicide, and suicide were the top three leading causes of death of people between 15 and 24 years of age. Note that unintentional injuries, cancer, and heart disease were the top three leading causes of death of people between 25 and 44 years of age.

## Table 1.1

### The 10 Major Causes of Death in the United States (Preliminary Data, 2009)

| Rank | Cause | Approx. Percentage of Deaths |
|------|-------|------------------------------|
| 1 | Heart disease | 24.6 |
| 2 | Cancer | 23.3 |
| 3 | Chronic lower respiratory diseases | 5.6 |
| 4 | Stroke | 5.3 |
| 5 | Accidents/unintentional injuries | 4.8 |
| 6 | Alzheimer's disease | 3.2 |
| 7 | Diabetes mellitus | 2.8 |
| 8 | Pneumonia/influenza | 2.2 |
| 9 | Kidney disease | 2.0 |
| 10 | Suicide | 1.5 |
| — | Other causes | 24.7 |

*Source:* Kockanek, K. D., et al. (2011): Deaths: Preliminary data for 2009. *National Vital Statistics Reports,* 59(4):1–68.

## Table 1.2

### Causes of Death: All Races, Selected Age Groups of American (Preliminary Data, 2009)

| *Ages 15–24* | |
|------|-------|
| Rank | Cause |
| 1 | Unintentional injuries |
| 2 | Homicide |
| 3 | Suicide |
| 4 | Cancer |
| 5 | Heart disease |

| *Ages 25–44* | |
|------|-------|
| Rank | Cause |
| 1 | Unintentional injuries |
| 2 | Cancer |
| 3 | Heart Disease |
| 4 | Suicide |
| 5 | Homicide |

*Source:* Kockanek, K. D., et al. (2011): Deaths: Preliminary data for 2009. *National Vital Statistics Reports,* 59(4):1–68.

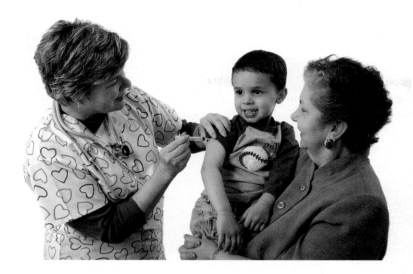

Over the past 100 years, Americans made great progress toward improving their health, well-being, and longevity. In 1900, the life expectancy of a newborn baby was less than 50 years. Compared to people who lived in the first half of the twentieth century, many Americans can now expect to live longer lives. This progress occurred largely because various government agencies provided greater access to health care, promoted preventive healthcare efforts, funded health education and research programs, and regulated the safety of the environment. For example, childhood vaccination programs have removed the threat of polio and controlled other infectious diseases such as measles, diphtheria, rubella, and tetanus. Food fortification programs have nearly eliminated nutritional deficiency diseases such as goiter, rickets, and pellagra. Efforts to educate the public concerning the importance of early and routine *prenatal care* (medical care for pregnant women) have helped reduce the infant death rate.

Although the life expectancy of Americans has increased, many people still die prematurely, that is, before they reach 75 years of age. According to health experts at the Centers for Disease Control and Prevention in Atlanta, actual causes of death are the underlying reasons that are not reported on death certificates. In 2000, for example, about 18% of all deaths were the result of tobacco use, including secondhand exposure to tobacco smoke; poor diet and lack of physical activity accounted for about 15% of deaths.[23] Leading causes of death tables such as Table 1.1, however, integrate those deaths within the number of deaths resulting primarily from heart disease, cancer, chronic lower respiratory diseases, and stroke. Health experts predict that the combination of poor diet and physi-

cal inactivity will soon replace tobacco use as the leading actual cause of death in the United States. In many instances, actual causes of death are associated with lifestyle choices, such as tobacco use or physical inactivity. By changing these and other health-related behaviors, people may avoid dying prematurely.

## Health Promotion: Development of *Healthy People 2020*

Health promotion is the practice of helping people become healthier by encouraging them to take more control over their health and change their lifestyles. Health promotional efforts strive to *prevent* rather than treat disease and injury. Federal, state, and local governments can help the population develop healthy lifestyles by funding and providing educational programs and preventive medical care services. When planning effective health promotional programs, public health experts and government officials need to identify which aspects of the population's health should receive the most attention. How does the federal government identify serious health concerns and monitor the health of its citizens? What is being done to improve the nation's health?

In the late 1980s, a team of concerned health experts, health educators, and U.S. government officials analyzed the results of reports, recommendations, and studies that provided data concerning the health status of Americans. In 1991, these experts published their findings in a report called *Healthy People 2000*.[24]

*Healthy People 2000* had three general goals: increase the healthy life span of Americans, improve the health status of American minorities, and extend the accessibility of preventive health services to all Americans. *Healthy People 2000* also established numerous health-related objectives that related to each goal, such as increasing the percentage of children who engaged in 20 minutes or more of vigorous physical activity at least 3 days a week. The overall aim was for Americans to achieve the health objectives by the year 2000; as more *Healthy People 2000* objectives were met, the overall health status of Americans would improve. By 2000, public health experts had collected and analyzed information about the population's progress toward achieving the health objectives, and the data were used for the publication of a revised set of goals and objectives. This process would be repeated approximately every 10 years. In 2000, the federal government released the second edition of the plan, *Healthy People 2010*. The analysis of data obtained from *Healthy People 2010* led to the publication of *Healthy People 2020*, the third and latest edition of the national health goals and objectives.

**Table 1.3** indicates the four main goals of *Healthy People 2020* and factors that will be measured to monitor progress toward meeting those goals. *Healthy People 2020* identifies 42 "objective topic areas," including "physical activity" and "injury and violence prevention" (see Appendix A) as well as nearly 600 health objectives. An *objective* identifies target populations and a specific health concern. One of the physical activity objectives, for example, is "Increase the proportion of adults who meet current Federal physical activity guidelines for aerobic physical activity and for muscle strengthening activity."

Staff of various federal, state, and local agencies are responsible for developing and implementing health education efforts, such as community and school-based programs to reduce the prevalence of childhood obesity, that support *Healthy People 2020* objectives. Additionally, staff will monitor Americans' progress in meeting these health objectives. You can learn more about *Healthy People 2020* by visiting the government's website www.healthypeople.gov/2020/default.aspx.

## Minority Health Status

For hundreds of years, immigrants from around the world have been changing the face of the United States as they settle in this country. Each new group of immigrants brings different cultural traditions and various ethnic identities with them (**Figure 1.5**). *Culture* consists of the unique social characteristics of a population, such as its customs, rituals, and health beliefs and practices, which are passed down from generation to generation. An ethnic group is one in which members share a common national, religious, racial, or ancestral identity. According to the U.S. Department of Health and Human Services, the major American racial/ethnic subpopulations are Caucasians (whites), African Americans (blacks), Latinos (Hispanics), American Indian/Alaska Natives, and Asian/Pacific Islanders. The same terms, however, are not used by all agencies. Throughout this textbook, terms such as *Caucasian* may be used in one context and *whites* in another; when reporting statistics or results of research studies, the text reflects the language of the agency or researcher.

In the United States, the majority of Americans have European ancestry, particularly northern European. The National Center for Health Statistics refers to this population as "white, nonHispanic." In 2005–2009, about 75% of the U.S. population identified itself as "white."[25]

Differences in death and illness rates between the nation's men and women, as well as among its diverse ethnic and racial groups, are major public health

### Table 1.3

### *Healthy People 2020:* Foundation Health Measures

| Main Goals of *Healthy People 2020* | Measures of Progress |
|---|---|
| **General Health Status** Attain high quality, longer lives free of preventable disease, disability, injury, and premature death | Life expectancy; healthy life expectancy |
| | Years of potential life lost |
| | Physically and mentally unhealthy days |
| | Self-assessed health status |
| | Limitation of activity |
| | Chronic disease prevalence |
| **Disparities and Inequity** Achieve health equity, eliminate disparities, and improve the health of all groups | Race/ethnicity |
| | Socioeconomic status |
| | Sex; sexual orientation |
| | Disability status |
| | Geography |
| **Social Determinants of Health** Create social and physical environments that promote good health for all | Social and economic factors |
| | Natural and built environments |
| | Policies and programs |
| **Health-Related Quality of Life and Well-Being** Promote quality of life, healthy development, and healthy behaviors | Self-reports of well-being and satisfaction |
| | Quality of life |
| | Participation in common activities |

*Source:* Adapted from U.S. Department of Health and Human Services, Office of Disease Prevention and Health Promotion. (2010). *Healthy People 2020*. Retrieved from http://www.healthypeople.gov/2020/TopicsObjectives2020/pdfs/HP2020_brochure.pdf

## Figure 1.5

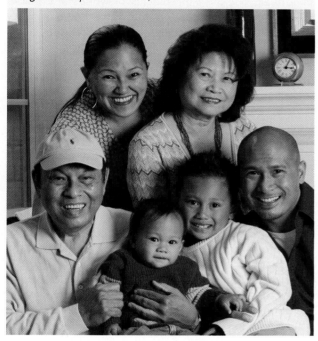

**An American Family.** Culture consists of the unique social characteristics of a population, such as its customs, rituals, and health practices. Immigrants who settle in the United States contribute much to the racial, ethnic, and cultural diversity of the population. © digitalskillet/ShutterStock, Inc.

concerns. For example, American men generally do not live as long as American women and are more likely to die from each of the 10 leading causes of death. Additionally, more African Americans die of cancers and diseases of the heart and blood vessels than members of other ethnic and racial groups. The reasons for these differences are unclear, but lifestyle choices, environmental conditions, and socioeconomic situations are major contributing factors.

Throughout this textbook, the Diversity in Health essays feature topics that concern a variety of populations in the United States as well as around the world. The Diversity in Health essay in this chapter, "Minority Health Status in the United States," discusses differences in the overall health of major minority groups in the United States.

## Genetics and Genomics

Your lifestyle and environment influence your health status, but your *genes* also play a role in determining your health. With the exception of red blood cells, all cells in your body contain genes. **Genes** are segments of *DNA*, a complex chemical compound that codes for the production of proteins. Cells use proteins for a variety of functions, including building, maintaining, and repairing structures, such as bones and other tissues. Mistakes in the genetic code can result in the production of faulty proteins that can cause disease and even death. Genes are *inherited*, that is, their coded instructions for protein synthesis are passed on to subsequent generations.

*Genetics* is the scientific study of genes and the way they pass certain traits, such as the risk of breast cancer, or medical conditions, such as birth defects, from one generation to another. Thus, genetics can help people understand how certain life-threatening medical conditions, including sickle cell anemia and cystic fibrosis, tend to "run in families." Scientists have developed tests to identify the gene or genes for hundreds of diseases, most of which are rare genetic disorders such as Duchenne muscular dystrophy, and certain breast and ovarian cancers.

Most of the 10 leading causes of death in the United States, particularly heart disease, cancer, stroke, diabetes, and Alzheimer's disease, have a genetic component. Unlike cases of rare genetic conditions, these common chronic diseases generally develop partly as a result of *multiple* genes interacting with behavioral and environmental risk factors, such as poor food choices, lack of physical activity, and exposure to tobacco smoke.

**Genomics** is the study of all a person's genes (*genome*), including the complex ways the genes interact with each other and the environment to influence the individual's health.[36] A person's genome can provide medical researchers with important biological clues about the individual's health status, disease risk,

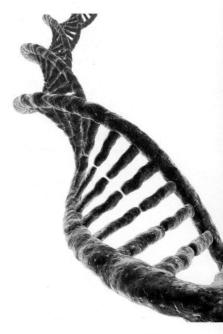

A gene is a segment of DNA.

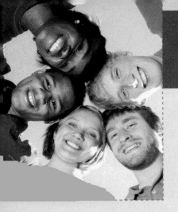

# Diversity in Health

## Minority Health Status in the United States

Did you know that African Americans are more likely to die of cancer than are whites? Did you know that Hispanics are more likely to die in accidents than as the result of strokes? The differences in death and illness rates for various population subgroups reflect numerous factors, such as socioeconomic status and access to health insurance and medical care. By investigating reasons for these differences, medical researchers have learned a great deal about the health of American minorities. A major goal of the U.S. Department of Health and Human Services is improving the health of all Americans through research, education, and better access to health care.

### Hispanic or Latino People

Hispanic, or Latino, people have immigrated to the United States or have ancestors from countries in which Spanish is the primary language, especially Mexico, Puerto Rico, Central and South America, and Cuba. Hispanics are the largest minority group in the United States, making up 15% of the population.[25]

In 2006, the leading causes of death for Hispanics were heart disease, cancer, accidental injuries, stroke, and diabetes.[26] Some Hispanic/Latino population groups have a high prevalence of asthma, obesity, chronic lung diseases, HIV infection, tuberculosis (TB), and diabetes.

Poverty, lack of health insurance, and poor education are barriers to good health for many Hispanics. About 23% of this minority lives in poverty.[25] Health disorders associated with poverty, such as tuberculosis and obesity, are more common in certain Spanish-speaking subgroups. In 2008, almost one-third of Hispanic Americans did not have health insurance.[25] Hispanic persons, especially those of Mexican ancestry, are more likely to be uninsured than non-Hispanic whites. Regardless of one's ethnic/racial background, not having health insurance is a major obstacle to obtaining good health care in the United States.

### African or Black Americans

In the United States, African Americans comprise 12% of the population; they are the second largest minority group.[27] Despite recent improvements, the health status of black Americans is generally poorer than that of other minorities. The life expectancies of whites and blacks reflect their health status. In 2009, the life expectancy of African American females was 77.4 years; the life expectancy of white American females was 80.9 years. At the same time, the life expectancy of African American males was 70.9 years, and that of white males was 76.2 years.[8]

The major causes of death of black Americans are similar to those of non-Hispanic whites. Although black Americans are less likely to die from chronic lung diseases, Alzheimer's disease, and suicide, members of this minority are more likely to die of homicide, cancer, stroke, diabetes, HIV infection, and heart disease than are white Americans.[28] Black women are more likely to die of breast, cervical, colon, and stomach cancers than white women are, and black men are more likely to die of lung, prostate, colon, and stomach cancers than white men are.[29]

Childbearing is riskier for an African American woman; in 2007, she was almost three times more likely to die during pregnancy or childbirth than a white woman was.[28] Additionally, black infants are more likely to die during the first month of life than other babies are. In 2009, the infant death rate among black infants was more than twice that of white babies.[8]

In 2005–2008, African Americans were more likely to have hypertension than non-Hispanic white Americans or Mexican Americans.[30] The reason for this high prevalence is unclear, but scientists think diet, genetics, stress, and smoking play roles. Overweight also increases the risk of hypertension. Black women are more likely to have excess body fat than are other Americans. In the period from 2005 to 2008, nearly 80% of non-Hispanic black women were too fat.[31]

### Asian and Pacific Islanders

As one of the fastest-growing minority groups, Asian Americans and Pacific Islanders (APIs) are a diverse group of people who immigrated to the United States from China, Japan, Vietnam, Korea, India, the Philip-

and responses to treatments. Scientific analysis of individual genomes may help explain why people who share similar environments or health-related behaviors do not always develop the same health conditions.

Genes play roles in a person's ability to achieve and maintain good health. Medical researchers use genetics to learn more about diseases that are caused by genes. Researchers use genomics to understand how multiple genes contribute to the development of com-

pines, and other Pacific Islands. In 2008, Asian Americans made up about 5% of the U.S. population.[32] Asian Americans generally have lower *age-adjusted* death rates for the 10 major causes of death than do whites and members of other minority groups.[7] This means that an average 30-year-old Asian American is less likely to die of any major cause of death, including heart disease and cancer, than is an average 30-year-old American who is a white person or a member of another minority population. Compared with other minority groups of Americans, Asian American women have the highest life expectancy.[32] Asian American women, however, are more likely to die from stomach cancer than other American women are.[29] Additionally, people who immigrated recently from Asia and the Pacific Islands are more likely to suffer from hepatitis, a serious liver disease, and tuberculosis than people who have lived in the United States for longer periods of time. Factors that contribute to the poor health status of some Asian Americans include language and cultural barriers; social disgrace (*stigma*) associated with certain conditions, especially mental illness; and lack of health insurance.[32]

## American Indians and Alaska Natives

American Indian and Alaska Natives (AI/ANs) is a diverse group of people comprising only about 1.5% of the American population in 2006.[33] About half of this minority live in designated areas such as reservations or reservation trust areas. AI/ANs generally have more health problems than do whites. Geographic isolation, poverty, inadequate sewage disposal, and cultural barriers are some of the reasons why health among AI/ANs is poorer than it is among other groups of Americans.[34]

American Indian/Alaska Native infants and children are more likely to die than other American infants and children.[33] AI/ANs are more likely to be smokers than members of other racial/ethnic groups, and binge drinking is a serious health concern of AI/ANs. Diabetes poses a health threat for many members of this minority. The rate of diabetes among AI/ANs is twice as high as the rate among whites.[35] In addition to diabetes, mental health problems and alcohol-related deaths such as accidents, homicides, and suicides are major health concerns for AI/ANs.

## The Impact of Social Conditions on Health Status

Although genetic factors may be the primary cause of many health problems, income level, health insurance coverage, educational attainment, and years living in the United States play major roles in determining a particular group's state of health. Many chronic diseases, such as tuberculosis and malnutrition, are associated with poor standards of living. Other health threats often associated with poverty include substance abuse, homicide, and lead poisoning. Poverty, however, is not limited to any single population group in the United States. Regardless of their racial or ethnic background, individuals who achieve a higher level of education usually have higher incomes and better health than those with less education.

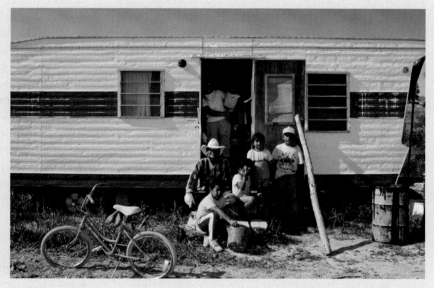

In the United States, many chronic diseases are associated with poor standards of living.

plex diseases and how these particular genes interact with other factors, such as lifestyle and environment. As a result of such analyses, medical researchers can develop better ways to prevent, diagnose, and treat diseases.

Genomics is a relatively new science, and genomic testing, which involves combinations of biochemical and molecular methods to analyze a cell's genes, has the potential to improve the health of individuals. However, the value of genomic testing for diagnos-

**motivation** The force or drive that leads people to take action.

**efficacy** (EF-fih-ka-see) Regarding health education, the belief that one is capable of changing his or her behavior.

ing, predicting, and treating common chronic diseases has not been established. Public health experts are concerned about *personal genomic tests* that are directly marketed to consumers through Internet and other media outlets. At present, very little scientific evidence supports the validity and usefulness of the results of such *direct-to-consumer* genomic tests.

More research is needed to establish the usefulness of adding information obtained by genomic testing to the standard medical history that healthcare practitioners routinely collect from their patients. The "Personal Health History" activity in the Student Workbook at the end of the book tracks your family's medical history. Maintaining a record of your health history can help you make a positive contribution to your medical care. How? When you share this information with your physicians, the medical practitioners can consider inherited factors to predict your risk of certain chronic diseases and develop ways (*interventions*) to help you prevent or forestall those diseases.

## Understanding Health-Related Behavior

Regardless of their cultural and ethnic background, not all Americans share the same level of concern for their health. How many times have you heard a smoker say, "I can stop smoking whenever I want to; now is just not a good time" or "You've got to die of something; it might as well be lung cancer." You may know people who eat too many fatty foods, do not exercise regularly, drink too much alcohol, and smoke cigarettes. You may know other people who follow a nutritious diet, walk at a brisk pace for 45 minutes nearly every day, and avoid drugs such as alcohol and tobacco. Why do some people adopt more positive health-related behaviors than others do?

### Changing Health-Related Behavior

"I wish I had the willpower to stop smoking." "I just can't seem to find the motivation to exercise more of-

ten." Do these statements sound familiar? Is having a lot of willpower the key to becoming healthier?

Health educators often refer to willpower as **motivation**, the force or drive that leads people to take action. Past experiences, perceived needs, and personal values influence one's motivation. For example, a person who has tried unsuccessfully to stop smoking several times and claims to enjoy smoking may have little motivation to make another attempt to quit.

Efficacy enhances motivation. **Efficacy** is the belief that one is capable of changing behavior. Various barriers such as poor education or lack of support from family members can interfere with someone's motivation to change behaviors.

Having knowledge about risky behaviors and the seriousness of a health-related condition does not necessarily motivate individuals to take appropriate actions. For example, most people know that seat belts reduce the possibility of a serious injury in an automobile accident and that most states require them to wear seat belts in a car. Nevertheless, individuals often make a variety of excuses to explain why they fail to buckle up. Additionally, many students enrolled in personal health classes can correctly identify behaviors that promote optimal health, yet they do not practice what they know. Acquiring knowledge about health is important, but becoming motivated to adopt a healthier lifestyle is essential if individuals are to make long-term changes that can benefit their health.

Taking an active role in achieving and maintaining good health depends on certain personal factors: degree of vulnerability, level of motivation (*willpower*), sense of control, and perceived value of the behavior. People are motivated to take action if they feel that a sufficient threat to their health exists and that the consequences of changing the behavior are worthwhile.

Assume, for example, that diabetes affects several members of your family. You have heard that diabetes may be inherited; therefore, you are aware that you have a good chance of developing this condition (*vulnerability*). You know that family members who have diabetes suffer from kidney damage, blindness, and premature heart disease. Because you want to avoid these consequences, you are motivated to change certain behaviors (*motivation*). Additionally, you believe that your actions influence the quality of your health (*sense of control*). Concerned, you decide to learn more about diabetes and determine what actions can reduce your risk of developing the disease. You now have a reason to take action because you believe it is important (*value*) to prevent this disease, even if it means making lifestyle changes now while you are still healthy.

# Making Positive Health-Related Decisions

### How I Quit Smoking

*About a month ago I was a smoker—about 10 cigarettes a day during the week and up to a pack a day on weekends. After thinking about quitting for about a year, it happened. Without even giving it any consideration, I was able to not buy a pack for 2 days. On day 3, I realized my success and told myself I would never buy a pack again. I miss it, especially after a drink or a meal, but I'm glad I've gone this far. There have been times when I've really wanted one, but that's when you realize how powerful of a drug it is. At least that's how I talk myself out of having one. Before, I never thought of myself as being addicted—too harsh of a word—but I was just like all of the other smokers out there. It's a filthy habit—I'm glad I stopped.*

Although this college student smoked less than a pack of cigarettes a day, he took about a year to quit smoking. He made the final decision to stop smoking while listening to other students' habit-breaking experiences in his health class. Some people take less time to make health-related decisions than others do, and some people have less difficulty making lifestyle changes than others do. **Figure 1.6** illustrates the complex process of decision making.

**Stages of Behavioral Change** According to many health education experts, the process of changing behaviors involves the five stages shown in **Figure 1.7**.[37] We use the example of smoking to illustrate this process. The first stage is *precontemplation*. In this stage, smokers show no interest in quitting tobacco use, do not see a need to quit, and may avoid discussing their smoking behavior with others. Smokers move into the *contemplation* stage when they realize or admit tobacco use is unhealthy, and they intend to quit smoking in the next 6 months. In the *preparation* stage of change, smokers may have made unsuccessful attempts to quit smoking, yet they express the desire to stop within the next month. Smokers in the *action* stage of change take

steps to quit smoking, such as "going cold turkey" or using a nicotine patch. They succeed in quitting for up to 6 months. Finally, smokers in the *maintenance* stage develop practices to avoid relapsing into using tobacco. Former smokers, for example, might socialize with nonsmokers or use exercise as a substitute for smoking. According to health education researchers, 40% of people who engage in risky behaviors such as smoking or being physically inactive are in the precontemplation stage, 40% are in the contemplation stage, and the remaining 20% are preparing to change the unhealthy behaviors.[38]

When people *relapse*, they return to an earlier stage of change and usually feel like failures as a result of their inability to maintain the new behaviors. In the case of smokers, they may even return to the precontemplation stage in which they stop thinking about quitting. However, the majority of people who relapse eventually decide to stop smoking again, and they tend to try a different method of quitting. People who seriously want to quit smoking, for example, typically make three to four efforts to stop before they actually succeed.[37]

When changing a behavior, people use various strategies to increase their chances of success, includ-

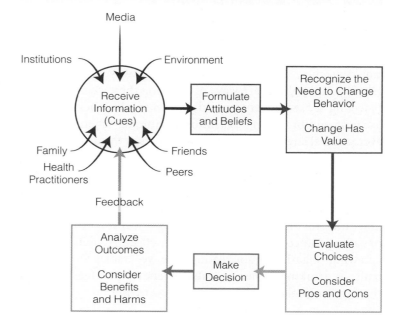

### Figure 1.6

**Decision-Making Model.** Decision making can be a complex process. Information, personal attitudes, and personal experiences influence your decision-making process. To change health-related behaviors, you must recognize the need to change, that the change has personal value, and that it is consistent with your beliefs.

## Figure 1.7

**Stages of Behavior Change.** According to many health education experts, the process of changing behaviors involves these five stages.

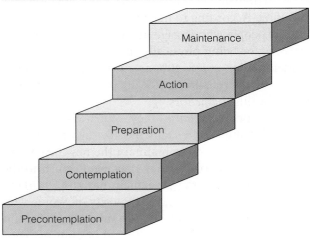

- Maintenance
- Action
- Preparation
- Contemplation
- Precontemplation

ing stimulus control, counterconditioning, rewards, and social support. *Stimulus control* involves altering cues to modify responses (behaviors). Cues can be sensory triggers, such as seeing a billboard advertisement for cigarettes or smelling someone else's cigarette smoke. Cues can also be emotional states or thoughts. For example, a person may smoke to relieve stress or because he or she associates smoking with celebrities or sophisticated people. As a result, this person is likely to light up a cigarette when tense or in certain social situations.

If you are a smoker who wants to quit, you may need to identify and eliminate the various cues that signal this unhealthy behavior. You may realize, for example, that seeing ashtrays and lighters are your smoking cues. Throwing out or giving away your ashtrays and lighters are ways of avoiding these cues. If feeling tense triggers your desire to smoke, then learning and practicing relaxation techniques whenever you feel stressed out may help you resist the urge to buy a pack of cigarettes.

*Counterconditioning* involves replacing unhealthy behaviors with less destructive or healthier ones. When you desire a cigarette, you may be able to eliminate the craving by exercising, taking a warm bath, or calling someone who supports your efforts to quit. Chewing sugarless gum, eating raw vegetables or fruit, or drinking a glass of water whenever you feel the urge to smoke may also reduce the craving.

Rewards are incentives for positive behaviors. Some former smokers keep a jar in which they save the money that would have been used to buy cigarettes. At the end of a week or two, they spend that money on something fun such as a movie, DVD, or another type of reward to help maintain the new behavior. Other former tobacco users are rewarded by the return of their sense of taste or the praise they receive from nonsmokers for adopting a smoke-free lifestyle.

Obtaining social support by enlisting the help of others is very important for changing a negative behavior and maintaining a positive one. If you are a smoker in the contemplation stage of change and most of your friends are smokers in the precontemplation stage, they are not likely to support your efforts to quit. Therefore, you may have to associate with nonsmokers or people in later stages of change to provide the help, encouragement, and positive reinforcement you need to quit tobacco use.

**A Decision-Making Model** In the Student Workbook, you will find a "Changing Health Habits" feature for each chapter. This feature uses a systematic model for the decision-making process that can help you improve your health and well-being. A model is a plan or pattern that can be used as a guide.

The first part of the decision-making process involves identifying a problem behavior that you want to change, a goal that you would like to reach, or a question that you would like to answer. For example, you might want to quit smoking, lose 20 pounds, or determine whether you are ready to end an abusive relationship. Because the process of altering a behavior can have its unpleasant aspects, particularly if you have to overcome side effects or cravings, it is important to determine your level of commitment. To determine if you are ready to change a behavior

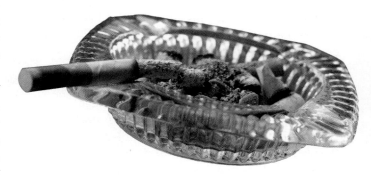

Cues are sensory triggers for behaviors, such as seeing cigarette butts is a cue for smoking.

or situation, it is helpful to make a list of the benefits, or pros, as well as the harms, or cons, of changing. After you make the list, think about each pro and con's value or importance to you. Assign a point value from 1 to 5 to each pro and con; a rating of 5 points would be the highest value. Then, find the sums of each list. If the sum of the cons list is greater than that of the pros list, you are probably in the precontemplation stage and not ready to make the change. On the other hand, if the sum of your pros is higher, you are likely in the contemplation stage and ready to make the change.

The second part of the process used in the decision-making model describes steps you can take to implement the change and evaluate your progress. After you decide to make a change, set a target date to begin the new behavior, reach the goal, or modify the situation. Mark that date on a calendar that is in an obvious place for you to notice, such as by your computer monitor or on your refrigerator or mirror. Then, make a list of factors that will increase the chances that you will be successful in making the change, such as enlisting the help of friends or obtaining advice from a medical expert. Because there are often barriers to making changes, make another list of factors that will hinder your chances for success, such as having little time to practice new behaviors or friends who will not support your decision to change.

The third major step in the process involves preparing an action plan that provides specific steps you will take to change your behavior or situation. You should be able to identify more than one way to reach your goal. To quit smoking, for example, you might quit "cold turkey," gradually reduce the number of cigarettes smoked over a 4-week period, or use a medically approved nicotine-containing product. At this point, you need to learn about the pros and cons of each method and consider the factors that can help or hinder your effort to change. How are you going to handle cravings or social situations that promote the behavior you are trying to change? Now you are ready to make the change by implementing your action plan. Keep a daily record of your progress, including strategies that are helpful and your feelings about the process. When you reach the goal date, analyze your success in attaining the goal. How well did your plan work? What can you learn from the experience?

To enjoy a long, healthy, and productive life, it is important for you to make numerous health-related decisions every day. If you act impulsively and base these decisions simply on cues, attitudes, and emotions, you may make poor choices. However, you are likely to make responsible choices if you follow a systematic method of decision making such as the one we describe. Changing habits often requires learning new information and practicing new skills. To practice making responsible health-related choices, complete the decision-making activities in the Student Workbook at the end of the book.

# The Goal of Prevention

A primary focus of health promotion is preventing diseases, infections, injuries, birth defects, and other serious health conditions. Preventing a health problem is a far better and less costly option than trying to treat it. In addition to adopting healthy lifestyle practices, you can take responsibility for preventing serious health problems by having routine physical examinations. The Managing Your Health box that follows provides recommendations for the frequency of routine screening procedures such as blood pressure, cholesterol, mammograms, prostate exams, and Pap smears (cervical cancer detection). Some examinations, such as testicular and breast self-exams, can be done in the privacy of your home. Many college students do not see the need for routine physical evaluations. Having regular medical checkups, however, enables you and your physician to monitor your physical and psychological health status. Furthermore, your physician may be able to identify a problem before it results in serious damage to your health and well-being.

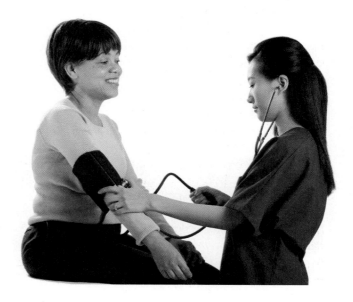

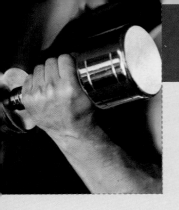

# Managing Your Health

## Routine Health Care for Disease Prevention: Adult Recommendations

The following recommendations apply to adults who have low risks of disease. People who have higher risks may need more frequent testing and to begin testing at an earlier age. Consult your personal physician for advice about routine testing and immunization schedules.

| Medical Test/Preventive Measure | Recommended Frequency* |
|---|---|
| Blood pressure | At least every 2 years |
| Cholesterol (fasting lipoprotein profile) | Every 5 years for people aged 20 and older |
| Glucose | Every 3 years starting at age 45 years |
| PSA and digital rectal exam (detects prostate cancer) | Discuss the need for testing with physician |
| Testicular exam | Some physicians recommend regular exams; discuss need for exam with physician |
| Skin exam (detects skin cancer) | Have physician check skin during routine general exams |
| Breast exam (detects breast cancer) | American Cancer Society recommends annual screen and clinical breast exams for healthy women aged 40 years and older; women between 20 and 39 years of age should undergo clinical breast exam every 3 years. Breast self-exam is an option for women |
| Pap test (detects cervical cancer) | Begin screening within 3 years of first sexual intercourse or by 21st birthday; yearly Pap test, or every 2 years if liquid form of test is used. Beginning at age 30 years, include human papillomavirus (HPV) test |

| Medical Test/Preventive Measure | Recommended Frequency* |
|---|---|
| Colon/rectal examination (detects cancer) | Have flexible sigmoidoscopy or colonoscopy at age 50 years; physician can decide which test is appropriate and how often testing should be repeated |
| Sexually transmitted infections | Sexually active people who are 25 years of age or younger should be tested annually for chlamydial infection; older women should be tested if they have new or multiple sex partners. Physician can decide which other tests are appropriate, such as for HIV infection |
| Immunizations§ | |
| Rubella | Nonpregnant women who lack immunity should be offered vaccine |
| Influenza | Recommended if risk factors are present (ages 19–49 years); annually after age 50 years |
| Tetanus | Every 10 years |
| Hepatitis B | Three doses |

*Recommendations vary among medical organizations.

§ U.S. Centers for Disease Control and Prevention. (2010, January 15). Quick guide: Recommended adult immunization schedule—United States, 2010. *Morbidity Mortality Weekly Report,* 59(1):1–4.

*Sources:* Data from Agency for Healthcare Research and Quality, The Guide to Clinical and Preventive Services, 2008. http://www.ahrq.gov/clinic/pocketgdo8/pocketgdo8.pdf; Centers for Disease Control and Prevention, http://hivtest.org/faq.cfm#stdtest; American College of Preventive Medicine, http://www.acpm.org; American Cancer Society, http://www.cancer.org. Accessed February 12, 2009.

## Can Good Health Be Prescribed?

No one has a crystal ball that predicts future health, and neither can anyone guarantee good health. Numerous factors contribute to an individual's chances of enjoying a long and productive lifetime of good health. Several of these factors are the result of lifestyle choices that people can make, while they are still young, to prevent or delay disease. You may know someone or have heard about individuals who avoided exercise, smoked a pack of cigarettes, and consumed a six-pack of beer each day, yet lived to a ripe old age. Such behavior defies nearly every reasonable prescription for good health. Perhaps these people inherited genes that foster the hardiness to withstand the effects of their risky lifestyles. You might wonder if these people enjoyed good health throughout their lives, or if they spent their last years in poor health. Would their lives have been even longer and healthier if they had followed more health-conscious behaviors?

### Healthy Living Practices

- To change your health-related behaviors, you must determine that you need to change and that you value the change.
- Use a decision-making plan as a tool to help you make responsible decisions.
- Take charge of your health by having regular physical examinations and monitoring your health.

## Analyzing Health Information

"Take antioxidants to live longer." "Drink red wine to prevent heart attacks." "Improve your memory with ginkgo." Every day Americans are barraged with a confusing array of health-related information in newspapers, magazines, television and radio shows, commercials, and infomercials. Family members, friends, medical professionals, and the Internet also supply information about health and health-related products. Are these sources reliable? Not necessarily. No laws prevent anyone from making statements or writing books about health, even if their information is false. The First Amendment to the U.S. Constitution protects freedom of speech and freedom of the press. This protection extends to talk show hosts and guests, authors, and salespeople in health food stores who might provide health misinformation.

Companies and individuals can make considerable amounts of money by selling untested remedies, worthless cures, unnecessary herbal supplements, and books filled with misinformation. Health frauds include the promotion or sale of substances or devices that are touted as being effective to diagnose, prevent, cure, or treat health problems, but the scientific evidence to support their safety and effectiveness is lacking.

Despite the regulatory activities of the Food and Drug Administration (FDA) and Federal Trade Commission (FTC), the sale of fraudulent products and services and the circulation of false or misleading health information continue to be concerns of medical experts. For information about the roles of the FDA and FTC in regulating health-related information, see the Consumer Health feature that follows.

## Becoming a Wary Consumer of Health Information

Maybe you have read an article or an ad about the health benefits of an herbal supplement or a weight loss device that you might buy. Perhaps you watched a physician promote his "anti-aging, high-energy" diet on a TV show. How do you know if health-related information and claims that are in the media and from other sources are true? Will the supplement, device, product, or diet do what its promoters claim? Or will you merely be wasting your money?

As shown in Figure 1.6, information is a crucial element of decision making. Although health information from some sources is based on scientific evidence and can be extremely useful, that from other sources may be unreliable. Relying on flawed information can waste time and money and can even be dangerous. To be a wary consumer of health information, you need to learn how to analyze it.

**Analysis Model** Analyzing something simply means breaking it down into its component parts for study. Analyzing information is easier to do if you follow a particular model of analysis. The following model is a series of questions that will help you evaluate health information and determine if it is reliable, regardless of its source.

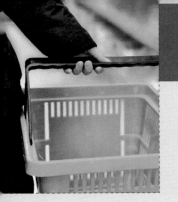

# Consumer Health

## Consumer Protection

The U.S. government has laws and agencies to protect consumers against health fraud.

The federal agencies that enforce consumer protection laws include the *Food and Drug Administration (FDA)* and the *Federal Trade Commission (FTC)*. The FDA protects consumers by regulating the information that manufacturers can place on food or drug product labels. In addition, FDA personnel alert consumers about fraudulent health practices and can seize untested or unsafe medical devices and drugs. The manufacturers of such products can be punished (usually fined) for their illegal practices. The FTC regulates claims made in advertisements for products and services. Both agencies regulate only products and services involved in interstate commerce. The FDA's website is www.fda.gov, and the FTC's website is www.ftc.gov.

To avoid being victims of health frauds, people must take the initiative and be very critical when judging the reliability of health-related information. If you suspect fraudulent activity, you can file a complaint with the local office of the FDA or your state's attorney general. You can also file a lawsuit if you have been injured as a result of following the advice or using the services or products of unscrupulous practitioners and manufacturers.

1. **Which statements are verifiable facts, and which are unverified statements or value claims?** In the context of this model, *verifiable facts* are conclusions drawn from scientific research. *Unverified statements* are conclusions that have no such support. *Value claims* are statements suggesting that something is useful, or effective, or has other worthwhile characteristics. Look for unverified statements and value claims; such information may or may not be true. Also, be wary of claims that "sound too good to be true."

Look for *red-flag* terms, expressions that indicate the possibility of irrelevant information or misinformation, such as "patented formula," "all-natural," "no risk," "chemical-free," "clinically tested," "scientifically proven," or "everyone is using." Claims that the product or service provides "quick," "painless," "effortless," or "guaranteed" cure or other desirable results are also red flags.

Ignore *anecdotes* and *testimonials*. **Anecdotes** are personal reports of individual experiences, such as "I take vitamin C and zinc pills, and I never get colds." **Testimonials** are claims individuals make concerning the value of a product. Advertisers often rely on paid celebrities to provide testimonials. Anecdotes may be interesting and testimonials may be persuasive, but these sources of information reflect the experiences of individuals and may not be true for most people. More compelling evidence, on the other hand, involves results of studies of hundreds or thousands of people. Such findings are more likely to be generalized to a wide population.

Look for *disclaimers* on product labels or in advertisements, such as "This statement has not been evaluated by the FDA," "This product is not intended to diagnose, treat, cure, or prevent disease," or "Results are not typical." In televised or written ads, disclaimers usually appear in small print near the end of the ad. Disclaimers may provide important information to consider.

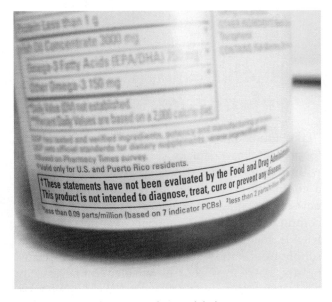

Disclaimer on a dietary supplement label.

2. **What are the credentials of the person who makes health-related claims? Does this person have the appropriate background and education in the topic area? What can you do to check the person's credentials?** Often it is difficult to tell if a health "expert" is qualified to make claims. Articles and books usually include the name and credentials of the author, but the credentials may be fraudulent. Anyone can call himself or herself a "nutritionist," "doctor," or "health expert." Therefore, a PhD or the title "Certified . . ." after someone's name is no guarantee that this person has had extensive training in a health or science field from an accredited educational institution. Individuals can buy certain doctorate degrees through the mail or Internet from unaccredited colleges called "diploma mills." To determine if a college or university is accredited, visit the U.S. Department of Education's website (www.ed.gov).

One way to investigate an author's medical or scientific expertise is to see if his or her work has been published in reputable journals. To conduct a literature search, use a site such as PubMed, which is sponsored by the National Library of Medicine (www.ncbi.nlm.nih.gov/pubmed/).

**Quackery** is the practice of medicine without having the proper training and credentials. *Quackwatch* is a website operated by retired psychiatrist Stephen Barrett, vice president of the Institute for Science and Medicine and a fellow of the Committee for Skeptical Inquiry. Quackwatch (www.quackwatch.com/) provides information about health-related frauds as well as people, popular books, and organizations that are sources of questionable health information.

3. **What might be the motives and biases of the person making the claims?** *Motive* is the incentive, purpose, or reason why someone promotes health misinformation. People profit from the sales of books as well as bogus treatments and products. Thus, ads are always written to motivate the consumer to buy the treatment, product, or service. A *bias* is the tendency to have a particular point of view. The author of a book or article, for example, may present information that supports his or her bias and ignores opposing views or research findings that do not support the bias. When analyzing health-related information, it is important to take into account the motives and biases of the people providing the information as you draw conclusions from it.

**anecdotes** Personal reports of individual experiences.

**testimonials** Individual claims about the value of a product.

**quackery** The practice of medicine without having the proper training and credentials.

4. **What is the main point of the article, ad, or claim? Which information is relevant to the issue, main point, product, or service? Which information is irrelevant?** The main point may be to provide practical information, but in many instances, it is to encourage you to buy a product or service. Ignore terms and information that are not pertinent or to the point; they will only confuse your analysis.

5. **Is the source reliable? What evidence supports your conclusion that the source is reliable or unreliable? Does the source of information present the pros and cons of the topic or the benefits and risks of the product?** Look for supporting or more in-depth information in scientific or medical journals because their articles are written and reviewed by scientists or medical experts. Articles in reputable scientific journals have been *peer reviewed*, meaning their content was critiqued by experts in that field before it was accepted for publication. If peer reviewers think a study was poorly designed or provides questionable conclusions, the article describing the study is likely to be rejected by the journal's editor.

Be wary of sources, such as magazines, books, and journals, that look like bona fide sources of health information but may not be. In many instances, they are actually designed to sell products or services. Such publications have articles about the benefits of healthcare products and include advertisements and instructions for ordering these products, often in the article or next to it.

Be skeptical of promoters, articles, or ads that do not present the risks along with the benefits of using a health product or service. For example, a reliable article about taking bee pollen supplements should present scientific evidence from peer-reviewed journals to support as well as refute health claims. Moreover, reliable sources of information often caution people about the hazards of using treatments, and they may include recommendations to seek the advice of more than one medical expert.

6. **Does the source of information attack the credibility of conventional scientists or medical authorities?** In some instances, people making health claims try to confuse readers by implying that evidence-based medicine is unreliable. For example, an ad for a treatment to relieve back pain may include claims that the technique is "unknown to Western medicine" or "used for centuries in China." Such claims suggest that conventional medical practitioners, including physicians, dietitians, and nurse practitioners, lag behind ancient systems of health care in finding cures or treatments. Statements that attack the reliability of conventional (scientific) medical practitioners are usually indications that the information is unreliable.

Finding reliable sources of health-related information can be challenging. You can usually obtain reliable answers to your questions from experts at state and local health departments, universities and colleges, local hospitals, and federal health agencies.

## Assessing Information on the Internet

The Internet can be a valuable source of health-related information. The U.S. government maintains websites for health-related information, including the sites of the Centers for Disease Control and Prevention (www.cdc.gov), Food and Drug Administration (www.fda.gov), and National Institutes of Health (www.nih.gov). Additionally, the Department of Health and Human Services sponsors www.healthfinder.gov, a general health information site that provides links to reliable sources, including government agencies, universities, and nonprofit health organizations.

Websites that are accredited by the Health on the Net (HON) Foundation (www.healthonnet.org/pat.html) are reliable sources of health-related or

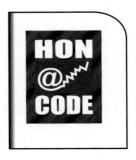

medical information. This nonprofit organization is headquartered in Switzerland and provides a widely recognized and accepted code of ethics. Websites can become certified by adhering to the HONcode. The HON site also provides a search engine to research trustworthy sources of health information (www.healthonnet.org/HONsearch/Patients/index.html).

Although HON monitors the websites it certifies, no organization regulates the quality and truthfulness of all the health information on the Internet. Many websites are sources of inaccurate and potentially harmful information. Therefore, you need to analyze the reliability of health information from websites as critically and carefully as you analyze health information from other sources. In addition, when researching a health topic, seek information from more than one Internet source and consult a medical professional before following advice from the Web.

When using a website as a source of health-related information, determine answers to the following questions to help you establish credibility of the site.

- **What is the source of the information?** Websites sponsored by individuals may give questionable advice that is based on personal experiences, biases, or opinions rather than medical expertise and scientific evidence, unless the individuals are credentialed experts. Commercial sites (.com) may or may not contain misinformation, but keep in mind that their purpose is generally commercial not educational. As with any commercial endeavor, the focus is usually selling products, so what is stated is meant to entice the buyer. Websites sponsored by organizations (.org) may or may not provide credible information as well. However, there are many good .com and .org sources of health-related information. Asking yourself the next questions will help you determine which of those sites likely provides reliable health-related information.

- **Is the site sponsored by a nationally known health or medical organization or affiliated with a well-known medical research institution or major university? If not, is the site staffed by well-respected and credentialed experts in the field?** Such sites usually provide accurate and timely health information. Some have independent review boards to ensure that the site maintains accuracy and timeliness. Websites providing credible health-related information usually include documentation of the expertise of the staff and the background of the institution or organization.

- **Does the site include up-to-date references from well-known, respected medical or scientific journals or links to reputable websites, such as nationally recognized medical organizations?** Such information generally helps support the claims or information on the site and provides ways to research the claims in-depth. Providing such references also shows that the information is based on published research.

- **Is the information at the website current?** Health information is constantly changing; the site should indicate when the information was posted and updated.

## Applying What You Have Learned

The Analyzing Health-Related Information features in this textbook provide examples of ads, articles, and websites to help you determine the value of health-related information. To sharpen your critical thinking skills, analyze the information in these features using the six points of the analysis model. When you analyze a website, use the questions posed in the previous section. If you determine that the website is highly credible, your analysis is completed. If, however, you are unsure of the credibility of the site after answering the Web analysis questions, then continue with the six Analyzing Health-Related Information questions. Additionally, the Consumer Health features in this and other chapters provide tips to help you become a better consumer of health information.

### Healthy Living Practices

- ☐ Use the model for analyzing health-related information and the questions for analyzing websites to evaluate information from the media and other sources.

**conventional medicine** The form of medicine that relies on modern scientific principles, modern technologies, and scientifically proven methods to prevent, diagnose, and treat health conditions.

**placebo** A sham treatment that has no known physical effects; an inactive substance.

To obtain reliable answers for your health-related questions, consult experts at clinics or hospitals, state and local health departments, universities and colleges, federal health agencies, and nationally recognized health associations and foundations.

## Conventional Medicine, Complementary and Alternative Medicine, and Integrative Medicine

**Conventional medicine** (scientific medicine) relies on modern scientific principles, modern technologies, and scientifically proven methods to prevent, diagnose, and treat health conditions. The notion that certain agents of infection such as bacteria and viruses cause many health disorders is accepted by conventional medical practitioners. To practice in their professions, conventional healthcare practitioners, such as physicians, nurses, dietitians, and dentists, must meet established national and/or state standards concerning their education and pass licensing examinations. To maintain their professional certification or licensing, many types of conventional healthcare practitioners must update their medical backgrounds regularly by participating in continuing education programs. Most Americans use the services of conventional medical practitioners.

Before adopting a method of treatment, conventional medical practitioners want to know if it is safe and effective. To determine the safety and effectiveness of a treatment, medical researchers usually conduct studies on animals before testing humans in *clinical studies*. A clinical study should contain at least 30 subjects, preferably hundreds or thousands, if possible. The greater the number of participants in the study, the more likely the findings did not occur by chance and are the result of the treatment.

In designing clinical studies, researchers take a group of volunteers with similar characteristics and randomly divide them into two groups: a treatment

## Sample Analysis of Health-Related Information

This statement has value claims that are not supported with scientific evidence.

No treatment contains everything each person needs to improve his or her health.

### For centuries, doctors in the Orient have known about the wonders of herbal medicines— nature's botanical cures for human ailments.

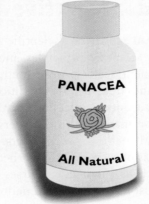

PANACEA

All Natural

This suggests that American scientists do not understand that medicines can be derived from plant sources, when, in fact, American researchers often rely on plants as sources of chemicals that have medicinal uses. No scientific evidence is cited to show that the herbs in Panacea have the touted properties. These two sentences, then, contain only value claims; thus, the information may be unreliable.

### Finally, American scientists are recognizing the healthful benefits of these herbs.

**SwayCon Pharmaceuticals** has developed a capsule that contains everything you need to reduce suffering, enhance health, and regain youthful vigor.

A team of medical experts from three major medical schools in the United States have clinical proof that the ingredients of Panacea are effective! Panacea contains a chemical-free mixture of natural enzymes and exotic herbs that

- relieve up to 80% more arthritis pain than aspirin;
- lower blood pressure by up to 20%;
- lower cholesterol by up to 45%;
- reduce lung cancer risk by as much as 50%, even in smokers;
- and reduce the risk of heart attack by 75%.*

**Other remarkable findings**

Taking Panacea for a few months can improve intelligence. R.P., a college student at a large East Coast university, reports, "At the beginning of the fall semester, I started taking three capsules of Panacea a day. My G.P.A. went from a 1.8 to a 3.4! Panacea has helped me get all A's!"

Reports are coming into our offices that Panacea acts as a sexual stimulant, increasing potency. S.D., a computer programmer in St. Louis, writes, "Thanks for saving my marriage. Before taking Panacea, my husband complained about my lack of interest in sex. One of my friends told me that Panacea can help. Just a few days after taking the capsules, our marriage turned into a perpetual honeymoon."

**Panacea is only available in fine health food stores. Order a three-month supply now, while supplies last**

### A PANACEA PILL A DAY KEEPS THE EXPENSIVE DOCTORS AWAY!

\* These statements have not been evaluated by the FDA.

Clinical proof is a red flag. The medical experts and medical schools where their research has been conducted are not identified. Objective testing could show the product is neither safe nor effective. The ad should cite the specific effects of the product, including negative ones.

"Chemical-free" is a red flag; all matter, including herbs and other plants, is composed of chemicals. Furthermore, scientific studies should be cited to provide evidence for these value claims.

A testimonial from an individual is not scientific evidence. This student's GPA my have risen for a variety of reasons. Studies conducted to show that a treatment is useful should contain at least 30 subjects.

Potency is a vague and undefined red-flag term. Again, this testimonial is a value claim that is unsupported by scientific evidence.

This is irrelevant information. Where the product is sold has nothing to do with its quality or characteristics. The authors of the ad are simply trying to make their product look superior to other similar products.

This statement gives the impression that consumers have no time to investigate the product thoroughly. It is intended to make consumers think that the product will sell out if they wait, and they will miss out on a good thing. Again, this information is irrelevant.

No scientific evidence is cited that a daily Panacea pill prevents serious illness. Additionally, this statement attacks conventional medical practitioners by implying that they are interested only in making money, which suggests that physicians cannot be trusted.

Disclaimer.

**Conclusion:** This ad is merely a collection of value claims that are not supported by scientific research. The ad further attempts to encourage the reader to purchase the product by suggesting that it is better (and less expensive) than conventional therapies. It claims to relieve a wide range of health conditions. The red-flag phrases and testimonials, lack of scientific evidence, and failure to caution consumers about potential hazards of the product all suggest the ad is an unreliable source of health-related information.

group and a control group. Subjects in the treatment group receive the experimental treatment; members of the control group are given a placebo. A **placebo**, often referred to as a "sugar pill," is a sham treatment that has no known physical effects. Because a person's positive expectations can result in positive findings, placebos help rule out the effects of such wishful thinking.

Researchers give subjects placebos to compare their responses to responses of subjects who receive the actual treatment. In *double-blind studies*, subjects and researchers are unaware of the identity of those taking placebos. Placebos can temporarily relieve subjective complaints, such as pain, lack of energy, and poor mood. Thus, subjects who are given placebos often report feeling better, even though the placebo did not provide any known physical effects. Scientists refer to these reports as the *placebo effect*. The placebo effect may be responsible for many claims of beneficial results from using unconventional medical therapies.

*Complementary and alternative medicine (CAM)* is an unconventional and diverse system of preventing, diagnosing, and treating diseases that emphasizes spirituality, self-healing, and harmonious interaction with the environment.[39] A treatment is *complementary* when it is used along with scientific medical care. A young man with liver cancer, for example, may use yoga and meditation to accompany the conventional medical treatments prescribed by his physician. An *alternative* therapy replaces conventional medical therapy. If the patient with liver cancer stops his prescribed treatments and substitutes fasting and coffee enemas in hopes of a cure, he is relying on alternative forms of medical care.

CAM can be classified as follows:

- *Alternative medical systems*, such as Ayurveda, traditional Chinese medicine, homeopathy, and naturopathy
- *Manipulative therapies*, such as spinal manipulation (chiropractics), osteopathy, reflexology, rolfing, and therapeutic massage
- *Mind–body interventions*, such as meditation, biofeedback, prayer, and creative arts healing (music therapy, for example)
- *Biologically based treatments*, such as aromatherapy, special foods (probiotic yogurt, for example), herbal teas, and large doses of vitamins
- *Energy therapies*, such as acupuncture, acupressure, and use of magnets

Certain CAM therapies have positive effects on the body and mind. For example, acupuncture (**Figure 1.8**) can relieve the nausea and vomiting that often occurs after surgery or that is associated with early pregnancy and lower back pain.[40] Although difficult to test scientifically, aromatherapy and therapeutic massage can be soothing and relaxing. **Table 1.4** provides information about popular CAM practices, including homeopathy and reflexology.

Promoters of certain CAM practices claim diseases can be prevented or cured by "cleansing" tissues, "eliminating toxins" from the body, and "balancing chi." To support claims of their method's effectiveness, promoters often use anecdotal reports and testimonials. Nevertheless, the effectiveness of most

### Figure 1.8

**Acupuncture.** Some physicians integrate acupuncture with conventional forms of medical care. Acupuncture may stimulate the body to release natural pain-relieving compounds, but its effectiveness is difficult to test scientifically.

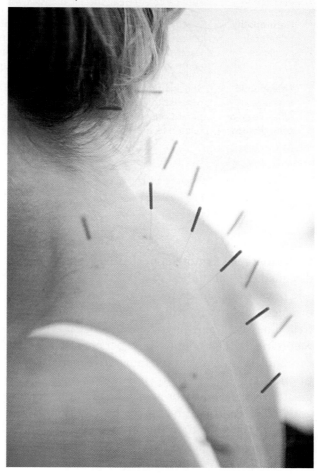

**Table 1.4**

## Common Alternative Medical Practices

| Type | Claims and Principles of Practice | Results of Scientific Research |
|---|---|---|
| Acupuncture | Used to treat a variety of common ailments. Based on an ancient Chinese medical practice in which thin needles are inserted into the skin or underlying muscles at specific places and stimulated to regulate the flow of "chi," the life force. | Testing acupuncture scientifically is difficult. It may relieve nausea and vomiting associated with "morning sickness," recovery from surgery, and cancer chemotherapy. Acupuncture may stimulate the body to release natural pain-relieving compounds. |
| Ayurvedic medicine | According to ancient Hindu religious beliefs, one achieves good health by meditating; eating grains, ghee (a form of butter), milk, fruits, and vegetables; and using herbs. Lack of balance between "energies" causes health problems. Fasting and enemas are used to treat severe ailments. | Meditation relieves stress; fruits, vegetables, and dairy products are nutritious foods; and some herbs have medicinal value. Ghee, however, can be fattening, and fasting can be dangerous for unhealthy people. Enemas are unnecessary for good health and should be used only under a physician's instructions. |
| Chiropractic medicine | According to some chiropractors, misaligned spinal bones cause disease. Spinal manipulation prevents or cures disease by correcting the spine. Other practitioners use spinal manipulation, but accept the germ theory of disease. | Can be effective in treating certain types of back pain, but some spinal conditions require medications and surgery that only a physician can provide. There is no scientific evidence that any disease can be treated by spinal adjustment.* |
| Homeopathy | Use of extremely dilute solutions of natural substances to treat specific illness symptoms. | Studies do not indicate that homeopathy is effective. |
| Naturopathy or natural medicine | Practice based on natural healing. Practitioners believe diseases occur as the body rids itself of wastes and toxins. Treatments include fasting, enemas, acupuncture, and "natural" drugs. | Lack of standardized medical training for practitioners called "naturopaths." |
| Therapeutic massage, reflexology, or zone therapy | Specific areas of the body correspond to certain organs. To alleviate pain or treat certain diseases, practitioners massage or press on the area that is related to the affected tissues. | The practice may stimulate the body to release pain-relieving compounds, but testing "touch" therapies scientifically is difficult. In general, scientific evidence does not indicate that pressing on body parts is an effective method of diagnosing or treating ailments. |

*Ernst, E. (2008). Chiropractic: A critical evaluation. *Journal of Pain and Symptom Management, 35*(5): 544–562.

CAM therapies is not supported by results of well-designed clinical studies.

Conventional medicine focuses on the "disease-oriented" approach, which seeks to diagnose and treat illnesses. Many physicians practice **integrative medicine**, which emphasizes personalized health care and disease prevention. Integrative medical practitioners focus on ways to encourage people to take greater responsibility for achieving and maintaining good health and well-being. Such practitioners also recognize the potential value of incorporating forms of alternative medicine that have scientific support into their preventive healthcare practices.

## Herbs as Medicines

Many Americans ingest pills or teas made from herbs and other plants because they think these products are natural and harmless ways to cure various disorders or achieve optimal health and well-being. The U.S. government classifies herbal products as *dietary supplements*. A **dietary supplement** is a product that is consumed to add nutrients, herbs, or other plant materials to a person's diet. Dietary supplements are not regulated by the FDA like medications are. As a result, the FDA does not require dietary supplement manufacturers to register their products and submit clinical evidence indicating that the products have been tested for safety and effectiveness prior to being marketed. In 2007, the FDA established a new rule that required manufacturers of dietary supplements to test the purity, strength, and composition of their products before marketing them to consumers. As a result, dietary supplements sold in the United States should be accurately labeled, contain the ingredients listed on the label, and provide standard amounts of the substances.

When the FDA determines that an ingredient contained in dietary supplements is dangerous, the agency can ban its use. Furthermore, the FDA can remove a dietary supplement from the market if its label states claims about the product's health benefits that are not supported by scientific evidence. The FDA permits herbal supplement manufacturers to include certain structure/function claims on the product's label. For example, the claims "maintains a healthy circulatory system" and "improves urine flow" describe how supplements can affect body functions. Unless given prior approval by the FDA, herbal supplement manufacturers cannot indicate on the label that a supplement can prevent, diagnose, treat, improve, or cure diseases. Results of clinical studies indicate that specific herbs can provide measurable health benefits. St. John's wort, for example, can relieve symptoms of mild to moderate depression and appears to be relatively safe when not combined with prescription medications.[41] Ginseng is a leading-selling dietary supplement in the United

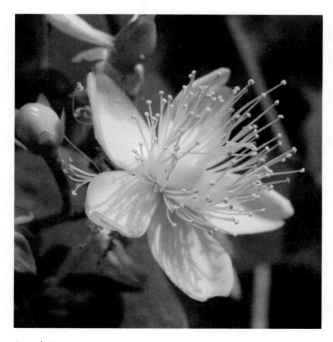

St. John's wort.

integrative medicine System of medical care that emphasizes personalized health care and disease prevention.

dietary supplement A product that is consumed to add nutrients, herbs, or other plant materials to a person's diet.

States. People use the herb for a variety of purposes, including as a sedative, antidepressant, and aphrodisiac. There is scientific evidence that taking *American ginseng* before meals may improve blood sugar values of people with type 2 diabetes.[43] Ingesting an extract made from the herb regularly may reduce the risk of respiratory tract infections, such as the common cold.[42] Although evidence that ginseng provides other healthful benefits is lacking, scientists continue to investigate the herb's potential uses.

Not every herbal product has measurable beneficial effects on health. Ginkgo is a popular dietary supplement, but scientific evidence to support claims that extracts made from ginkgo leaves improve memory is weak or inconsistent.[43] Many people take echinacea to prevent or treat the common cold, but the usefulness of this practice does not have widespread scientific support.[44] More research is needed to determine whether taking ginkgo, echinacea, and many other dietary supplements has measureable health benefits.

A "natural" therapy is not necessarily a safe one. Many plants, including comfrey, chaparral, pennyroyal, kava, birthwort, snakeroot, and germander, contain chemicals that can be harmful and even deadly when consumed. Ingesting *kava*, an herb that is promoted for relieving anxiety, can result in serious liver damage.[45] In 2004, the FDA banned the sale of most dietary supplements that contained *ephedra*, a naturally occurring stimulant drug that is often called ma huang. Traditional Chinese remedies and herbal teas that contain ephedra were exempt from the ban. Consuming ephedra can result in stroke, heart attack, and death.[46] In 2003, a weight-loss supplement that contained the toxic herb contributed to the sudden death of Steve Bechler, a 23-year-old professional pitcher for the Baltimore Orioles baseball team.

Consumers need to be aware that medicinal herbs may interact with prescription medications or other herbs, producing serious side effects. Additionally, these products may be contaminated with pesticides or highly toxic metals. Many dietary supplements are expensive and useless in promoting good health. *Table 1.5* includes information about the safety and

## Table 1.5

### Popular Herbal Supplements

| Supplement | Common Claims | Research Findings | |
| --- | --- | --- | --- |
| | | Uses | Risks |
| St. John's wort | Relieves depression | May reduce mild to moderate depression symptoms; no value for major depression | Can interfere with birth control pills and other prescribed medicines, increase sensitivity to sunlight, and cause stomach upset |
| Saw palmetto | Improves urine flow | May reduce symptoms of prostate enlargement that are not caused by cancer | May interfere with prostate-specific antigen (PSA) test to detect prostate cancer |
| Feverfew | Relieves headaches, fever, arthritis pain | Contains a chemical that may prevent migraines or reduce their severity | May cause dangerous interactions with aspirin or Coumadin (warfarin; a prescribed drug) |
| Echinacea | Prevents colds and influenza | Does not prevent colds or reduce their severity | May cause allergic response and be a liver toxin |
| Ginkgo biloba | Enhances memory and sense of well-being; prevents dementia | Weak or inconsistent scientific evidence to support claims | May interfere with normal blood clotting, cause intestinal upset, and increase blood pressure |
| Ginseng | Enhances sexual, mental, and exercise performance; increases energy; relieves stress and depression | Has no mood-enhancing effects. May reduce risk of respiratory infections and improve blood sugar values of people with diabetes | Can cause "jitters," insomnia, hypertension, and diarrhea and can be addictive; can be contaminated with pesticides and the toxic mineral lead |
| Yohimbe | Enhances muscle development and sexual performance | Dilates blood vessels but has no beneficial effects on muscle growth or sex drive of humans | Can produce abnormal behavior, high blood pressure, and heart attacks |
| Guarana | Boosts energy and enhances weight loss | Acts as a stimulant drug | May cause nausea, anxiety, and irregular heartbeat |
| Kava | Relieves anxiety and induces sleep | Acts as a depressant drug | May cause serious liver damage; do not use when driving |

effectiveness of some popular herbal supplements. Chapters 9 and 11 also provide information about dietary supplements. For reliable information about herbs and other dietary supplements, check the following government websites: http://nccam.nih.gov/health/atoz.htm and www.ods.od.nih.gov.

Some herbal supplement manufacturers claim their products have been clinically tested and shown to provide health benefits. The reliability of these claims may be questionable, however, because they are often based on results obtained from animal research or few, poorly designed human studies. Given the lack of scientific evidence that most medicinal herbs are safe and effective, the amount of money consumers pay for these products is astonishing. In 2009, for example, Americans spent more than $5 billion on herbal supplements.[47]

## CAM Therapies in Perspective

National surveys provide estimates of the extent to which Americans use unconventional medical therapies. According to the National Health Interview Survey, 38% of adults used forms of CAM in 2007.[48] Other commonly used CAM treatments were natural products, deep breathing exercises, meditation, and chiropractic care. In most cases, CAM was used to treat back, neck, and joint problems; colds; anxiety; and depression.

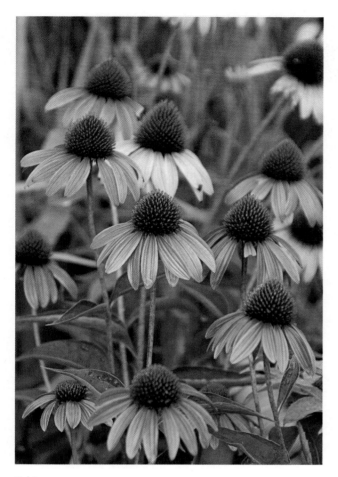

Echinacea.

The natural or exotic nature of many alternative therapies such as herbal pills and teas, coffee enemas, shark cartilage, and reflexology may appeal to people who distrust modern technology or have lost faith in conventional medical care. Others use alternative therapies to prevent or treat ailments because they want to take more control over their health. Conventional medical practitioners are concerned when persons with serious conditions forgo or delay conventional treatments and rely instead on questionable alternative therapies. These could be life-threatening decisions. Many forms of cancer, for example, respond well to conventional treatments, particularly if the disease is in an early stage. Many adults who use alternative medical therapies choose them to complement rather than replace conventional treatments.[48]

Regardless of treatment, people suffering from acute conditions such as low back pain, common colds, and gastrointestinal disturbances generally recover with time. Individuals with chronic health problems such as osteoarthritis and multiple scle-rosis often report *remissions*, times when their conditions improve. If people use alternative therapies when they are recovering or their illnesses are in remission, they are likely to think the nonconventional treatment cured or helped them. Additionally, people who combine alternative therapies with conventional medical care may attribute any improvement in their health only to the alternative treatments.

Conventional medical practitioners are likely to be skeptical of CAM techniques if they have not been shown scientifically in large-scale clinical studies to be safe or more helpful than placebos. The National Center for Complementary and Alternative Medicine within the National Institutes of Health funds research to determine the safety and effectiveness of alternative medical practices. Until supportive data are available from well-designed studies, consumers should be wary of CAM practices.

Before using alternative therapies, discuss your options with your physician and consider taking the following steps to protect yourself:

- Contact a variety of reliable sources of information to determine the risks and benefits of the treatment. For example, ask people who have used the treatment to describe its effectiveness and side effects. Conduct a review of medical literature, and recognize that popular sources of information such as health magazines and the Internet may be unreliable. Look for articles in medical journals or news magazines that have information concerning the usefulness of conventional as well as alternative medical approaches to care.

- Ask people who administer the treatment to provide proof of their medical training. Investigate the validity of their educational credentials. People who promote certain alternative medical practices often have little or no medical and scientific training.

- Determine the cost of treatment and whether your health insurance covers the particular alternative therapy. If it does not, find out why. You may find that your health insurer considers the treatment risky or ineffective.

- Ask your primary care physician for his or her opinion of the treatment. If you still have questions about the treatment, seek a "second opinion" from one or more other physicians.

- If you decide to use an alternative therapy, do not use it along with conventional therapy or abandon conventional treatment for any medical problem without consulting your physician.

- Investigate the possibility that the alternative medicine or herbal supplement can interact with conventional medications that you take and produce serious side effects. Additionally, investigate the possibility that taking combinations of herbal supplements can be harmful.

- If you are pregnant or breastfeeding, do not use herbal supplements or alternative therapies without consulting your physician.

- Do not give herbal supplements or alternative therapies to children.

 **Healthy Living Practices**

☐ Before using an herbal supplement or alternative therapy, obtain reliable information concerning the pros and cons of the treatment and discuss your options with your physician.

## Choosing Conventional Medical Practitioners

Scientific research, technological advancements, and a systematic approach to medical education make the conventional healthcare system in the United States among the best in the world. Conventional medicine, however, has its limitations; not every condition can be prevented, managed, or cured.

Americans generally consider conventional medical care practitioners, such as physicians, dentists, nurses, and dietitians, to be experts in their fields. How do you choose the best medical professionals? A good way is to ask family and friends for their recommendations. If you are enrolled in certain health insurance plans, you generally must select from approved lists of providers. After you obtain some names of physicians or other conventional practitioners, check your health insurance plan's list of healthcare providers to determine whether the recommended individuals are listed.

To help ensure high-quality conventional health care, consumers should choose physicians who have certain personal and professional characteristics, in-

**Table 1.6**

### Characteristics of Good Personal Physicians

**A good personal physician:**

- Is intelligent and well qualified in his or her field of practice
- Spends adequate time with patients and listens to patients' concerns
- Is willing to modify treatment to meet patients' concerns and values
- Is caring and sympathetic
- Enlists patients' active participation in health-related decisions
- Is willing to admit when his or her medical knowledge is lacking
- Recognizes the limitations of his or her expertise and is willing to refer patients to other medical professionals when necessary
- Provides thorough physical examinations and orders appropriate testing, such as blood tests or x-rays
- Is available for telephone consultations when necessary
- Is available to handle emergencies or has a competent backup physician to take care of such situations
- Does not delay in seeing patients with urgent care needs
- Is on staff at one or more nearby accredited hospitals
- Keeps up to date by attending professional educational meetings or reading medical journals
- Has a well-managed, well-equipped office with friendly, courteous staff

cluding appropriate training and excellent medical credentials (**Table 1.6**). For example, a physician who is *board certified* or *board eligible* in a specialty, such as internal medicine, is well trained in that particular field of practice. In addition to considering a prospective physician's qualifications, you should evaluate his or her personality and office conditions. Make an appointment to meet with the physician and prepare a list of questions to ask him or her. For example, which health insurance plans are accepted? Where did the practitioner receive his or her medical training? With which hospitals does the physician have affiliations? When you are in the practitioner's waiting room, observe its cleanliness and the staff's attitude and friendliness. When you interview the physician, observe his or her body language and judge the person's verbal responses to your questions. After the interview, evaluate the physician's level of comfort with you, his or her answers to your questions, and office conditions. Was the physician friendly and interested in you and your health history? Did he or she provide satisfactory answers to your questions? Was the office clean and staff courteous? If you answered "yes" to these questions, you are likely to enjoy a good relationship with this physician and receive good medical care.

Ideally, people should be able to form a trusting relationship with their conventional medical practitioners, including physicians. To develop these relationships, patients need to acknowledge that they are largely responsible for their health status. For example, patients should adopt healthy lifestyles, obtain regular checkups, and seek medical attention for ailments that do not improve within a few days or have serious signs or symptoms. Moreover, patients should follow their healthcare practitioners' advice and communicate with them should concerns about their medical care arise.

Healthcare practitioners can foster positive relationships with patients by spending adequate time with them, listening to their concerns carefully, and showing an interest in knowing more about them, not just their physical signs and symptoms. Additionally, it is important for practitioners to be caring, sensitive, and understanding; to modify treatment to meet the patient's concerns and values; and to enlist the patient's active participation in health-related decisions.

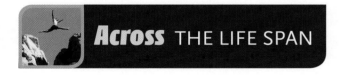

**Across** THE LIFE SPAN

## HEALTH

Although the focus of this text is adult health, the Across the Life Span feature in each chapter briefly describes health concerns that are specific to other stages of life, such as infancy, childhood, adolescence, and the older adult years. **Table 1.7** indicates the approximate age groupings for these life stages.

Why should college students learn about health conditions that can affect very young or very old members of the population? This information is relevant because many college students have younger siblings, some students have children, and those who are not parents may have children in the future. Ad-

| **Table 1.7** | |
|---|---|
| **Life Stages** | |

| Stage | Approximate Age |
|---|---|
| Prenatal period | Conception to birth |
| Infancy | Birth to 1 year |
| Childhood | 1 to 12 years |
| Adolescence | 13 to 20 years |
| Adulthood | 21 to 65 years |
| Older adult | Older than 65 years |

*Source:* Adapted from Smith, R. E. (1993). *Psychology.* Minneapolis/St. Paul, MN: West Publishing Company, p. 120

ditionally, many college students are middle-aged or have elderly parents and grandparents. The following information highlights some major life cycle health concerns of Americans.

In the United States in 2009, about 6 babies in 1,000 died during the first year after birth.[8] Most of these deaths were due to birth defects, low birth weights, and breathing difficulties that arose from *prematurity*, being born too early (**Figure 1.9**). Public health efforts aimed at educating and providing medical care for pregnant women can reduce the number of infant deaths.

Unintentional injuries are the major health threat to children between 1 and 14 years of age. Most deaths from unintentional injuries are preventable, such as deaths due to motor vehicle crashes, drownings, and house fires. Appendix B, "Injury Prevention and Emergency Care," provides information concerning safety.

Adolescence is a time when youngsters establish behaviors that may last a lifetime and when experimentation with risky behaviors usually begins. In 2009, about 10% of high school students reported driving a car or other vehicle after consuming alcohol, and about 18% had carried a weapon on at least one day during the 30 days preceding the survey.[49] Almost 10% reported that they had been physically abused intentionally by a boyfriend or girlfriend. About 28% of these students reported being too fat. Unintentional injuries (accidents), homicide, and suicide are major causes of death for people aged 15 to 24. In 2009, motor vehicle accidents accounted for

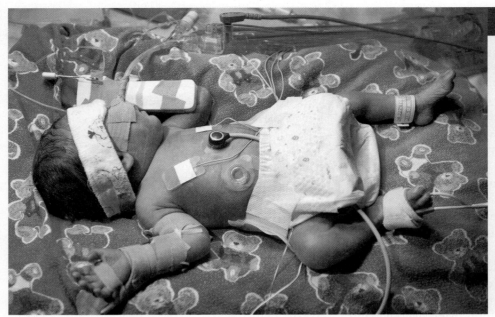

**Figure 1.9**

**Premature Newborns.** Infants born prematurely have a greater risk of serious health problems than do healthy full-term infants.

almost two-thirds of deaths resulting from unintentional injuries for Americans in this age group.[8]

In 2009, the teenage birth rate declined to its lowest level in nearly 70 years of recordkeeping in the United States.[50] However, sexually transmitted infections (STIs) continue to be major health problems for adolescents. People between 15 and 24 years of age contract about 50% of all new cases of sexually transmitted infections.[51] AIDS is primarily a sexually transmitted infection; sexually active adolescents are at risk of becoming infected with HIV, the virus that causes AIDS.

In 2009, people 65 years of age and older made up nearly 13% of the U.S. population. The percentage of older adults in the population is expected to increase rapidly over the next 40 years.[52] Chapter 15 discusses the health-related concerns of older adults.

# CHAPTER REVIEW

## Summary

Lifestyle includes behaviors that promote or deter good health and well-being. Optimal wellness is an optimal degree of health. The holistic approach to health integrates physical, psychological, social, intellectual, spiritual, and environmental dimensions. Contemporary definitions of *health* reflect not only how an individual functions, but also what that person can achieve, given his or her circumstances.

Heart disease and cancer are the major killers of Americans. Lifestyle choices contribute to the development of these and many other life-threatening diseases. The distribution of health problems differs among the various ethnic and racial groups in the United States. Poverty and cultural differences are often barriers to good health care.

Experiences, knowledge, needs, and values affect one's motivation to change health-related behaviors. People are motivated to take action if they feel that a sufficient threat to their health exists and that the results of changing their behavior will be worthwhile.

Although no one can guarantee good health, many factors contribute to one's chances of enjoying a long and productive lifetime of good health. Several of these factors are the result of lifestyle choices that people can make, while they are still young, to prevent or delay disease. Responsible health-related lifestyle choices involve a systematic approach to decision making.

People can become more careful consumers of health-related information, products, and services by learning to recognize misinformation. To obtain reliable health-related information, check with experts in federal, state, and local agencies and organizations.

Conventional medicine relies on modern scientific principles, modern technologies, and scientifically proven methods to prevent, diagnose, and treat health conditions. Complementary and alternative medicine (CAM) is an unconventional and diverse system of preventing, diagnosing, and treating diseases that emphasizes spirituality, self-healing, and harmonious interaction with the environment. Conventional medical practitioners are likely to be skeptical of CAM techniques that have not been shown scientifically to be safe and effective. Until supportive data are available, consumers should be wary of CAM practices.

Throughout the life span, health concerns vary. The most common causes of infant deaths are birth defects, low birth weights, and prematurity. Preventable injuries are the major causes of death for children and youth. Additional serious public health concerns for adolescents are suicide, homicide, drug abuse, obesity, pregnancy, and sexually transmitted infections (including HIV).

## Applying What You Have Learned

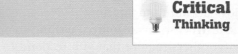

Critical Thinking

1. Develop a plan to improve your health. **Application**
2. Analyze a health-related advertisement or article to determine the validity of its information. **Analysis**
3. Identify sources of health information that you have used in the past year. Explain why you think each source is reliable or unreliable. **Synthesis**
4. Think of a health-related decision that you made recently. For example, did you decide to turn

down an offer to use a mind-altering drug, wear a helmet while riding a motorcycle, lose a few pounds, or use an herbal product to treat a condition? When you made this decision, did you use the decision-making process described in this chapter or did you act impulsively? Explain why you would or would not make the same decision today. **Evaluation**

| **Key** | **Application** using information in a new situation. | **Analysis** breaking down information into component parts. | **Synthesis** putting together information from different sources. | **Evaluation** making informed decisions. |

# *Reflecting on Your Health*

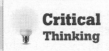

A reflective journal is a personal record of your thoughts and expressions of your feelings. The purposes of keeping this journal are to stimulate your thinking about what you have learned about health and to help you understand how your thoughts and feelings about your health might have changed over the semester. Thinking about new information can help you determine its usefulness, which can influence your attitudes and behaviors.

The Reflecting on Your Health questions at the end of each chapter are designed to guide your thinking. If you want to write about something else that is related to the contents of the chapter, feel free to do so, but make sure to identify the topic in your opening sentence. Write your journal entries in the first person, using "I" statements to express your thoughts, as though you were talking to a close friend. Do not worry about your spelling, punctuation, or grammar—just let your thoughts flow.

Some instructors make journal writing an optional activity; others require that you respond to all of the questions, and they grade journals. Still other instructors simply check to see if students are doing the assignment. Refer to the course syllabus or ask your instructor about his or her grading practices and other instructions concerning the journal.

## Journal Questions

1. What does the term *health* mean to you?
2. What do you think of the idea that people should strive to achieve optimal health?
3. What impact does spiritual health have on your sense of well-being? If spiritual health is important to you, describe the role it plays in your life.
4. Do you agree with the idea presented in the chapter that social health influences your physical health? Why or why not?
5. What factors influence your health-related behaviors?
6. Under what circumstances would you consider using alternative therapies?

# References

1. U.S. Centers for Disease Control and Prevention. (2010). Physical Activity Statistics. 1988–2008 No Leisure-Time Physical Activity Trend Chart. Retrieved on February 1, 2011, from http://www.cdc.gov/nccdphp/dnpa/physical/stats/leisure_time.htm

2. U.S. Centers for Disease Control and Prevention. (n.d.). Behavioral Risk Factor Surveillance System: Prevalence and trends data. Retrieved on February 20, 2011, from http://apps.nccd.cdc.gov/brfss/

3. Beck, L. F., & West, B. A. (2007, January 7). Vital signs: Nonfatal, motor vehicle-occupant injuries (2009) and seat belt use (2008) among adults—United States (2011). *Morbidity and Mortality Weekly Report, 59*(51):1681–1686. Retrieved on February 1, 2011, from http://www.cdc.gov/mmwr/preview/mmwrhtml/mm5951a3.htm?s_cid=mm5951a3_w

4. U.S. Department of Agriculture, Agricultural Research Service. (2010, August). Data tables from: *What we eat in America, NHANES 2001–2002.* Nutrient intakes: Mean amount consumed per individual, one day, 2001–2002. Retrieved on February 3, 2011, from http://www.ars.usda.gov/SP2UserFiles/Place/12355000/pdf/0102/Table_1_BIA.pdf

5. U.S. Department of Agriculture, Agricultural Research Service. (2010, August). Data tables from: *What we eat in America, NHANES 2007–2008.* Nutrient intakes: Mean amounts consumed per individual, by gender and age, in the United States, 2007–2008. Retrieved on February 3, 2011, from http://www.ars.usda.gov/SP2UserFiles/Place/12355000/pdf/0708/Table_1_NIN_GEN_07.pdf

6. U.S. Centers for Disease Control and Prevention. (n.d.). U.S. cancer statistics: An interactive atlas. Retrieved on February 18, 2011, from http://apps.nccd.cdc.gov/DCPC_INCA/DCPC_INCA.aspx

7. Centers for Disease Control and Prevention, National Center for Health Statistics. (2010). *Health, United States, 2010*: Data table for figure 1 (page 73). Retrieved on February 10, 2011, from http://www.cdc.gov/nchs/data/hus/hus10.pdf

8. Kochanek, K. D., Xu, J., Murphy, S. L., Miniño, A. M., & Kung, H.-C. (2011). Deaths: Preliminary data for 2009. *National Vital Statistics Reports, 59*(4). Retrieved on March 17, 2011, from http://www.cdc.gov/nchs/data/nvsr/nvsr59/nvsr59_04.pdf

9. U.S. Centers for Disease Control and Prevention. (2010). Vital signs: Current cigarette smoking among adults aged ≥ 18 years—United States, 2009. *Morbidity and Mortality Weekly Report, 59*(35):1135–1140. Retrieved on February 2, 2011, from http://www.cdc.gov/mmwr/preview/mmwrhtml/mm5935a3.htm?s_cid=mm5935a3_w

10. U.S. Centers for Disease Control and Prevention. Smoking and tobacco use: Consumption data: Total and per capita adult yearly consumption of manufactured cigarettes and percentage changes in per capita consumption—United States, 1900–2006. Retrieved on February 2, 2011, from http://www.cdc.gov/tobacco/data_statistics/tables/economics/consumption/index.htm

11. U.S. Census Bureau. (n.d.). *Statistical Abstract of the United States: 2011.* Table 1112. Alcohol involvement for drivers in fatal crashes: 1998 and 2008. Retrieved on February 2, 2011, from http://www.census.gov/compendia/statab/2011/tables/11s1112.pdf

12. Centers for Disease Control and Prevention. (2010). Vital signs: Binge drinking among high school students and adults—United States, 2009. *Morbidity and Mortality Weekly Report, 59*(39):1274–1279. Retrieved on February 3, 2011, from http://www.cdc.gov/mmwr/preview/mmwrhtml/mm5939a4.htm?s_cid=mm5939a4_w

13. National Institute on Alcohol Abuse and Alcoholism. (2010, July). A snapshot of annual high-risk college drinking consequences. Retrieved on February 3, 2011, from http://www.collegedrinkingprevention.gov/StatsSummaries/snapshot.aspx

14. Krebs-Smith, S. (2010). Americans do not meet federal dietary recommendations. *Journal of Nutrition, 140*(10):1832–1838.

15. Ogden, C., & Carroll, M. (2010). Division of Health and Nutrition Examination Surveys. Prevalence of obesity among children and adolescents: United States, trends 1963–1965 through 2007–2008. Retrieved on February 18, 2011, from http://www.cdc.gov/nchs/data/hestat/obesity_child_07_08/obesity_child_07_08.htm

16. U.S. Centers for Disease Control and Prevention, National Center for Health Statistics. (2009). Health E-Stat: Prevalence of overweight, obesity and extreme obesity among adults: United States, trends 1960–1962 through 2005–2006 Retrieved on February 18, 2011, from http://www.cdc.gov/nchs/data/hestat/overweight/overweight_adult.htm

17. U.S. Centers for Disease Control and Prevention. (2011). Obesity: Halting the epidemic by making health easier: At a glance 2010. Retrieved on February 3, 2011, from http://www.cdc.gov/chronicdisease/resources/publications/AAG/obesity.htm

18. World Health Organization. (1948). *Official records of the World Health Organization, no. 2. Proceedings and final acts of the international health conference held in New York from 19 June to 22 July 1946.* New York, NY: United Nations WHO Interim Commission.

19. World Health Organization. (1986). *Ottawa charter for health promotion.* Copenhagen, Denmark: Author.

20. Hochbaum, G. M. (1979). An alternative approach to health education. *Health Values, 3*:197–201.

21. U.S. Department of Health and Human Services, Centers for Medicare and Medicaid Services. (2010, August). National health expenditure data, updated NHE projections 2009–2019, forecast summary and selected tables. Retrieved on February 10, 2011, from http://www.cms.gov/NationalHealthExpendData/downloads/NHEProjections2009to2019.pdf

22. Cohen, R. A., Martinez, M. E., & Ward, B. W. (2009). Health insurance coverage. Early release of selected estimates based on data from the 2009 National Health Interview Survey, tables 1.1a-b, 1.2b. Retrieved on February 10, 2011, from http://www.cdc.gov/nchs/data/nhis/earlyrelease/insur201006.pdf

23. Mokdad, A. H., et al. (2004). Actual causes of death in the United States, 2000. *Journal of the American Medical Association, 291*(10):1238–1245. [Published correction appears in *Journal of the American Medical Association, 293*(3):293–294.]

24. U.S. Department of Health and Human Services, Public Health Service. (1991). *Healthy People 2000*: National health promotion and disease prevention objectives. Washington, DC: Government Printing Office.

25. U.S. Census Bureau. (n.d.). 2005–2009 American community survey. Retrieved on February 12, 2011, from http://factfinder.census.gov /servlet/ACSSAFFFacts?_event=&geo_id=01000US&_geo Context=01000US&_street=&_county=&_cityTown=&_state=& _zip=&_lang=en&_sse=on&ActiveGeoDiv=&_useEV=&pctxt =fph&pgsl=010&_submenuId=factsheet_1&ds_name= DEC_2000_SAFF&_ci_nbr=002&qr_name=DEC_2000_SAFF _R1010&reg=DEC_2000_SAFF_R1010%3A002&_keyword=&_ industry=

26. U.S. Centers for Disease Control and Prevention, Office of Minority Health and Health Disparities. (2010, November). Hispanic or Latino populations. Retrieved on February 20, 2011, from http://www .cdc.gov/omhd/Populations/HL/HL.htm#high

27. U.S. Centers for Disease Control and Prevention, Office of Minority Health and Health Disparities. (2010, November). Black or African American populations. Retrieved on February 13, 2011, from http://www.cdc.gov/omhd/Populations/BAA/BAA.htm

28. Centers for Disease Control and Prevention, National Center for Health Statistics. (2010). *Health, United States, 2010*: Table 24. Retrieved on February 10, 2011, from http://www.cdc.gov/nchs/data /hus/hus10.pdf

29. National Cancer Institute. (2011, January 7). SEER Cancer Statistics Review 1975–2007. Retrieved on February 20, 2011, from http:// seer.cancer.gov/csr/1975_2007/index.html

30. Centers for Disease Control and Prevention, National Center for Health Statistics. (2010). *Health, United States, 2010*: Table 67. Retrieved on February 20, 2011, from http://www.cdc.gov/nchs/data /hus/hus10.pdf

31. Centers for Disease Control and Prevention, National Center for Health Statistics. (2010). *Health, United States, 2010*: Table 71. Retrieved on February 20, 2011, from http://www.cdc.gov/nchs/data /hus/hus10.pdf

32. U.S. Centers for Disease Control and Prevention, Office of Minority Health and Health Disparities. (2010, October). Asian American populations. Retrieved on February 21, 2011, from http://www.cdc .gov/omhd/Populations/AsianAm/AsianAm.htm

33. U.S. Department of Education, National Center for Education Statistics, Education Sciences. (n.d.). Status and trends in the education of American Indians and Alaska Natives: 2008. Retrieved on February 21, 2011, from http://nces.ed.gov/pubs2008/nativetrends /highlights.asp

34. U.S. Centers for Disease Control and Prevention. (2011). CDC health disparities and inequalities report—United States, 2011. *Morbidity and Mortality Weekly Report, 60*(Suppl):1–116. Retrieved on February 21, 2011, from http://www.cdc.gov/mmwr/pdf/other /su6001.pdf

35. U.S. National Institute of Diabetes and Kidney and Digestive Diseases, National Diabetes Information Clearinghouse (NDIC). (2011). National diabetes statistics, 2011. Retrieved on February 21, 2011, from http://www.diabetes.niddk.nih.gov/dm/pubs/statistics/#fast

36. National Institutes of Health, National Human Genome Research Institute. (2010, November). Frequently asked questions about genetic and genomic science. Retrieved on April 15, 2011, from: http://www.genome.gov/19016904

37. Norcross, J. C., & Prochaska, J. O. (2002). Using the stages of change. *Harvard Mental Health Letter, 18*(11):5–7.

38. Prochaska, J. O., & Velicer, W. F. (1997). The transtheoretical model of health behavior change. *American Journal of Health Promotion, 12*(1):38–48.

39. Eskinazi, D. P. (1998). Factors that shape alternative medicine. *Journal of the American Medical Association, 280*(18):1621–1623.

40. Vanderploeg, K., & Yi, X. (2009). Acupuncture in modern society. *Journal of Acupuncture and Meridian Studies, 2*(1):26–33.

41. U.S. National Institutes of Health, National Center for Complementary and Alternative Medicine. (2010). *St. John's wort*. Retrieved on February 24, 2011, from http://nccam.nih.gov/health/stjohnswort /ataglance.htm

42. U.S. National Institutes of Health, National Library of Medicine, MedlinePlus. (2011, February). *Ginseng, American*. Retrieved on February 24, 2011, from http://www.nlm.nih.gov/medlineplus /druginfo/natural/967.html

43. Fransen, H. P., Pelgrom, S. M., Stewart-Knox, B., de Kaste, D., & Verhagen, H. (2010). Assessment of health claims, content, and safety of herbal supplements containing *Ginkgo biloba Food & Nutrition Research, 54*:5221. doi:10.3402/fnr.v54i0.5221

44. Barrett, B., et al. (2010). Echinacea for treating the common cold. A randomized trial. *Annals of Internal Medicine, 153*(12):769–777.

45. U.S. National Institutes of Health, National Center for Complementary and Alternative Medicine. (2010). Kava. Retrieved on February 24, 2011, from http://nccam.nih.gov/health/kava/

46. U.S. National Institutes of Health, National Center for Complementary and Alternative Medicine. (2010). Ephedra. Retrieved on February 24, 2011, from http://nccam.nih.gov/health/ephedra/

47. American Botanical Council. (2010). Herbal supplement sales increase in U.S. in 2009. Retrieved on February 24, 2011, from http://cms.herbalgram.org/press/2009_Market_Report.html

48. Barnes, P. M., et al. (2008). Complementary and alternative medicine use among adults and children: United States, 2007. *National Health Statistics Reports*, No. 12. Hyattsville, MD: National Center for Health Statistics.

49. U.S. Centers for Disease Control and Prevention. YRBSS: Youth Risk Behavior Surveillance System, 2009 results. Retrieved on February 24, 2011, from http://www.cdc.gov/healthyyouth/yrbs/index.htm

50. Ventura, S. J., & Hamilton, B. E. (2011). U.S. teenage birth rate resumes decline. *NCHS Data Brief, 58*. Retrieved on February 24, 2011, from http://www.cdc.gov/nchs/data/databriefs/db58.pdf

51. Centers for Disease Control and Prevention. (2010, November). Sexually Transmitted Disease Surveillance, 2009: STDs in adolescents and young adults. Retrieved on February 24, 2011, from http://www.cdc.gov/std/stats09/adol.htm

52. U.S. Census Bureau. Fact Sheet. (n.d.). 2005–2009 American Community Survey 5-year estimates United States. Retrieved on February 24, 2011, from http://factfinder.census.gov/servlet/ACSSAFFFacts?_submenuId=factsheet_0&_sse=on

go.jblearning.com/alters6e

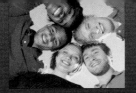
**Diversity in Health**
American Indians and
Psychological Health

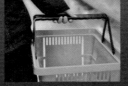
**Consumer Health**
Locating and Selecting
Mental Health Therapists

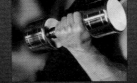
**Managing Your Health**
Resolving Interpersonal
Conflicts Constructively

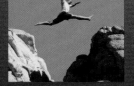
**Across the Life Span**
Psychological Health

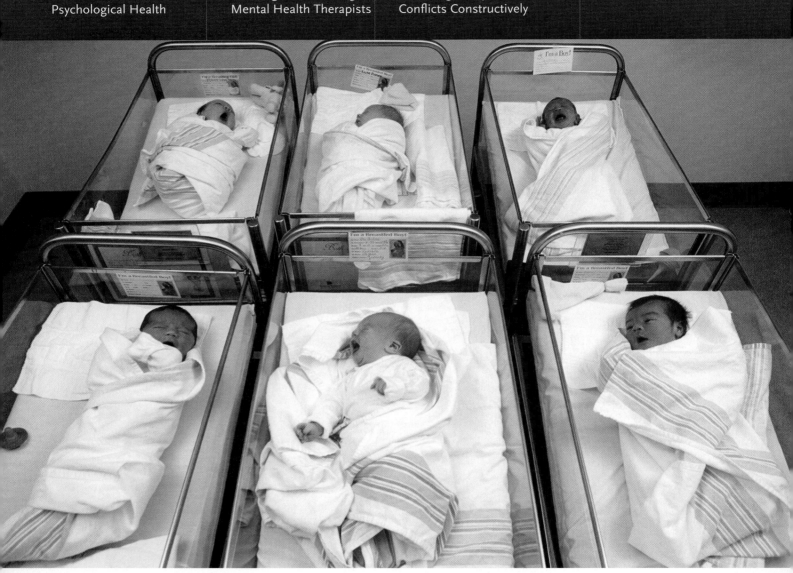

# Chapter Overview

How your nervous system affects your psychological health

How biological, social, and cultural forces interact to mold
personality

How psychological adjustment leads to psychological
growth

How to identify common psychological disorders

How to recognize suicidal behavior and prevent suicide

# Student Workbook

Self-Assessment: Self-Esteem Inventory

Changing Health Habits: Are You Ready to Improve Your
Psychological Health?

# Do You Know?

If you are psychologically healthy?

Why emotions are useful?

How to resolve conflicts in a healthy manner?

## CHAPTER 2

# Psychological Health

Observing newborn infants in a hospital nursery is a fascinating experience. While some of the babies sleep peacefully, others are awake, calmly gazing around at their surroundings while gently sucking their pacifiers. A few of the newborns are restless. Although tightly wrapped in swaddling, one infant tries to stretch her hand into the air as though she were reaching for something hanging above the bassinet. Another fussy baby frowns and closes his eyes tightly before spitting out his pacifier, kicking his feet, and howling in pain. Moments later, several other babies begin to grow fussy. Soon a chorus of crying babies shatters the calmness of the nursery. The infants' caregivers scurry to each bassinet, trying to determine which babies are truly in need of their attention and the reasons why. Why do some newborns respond differently when all of them are in the same situation?

Each newborn is a unique person. All infants, however, have basic physical needs that must be met if they are to survive. These needs include nutritious food and a safe environment. Additionally, children have psychologi-

> *"Each newborn is a unique person."*

**psychology** The study of the mental processes that influence human behavior.

**physiology** The study of bodily functions.

**central nervous system (CNS)** Of the two primary divisions of the nervous system, the one that consists of brain and spinal cord.

**peripheral nervous system (PNS)** Of the two primary divisions of the nervous system, the one that consists of nerves, which relay information to and from the CNS.

**neurotransmitters** Chemicals produced and released by nerves that convey information between most nerve cells.

cal needs for belonging, love, social acceptance, and respect that must be met if they are to mature into healthy adults. What if there was a crystal ball in the nursery that would enable you to predict each baby's future? Which of these infants will be psychologically healthy, achieving personal fulfillment and being satisfied with themselves and their lives? Which ones will be emotionally distressed and lead troubled lives?

**Psychology** is the study of the thinking or mental (cognitive) processes that influence human behavior. As defined in Chapter 1, psychological (mental) health involves the ability to deal effectively with the psychological challenges of life. Psychological health is dynamic, becoming more positive or negative as a person responds to a constantly changing environment. Many individuals, however, manage to maintain high degrees of positive psychological functioning throughout their lives. People with positive mental health are able to deal effectively with the psychological challenges of life. Such people accept themselves, have realistic and optimistic outlooks on life, function independently, form satisfying interpersonal relationships, and cope effectively with change (**Table 2.1**). In addition to these traits, psychologically healthy individuals resolve their problems without resorting to substance abuse or violence, and they assert themselves in social situations.

The quality of one's psychological health often affects the other components of health, such as social, spiritual, and physical health. This chapter discusses factors that influence positive psychological health as well as those that contribute to the development of psychological disorders. Chapter 3 examines the impact of psychological stress on health; Chapter 4 focuses on the effects of violence on health, including stress.

## The Basics of Psychological Health

Understanding psychological health involves learning about **physiology**, the study of body functions, and psychology. Cognitive processes such as thinking, decision making, and remembering rely on the functioning of the nervous system. The nervous system is an elaborate biological communications network that contains billions of nerve cells, or neurons, which are designed to receive, send, and interpret messages in your body by means of electrical and chemical signals. As you can see in **Figure 2.1**, this network consists of two interrelated parts: the **central nervous system (CNS)**, the brain and spinal cord; and the **peripheral nervous system (PNS)**, nerves that relay information to and from the CNS.

Most nerves produce and release **neurotransmitters**, chemicals such as acetylcholine, dopamine, and serotonin that convey information between nerve cells. By altering the levels of various neurotransmitters, the nervous system transmits information and produces physical responses, thoughts, and emotions.

Emotions are a way of communicating our moods to others. Emotions are associated with typical behavioral and physical responses, including changes in speech patterns as well as facial expressions and other forms of body language. Happiness, sadness, anger, and fear are among the basic emotions that we often

## Figure 2.1

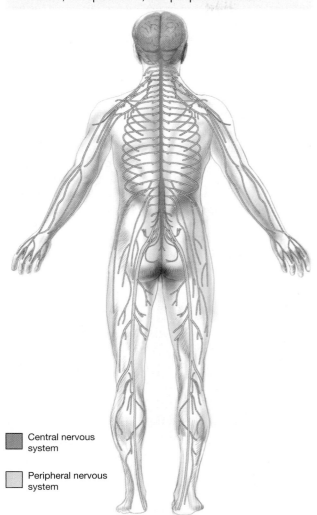

**The Nervous System.** The nervous system consists of the brain, the spinal cord, and peripheral nerves.

■ Central nervous system

□ Peripheral nervous system

alistic thoughts, and *maladaptive* behaviors occur. Maladaptive behaviors interfere with one's ability to be productive, interact well socially, and adjust to the demands of everyday living. In many instances, treating these conditions involves taking medication that corrects abnormal neurotransmitter levels as well as learning how to change distorted ways of thinking.

## Personality Development

**Personality** is a set of distinct thoughts and behaviors, including emotional responses, that characterizes the way a person responds to situations. Many factors, including biological, cultural, social, and psychological forces, interact to mold personality.

**Biological Influences Heredity** is the transmission of biological information, coded within genes, from parents to offspring. This information determines, in part, an individual's physical, emotional, and intellectual characteristics. Much of a person's **temperament**, the predictable way an individual responds to the environment, is inherited. Soon after birth, parents can usually describe their children's temperamental styles, such as irritable, fearful, or pleasant. As children mature, social and cultural influences modify their temperaments.

**Social and Cultural Influences** From the moment of birth, the social environment, such as interactions with parents and other family members, influences the psychological development of an individual. Most people learn how to respond to situations in socially and culturally acceptable ways when they are children. The circumstances surrounding a situation influence the kind and extent of an emotional display. Consider, for example, emotions that are appropriate to express while attending the funeral of a child.

A person's cultural and ethnic background can influence his or her responses to situations and perceptions of mental health disturbances. Although psychological problems affect people from every culture, symptoms of these problems may differ among cultures. The Diversity in Health essay "American Indians and Psychological Health" discusses a traditional American Indian concept of health, the *medicine wheel*, and healing methods.

call *feelings*. A psychologically healthy person is able to express his or her emotions appropriately. Much of the disability that is associated with psychological illness results from abnormal or extreme emotional responses to situations.

Parts of the brain, collectively referred to as *the mind*, process various types of information received from the rest of the body and the environment. As a result, the mind thinks about what takes place, finds meaning in events, considers actions, makes decisions, directs responses, evaluates and remembers consequences, and plans for the future. These activities involve neurotransmitters in the brain. Certain conditions can negatively affect the mind by altering neurotransmitter levels and disrupting normal brain chemistry and functioning. As a result, inappropriate moods, unre-

The Basics of Psychological Health  **41**

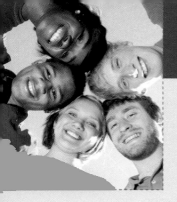

# Diversity in Health

## American Indians and Psychological Health

The Diversity in Health essay in Chapter 1 discussed major health concerns affecting American Indians (AIs), including problems associated with poor psychological health such as alcoholism, suicide, and accidents. According to the results of a major survey conducted from 2000 to 2004, AI adults were more likely to have experienced serious psychological distress—feeling sad, restless, hopeless, nervous, or worthless—during the past 30 days than adults of other racial or ethnic groups. A study of more than 3,000 Northern Plains and Southwest tribal members indicated that alcoholism and major depression were common among subjects. Factors that may contribute to AIs' generally poor mental health status include poverty, low educational level, exposure to violence, and discrimination. AIs can obtain professional help for mental health problems through the Indian Health Service (IHS). However, many AIs have more confidence in traditional healing practices than therapies provided by conventional medical practitioners.

The traditional AI concept of health involves the *medicine wheel*, a circle divided into four equal parts representing the major aspects of health: context (natural environment and social setting), mind, body, and spirit. When the four components of the medicine wheel are balanced with each other, people enjoy wellness or "harmony." When people are not in harmony with nature, their community, or themselves, they suffer from physical and psychological illnesses. According to some traditional AI beliefs, an emotionally disturbed individual is in a state of disharmony with the rest of nature or in a hopeless state of health. In other AI traditions, the symptoms of mental illnesses result from supernatural forces exerting control over the person.

Traditionally, AIs view alcohol abuse and other mental health problems as imbalances in the spiritual component of the medicine wheel. Because spiritual health is linked closely with psychological health, treatments are spiritual in nature and may involve prayer, sweat lodges, or purification ceremonies led by natural healers. Efforts to restore spiritual balance may also include participa-

tion in activities that increase cultural identity and self-esteem, such as crafts, storytelling, and making drums and baskets. In addition to relying on traditional healing methods, many AI accept conventional forms of treatment, especially for serious psychological disturbances.

In the United States, conventional mental health practitioners have been taught to identify normal and abnormal behaviors and diagnose mental illness by using an established set of standards. Often, these healthcare providers do not consider the importance of culture when treating patients who are members of minority groups, particularly AIs. Medical practitioners need to recognize the importance of cultural traditions when treating an AI or any individual. Furthermore, mental healthcare providers can often gain the trust and respect of clients from various cultural backgrounds by learning about traditional healing methods. As a result, patients are more likely to accept the healthcare provider's advice and suggestions for conventional treatment.

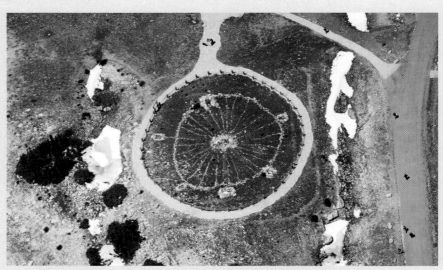

Aerial view of Medicine Wheel, Bighorn National Forest, Wyoming.

*Sources:* Centers for Disease Control and Prevention. (2006). Quickstats: Percentage of adults with self-assessed symptoms of serious psychological distress, by sex and race—United States, 2000–2004. *Morbidity and Mortality Weekly Report, 55*(29):801. Retrieved from http://www.cdc.gov/mmwr/preview/mmwrhtml/mm5529a5.htm; Beals, J., et al. (2005). Prevalence of *DSM-IV* disorders and attendant help-seeking in 2 American Indian reservation populations. *Archives of General Psychiatry, 62*(1):99–108; Walls, M. L., et al. (2006). Mental health and substance abuse services preferences among American Indian people of the Northern Midwest. *Community Mental Health Journal, 42*(6):521–535; and Cross, T., et al. (2000). Cultural strengths and challenges in implementing a system care model in American Indian communities. *Systems of care: Promising practices in children's mental health* (2000 series, Vol. 1). Washington, DC: Center for Effective Collaboration and Practice, American Institutes for Research.

# Theories of Personality Development

**Freud's Framework of Personality** More than 100 years ago, physician Sigmund Freud pioneered modern approaches to the diagnosis and treatment of psychological disturbances. Freud observed that people have an element of the mind that lacks awareness of certain thoughts, feelings, and impulses. He proposed that this "unconscious" component of the mind influences much of an individual's behavior. The unconscious mind, for example, engages various defense mechanisms such as repression and avoidance to cope with anxiety and guilt.

**Defense mechanisms** are ways of thinking and behaving that reduce or eliminate anxiety and guilt feelings by altering the individual's perception of reality. Nearly everyone uses defense mechanisms to protect their minds against psychological conflicts and threats. A basic defense mechanism is *repression,* the unconscious forgetting of anxiety-producing feelings, thoughts, or impulses. For example, adults who were sexually or physically abused as children may repress the memories of the abuse. Students who blame teachers for their lack of academic success, instead of themselves for skipping classes or not

studying, may be using *rationalization* as a defense mechanism. **Table 2.2** lists repression, projection, and some other common defense mechanisms and describes instances in which the unconscious mind employs them. Although these strategies may protect the mind and reduce anxiety in the short run, defense mechanisms usually do not provide long-term solutions to problems.

Freud believed that unconscious desires or drives, particularly the *libido*, or sex drive, control human behavior by creating psychological tension. Relieving this tension produces pleasurable sensations. However, members of society establish *moral values*, rules for good and bad behavior that often prevent individuals from satisfying all of their desires. If a person who accepts the moral values of society acts or thinks in ways that conflict with these rules, he or she usually feels anxious and guilty. Many people use moral values as guidelines to judge their behavior, themselves, and others.

**Erikson's Psychosocial Stages of Development** Psychoanalyst Erik Erikson modified Freud's

> **defense mechanisms** Ways of thinking and behaving that reduce or eliminate anxious and guilt feelings.

## Table 2.2

### Defense Mechanisms

| Defense Mechanism | Behavior | Example |
|---|---|---|
| Repression | Blocking unpleasant thoughts or feelings | A woman suppresses the memory of being sexually abused as a child. |
| Rationalization | Making up false or self-serving excuses for unpleasant behavior or situations | A man makes excuses for not being hired for a job. |
| Denial | Refusing to acknowledge unpleasant situations or feelings | A young man does not accept the fact he has been diagnosed with a terminal illness. |
| Projection | Attributing unacceptable thoughts, feelings, or urges to someone else | A woman accuses her boyfriend of being unfaithful while repressing her desire to have an affair. |
| Displacement | Redirecting a feeling or response toward a target that usually is less of a threat | An abused wife does not fight back but mistreats her child instead. |
| Avoidance | Taking action to prevent situations that produce powerful feelings | A woman will not date because she is afraid of falling in love. |
| Regression | Reducing anxiety by acting immature to feel more secure | A 6-year-old child begins to suck his thumb after the birth of his baby brother. |

### Table 2.3

### Erikson's Psychosocial Stages of Personality Development

| Conflicts | Approximate Age Ranges |
| --- | --- |
| Trust vs. mistrust | Birth to 1 year |
| Autonomy vs. doubt and shame | 1 to 3 years |
| Initiative vs. guilt | 3 to 6 years |
| Industry vs. inferiority | 6 to 12 years |
| Identity vs. identity confusion | 12 to 18 years |
| Intimacy vs. isolation | Young adulthood |
| Generativity vs. stagnation | Middle age |
| Integrity vs. despair | Old age |

ideas by proposing that social influences play a greater role in shaping personalities than do sexual drives.[1] According to Erikson, individuals progress through eight psychosocial stages during their lifetimes (**Table 2.3**). Each stage has major social crises or conflicts that people must manage or resolve to achieve a sense of emotional well-being.

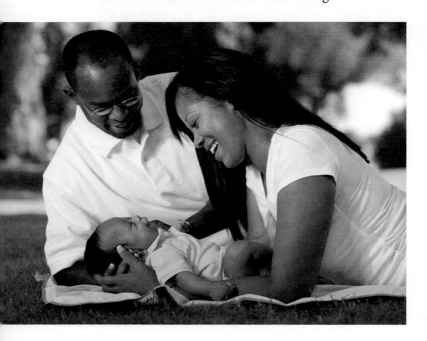

Establishing trusting relationships with loving adults enables infants to begin developing psychological well-being.

Infants require a considerable amount of care and nurturing from adults to survive and to develop normally. Erikson thought that babies learn to *trust* other individuals if their parents or other caregivers meet their basic physical and emotional needs. Establishing trusting relationships with caring and loving adults enables infants to begin the process of developing high degrees of psychological well-being later in life.

Erikson viewed adolescence as a critical period in which youth develop a sense of *identity*. During this stage, adolescents become increasingly responsible for making their own decisions. They begin to function separately from their families and define who they are as well as what their future roles will be. According to Erikson, the three major areas of concern that adolescents must clarify relate to their sexuality, future occupation, and social conduct. Adolescents begin to establish their identities when they begin to clarify their feelings and positions about their roles in life. Identity confusion results when they are unable to develop sound self-concepts and function independently of their families.

As adolescents mature into young adulthood, they face the challenge of *intimacy*, forming close and loving relationships with others. Adults who did not develop a sense of trust earlier in their lives or have not clarified their identities may be unable to establish intimate relationships and thus feel isolated. During middle age, individuals who have mastered previous developmental tasks often focus on meeting the needs of others through activities such as raising families and performing community service. Erikson coined the term *generativity* to refer to these psychosocial tasks. In the final stage of life, people seek *integrity*, a feeling that their lives have been fulfilling and complete.

**Maslow's Hierarchy of Human Needs** According to psychologist Abraham Maslow, individuals behave in response to their values rather than to their unconscious drives.[2] Maslow thought that healthy people value the freedom to achieve personal fulfillment by developing their talents and competencies. This freedom becomes a psychological need that drives personality development. Maslow created a hierarchy of five human needs, from the most basic biological requirements that contribute to human survival to the one that is most essential for psychological fulfillment, self-actualization (**Figure 2.2**). To achieve *self-actualization*, each level of needs from the base to the top of the hierarchy must be met, in order.

Self-actualized persons are psychologically healthy and mature. They feel free to pursue their creative and intellectual capabilities. The possibility of self-actualization exists in all people, but unless the prerequisite needs are met, individuals can never fully realize their potential. According to Maslow and others, only about one person in a hundred will reach the top of the human needs hierarchy. Nevertheless, Maslow admitted that many people are satisfied with their lives even if they have not achieved self-actualization.

## Adjustment and Growth

Each day, individuals respond to the demands of other people, their physical environment, and themselves. Throughout life, these demands are changing constantly. Being in college is especially demanding, but consider how your life will change after you graduate. What do you think your life will be like 10, 20, or 30 years after graduation? What kinds of adaptations do you expect to make over your lifetime?

Adapting to change, which is called *adjustment*, involves the responses people make to cope with the demands of life. **Psychological adjustment** occurs when an individual learns that certain responses meet these demands more effectively than others do. For example, one way a new student might psychologically adjust to college life is by scheduling time each week for various tasks, such as studying, attending classes, and going to work. Maintaining the new schedule may be challenging, particularly if the student followed a less structured lifestyle in the past.

**Psychological growth** occurs when a person discovers that certain adjustment strategies, such as studying more or planning for the future, enhance one's sense of freedom and control over oneself and the environment. To adjust in beneficial ways and to experience psychological growth, an individual needs to obtain reliable information, set realistic goals, plan effective ways to achieve those goals, take actions that are based on reasonable judgments and decisions, and evaluate the consequences of his or her choices.

If not managed effectively, interpersonal conflicts can hinder psychological adjustment and growth. Such conflicts often arise when people do not share opinions, values, needs, or beliefs. In these situations, many individuals respond by expressing anger or aggression. *Aggressive* reactions often injure other people physically or psychologically; therefore, these responses do not facilitate social interactions.

*Assertiveness* is a way of reacting to social situations by maintaining one's rights without interfering with the rights of other people and without harming them. Consider how students respond to an instructor who failed to consider certain possible answers to an essay question. An aggressive student might take class time to argue a point, verbally lashing out at the teacher. An assertive student might arrange to meet with the instructor after

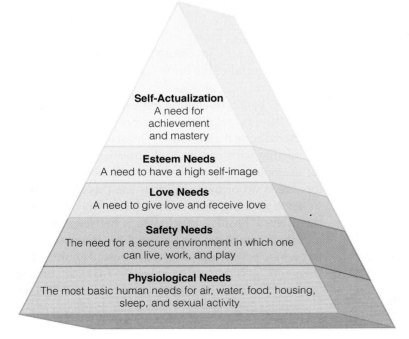

**Figure 2.2**

**Maslow's Hierarchy of Human Needs.** Maslow created a hierarchy of five human needs, from the basic biological survival requirements to psychological fulfillment (self-actualization). Before achieving self-actualization, a person must satisfy all of the preceding needs.

**Self-Actualization**
A need for achievement and mastery

**Esteem Needs**
A need to have a high self-image

**Love Needs**
A need to give love and receive love

**Safety Needs**
The need for a secure environment in which one can live, work, and play

**Physiological Needs**
The most basic human needs for air, water, food, housing, sleep, and sexual activity

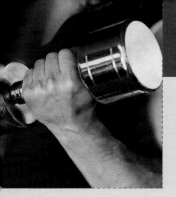

# Managing Your Health

## Resolving Interpersonal Conflicts Constructively

In addition to compromise, consider using the following tips to resolve conflicts constructively:

1. Focus on one issue; state your perception of the problem as clearly as possible.
2. Consider the feelings of others; avoid criticizing, name-calling, threats, or sarcasm.
3. Use "I feel" statements. "You" statements make others defensive. For example, say, "I feel angry when you . . ." instead of "You make me angry."
4. Do not assume how other people feel, what they believe, or how they will react.
5. Discuss the current concern; avoid dredging up past arguments.
6. Think before you speak; choose your words carefully to avoid confusion.
7. Listen carefully to others; avoid interrupting them while they talk.
8. Accept responsibility for your actions. Apologize for making mistakes.
9. Offer reasonable solutions.
10. Give others time to consider, accept, or reject your ideas.
11. Be patient; keep the door open for future communication.

---

class, using the time to discuss his or her case in a more thoughtful and rational manner.

Another way healthy people constructively resolve interpersonal conflicts is by using compromise. An individual who disagrees with a friend over an issue, for example, may decide that preserving the friendship is more valuable in the long run than "winning" the argument. This person is willing to compromise by modifying his or her attitudes. The Managing Your Health feature in this chapter provides additional suggestions for resolving conflicts constructively.

Psychological growth fosters the development of **autonomy**, or self-control. People with a high degree of autonomy function independently. Autonomy is associated with **self-esteem**, the extent to which a person feels worthy and useful.

## Self-Esteem

Self-esteem is a key component of personality that influences an individual's thoughts, actions, and feelings. Positive self-esteem is a characteristic of psychologically healthy people. Individuals who have positive or high self-esteem:

- Have a high degree of autonomy
- Are self-confident and have self-respect
- Are satisfied with themselves
- Accept challenges and work well with others
- Seek supportive and loving relationships

- Adjust easily to change
- Accept responsibility for actions when they make mistakes

People with low self-esteem:

- Have difficulty making decisions
- Resist changing their behavior
- Resent any form of criticism, even if it is constructive
- Put down others to make themselves look or feel better

The "Self-Esteem Inventory" in the Student Workbook at the end of the book can help you assess your self-esteem.

People begin developing self-esteem early in childhood. Parents and other caregivers play a crucial role in determining their children's level of self-esteem. By interacting with parents and other family members, for example, young children learn that certain behaviors are good or bad. Children use this information to begin forming their *self-image*, the way they view themselves. Positive relationships between children and their caregivers are essential for the youngsters to become psychologically well-adjusted adults. Children with positive self-images have high self-esteem because they see themselves as being good, lovable, and possessing many worthwhile and valuable characteristics such as honesty and sensitivity.

When children enter school, their social environment enlarges to include more children, teachers, and other members of the community. These individuals provide new learning experiences that can have positive or negative impacts on the personality, self-image, and self-esteem of children. If a child who has a negative self-image enters school and has experiences, such as being bullied, that reinforce this perception, emotional disturbances can develop that persist into adulthood. With the help of others, children can develop positive self-concepts that establish the foundation for a lifetime of wellness. Parents and other adults help children feel good about themselves by spending time with them, listening to their concerns, and treating them with respect.

During adulthood, experiences at school, work, and home and a variety of social factors, including relationships, influence self-esteem. Relationships and experiences that are rewarding, enriching, and satisfying support positive self-esteem. In addition to having self-respect, people with a high degree of self-esteem gain the respect and approval of colleagues and others.

Self-esteem is a deep-rooted aspect of an individual. Although self-esteem may rise or fall over the course of a day, its basic nature remains fairly stable over longer periods. Individuals with persistent low self-esteem can improve their negative thoughts and feelings about themselves. By analyzing their situations, these people can determine factors that contribute to their poor self-concepts. For example, working in a dull job or remaining in an abusive relationship can affect self-esteem negatively. In these instances, people may improve their situations and feelings of self-worth by finding new jobs or ending the self-destructive relationships.

To feel better about themselves, persons with low self-esteem can learn to identify and appreciate their positive traits and abilities, instead of focusing on their negative characteristics and shortcomings. It can also help if the individual recognizes that not all criticism is destructive and insensitive. Accepting *constructive criticism* can support personal growth. Making a few lifestyle changes, such as developing new interests, changing some bad habits, exercising regularly, or taking an assertiveness training class, can improve a person's psychological outlook. To overcome low self-esteem, psychological counseling may be necessary to help individuals develop the ability to evaluate themselves realistically and form accurate self-perceptions.

**autonomy** Sense of independence and self-control.

**self-esteem** The extent to which a person feels worthy and useful.

# Improving Your Psychological Health

What can you do to improve your psychological health? You can enhance the quality of your mental health primarily by improving the other dimensions of your health. Exercising regularly may boost your mood.[3,4] Getting enough sleep, eating a nutritious diet, and maintaining a healthy weight for your height may also enhance psychological health by improving physical health. In addition to taking good care of your physical needs, fostering positive social contacts, whether with family, friends, or colleagues, is very important. Everyone needs to communicate with other people on a regular basis. For example, one goal to improve your psychological health could be to make and maintain at least one new social contact each year. You can improve your intellectual health by reading challenging books, playing mind-stimulating games such as crossword puzzles or chess, or serving as a tutor. Some people find that keeping a journal or diary in which they record their most private feelings helps them cope with the challenges of daily life. Attending to your spiritual needs can provide personal fulfillment also. For example, you can volunteer to serve as a mentor for troubled children or become involved in your religious organization. Finally, taking an active role in ensuring and protecting the quality of your environment will support all dimensions of your health.

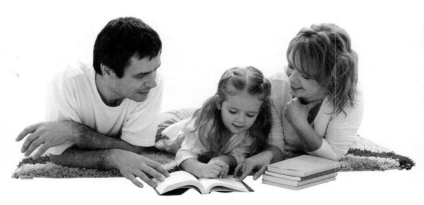

Caregivers play a crucial role in determining children's level of self-esteem.

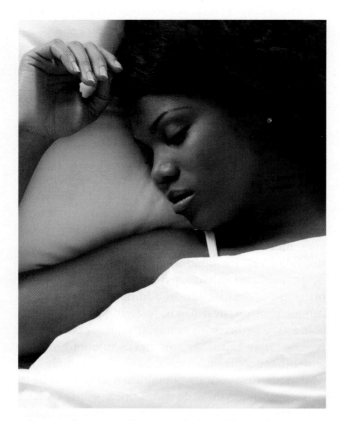

Adequate sleep can enhance psychological health by improving physical health.

## Healthy Living Practices

☐ To experience psychological adjustment and growth, set realistic goals, plan effective ways to achieve those goals, take actions that are based on reasonable judgments and decisions, and evaluate the consequences of your choices.

☐ To facilitate your psychological adjustment, learn ways to manage interpersonal conflicts constructively, without being aggressive. When such conflicts arise, decide when it is best to compromise or assert your position.

☐ To improve your self-esteem, avoid making negative statements about yourself. Identify and be realistic about your strengths and weaknesses; focus on your accomplishments and positive characteristics.

☐ To improve your psychological health, take steps to improve the quality of the other dimensions of your health.

# Understanding Psychological (Mental) Illness

Having "the blues," feeling "scared to death," or being "worried sick"—perhaps you can recall situations in which you experienced these strong emotions or uncomfortable sensations. Occasionally, healthy people have disturbing thoughts, experience unpleasant feelings, or display inappropriate behaviors. In most instances, these are normal responses and adaptive reactions to unpleasant or threatening situations. For example, it is normal to be sad after learning about the death of a friend or to be afraid when a snake crosses your path. Given a reasonable amount of time, however, the strong emotional responses or unpleasant thoughts and feelings resolve, and you regain your sense of well-being.

The observable physical and behavioral changes that signal an emotional state are referred to as **affect**, or mood. Expressing emotions appropriately is a characteristic of a psychologically healthy individual; extreme or improper emotional responses can indicate a serious psychological disturbance. The key features that distinguish a normal emotional response from an abnormal one are the intensity and duration of the feelings. Mentally ill individuals experience abnormal feelings, thoughts, and behaviors that persist, interfere with daily life, and hinder psychological adjustment and growth.

A *psychosis* is a severe type of mental illness characterized by disorganized thoughts and unreal perceptions that result in strange behavior, isolation, delusions, and hallucinations. **Delusions** are inaccurate and unreasonable beliefs that often result in decision-making errors. For example, a person suffering from a delusion might think that he or she can fly, so this individual jumps off a tall building. **Hallucinations** are false sensory perceptions that have no apparent external cause, but they are real to the psychotic individual. Examples of hallucinations include hearing instructions from pictures, seeing ghostly images, or feeling insects crawling underneath skin. Psychotic conditions (psychoses) can be acute or chronic, and they can result from brain damage, chemical imbalances in the brain, or substance abuse.

Situations and cultures provide the context in which behaviors are judged as normal or abnormal. If a person who is living in a country torn apart by civil war bombs a crowded marketplace, people may view this individual as a terrorist or a hero, but not necessarily mentally ill. However, if this bombing occurs in an American shopping mall, and the bomber says that a dog gave the order to perform the deed, you might suspect that this person is psychotic.

## The Impact of Psychological Illness

Why is it important to learn about psychological illness? Most Americans have one or more family members who suffer from a psychological illness. Between 2005 and 2009, about 1 in 10 adult Americans reported experiencing "frequent mental distress" for 14 or more days during the previous 30 days.[5] According to data from the National Comorbidity Survey Replication, depression and alcohol dependence are the most common psychological disturbances that affect Americans (**Table 2.4**).[6] Throughout the world, mental illnesses are prevalent and often not treated adequately.[7]

The emotional and economic costs of mental illness are high not only for affected individuals and their families but also for society. People may drop out of college or abuse alcohol and other drugs because of unresolved emotional problems or underlying psychological disorders. Mental illness frequently has a negative impact on the quality of life and the productivity of workers.

In the past, psychologically disturbed individuals were often misunderstood and mistreated. Having a mental illness was considered disgraceful by people who associated the condition with bizarre behaviors, violent acts, and long stays in mental healthcare facilities. Today, being diagnosed with a psychological disorder is no longer a hopeless situation, because scientists are understanding more about the various biological, environmental, and social factors that influence behaviors. Nevertheless, these disorders do not receive the kind of interest and concern from public health officials that conditions such as heart disease, cancer, and stroke generate. Why? Mental illnesses may not get much attention because of the stigma associated with them and the lack of major risk factors that can be modified to prevent them.

Although mental health disorders are common and can be quite disabling, fewer than 50% of Americans who have these conditions seek treatment.[8] Because negative attitudes toward mental illness persist, many psychologically disturbed people are reluctant

**affect** Observable expressions of mood.

**delusions** Inaccurate and unreasonable beliefs that often result in decision-making errors.

**hallucinations** False sensory perceptions that have no apparent external cause.

to seek beneficial therapy; they live in misery, hiding their illness from others. Seeking professional help for psychological problems is a sign of personal strength, not weakness.

### Table 2.4

### Lifetime Prevalence of Mental Health Disorders

| Disorder | Percentage of Americans Affected* |
|---|---|
| Any mental health disorder | 46.4 |
| Any anxiety disorder | 28.8 |
| Panic disorder | 4.7 |
| Specific phobia | 12.5 |
| Social phobia | 12.1 |
| Generalized anxiety disorder | 5.1 |
| Obsessive-compulsive disorder | 1.6 |
| Impulse control disorders | 24.8 |
| Attention-deficit hyperactivity disorder | 8.1 |
| Any substance abuse/ dependence | 14.6 |
| Alcohol abuse | 13.2 |
| Alcoholism | 5.4 |
| Drug dependence other than alcoholism | 3.0 |
| Any mood disorder | 20.8 |
| Major depressive episode | 16.6 |
| Bipolar disorders | 3.9 |

*The sum of these percentages is more than 100 because many individuals suffer from more than one disorder.

*Source:* Data from Kessler, R. C. et al. (2005). Lifetime prevalence and age-of-onset distributions of *DSM-IV* disorders in the National Comorbidity Survey Replication. *Archives of General Psychiatry, 62*(6):593–602.

# What Causes Psychological Disorders?

There are numerous psychological disorders, and in each case, it may be impossible to determine a single cause. Alterations in the normal chemical and physical environment of the brain often produce mental illness. In many instances, these alterations are the result of genetic defects that adversely affect neurotransmitter levels. Additionally, people whose brains have been physically damaged by injuries, tumors, or infections often display abnormal behavior. When introduced into the body, drugs such as cocaine can interfere with the brain's ability to produce, use, or eliminate neurotransmitters. Furthermore, pollutants such as pesticides and toxic minerals, including lead, mercury, and arsenic, can damage the brain.

Scientists note that certain mental illnesses such as schizophrenia and most major mood disorders tend to occur within the same family. These observations support the role of inheritance in their development.

Genetic factors alone, however, do not explain the development of every psychological disorder. Several members of a family could develop similar forms of mental illness because they are more likely to experience the same physical, economic, and social environments than unrelated individuals.

Environmental conditions influence the expression of many inborn traits, including psychological responses. Children, for example, often learn ways of reacting to situations by observing their parents. Think about how you respond when angered or frustrated. Are your responses like those of your mother or father?

Personal experiences can trigger the onset and influence the severity of some psychological disturbances. Some experts think that a child's brain can be altered by exposure to extremely stressful situations, increasing the youngster's risk of developing depression later in life. However, researchers have yet to understand completely the extent to which biological, social, and environmental factors interact to influence psychological health.

## Table 2.5

### Major Types of Mental Health Therapists

| Therapist | Training and Degrees |
|---|---|
| Counseling and clinical psychologists | M.A., Ph.D., or Psy.D. in psychology; 5 or more years in psychotherapy methods, research, and assessment |
| Psychiatrists | Medical (M.D. or O.D.) degree and at least 3 years of specialized training in psychiatry |
| Psychoanalysts | Have undergone personal psychoanalysis and completed 7 to 10 years of part-time psychoanalytic training (most are psychiatrists) |
| Psychiatric social workers | MSW; most states require certification by the Academy of Certified Social Workers |
| Clinical mental health counselors | Master's degree (or equivalent) and 2 years of counseling experience; certified by National Academy of Certified Clinical Mental Health Counselors |
| Psychiatric nurse practitioners | Registered nurses with additional education and experience working in psychiatric settings |
| Marital and family therapists | Master's degree. Licensed or certified in about one-half of the states; member of the American Association for Marriage and Family Therapy |
| Sexual therapists | Minimum of a master's degree, a license in related field, specialized sex education and sex-therapist training, extensive supervised individual and group therapy experience; the American Association of Sex Educators, Counselors and Therapists provides certification |
| Abuse counselors | Substance abuse training; often counselors are recovering substance abusers |
| Clergy | Religious training; may have spiritual and family counseling training |

Source: Data from Cornacchia, H. J., & Barrett, S. (1993). Consumer health. St. Louis, MO: Mosby.

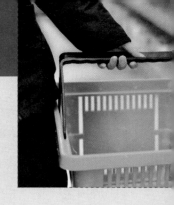

## Locating and Selecting Mental Health Therapists

The following tips can help you find and select qualified mental health specialists:

- Discuss psychological health concerns with your personal physician or with medical staff at your student health center. These individuals can assess your health and refer you to qualified mental health specialists if necessary.
- Contact local mental health associations or agencies for information about psychological health.

Members of these associations can give you information about local support groups and mental health services.

- Contact your state's social welfare department or the social services department of a local hospital to identify qualified therapists.
- Interview therapists before making any agreements for services.
- Ask therapists about treatment philosophies, methods, insurance coverage, and payment expectations before agreeing to use their services.

## Treating Psychological Disorders

Many people with psychological disorders respond well to treatment. Treating these conditions involves the cooperation of the affected individuals and their families and, in many instances, the assistance of mental health therapists who have specialized training. **Table 2.5** lists the major types of mental health therapists and some information concerning their qualifications.

Many people learn to cope with various psychological problems, such as drug addictions or the loss of loved ones, by joining *support groups*. The support group is an informal approach to treatment. Support group participants have regular meetings in which they can discuss personal adjustment problems. Group members usually conduct these meetings rather than mental health therapists. In addition to attending regular meetings, some group members may need to obtain professional counseling.

Mental health therapists can offer a variety of effective psychotherapies (treatments) that enable many individuals with psychological disorders to lead normal, productive lives. Psychotherapy often includes counseling, including *cognitive behavioral therapy*, group therapy, and medications. Cognitive behavioral therapy can help anxious, angry, or depressed people identify and change negative or inaccurate ways in which they think about themselves and their situations. As mentioned earlier, medication can correct neurotransmitter imbalances in the brain.

More than one form of treatment may be necessary to alleviate or control the disorder. In severe cases,

psychologically disturbed people may require hospitalization for treatment and to prevent self-injury or harm to others. If you or someone you know needs mental health care, the Consumer Health box titled "Locating and Selecting Mental Health Therapists" provides some suggestions for finding and choosing qualified help.

### Healthy Living Practices

- Many psychological problems respond well to treatment. If you think you may have a mental health disorder, ask your personal physician or the medical staff at your campus health center for help.

## Common Psychological Disorders

### Anxiety Disorders

Do you feel uneasy when you ride in an elevator, enter a classroom to take a test, or give a speech? Nearly everyone experiences anxiety, the uncomfortable feeling of apprehension or uneasiness that results while expecting a vague threat. The physical changes associated with anxiety states include increased heart rate, rapid breathing, and elevated blood pressure. Anxious people may report feeling tense, distressed, or worried; and they may be emotionally upset, sweating, and trembling. Anxiety disorders are common; according to the results of the National Comorbidity Survey Replication, nearly 30% of Americans suffer from these conditions at some time in their lives.[6]

**Generalized Anxiety Disorder** When you perceive a threat, it is normal to feel mildly anxious as your body physically prepares to deal with the danger. However, if the anxiety interferes with your ability to perform daily activities, the condition is abnormal. During their lifetimes, about 5% of the population suffers from **generalized anxiety disorder**, a condition characterized by uncontrollable chronic worrying, anxiousness, and nervousness. People with this disorder have unrealistic and excessive concerns about their jobs, children, health, or minor situations such as making home repairs. They are tense, irritable, and restless, and they often experience sleeping problems. Treatment usually includes antianxiety and antidepressant medications as well as cognitive behavioral therapy.

**Phobias** A **phobia** is an intense and irrational fear of a situation or object. *Agoraphobia* is the fear of open places or public areas. *Social phobias* are fears of performing in situations that involve people, such as giving speeches or taking tests. *Specific phobias* (formerly called simple phobias) are fears of certain objects or situations, such as snakes or flying. According to the results of the National Comorbidity Survey Replication, phobias are among the most common psychological disturbances in the United States.[6] About 12% of Americans report having social phobias, and about 12.5% of Americans report experiencing specific phobias. It is not uncommon for a person to be affected by more than one phobia. Although people who suffer from phobias know that their behavior is irrational, they still become anxious in the situations that arouse their fears (**Figure 2.3**).

Most cases of phobia are mild; affected individuals often learn to live with this condition by avoiding situations that arouse the anxiety. Severe phobias can interfere with normal social functioning. For example, people with agoraphobia may refuse to leave their homes. Individuals who are severely affected by phobias can seek professional treatment that includes behavioral therapy and medications to control irrational feelings and reduce anxiety.

**Panic Disorder** An estimated 3 million Americans suffer from **panic disorders** that feature *panic attacks*, unpredictable episodes of extreme anxiety and loss of emotional control. During a panic attack, people usually experience shortness of breath, shakiness, faintness, nausea, and a rapid, pounding heartbeat. Affected individuals often feel terrified because they think they are becoming insane or having a heart attack. Severe phobias, certain drugs, or frightening experiences may trigger panic attacks, but they can occur spontaneously.

Therapists often combine cognitive behavioral therapy and medications to treat panic disorders. People who have frequent panic attacks should seek medical help because studies indicate that they are at risk of committing suicide.

**Post-Traumatic Stress Disorder** Individuals who survive extraordinary life events such as a sexual assault, military combat, or a natural disaster may develop *post-traumatic stress disorder* (*PTSD*) (**Figure 2.4**). Nevertheless, some people suffer from PTSD even after being in an auto accident or abusive relationship. About 7% of Americans experience PTSD during their lifetime.[6]

Symptoms of PTSD may take months to develop fully and include having disturbing rec-

## Figure 2.3

**Phobias.** Phobias are intense and irrational fears of certain situations or objects that can interfere with functioning. Many people have a fear of flying.

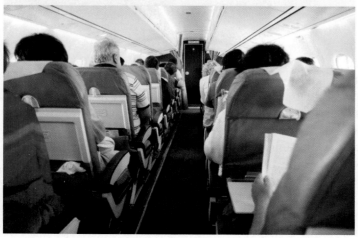

ollections or nightmares of the event, and in severe cases, feeling emotionally "numb." Affected people often avoid thinking about or discussing the traumatic experiences, and they may smoke heavily, overeat, or abuse drugs as a way of coping. Treatment of PTSD includes antianxiety medication and counseling that encourages survivors to talk about the traumatic events with others.[9]

**Obsessive-Compulsive Disorder** Although the experts disagree, *obsessive-compulsive disorder (OCD)* is generally classified as an anxiety disorder. An **obsession** is a persistent, inappropriate, and repetitive thought or impulse that produces anxious feelings. Obsessions are often related to self-doubt or fears. A **compulsion** is the behavior that usually follows the obsessive thoughts or impulses. Compulsive behaviors reduce the obsessed individual's anxiety. A young person, for example, might have recurring thoughts of injuring a family member. This individual may wash his or her hands hundreds of times a day and take numerous long showers to reduce anxious feelings. Other typical compulsive behaviors include hoarding cats and dogs or useless items like plastic containers or making repetitive actions such as checking the oven frequently to see if it is turned off. Affected individuals often think that their obsessions and compulsions are repulsive or troublesome, but efforts to stop create more anxiety. Treatment includes medication and psychological counseling. In most cases, the longer the obsessive-compulsive behavior pattern has been in place, the more difficult the disorder is to treat.

**obsession** A repetitive thought that produces anxious feelings.

**compulsion** The behavior that follows obsessive thoughts and reduces anxiety.

# Impulse Control Disorders

Impulse control disorders are behaviors that interfere with a person's relationships, school or job performance, and well-being. The affected person typically acts without thinking about the negative consequences of his or her behavior. *Attention-deficit hyperactivity disorder (ADHD)* is one of the more common impulse control disorders. Although the condition is generally diagnosed and treated during childhood, the behavior can persist into adulthood.

**Attention-Deficit Hyperactivity Disorder** ADHD is characterized by short attention span and/or hyperactivity-impulsivity that results in serious social impairment. An estimated 4.4% of American adults have ADHD; men are more likely to be diagnosed with ADHD than are women.[10] The causes of ADHD are unclear, but genetics plays a role in the development of the condition.

People with ADHD have difficulty focusing and maintaining their attention on tasks, such as performing work-related responsibilities, studying, or completing assignments. Unemployment, sleep disturbances, accident proneness, and cigarette smoking are associated with adult ADHD.[10]

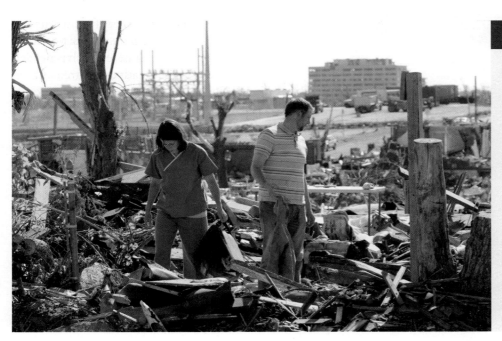

### Figure 2.4

**Surviving a Disaster.** This couple is searching through the rubble of their home a few weeks after an EF-5 tornado destroyed it and thousands of other homes in Joplin, Missouri on May 22, 2011.

There is no generally accepted test for diagnosing adult ADHD, and the condition is often more difficult to recognize in adults than in children because the signs are less obvious.[10] Adults with ADHD frequently suffer from anxiety, mood, and drug abuse disorders. Treatment may include stimulants such as methylphenidate (Ritalin) and psychological counseling. According to the results of one survey, only about 10% of adults with ADHD reported receiving treatment for the condition during the past 12 months.[10] More consumer and physician awareness programs are needed to alert the public about adult ADHD and its treatments. If you would like more information about ADHD, visit the Centers for Disease Control and Prevention's website at www.cdc.gov /ncbddd/adhd/.

**Problem Gambling** Nearly every state permits some form of gambling, such as lotteries, track racing, or casinos. For most people who place bets, the activity is entertaining, occasional, and controllable. However, about 1% of adult Americans are problem gamblers who gamble compulsively, excessively, and at the expense of their families, jobs, and relationships.[11] Men are more likely to be compulsive gamblers than women are. Psychological disorders,

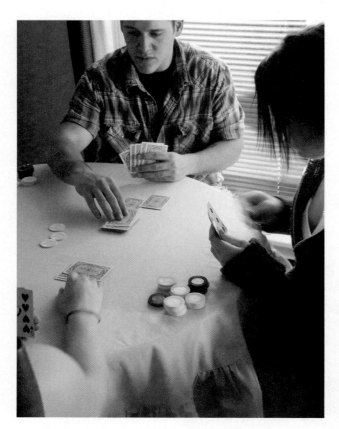

Do you know someone who is a problem gambler?

## Table 2.6

## Typical Features of Problem Gambling

**The problem gambler:**

- Seems to think only about gambling or how to get money to gamble
- Loses friends, family members, and jobs because of his or her behavior
- Gambles more often over time
- Has no control over the impulse to gamble
- Becomes restless, angry, or agitated when he or she tries to gamble less often (withdrawal)
- Gambles to escape problems or cope with depression, guilt, or anxiety
- Gambles again, trying to recover losses
- Lies to cover up the behavior
- Has others financially bail him or her out
- Resorts to illegal acts, such as forging checks and stealing money, to obtain money for gambling
- Abuses mind-altering drugs

including depression and anxiety disorders, and risky behaviors such as binge drinking and illegal drug use often accompany problem gambling behavior. **Table 2.6** lists typical features of problem gamblers.

Gamblers Anonymous is a self-help group that can enable problem gamblers to control their troublesome behavior (www.gamblersanonymous.org). Many problem gamblers, however, do not remain in treatment. Some counselors have certification to treat compulsive gambling, but health insurance providers may not cover their services. More research is needed to determine effective ways to prevent as well as treat this condition.

## Mood Disorders

*Until a few years ago, the two words that best described my life were fear and loneliness. As a child, I experienced physical, emotional, and verbal abuse from my parents. There were some instances when the beatings were so severe, I just forgot about them. I married a man who also physically abused me. Having no savings or college degree, I lacked the self-confidence to walk out of the marriage. I felt trapped. Deep depression set in; I cried a lot of the time and felt guilty because I was unable to carry out the normal daily responsibilities of cooking and cleaning the house. I began to think suicidal thoughts.*

*Finally, I entered a hospital that had a stress unit. Between the group sessions and private therapy, I learned a lot about those who abuse others and how to handle stress. However, spending three weeks in the hospital did not cure my depression. I realized that the only thing that would do that would be to remove myself from its cause. I separated from my husband and started college.*

*It has been a struggle financially, but I am determined to make it. I am preparing to graduate this semester with a Bachelor of Arts degree, and I plan to continue on to get a Master of Arts degree. The best change is my new self-confidence gained from overcoming the obstacles and becoming independent.*

This middle-aged college student's case not only illustrates the harsh origins of her depression, but also how an emotionally resilient person can recover from depression, resolve problems, and regain self-esteem. How can you distinguish a normal period of sadness from one that signals a major depressive disorder?

It is normal for people to feel "down" after a loss or disappointment. After a significant loss, such as the death of a close friend or relative, one normally feels grief, an intense sadness that may persist up to a year after the loss. Most grieving individuals soon recover their emotional balance and resume their usual activities. Grieving people are probably severely depressed if they become so profoundly sad that they withdraw and isolate themselves for several months and harbor feelings of guilt, low self-worth, and suicide. Enduring other stressful experiences, such as a difficult relationship or experiencing severe physical or emotional trauma, can trigger the first episode of depression in susceptible persons.

People suffering from **major depressive disorder** generally experience the following:

- Persistent sad, "empty," or hopeless feelings
- Feelings of guilt, worthlessness, or helplessness
- Loss of interest or pleasure in activities that used to be enjoyed
- Unexplainable fatigue
- Difficulty concentrating, remembering, or making decisions
- Frequent insomnia, early-morning wakening, or oversleeping
- Changes in appetite resulting in weight loss or gain

> **major depressive disorder** A mood disorder characterized by persistent and profound sadness, hopelessness, helplessness, and feelings of worthlessness; lack of energy; loss of interest in usual activities; loss of the ability to concentrate; suicidal thoughts; and appetite and sleep disturbances.

- Restlessness
- Physical complaints that do not respond to treatment, such as chronic headaches, intestinal tract disturbances, and pain
- Thoughts about death, suicide, or attempting suicide

These symptoms last for 2 weeks or more and interfere with relationships and responsibilities related to school, work, and home. Depressed people may be anxious and irritable, and they often use alcohol or illegal drugs to alter their emotional state. Self-mutilation (for example, "cutting") can also be a sign of depression. Depression can be devastating for individuals and their families. About 7% of men with a history of depression commit suicide, whereas only

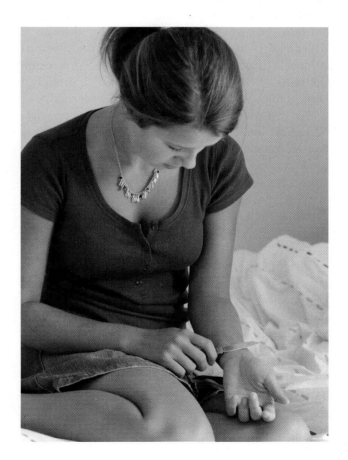

"Cutting" can be a sign of depression.

1% of women with a history of depression will take their own lives.[12]

According to results of a survey conducted in 2006–2008, almost 10% of U.S. adults were depressed at the time of the study, and about one-third of those persons were suffering from *major* depression.[13] The people who were most likely to have major depression were:

- Between 45 and 64 years of age
- Women
- Blacks and Hispanics
- People who had dropped out of high school
- Divorced persons
- People who were unable to work or find work
- People without health insurance coverage

**What Causes Depression?** Depressive illnesses are disorders of the brain that have no single cause. The condition probably results from a complex combination of genetic, biochemical, and environmental factors as well as learned behavioral responses to situations. Some types of depression tend to run in families; however, depression also occurs in people who do not have family histories of the disorder.[14] Researchers have detected abnormal neurotransmitter levels in depressed people's brains.[14] As a result, the parts of the brain that regulate mood, thoughts, sleep, appetite, and behavior function abnormally.

For reasons that are unclear but that may be related to hormonal fluctuations, women are more likely to become depressed than are men. Men, however, tend to experience depression differently from how women experience it. Men are more likely to be irritable, report lack of interest in formerly pleasurable activities, be unusually fatigued, and have sleep disturbances; women are more likely to report feeling sad, worthless, and guilty.[14]

Like diabetes and high blood pressure, depression is a chronic but treatable disease. Many severely and chronically depressed people can obtain dramatic relief from their disabling symptoms by receiving therapies that include prescribed antidepressant medications. However, physicians who are not psychiatrists often fail to diagnose the condition in their patients. As a result, many depressed individuals are not treated or are improperly treated.[15,16] Depressed people who are 18 to 25 years of age are less likely than older adults to receive mental health treatment.[16]

Alternative remedies for depression are becoming popular in the United States. The herb St. John's wort may be helpful as a treatment for mild to moderate depression.[17] St. John's wort has been reported to interact with certain prescription drugs and cause side effects, so individuals should not take this substance without consulting a physician.

Depressed individuals often feel better by engaging in regular physical activity. According to the Surgeon General's report *Physical Activity and Health*,[18] a moderate amount of physical activity each day may reduce symptoms of anxiety and depression and improve mood and a sense of well-being.

**Managing Mild Depression** If you experience mild depression, you can help yourself by:

- Setting priorities at work, home, or school
- Avoiding excess responsibilities
- Maintaining social contacts and confiding in someone you can trust
- Participating in a few enjoyable activities, especially if they are social and improve your mood
- Exercising regularly
- Relaxing
- Focusing on positive rather than negative thoughts
- Volunteering to help others in need

By taking these actions, your mood should gradually improve. If you still feel depressed after a couple of weeks, or your mood worsens, seek professional help. For more information about depression, visit the National Institute of Mental Health's website: www .nimh.nih.gov/publicat/depression.cfm#ptdep3.

**Bipolar Disorder** *Bipolar disorder*, formerly called manic depression, is characterized by unusual shifts in mood, energy and physical activity levels, and ability to carry out daily tasks. A person with bipolar disorder typically experiences distinct episodes of intense positive and negative emotional states. The extremely happy and excited emotional state is called *mania*. Individuals with mania typically brag about themselves and their accomplishments, engage in excessive physical activity and rapid talking, and sleep very little. Another characteristic of mania is excessive participation in pleasurable and risky activities that can lead to unwelcome consequences, such as careless sexual encounters or costly shopping sprees. After the manic episode subsides, the person's behavior and mood become more "normal." In time, however, his or her emotional state swings to the negative mood (severe depression) state, and this person feels extremely sad and hopeless.

## Table 2.7

### Typical Symptoms of Bipolar Disorder

| Mania Symptoms | Depressive Symptoms |
|---|---|
| Experiences an unusually long period of acting "high" or being extremely happy or outgoing | Experiences an unusually long period of feeling worried or empty |
| Is extremely irritable; appears jumpy or "wired" | Loses interest in activities that he or she had enjoyed |
| Talks very fast, jumps from one idea to another, has "racing" thoughts | Feels tired or in "slow motion" |
| Is easily distracted | Has difficulty concentrating, remembering, and making decisions |
| Takes on several new projects but does not complete them or performs poorly | Is restless and irritable |
| Is restless and sleeps very little | Experiences changes in usual eating, sleeping, and other habits |
| Has unrealistic beliefs about his or her abilities | Thinks about death or suicide, or attempting suicide |
| Behaves impulsively and engages in risky behaviors | |

During each phase of bipolar disorder, the mood of the affected person gradually reaches an extreme level, and the affected person may not be able to function normally. When this occurs, the person with bipolar disorder may become suicidal and require hospitalization.

In addition to the extremes of mania and severe depression, bipolar disorder can cause a range of moods. People with bipolar disorder may develop *hypomania*, an emotional state that is characterized by increased energy and activity levels, which are not as excessive as in the manic state. A person with hypo-

mania tends to feel very well and be highly productive. Although close associates of this individual may recognize that he or she is not behaving and functioning normally, the affected person may feel fine. Unless people with hypomania receive proper treatment, they may develop severe mania or depression. **Table 2.7** lists typical symptoms of manic and depressive states, and **Figure 2.5** shows the cyclic pattern of bipolar disorder.

Bipolar disorder tends to develop during the late teens or young adult years—before 25 years of age. People with the bipolar disorder tend to have a family

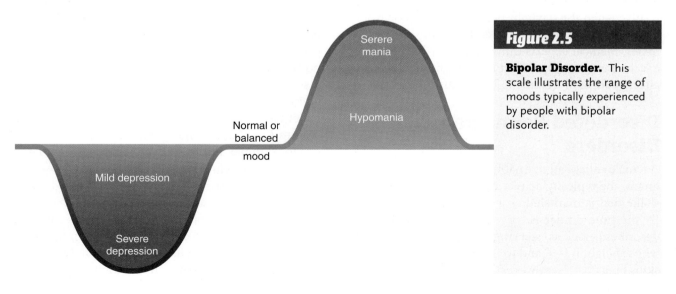

### Figure 2.5

**Bipolar Disorder.** This scale illustrates the range of moods typically experienced by people with bipolar disorder.

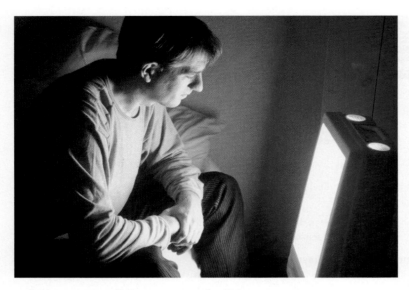

Light therapy is an effective treatment for SAD.

history of the illness, so medical researchers suspect the condition may be inherited.[19]

The cyclic mood shifts that characterize the bipolar disorder may recur several times during an individual's life. In many cases, however, the symptoms are not easy to recognize or distinguish from normal emotional responses. As a result, the illness may not be diagnosed or treated properly. There is no cure for bipolar disorder, but in many cases, the condition can be managed with medications.

**Seasonal Affective Disorder** Besides bipolar disorder, other mood disorders occur in cycles. People with *seasonal affective disorder (SAD)* become depressed around mid- to late fall, and their depression ends in late winter or early spring. Besides feeling depressed and tired, people with SAD also report craving sweets and gaining weight. Because these symptoms resolve when the daylight period lengthens or when people with the condition spend time in sunnier climates, medical experts think SAD may be related to a lack of exposure to bright light. Light therapy is an effective form of treatment for this disorder.[20]

## Disordered Eating and Eating Disorders

A female college athlete habitually skips breakfast. For lunch, she typically drinks an 8-ounce canned milkshake that is marketed as a weight loss supplement. By the time dinner is served in her dormitory, she describes herself as "starving." A male college student whose height is 5' 9" and weight only 125 pounds also skips breakfast. Nearly every day, he eats cheeseburg-

ers and french fries from a fast-food restaurant that is within walking distance of his campus. He rarely eats fruits or green vegetables. A young man who describes himself as a vegetarian eats only brown rice, fruit, and tea. Are these behaviors examples of eating disorders?

Occasionally, most people engage in unusual eating practices, such as skipping meals, fasting, or avoiding sweets in an effort to lose a few pounds. *Disordered eating* practices are mild and often temporary changes in an individual's otherwise normal food-related behaviors. In many instances, a person uses these behaviors to improve health or appearance. Disordered eating practices, however, can become eating disorders. **Eating disorders** are persistent, abnormal eating patterns that can threaten a person's health and well-being. Each year, millions of American lives are disrupted by the three major eating disorders—bulimia nervosa, anorexia nervosa, and binge eating disorder. These conditions often develop in adolescence or young adulthood, and they are more likely to affect females than males. An estimated 85% to 95% of the people with anorexia nervosa and 65% of those suffering from bulimia nervosa are female.

Hormonal, genetic, psychological, and sociocultural factors influence the development of eating disorders. Risk factors include family history, childhood abuse, depression and anxiety, low self-esteem, and family conflict.[21] Additionally, homosexual males may have a higher risk of eating disorders than heterosexual males.[21]

Although it is true that excess body fat is not healthy, a society that emphasizes thinness as a sign of physical attractiveness makes many young people overly concerned about and dissatisfied with their body size and shape, even when it is normal. As a result of societal influences, many American females admire the bodies of actresses, fashion models, and ballet dancers who look as though they are starving (**Figure 2.6**). Young males, on the other hand, may equate optimal health and attractiveness with the massive, well-defined muscles of action heroes that are typically portrayed in comic books and movies. Such efforts to achieve an ideal body shape can evolve into a disastrous and obsessive preoccupation with body weight and composition, food intake, and physical activity level. It is interesting to note that eating disorders are uncommon in regions of the world

## Figure 2.6

**Anorexia Nervosa.** Isabelle Caro, a young Italian model and actress, died in 2010 from a long-term illness. This photo was taken in 2008, when Caro weighed only about 66 pounds.

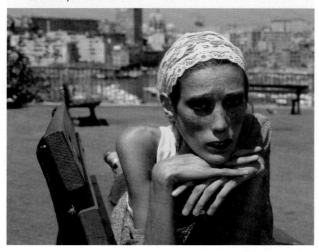

**eating disorders** Persistent, abnormal eating patterns that can threaten a person's health and well-being.

**anorexia nervosa** A severe psychological disturbance in which an individual refuses to eat enough food to maintain a healthy weight.

where the food supply is limited and starvation is an everyday occurrence.

Although usually considered nutritional problems, eating disorders are often associated with psychological disturbances, including obsessive-compulsive and mood disorders as well as substance abuse. Goals of counseling include encouraging patients to cooperate in their recovery and change their unhealthy attitudes toward food and their bodies. Treating underlying psychological and family-related problems may help resolve the eating disorder or reduce the frequency of the abnormal eating behavior, but many people with severe eating disorders do not respond to treatment.

**Anorexia Nervosa** Occasionally, nearly everyone has *anorexia*, appetite loss that can occur under various circumstances, such as excitement or fever. **Anorexia nervosa**, however, is a severe psychological disturbance in which an individual refuses to eat enough food to maintain a healthy body weight. People with anorexia nervosa have an irrational fear of becoming fat, usually maintain strict control over their food intake, and are preoccupied with calorie counting and food preparation. As mentioned earlier, females are more likely to suffer from anorexia nervosa than males are. During their lifetimes, an estimated 0.3% to 3.7% of American females suffer from this condition.[21]

People with anorexia nervosa have a distorted image of their bodies. They deny that they are severely underweight even though they weigh 15% or more below normal for their height. Typically, females with this condition do not have normal menstrual cycles and feminine body contours. Without an adequate supply of fat to insulate their bodies against heat loss, anorexics feel cold easily and often wear layers of clothing to provide extra warmth.

Some people suffering from anorexia nervosa occasionally lose control over their food intake and eat excessive amounts of food (*bingeing*). To avoid gaining weight, these individuals induce vomiting, give themselves frequent enemas, or abuse laxatives (*purging*). Additionally, people with anorexia nervosa often exercise excessively to "burn up" calories. **Table 2.8** lists these and other typical signs of anorexia nervosa.

Treatment for anorexia nervosa includes individual and family counseling; patients must reach about

## Table 2.8

### Typical Signs of Anorexia Nervosa

**In addition to refusing to gain weight despite weighing 15% or more below that which is healthy, a person who has anorexia nervosa typically:**

- Has an intense drive to achieve a thin body
- Seems unaware that body size has changed
- Denies malnourished appearance
- Derives little satisfaction from his or her body shape
- Fears losing control over appetite
- Becomes full after eating small amounts of food
- Is a "picky" eater; avoids foods that contain fat, starch, or sugar
- Exercises excessively
- Lacks menstrual periods (females)
- Is depressed
- Has low self-esteem
- Has perfectionist tendencies

*Source:* Adapted from Garfinkel, P. (1992). Classification and diagnosis. In K. A. Halmi (Ed.), *Psychobiology and treatment of anorexia nervosa and bulimia nervosa*. Washington, DC: American Psychiatric Press.

**bulimia nervosa** An eating disorder characterized by a craving for food that is difficult to satisfy.

**binge eating disorder** A pattern of eating excessive amounts of food in response to distress such as anxiety or depression.

85% of their normal body weight before antidepressant therapy is useful. In severe cases, people with anorexia nervosa can die unless they are given special feedings and monitored closely in hospitals. Earlier estimates of the percentage of deaths that resulted from anorexia nervosa may have been too high. According to a review of studies in which the long-term outcomes of nearly 5,600 patients with anorexia nervosa were analyzed, about 5% of the patients died, in most instances from suicide, and less than 50% recovered completely.[22] The remaining individuals with anorexia nervosa were improved or remained chronically ill with the disorder.

**Bulimia Nervosa** Whereas people with anorexia nervosa are so thin they are easy to identify, those with bulimia nervosa may be more difficult to recognize because their weights are often normal. **Bulimia nervosa** is a craving for food that is difficult to satisfy; bulimic people typically eat excessive amounts of food at one time because they are depressed or anxious rather than hungry (**Table 2.9**). Some bulimic persons are able to maintain normal body weights because after bingeing, they purge by fasting, practicing

## Table 2.9

## Typical Signs of Bulimia Nervosa

- Evidence of consuming excessive amounts of food in short periods, such as empty food containers, without gaining weight
- Evidence of efforts to avoid digesting large amounts of food
- Spending time in the bathroom during meals or immediately after eating
- Odor of vomit in bathroom
- Presence of empty laxative or diuretic packages
- Sores or scars on knuckles that result from self-induced vomiting
- Dental decay from frequent contact with acidic stomach contents
- Preoccupation with obtaining food and exercising
- Social withdrawal

self-induced vomiting, taking laxatives and diuretics, or exercising excessively. Vomiting prevents the body from absorbing and using the nutrients in food and beverages. Laxatives speed up the movement of the intestinal tract and can lead to watery diarrhea; diuretics increase urine production and elimination. Vomiting and abusing laxatives and diuretics can seriously disrupt the body's normal fluid and chemical balance, which can be life threatening.

Occasional episodes of bulimic behavior are common among young women who are trying to control their weight. It is estimated that about 1% to 4% of females suffer from bulimia nervosa during their lifetimes.[21] Men may also have bulimia nervosa if they regularly consume too much food along with excessive amounts of alcohol and then vomit afterward. Furthermore, some young men who participate in sports that require maintaining a particular weight, such as wrestling and gymnastics, practice the behaviors associated with bulimia nervosa to remain competitive.

Many people who binge eat and follow up with purging are disgusted with their disordered eating behavior, and they hide it from roommates, friends, and family members. Some people practice bingeing and purging twice a week; in severe cases, affected individuals engage in these behaviors several times a day. Severely bulimic people can become so preoccupied with eating that they shoplift food to supply their binges and experience legal problems as a consequence. College students with bulimia nervosa frequently encounter academic problems after they neglect to attend their classes.

Typically, bulimic individuals are more socially outgoing than people with anorexia nervosa, yet they experience low self-esteem, anxiety, and depression. Eating temporarily relieves the bulimic person's anxiety. Although antidepressant medications and psychotherapy are useful treatments, people with bulimia nervosa often do not seek help for their behavior. Affected women tend to improve over time, but 10 years following diagnosis, about 30% still suffer from the condition.[21]

**Binge Eating Disorder** About one-third of overweight people engage in regular episodes of binge eating that are rarely followed up with purging or heavy exercise.[23] This behavior is called **binge eating disorder**. Some binge eaters report *blackouts*, periods of time that they cannot recall when they had overeating episodes, but empty food containers provide them with evidence of the incidents. Like persons with bulimia nervosa, binge eaters have poor self-esteem, and they often feel disgusted, depressed, and guilty about their eating behavior and physical appearance. These feelings may trigger additional episodes of overeating. *Night eating syndrome*, which is more common among obese than normal-weight persons, may be a variation of binge eating disorder. People with night eating syndrome are not hungry during the day, but have difficulty staying asleep at night; they awake often and frequently get out of bed to eat large amounts of food.

If you or someone you know suffers from an eating disorder such as bulimia nervosa or binge eating, ask the staff at your campus health center or your personal physician to recommend conventional mental health practitioners, such as psychiatrists, who specialize in treating these conditions. Additionally, check hospitals in your area because many have self-help groups for people with eating disorders.

**Other Disordered Eating Conditions** Athletes involved in sports that tend to emphasize leanness, such as gymnastics, wrestling, light-weight rowing, horse racing, figure skating, body building, and distance running, have an increased risk of developing eating disorders. As many as 62% of female athletes and 33% of male athletes suffer from eating disorders.[24] A relatively small number of female athletes develop the *female athlete triad*, a condition characterized by low energy intake, menstrual cycle abnormalities, and bone mineral irregularities, such as *osteopenia* (low bone density). Osteopenia is generally associated with postmenopausal women, not healthy young women.

Although most females with the female athlete triad do not show every sign of illness associated with anorexia nervosa or bulimia nervosa, their food-related practices, such as bingeing and self-induced vomiting, are similar. To prevent this condition, it is important to teach young athletes about healthy eating practices and body weights. Furthermore, parents need to be aware of factors that contribute to the triad, such as having low self-esteem and few friends, identifying thin physiques with ideal body shapes, being preoccupied with weigh-ins, and having overly demanding coaches who criticize the young athlete for being "fat" and insist on weight loss.

In the United States, many men experience social pressure to attain larger, more muscular body builds. *Muscle dysmorphia* ("bigorexia") is a psychological condition that affects weightlifters, particularly bodybuilders.[25] Despite their very muscular body builds, people suffering from this condition are not satisfied with the size of their bodies, and as a result, they spend hours working out each day, particularly lifting weights. Moreover, they are ashamed of their bodies and reluctant to expose themselves in public places such as beaches. Individuals with muscle dysmorphia are obsessed with the need to gain muscle without adding body fat; they have a high risk of eating disorders and abuse of *anabolic steroids*, drugs that can increase muscle size. At this point, little is known about the prevalence of muscle dysmorphia or effective ways to treat the condition.

## Schizophrenia

An estimated 1% of Americans suffer from **schizophrenia**, a type of psychosis.[26] Laypeople often believe schizophrenia means "split" or "multiple personalities," but actually, people with schizophrenia experience extremely disorganized thought processes, including hallucinations and delusions. People with *paranoid* delusions may think someone is trying to harm them. Individuals with schizophrenia often display strange behavior and inappropriate emotions. Communicating with some affected individuals is difficult because their speech often consists of words strung together into meaningless sentences. *Table 2.10* lists common symptoms of schizophrenia.

The brains of people with schizophrenia tend to have biochemical or structural defects that many medical

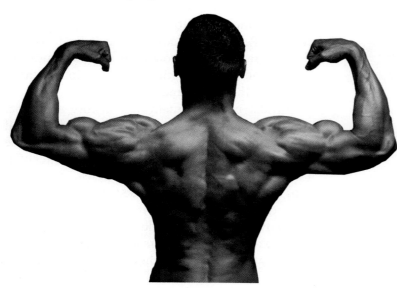
Could this be a case of muscle dysmorphia?

## Table 2.10

### Common Symptoms of Schizophrenia

- Hallucinations, particularly hearing "voices" (auditory hallucinations)
- Delusions, including bizarre beliefs or paranoid beliefs
- Difficulty organizing thoughts; illogical thoughts
- Garbled speech and use of meaningless words
- Agitated body movements
- Dull, monotonous voice
- Little or no speaking
- Neglect of personal hygiene
- Inability to focus attention
- Difficulty using recently learned information

experts think are inherited. A person who has a parent with schizophrenia has a 10% likelihood of developing the condition.[26] If a person has an identical twin with schizophrenia, he or she has a 45% to 65% chance of developing the illness.

Schizophrenia usually develops early in adulthood. Some affected people have one schizophrenic episode and recover, but others experience recurrent episodes and require long-term treatment. By taking special medications, many people with schizophrenia experience relief from their symptoms and live as productive members of society. Individuals with severe forms of schizophrenia must live in mental healthcare facilities because their behavior is unmanageable or dangerous to themselves or others.

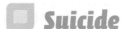

### Healthy Living Practices

☐ If you or someone you know has an eating or other psychological disorder, seek help from the medical staff at the campus health center or from your personal physician.

## Suicide

Suicide, the deliberate ending of one's own life, is not a mental illness. However, such extreme violence against oneself is often the behavioral consequence of a severe psychological disorder. Most people who choose to end their lives feel overwhelmed by the demands of life; they are unable to solve their problems or adapt to their situations.

Overall, suicide accounts for only a small percentage of deaths in the United States. In 2009 about 1.5% of deaths were attributed to suicide.[27] Suicide was the third leading cause of death for Americans between 18 and 24 years of age. Males are almost four times more likely to kill themselves than are females.[28]

Despite what many people believe, the Christmas holiday season is not the time that suicide rates peak; intentional deaths are generally low in winter, and high in late spring and early summer.[29] Although women are more likely to attempt suicide, men are more likely to complete the act of killing themselves. Most people use a firearm to end their lives; however, taking drug overdoses and crashing motor vehicles are also frequent suicide methods. Thus, it is difficult to determine the actual number of suicides that occurs each year.

## Preventing Suicide

Suicide victims often suffer from a psychological disturbance, particularly a mood disorder that may have included substance abuse.[28] Other characteristics associated with a high risk of committing suicide are previous suicide attempts, family history of suicide, being abused as a child, loss (relational, work, or financial), illness, and feeling socially isolated.[30] Some individuals with severe or terminal health problems seek the help of others, particularly family members or physicians, to commit suicide. (Chapter 15 discusses the "right to die" and physician-assisted suicide.) People who know or treat individuals with these characteristics or conditions should be aware of their suicide risk and initiate intervention methods to prevent them from ending their lives.

Suicidal persons usually feel intense emotional strain, are preoccupied with thoughts of death, and often communicate their intentions to others. These individuals might say "everyone would be better off if I were dead" or "I am going to kill myself," discuss the pros and cons of various suicide methods, and make unsuccessful suicide attempts. After deciding to kill themselves, suicidal individuals often seem cheerful and relaxed. When survivors recall the positive emotional state of the victims, they may report that these persons showed no signs of distress prior to dying.

## Table 2.11

### Behavioral Warning Signs of Suicide

**Behavior and examples:**

- Discussing, joking, or writing about suicide or death
- Giving away prized possessions
- Making final arrangements: planning a will or making funeral plans
- Displaying severe depressive symptoms
- Reporting feelings of hopelessness and helplessness
- Performing risky behaviors: playing with guns, driving while drunk, or performing daredevil stunts
- Injuring oneself by cutting, burning, or hitting
- Behaving in a manner that is different from usual: showing no interest in usual activities, becoming socially withdrawn
- Planning the suicide: buying a gun or hoarding a supply of barbiturates
- Expressing anxiety over an impending action: worrying about a divorce, dropping out of school, or losing a job
- Showing physical signs of a previous suicide attempt: cut or scarred wrists, neck bruises

*Table 2.11* lists these and other behavioral warning signs of suicidal persons.

It is always important to take suicidal conversations or gestures seriously and obtain suicide prevention counseling for these individuals immediately. Most major metropolitan areas have mental health centers with trained counselors who provide 24-hour crisis intervention services. The Yellow Pages of local telephone books usually list these facilities under "suicide prevention centers." For more information, call the National Suicide Prevention Lifeline at 1-800-273-TALK (8255).

## Healthy Living Practices

☐ If you are or someone you know is suicidal, immediately contact a suicide prevention center to obtain specific instructions concerning ways to prevent yourself or another from committing this act.

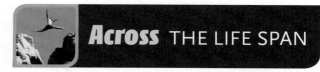

# Across THE LIFE SPAN

## PSYCHOLOGICAL HEALTH

Children and adolescents establish the foundation for a lifetime of good mental health by developing positive self-concepts. Parents can help their children feel good about themselves by spending time with them, listening to their concerns, and helping them learn to adjust to a changing world (**Figure 2.7**).

School-age children who live in dysfunctional families are vulnerable to developing emotional disorders such as depression and school anxiety. However, childhood depression can occur in any child

## Figure 2.7

**Establishing Good Mental Health.** Parents can help their children feel good about themselves by spending time with them.

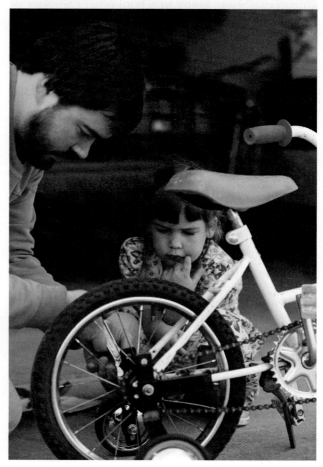

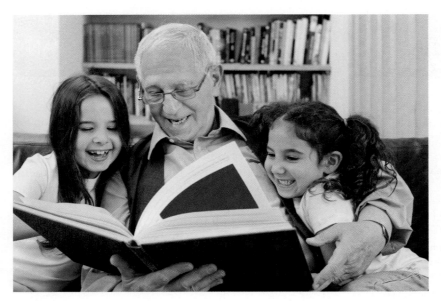

Older adults who approach the end of their lives with a sense of satisfaction about their accomplishments are likely to feel emotionally fulfilled.

and defiant. Not surprisingly, children with ADHD frequently have low self-esteem and conflicts with their family members, peers, and teachers.

In addition to prescribing medications, many physicians recommend behavioral and family counseling to treat the disorder. Recently, some people expressed concerns that ADHD is overdiagnosed and that too many children are being treated with stimulant medications, such as Ritalin, in the United States. Additionally, questions were raised about the negative effects of stimulants on children's growth and the potential for substance abuse among children treated with these medications. Although some studies indicate stimulants can mildly suppress the growth rates of children with ADHD, more long-term research is needed.

During the maturation process, an adolescent undergoes numerous hormonal, physical, social, and other changes necessary to become an independent adult. Many youth make this transition smoothly with a minimum of serious problems, but for some, the teenage years are filled with emotional turmoil and family conflict. Certain forms of mental illness, including major depression and eating disorders, are likely to develop during this period. As mentioned earlier, suicide is a major cause of death for adolescents.

By the time people reach late adulthood, they may have raised a family, retired from working outside of the home, and maintained a network of friends and family. Older adults who approach the end of their lives with a sense of satisfaction with their accomplishments are likely to feel emotionally fulfilled. Many elderly people, however, suffer from sleep disturbances and depression after the death of a spouse and friends, family separation or disintegration, financial instability, or a disabling physical illness. It is important for older adults and their families to recognize the symptoms of depression and obtain professional help. Chapter 15 discusses the health concerns of older adults.

who experiences a traumatic event, such as the loss of a parent through death or divorce. Children who are anxious about going to school often complain of morning headaches and stomach upsets before leaving for school, and they return home in a distressed state. Parents and teachers need to recognize the symptoms of childhood depression and anxiety. By receiving individual and family counseling, many distressed children and their families can learn positive ways of handling crisis situations.

Attention-deficit hyperactivity disorder (ADHD) is a common childhood behavioral disorder. In 2007, nearly 10% of American school-age children, mostly boys, were reported to have ADHD.[31] This condition is characterized by an inability to focus and maintain attention on tasks, such as doing homework or following simple instructions. Children with ADHD also display excessive levels of physical activity and restlessness. They cannot sit still; they rush through meals, dash away from their caregivers, and resist efforts to relax or fall asleep. Their attention spans are so short, they are often unable to follow instructions or complete tasks. Additionally, children with this condition demonstrate impulsive behaviors such as interrupting conversations, talking when it is inappropriate, and acting before thinking. Some children with ADHD are aggressive, argumentative,

# Analyzing Health-Related Information

The following ad promotes a series of compact discs designed to improve mood and reduce anxiety. Read the advertisement and evaluate it using the model for analyzing health-related information. The main points of the model are noted here; the model is fully explained in Chapter 1.

1. Which statements in the ad are verifiable facts, and which are unverified statements or value claims?
2. What might be the motives and biases of the person making the claims?
3. What is the main point of the ad? Which information is relevant to the product? Which information is irrelevant?
4. Is the source of information reliable? What evidence supports your conclusion that the source is reliable or unreliable? Does the source of information present the benefits and risks of the product? Does the ad include a disclaimer?
5. Does the source of information attack the credibility of conventional scientists or medical authorities?

Based on your analysis, do you think that this ad is a reliable source of health-related information? Explain why you would or would not buy the CDs. Summarize your reasons for coming to this conclusion.

---

ADVERTISEMENT    ADVERTISEMENT    ADVERTISEMENT    ADVERTISEMENT

## Feeling sad? Hopeless? Anxious?
## Have you lost interest in usual activities? If you answered "yes" to one or more of these questions. You are depressed.

Fortunately, you can learn how to cure depression and prevent anxiety from ruining your life. Now you can benefit from the latest discovery in subliminal microtechnology that produces phenomenal advances in brain functioning. Scientists from around the world are predicting that this incredible breakthrough will be the greatest medical discovery of the 21st century!

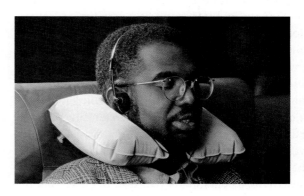

> "How can I ever thank you? I've tried three other neurotechnology products, but BRAINFIT was the only one that worked." B. J., London, England
>
> "Please send another copy of the miraculous BRAINFIT CD—my sister took mine and won't return it!" S. A., New Delhi, India

Our amazing new **BRAINFIT CD** can improve your mood without the need for potentially harmful drugs. Listening to the CD has been scientifically proven to decrease anxiety by up to 35%, enhance positive feelings by up to 28%, and boost enthusiasm for

living by up to 55%.* Millions of people in 60 countries report that BRAINFIT really works!

For the first time, BRAINFIT is available in the United States. Order your copy now. We guarantee that BRAINFIT will improve your mental health, and we'll add our clinically tested antianxiety pillow to your order—free! BRAINFIT is easy to use at home, work, or even as you drive your car!

For your personalized copy of BRAINFIT, send a money order for $69.95 to: BRAINFIT

* This statement has not been evaluated by the Food and Drug Administration.

# CHAPTER REVIEW

## Summary

A person's psychological health affects and is affected by other wellness components such as physical and social health. Psychological health is dynamic, becoming healthier or unhealthier as an individual responds to a constantly changing environment. Psychologically healthy people accept themselves, are assertive, have realistic and optimistic outlooks on life, function independently, form satisfying interpersonal relationships, cope with change, and find effective solutions to their problems.

Understanding mental health involves the study of physiology and psychology. Biochemical changes in the brain elicit myriad human responses, including thoughts, emotions, and behaviors. Conditions that alter normal brain chemistry can disrupt the mind, producing negative moods or abnormal behaviors.

Personality is a set of distinct thoughts and behaviors, including emotional responses that characterize the way an individual responds to situations. Biological, cultural, social, and psychological forces interact to mold a person's personality.

Over the past 100 years, numerous psychologists, including Freud, Erikson, and Maslow, provided valuable insights into human behavior, laying the foundation for our present understanding of personality development. Freud thought unconscious drives control human behavior. Erikson identified eight stages of the life span in which different social forces influence personality. Maslow believed that the freedom to achieve personal fulfillment is a psychological need that motivates human behavior.

Psychological adjustment and growth occur when one adapts effectively to the demands of life by altering one's thoughts, attitudes, and responses. Self-esteem, a feeling of self-worth, is a key component of personality. Positive self-esteem is a characteristic of psychologically healthy people.

Intensity and duration are the key features that distinguish a normal emotional response from an abnormal one. Mentally ill individuals experience abnormal feelings, thoughts, and behaviors that persist, interfere with daily life, and hinder psychological adjustment and growth.

There are numerous psychological disorders; each may have multiple causes. Alterations in the normal chemical and physical environment of the brain often produce mental illness. These alterations may be the result of genetic defects, injuries, tumors, infections, or exposure to certain drugs or pollutants. Additionally, social interactions, including those with one's family, contribute to the quality of an individual's psychological health.

In many cases, medications and/or behavioral therapies are effective treatments for mental health problems. People can learn to cope with various problems by seeking the help of conventional mental health therapists or by joining self-help groups.

It is common for individuals to experience phobias, anxiety, panic attacks, or mood disorders at some time in their lives. In many cases, these disorders are mild and do not interfere with the affected person's ability to function in society. In other instances, psychological illnesses such as schizophrenia, generalized anxiety, or major depression impair functioning to the extent that affected individuals require professional treatment.

Eating disorders are often symptoms of underlying mental illnesses, particularly depression and obsessive-compulsive disorders. Self-imposed starvation and denial of thinness characterize anorexia nervosa. Bulimic individuals and some people with anorexia nervosa engage in food bingeing and purging practices. Binge eaters overeat but rarely follow up with purging.

Suicide is not a mental illness, but in many instances suicide is the behavioral consequence of a major depressive illness that includes substance abuse. Individuals who are contemplating suicide often discuss their feelings and intentions with others. Thus, people should take someone's suicidal conversations or gestures seriously and assist the individual by obtaining immediate intervention.

Parents can help their children feel good about themselves by spending time with them, listening to their concerns, and helping them learn to adjust to a changing world. Some children develop psychological disturbances, particularly anxiety and depression. Attention-deficit hyperactivity disorder is a common childhood behavioral disorder. Most adolescents experience relatively few emotional problems as they mature into adults, but for some, the teenage years are filled with turmoil. Certain forms of mental illness, including major depression and eating disorders, are likely to develop during this period of life. Older adults who approach the end of their lives with a sense of satisfaction with their accomplishments are likely to feel emotionally fulfilled.

## Applying What You Have Learned

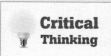
**Critical Thinking**

1. Develop at least three recommendations for parents to follow that would build their children's self-esteem. **Application**
2. Analyze your present situation to determine your position on Maslow's human needs hierarchy. Explain how you determined your position. **Analysis**
3. Many persons have negative feelings about people with mental illness. Explain how the media contribute to these feelings. **Synthesis**
4. Consider your current state of psychological health. Rate your psychological health as excellent, good, fair, or poor. Explain how you determined this rating. **Evaluation**

**Application**
using information in a new situation.

**Analysis**
breaking down information into component parts.

**Synthesis**
putting together information from different sources.

**Evaluation**
making informed decisions.

**Key**

# Reflecting on Your Health

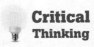

**Critical Thinking**

1. As described in this chapter, self-esteem develops during childhood. When you were a child, how did your interactions with family members, peers, and teachers influence the development of your self-esteem?

2. Using Table 2.1, Characteristics of Psychologically Healthy People, identify the characteristics that describe you best. Why did you choose those traits?

3. What have you done to boost your psychological health by improving your physical, social, intellectual, spiritual, and environmental health? How did your actions help?

4. As mentioned in this chapter, people often have negative feelings toward psychologically disturbed persons. How would you feel if you, a close friend, or a family member were diagnosed with a psychological disorder? If you, a close friend, or a family member has a serious psychological disorder, how does it affect you?

5. People older than 65 years of age have a high risk of depression. What could you do or have you done to enhance the psychological health of an elderly person whom you know, such as a grandparent?

# References

1. Erikson, E. H. (1982). *The life cycle completed.* New York, NY: Morton. (Original work published 1964)

2. Maslow, A. H. (1968). *Toward a psychology of being* (2nd ed.). New York, NY: Van Nostrand Reinhold.

3. Mead, G. E., et al. (2009, July 8). Exercise for depression. *Cochrane Database Systematic Reviews,* 3:CD004366.

4. Martin, C. K., et al. (2009). Exercise dose and quality of life: Results of a randomized controlled trial. *Archives of Internal Medicine,* 169(3):269–278.

5. U.S. Centers for Disease Control and Prevention, National Center for Chronic Disease Prevention and Health Promotion. (2011, February 25). Health-related quality of life, BRFSS trend data, annual trend data. Retrieved from http://apps.nccd.cdc.gov/HRQOL/

6. Kessler, R. C., Berglund, P., Demler, O., et al. (2005). Lifetime prevalence and age-of-onset distributions of *DSM-IV* disorders in the National Comorbidity Survey Replication. *Archives of General Psychiatry,* 62(6):593–602.

7. Demyttenaere, K., et al. (2004). Prevalence, severity, and unmet need for treatment of mental disorders in the World Health Organization world mental health surveys. *Journal of the American Medical Association,* 291(21):2581–2590.

8. U.S. Department of Health and Human Services, Substance Abuse and Mental Health Services Administration, Office of Applied Studies. (2009). Serious psychological distress and receipt of mental health services. Retrieved from http://www.oas.samhsa.gov/2k9/SPDtx/SPDtx.cfm

9. U.S. Department of Veterans Affairs, National Center for PTSD. (2010). Treatment of PTSD. Retrieved from http://www.ptsd.va.gov/public/pages/treatment-ptsd.asp

10. Kessler, R. C., et al. (2006). The prevalence and correlates of adult ADHD in the United States: Results from the National Comorbidity Survey Replication. *American Journal of Psychiatry,* 163(4):716–723.

11. Kessler, R. C., et al. (2008). The prevalence and correlates of *DSM-IV* pathological gambling in the National Comorbidity Survey Replication. *Psychological Medicine,* 38(9):1351–1360.

12. U.S. Department of Health and Human Services. Does depression increase the risk of suicide? Retrieved from http://answers.hhs.gov/questions/3200

13. Gonzalez, O., et al. (2010). Current depression among adults—United States, 2006–2008. *Morbidity and Mortality Weekly Report,* 59(38):1229–1235.

14. National Institute of Mental Health. (2010). *Depression.* Retrieved from http://www.nimh.nih.gov/health/publications/depression/complete-index.shtml#pub5

15. Kocsis, J. H., et al. (2008). Chronic forms of major depression are still undertreated in the 21st century: Systematic assessment of 801 patients presenting for treatment. *Journal of Affective Disorders,* 111(1–2):55–61.

16. U.S. Department of Health and Human Services, Substance Abuse & Mental Health Services Administration, Office of Applied Studies. (2009, July). *The NSDUH report—serious psychological distress*

and receipt of mental health services. Retrieved from http://www
.oas.samhsa.gov/2k9/SPDtx/SPDtx.cfm

17. Sharpley, C. F., & Bitsika, V. (2010, December 11). Joining the dots: Neurobiological links in a functional analysis of depression. *Behavioral and Brain Functions, 6*:73. doi:10.1186/1744-9081-6-73

18. National Center for Complementary and Alternative Medicine. (2010, July). Herbs at a glance. St. John's wort. Retrieved from http://nccam.nih.gov/health/stjohnswort/ataglance.htm

19. Centers for Disease Control and Prevention. (1996). *Physical activity and health: A report of the Surgeon General.* Atlanta, GA: Author. Retrieved from http://www.cdc.gov/nccdphp/sgr/summary.htm

20. National Institute of Mental Health. (2010). *Bipolar disorder.* Retrieved from http://www.nimh.nih.gov/health/publications/bipolar-disorder/complete-index.shtml

21. Howland, R. H. (2009). Somatic therapies for seasonal affective disorder. *Journal of Psychosocial Nursing and Mental Health Services, 47*(1):17–20.

22. American Psychiatric Association Work Group on Eating Disorders. (2006). *Treatment of patients with eating disorders* (3rd ed.). Washington, DC: American Psychiatric Association.

23. National Institute of Mental Health. (2010). *Eating disorders.* Retrieved from http://www.nimh.nih.gov/health/publications/eating-disorders/complete-index.shtml

24. Grucza, R. A., et al. (2007). Prevalence and correlates of binge eating disorder in a community sample. *Comprehensive Psychiatry, 48*(2):124–131.

25. Bonci, C. M., et al. (2008). National Athletic Trainers' Association position statement: Preventing, detecting, and managing disordered eating in athletes. *Journal of Athletic Training, 43*(1):80–108.

26. Knoesen, N., et al. (2009). To be superman: The male looks obsession. *Australian Family Physician, 38*(3):131–133.

27. National Institute of Mental Health. (2010). *Schizophrenia.* Retrieved from http://www.nimh.nih.gov/health/publications/schizophrenia/complete-index.shtml

28. Kochanek, K. D., et al. (2011). Deaths: Preliminary data for 2009. *National Vital Statistics Reports, 59*(4). Retrieved from http://www.cdc.gov/nchs/data/nvsr/nvsr59/nvsr59_04.pdf

29. National Institute of Mental Health. (2010, September). Suicide in the U.S.: Statistics and prevention. Retrieved from http://www.nimh.nih.gov/health/publications/suicide-in-the-us-statistics-and-prevention/index.shtml

30. Voracek, M., et al. (2007). Facts and myths about seasonal variation in suicide. *Psychological Reports, 100*(3 Pt 1):810–814.

31. Centers for Disease Control and Prevention. (2008). Suicide prevention, scientific information: Risk and protective factors, risk factors for suicide. Retrieved from http://www.cdc.gov/Violence Prevention/suicide/riskprotectivefactors.html

32. U.S. Centers for Disease Control and Prevention. (2011, March 9). Rates of parent-reported ADHD increasing. Retrieved from http://www.cdc.gov/Features/dsADHD/

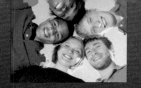
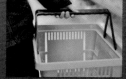
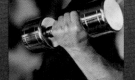
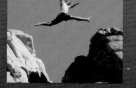

**Diversity in Health**
Stress and Asian Americans

**Consumer Health**
Herbal Remedies for Stress Symptoms

**Managing Your Health**
A Technique for Progressive Muscular Relaxation

**Across the Life Span**
Stress

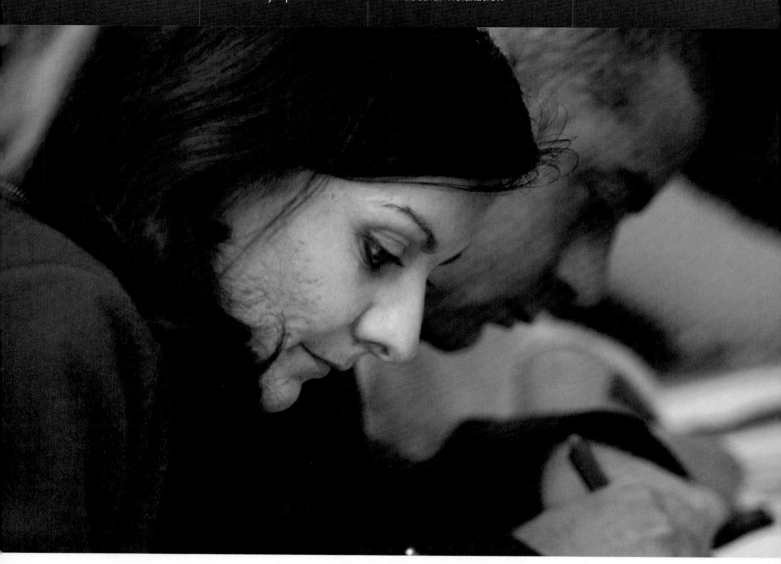

# Chapter Overview

The different meanings of stress

The ways your body responds to stress

How stressful life events can affect your health

Strategies for coping with stress

Skills that can help you manage stress

# Student Workbook

Self-Assessment: How Much Stress Have You Had Lately?

K6 Serious Psychological Distress Assessment

Changing Health Habits: Taking Steps to Reduce Your Stress

# Do You Know?

An easy way to manage your time more effectively?

If having a pet can reduce stress?

How to relax within just a few minutes?

## CHAPTER 3

# Stress and Its Management

I f you ask students to identify what makes college life stressful, you will receive a long list of situations, including taking exams, preparing term papers and lab reports, applying for loans, and juggling hours to fit part-time jobs into their class schedules. College students probably cannot imagine any other period in their lives that will demand so much of their time, energy, and finances.

How would you respond to the question, "What was the most stressful situation that you've experienced in the past year?" Three college students enrolled in a health course wrote the following answers to this question.

*The most stressful situation I've encountered in the past 12 months must be the discovery that my wife was pregnant and our financial security was at risk because the only source of income for us is her wages. I'm wondering if I will be able to continue pursuing my degree after the baby is born—this adds to my stress day by day.*

> "Going to college places considerable demands on your time and mind..."

**stress** A complex series of psychological and physical reactions that occur as one responds to a situation.

**stressors** Events that produce physical or psychological demands on an individual.

*I went away to a university last year and was the victim of a rape. The whole ordeal of talking to the police, confronting the man who did it, and telling my boyfriend was horrible, but the most stressful part was having to tell my parents.*

*The most stressful situation was the death of both of my grandparents within 6 months of each other. I watched them suffer as they passed away. It was very difficult. Also, my choice of a major was a mistake; I've had to change it.*

Each of these students had to cope with a different stressful situation. You may have had to cope with similar distressing events. Although going to college places considerable demands on your time and mind, you can expect stressful situations to arise during every phase of your life.

What is stress? What effects can it have on your health and well-being? Can stress be good for you? What factors make a situation stressful? Is it possible to reduce the negative effects that stress can have on your health? This chapter examines the nature of stress, how it can affect you, and how you can manage your stress.

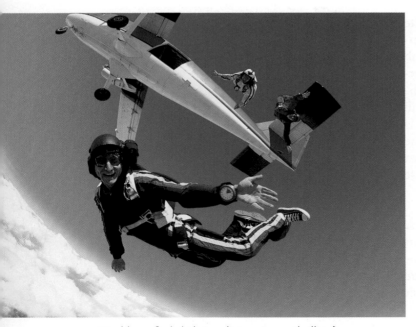

Would you find skidiving distressing or thrilling?

# What Is Stress?

Stress can refer to the situations that threaten or place demands on your mind and body. Stressful situations can be real, such as being confronted by an angry dog, or imaginary, such as worrying over your future employment possibilities. Stress can also describe your responses to a threatening situation; you *feel* stress. Imagine that a vicious dog attacks you. How would you feel?

Many experts define **stress** as a complex series of psychological and physical reactions that occur as a person responds to a demanding or threatening situation. However, each person views and appraises the situation to determine whether it will have positive, negative, or neutral consequences. Additionally, an individual determines his or her ability to manage the situation according to his or her previous experiences and personality characteristics. For example, how would you respond if a friend were to ask you to go skydiving with him? If you have never skydived but have no concerns about the safety of skydiving and are curious by nature, you might accept your friend's invitation. However, if jumping out of a plane with only a parachute to keep you from free falling is not something you would look forward to doing, you probably would be very "stressed out" in anticipation of the activity and would turn down your friend's request. On the other hand, if you have skydived before and found the activity thrilling and enjoyable, you would likely be excited to accompany your friend. Thus, it is possible for different individuals to form different appraisals of the same event; as a result, each person can have a different stress response.

## Stressors

**Stressors** are situations that create stress. Physiologic (physical) stressors include engaging in exercise; experiencing illness, pain, or injury; and being exposed to dangerous pollutants or extreme temperature changes. *Psychological stressors* include managing extreme emotions, handling difficult social situations, and dealing with troublesome thoughts and relationships. Certain psychologically demanding situations can add just enough stress to make life more challenging and interesting, but enduring too much stress, physical or psychological, can have negative effects on health and well-being. This chapter focuses on the impacts of psychological stressors.

The nature of a psychological stressor has a major role in determining its impact on health. When people think of stress, they usually think of **distress**, that is, events that are difficult to control and that have unwanted or negative outcomes. Distressing experiences include having problems with one's education, job, family, and relationships. Other situations create positive stress, or **eustress**. Becoming a new parent, competing in an athletic event, and accepting a desired job are examples of events that can have positive outcomes by making people feel happy, challenged, or successful.

Experiencing stressors with positive psychological consequences may reduce the unhealthy effects of negative stressors. Eustress, however, still has negative effects on the body and mind because any event that creates stress requires specific physical and psychological adjustments. These changes can damage the body and disturb the mind. In this chapter, the terms stress and distress are used interchangeably when referring to negative psychological stressors.

According to the results of a nationwide survey conducted in 2006, almost half of American adults reported concern over their financial situations as a major stressor.[1] Other major sources of stress included health problems, employment concerns, and relationships. The following section describes the stress response and its effects on health.

**distress** Events or conditions that produce unwanted or negative outcomes.

**eustress (YOU-stress)** Events or conditions that create positive effects, such as making one feel happy, challenged, or successful.

**hormones** Chemical messengers that convey information from a gland to other cells in the body.

**endocrine system** A group of glands that produce hormones.

## ☐ Stress Responses

## Physical Responses

The environment constantly exposes people to stressful situations; to survive, they must deal physically with these stressors. The body has a variety of ways to manage stressors, including the release of certain *hormones*. **Hormones** are chemical messengers that convey information from a gland to other cells in the body. The glands of the **endocrine system** produce several different hormones and secrete them directly into the bloodstream (**Figure 3.1**). Some endocrine hormones regulate growth and development. Other

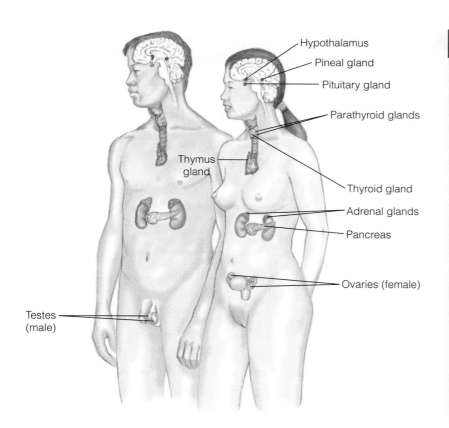

Hypothalamus
Pineal gland
Pituitary gland
Parathyroid glands
Thymus gland
Thyroid gland
Adrenal glands
Pancreas
Ovaries (female)
Testes (male)

### Figure 3.1

**The Endocrine System.** The glands of the endocrine system produce chemical messengers called hormones, which enter the bloodstream via small ducts.

**fight-or-flight response** The physical responses to stressful situations that enable the body to confront or leave dangerous situations.

**general adaptation syndrome (GAS)** The three-stage manner in which the human body responds to stress: alarm, resistance, and exhaustion.

hormones regulate body processes, including those necessary to function during stress.

In emergencies, a person's nervous system instantly activates the adrenal glands that are on top of the kidneys to release *cortisol*, epinephrine (adrenaline), and norepinephrine (noradrenaline). These hormones are often referred to as the "stress hormones" because they can prepare the body to respond rapidly when danger threatens. As a result, the person's body is able to confront or leave the dangerous situation quickly (the **fight-or-flight response**).

Stress hormones increase heart rate, blood pressure, central nervous system (CNS) activity, and blood flow to the heart and skeletal muscles. These hormones also increase the metabolic rate, the rate at which cells use energy. At the same time, the stress hormones reduce blood flow to the skin, kidneys, and intestinal organs. Under the influence of cortisol, certain cells release fat and *glucose* (blood sugar) into the bloodstream, which transports these energy nutrients to active muscle or nerve cells.

The nervous system also participates directly in the body's response to stressors. When the body is exercising or under emotional stress, the CNS produces and releases a group of chemical messengers that have pain-killing properties, including *endorphins*. Being less able to feel pain may be a valuable adaptation during stressful situations, especially if an injured person has to react quickly when threatened. ***Table 3.1*** lists major immediate or short-term physical adaptations to stress and their possible survival value.

**Selye's General Adaptation Syndrome** The classic research of Hans Selye paved the way for our understanding of the relationship between the mind and body.[2] Selye first used the term *stress* to describe the responses that allow a person to adapt physically or psychologically to any demand. As a result of his classic observations, Selye developed a three-stage description of the physical responses to stressors, the **general adaptation syndrome (GAS)**. Selye identified the three GAS stages as alarm, resistance, and exhaustion; he described the physical status of the body in each stage.

When you think about or see a stressor, your brain sends an alarm through your nerves to your adrenal

## Table 3.1

### Acute Physical Adaptations to Stress

| Physical Change | Immediate or Short-Term Effect |
| --- | --- |
| Central nervous system activity increases | Increases mental alertness and reduces reaction times |
| Pupils enlarge | Improves vision |
| Energy nutrients released from storage | Supplies fuels for muscular activity |
| Heart rate increases | Pumps more blood and faster |
| Blood pressure increases | Provides more pressure to circulate blood |
| Blood clots more easily | Prevents bleeding |
| Skeletal muscles become tense and can work longer | Allows for fighting or escaping threats |
| Sweating increases | Removes extra heat created by muscular activity |
| Saliva flow decreases | Avoids wasting valuable body water |
| Respiratory tract (the smaller airways) dilates | Allows more air to move into and out of lungs, supplying more oxygen for energy and removing more carbon dioxide waste |
| Gastrointestinal tract movements decrease | Shifts blood to skeletal muscles for their more critical needs |
| Endorphin levels increase | Reduces sensations of pain |

# Diversity in Health

## Stress and Asian Americans

In the United States, the majority of recent Asian American immigrants are from China, the Philippines, India, Korea, and Vietnam. The new immigrants to this country often face a variety of unfamiliar situations, as well as new and conflicting demands. Many of the immigrants must cope with being separated from friends and family members who remain in their homeland, learning an unfamiliar language, and adjusting to a very different culture.

The cultural "shock" that often results after settling in the United States creates numerous psychological conflicts for the immigrants. Many members of this population experience homesickness, discrimination, unemployment, racial stereotyping, language barriers, and social isolation. The stress of immigrating and adjusting to a new culture may lead to depression.[4]

Asian Americans who espouse traditional beliefs think that fate determines much of what occurs in their lives, and they often deny or hide feelings of sadness, disappointment, and anxiety. As a result, Asian Americans may avoid expressing negative feelings.

Recent immigrants from Asia tend to follow traditional gender-specific roles. Men are accustomed to having a dominant role over women, especially in making decisions, and they expect their wives to maintain households and take care of children. Although wives may work outside the home, their incomes often are not crucial for supporting their families. In the United States, people who are descendants of immigrants who came to this country several decades ago tend to accept more equitable roles at work and home for men and women. Therefore, many women who recently immigrated to this country from Asia perceive their status in society as very low, and they experience much psychological stress as a result.[5]

Instead of seeking treatment for anxiety or depression, distressed Asian American women often visit conventional medical practitioners, such as their personal physicians, for treatment of various physical symptoms such as appetite loss, headaches, and fatigue.[6] The effects of unrecognized and untreated stress can be devastating. Suicide is the second leading cause of death for Asian American women who are between 15 and 24 years of age.[7]

Regardless of one's ethnic/racial background, the unwillingness to reveal conflicting feelings can produce stress. The serious effects of stress on the health and well-being of Asian American immigrants underscore the need for conventional medical practitioners to be culturally sensitive and recognize symptoms of emotional distress in members of this minority group.

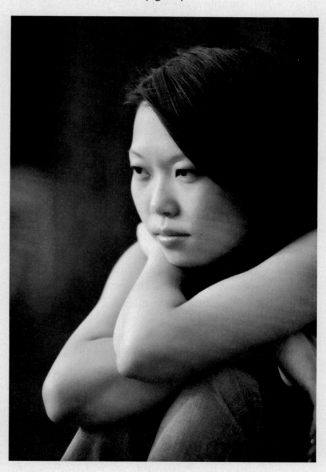

glands. Almost immediately, these glands release stress hormones to prepare your body to deal with the stressful event (*alarm stage*). In the alarm stage, your entire body undergoes the dramatic physical changes listed in Table 3.1. Consider, for example, how quickly you respond to an unexpected loud noise that sounds like a gun shot.

If you manage to survive the initial encounter but the stressor persists, your body enters the *resistance phase* of the response. During this stage, your body maintains its protective physical reactions to the stressor. As the threatening situation eases, your body recovers its normal physical state. Generally, by resting and avoiding additional exposure to stressors, your body can repair any damage that has occurred.

If the stressful situation persists, your body will not be able to maintain its resistance, and it will enter the *exhaustion stage*. In this stage, physical stress defenses are weakened, and you become more susceptible to infections. Prolonged exposure to stress may lead to death, if the body depletes its response mechanisms.

The stress response evolved to enable humans to react immediately to physical threats. Indeed, when people are in life-threatening situations, these dramatic physical changes may be essential for their survival. The same dramatic adaptations, however, take place when people deal with everyday hassles and concerns. Although these situations may be worrisome, they usually do not represent direct or serious threats to people's physical well-being. Nevertheless, such stressors elicit the unnecessary release of stress hormones into the bloodstream.

People with higher than normal levels of stress hormones, fat, and glucose in their blood are likely to develop chronic high blood pressure and other diseases of the heart and blood vessels. Enhanced blood clotting is a beneficial adaptation to an immediate, life-threatening situation. Blood clots, however, pose a serious danger when they form too easily and block blood flow in arteries and veins. Stress hormones also increase appetite; elevated cortisol levels are associated with increased body fat and weight gain.[3] The Diversity in Health feature in this chapter discusses the effects of severe stress on the psychological health of Asian immigrants, particularly Asian women, in the United States.

**Psychological Responses** Stressful situations affect the mind as well as the body, but the psychological impacts are not easy to test, observe, or measure. To determine your level of distress over the past 30 days, take the "K6 Serious Psychological Distress" assessment in the Student Workbook at the end of the book. Chapter 2 describes several mental health conditions, including post-traumatic stress disorder and depression, which have direct links to stressful life events.

Distressed individuals are more likely to report psychological symptoms such as frustration, anxiety, and anger. They may be irritable most of the time, eat too much food, or abuse drugs. "Stressed-out" people often have difficulty focusing their attention, making decisions, and sleeping.

*Burn-out* can be a consequence of experiencing too much psychological stress. People who are burned out feel as though they have exhausted their physical and psychological abilities to cope with stressors.[8] Typical signs and symptoms of burn-out are loss of enthusiasm for job, school, or others; increased feelings of dissatisfaction, irritation, frustration, and pessimism; loss of concern for others; and anxiety and depression. Burn-out often results from unrealistic beliefs or expectations concerning one's occupation and workplace situation, but caregivers and college students can also experience the condition. The stress management skills presented in this chapter, especially coping mechanisms based on social support, can help reduce the effects of burn-out.

To some extent, stress can have positive effects on the mind. Low levels of psychological stress can enhance performance by increasing one's effort and attention to the task. As the degree of stress increases, however, the individual may respond by worrying too much about performance, which creates even more psychological stress. This response can reduce the ability of actors, athletes, and college students to concentrate on and perform tasks. Stage fright affects the best veteran actors, and many superb athletes "choke" under competitive pressure.

Taking tests is stressful for many college students, but students with test anxiety overreact emotionally to the testing situation. As a result, such students have difficulty recalling information and concentrating on test questions. To avoid becoming overwhelmed by anxiety, students can learn to relax before and during exams by using the stress management skills presented later in this chapter.

## The Impact of Stress on Health

### Stressful Life Events

In 1967, Thomas Holmes and Richard Rahe introduced the Social Readjustment Rating Scale (SRRS), maintaining that people who experience numerous major life events within a short time span are likely to develop illnesses.[9] Holmes and Rahe developed this scale by asking nearly 400 people to rate life events according to the average amount of social change the individuals thought would be needed to deal with the situation. Death of a spouse, for example, received the maximum score of 100 points (see **Table 3.2**). In studies using the SRRS, Rahe found that subjects who accumulated higher scores, because they had experienced more major life events in a year, were more

## Table 3.2

### Social Readjustment Rating Scale

| Rank | Life Event | Value | Rank | Life Event | Value |
|------|-----------|-------|------|-----------|-------|
| 1 | Death of spouse | 100 | 23 | Son or daughter leaving home | 29 |
| 2 | Divorce | 73 | 24 | Trouble with in-laws | 29 |
| 3 | Marital separation | 65 | 25 | Outstanding personal achievement | 28 |
| 4 | Jail term | 63 | 26 | Wife begins or stops work | 26 |
| 5 | Death of close family member | 63 | 27 | Begin or end school | 26 |
| 6 | Personal injury or illness | 53 | 28 | Change in living conditions | 25 |
| 7 | Marriage | 50 | 29 | Revision of personal habits | 24 |
| 8 | Fired at work | 47 | 30 | Trouble with boss | 23 |
| 9 | Marital reconciliation | 45 | 31 | Change in work hours or conditions | 20 |
| 10 | Retirement | 45 | 32 | Change in residence | 20 |
| 11 | Change in health of family member | 44 | 33 | Change in schools | 20 |
| 12 | Pregnancy | 40 | 34 | Change in recreation | 19 |
| 13 | Sexual difficulties | 39 | 35 | Change in religious activities | 19 |
| 14 | Gain a new family member | 39 | 36 | Change in social activities | 18 |
| 15 | Business readjustment | 39 | 37 | Mortgage or loan less than $10,000 | 17 |
| 16 | Change in financial state | 38 | 38 | Change in sleeping habits | 16 |
| 17 | Death of close friend | 37 | 39 | Change in number of family get-togethers | 15 |
| 18 | Change to different line of work | 36 | 40 | Change in eating habits | 15 |
| 19 | Change in the number of arguments with spouse | 35 | 41 | Vacation | 13 |
| 20 | Mortgage over $10,000 | 31 | 42 | Christmas | 12 |
| 21 | Foreclosure of mortgage or loan | 30 | 43 | Minor violations of the law | 11 |
| 22 | Change in responsibilities at work | 29 | | | |

Source: Holmes, T. H., & Rahe, R. H. (1967). The social readjustment rating scale. *Journal of Psychosomatic Research, 11*:213–218. Reprinted with permission from Elsevier Science.

likely to become ill at some time in the following year.

Although a few items on the original SRRS are out-dated, such as "mortgage over $10,000," this scale has been a popular measurement of stress levels. Many stress experts, however, question the scale's ability to predict the onset of illness. Using the SRRS as a model, Martin Marx and his colleagues developed the College Schedule of Recent Experience to assess the level of stress experienced by college freshmen (see the assessment activity "How Much Stress Have You Had Lately?" in the Student Workbook).[10] First-year college students often have difficulty coping with the unfamiliarity and demands of college life. Not surprisingly, these individuals have a high dropout rate. Concerned with the negative impact of change on first-year students, college administrators often establish academic, social, and counseling programs

## Figure 3.2

**The Immune System.** The immune system defends the body against disease-causing agents. The organs of the immune system include the thymus gland, spleen, and lymph nodes.

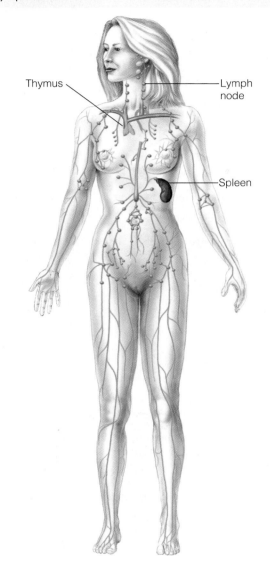

Thymus

Lymph node

Spleen

to ease the stress new students feel during their first year in school.

Medical experts generally agree with the idea that stressful life events are related to illness. However, observing an association between stressful events and the onset of illnesses does not mean that stress *causes* health problems. Distressed people may follow unhealthy lifestyles. They may not exercise regularly, eat nutritious foods, or get enough sleep. Such behaviors are likely to result in poor health. The following section explores the connections between psychological stress and physical health.

## The Mind–Body Relationship

**Psychoneuroimmunology**, the study of the relationships among the nervous, endocrine, and immune systems, is the field of medical research that explores the connection between mind and body. The **immune system**, which includes the red bone marrow, spleen, lymph nodes, white blood cells, and thymus gland, defends the body against disease-causing agents (**Figure 3.2**). The white blood cells are the key soldiers of the immune system, serving as the body's internal scouts and commandos. These special cells find, identify, and destroy many agents that can endanger one's health. *Inflammation* is a normal result of the immune system's response to infection or injury and can assist in the recovery process (see Chapter 14).

The immune system does not function independently of the other body systems. By using nerves and neurotransmitters, the brain relays information about the person's emotional state to the places where white blood cells are made and located in the body. These specialized cells produce their own chemical messengers that enable them to communicate information about the state of the body back to the brain and the endocrine system.

Scientists have discovered links between the nervous and immune systems that explain how some emotional responses affect physical health. Stress alters the normal functioning of the brain, which in turn, affects immune system functioning. Stress depresses some aspects of the immune system, resulting in delayed wound healing and increased susceptibil-

ity to infection. Stress may also stimulate other components of the body's immune response, resulting in inflammation. Immune system cells produce *cytokines*, a group of compounds that regulate the immune response and communicate with the nervous system. Stress increases the production of cytokines that promote inflammation. Under these circumstances, the inflammatory processes are not necessary and cause harmful effects on the body. Chronic mild inflammation is thought to be associated with the development of many serious diseases, including heart and other

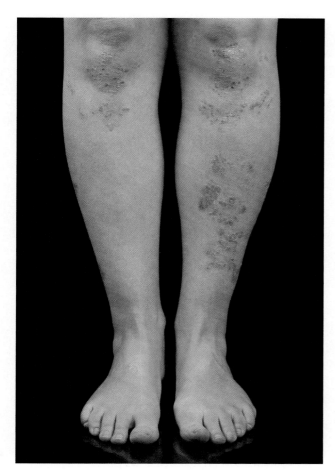

Psoriasis.

group-based stress management program lived longer than participants who did not receive the stress reduction training.[15] A later section of this chapter describes stress reduction techniques.

## Personality and Stress

Although exposure to any stress can increase an individual's susceptibility to illnesses, the same stressful situation can have a different impact on different individuals. Why do people often respond differently to a stressor? Each person's unique combination of personality traits and background experiences contributes to his or her stress response.

People who see only the negative aspects of a stressor may view a difficult situation as impossible to overcome and be more vulnerable to stress than those who make positive appraisals of the situation. As a result, vulnerable people are more likely to become anxious, angry, and depressed and to make poor decisions. By making poor decisions, people often create more stress for themselves. Additionally, distressed individuals may adopt lifestyles that undermine their health, such as obtaining insufficient sleep, smoking cigarettes, or abusing drugs.

People who are less vulnerable to the negative effects of stress may have personalities that act as buffers. These stress-resistant ("hardy" or resilient) people are committed to achieving their goals, have

blood vessel diseases, obesity, diabetes, smoking, rheumatoid arthritis, inflammatory bowel disorders, certain cancers, and Alzheimer's disease.[11-13]

*Autoimmune diseases* occur when the immune system malfunctions and the system's defense mechanisms become aimed at the body's own healthy cells. Rheumatoid arthritis, "lupus," celiac disease, psoriasis, type 1 diabetes, and multiple sclerosis are autoimmune diseases. Although these chronic health problems have a genetic component, stress may contribute to their development.

Psychological stress can cause existing conditions to flare or worsen (*Table 3.3*). For example, people with chronic health problems such as asthma, rheumatoid arthritis, migraines, and genital herpes report that the signs and symptoms of their illness tend to recur or worsen during stressful periods.[14]

Psychological, environmental, and biological forces can influence health in complex ways. Many people can reap major health benefits by modifying the way they respond to stress. For example, a group of women with heart disease who participated in a

| Table 3.3 |
| --- |
| **Common Disorders Linked to Psychological State** |

| | |
| --- | --- |
| Eating disorders | Itchy skin |
| Tension headaches | Rapid or irregular heart rate |
| Migraines | |
| Muscle spasms | Intestinal ulcers |
| Chest pains | Nausea and vomiting |
| Excessive menstrual cramps | Frequent urination |
| | Irritable bowel syndrome |
| Acne | Rheumatoid arthritis flare-ups |
| Recurring herpes simplex | |
| | Asthma attacks |
| Chronic fatigue syndrome | Premenstrual syndrome (PMS) |
| Fibromyalgia syndrome | |

a sense of control over their lives, and view stressful situations as challenges rather than threats.[16] Although stress-resistant people view the need to change as a challenge, they recognize that change is a part of life. Resilient individuals are more likely to express positive emotions (for example, recalling happy memories) when experiencing stressful situations than people who do not have such personalities.[16] Other stress-resistant characteristics include having an "easy-going" temperament and optimistic outlook. Some aspects of the stress-resistant personality may be inherited. However, children who experience trusting, warm, and close relationships with parents or other adults are likely to be more stress resistant than are children who lack such relationships.[16]

## Stress and Chronic Health Problems

As mentioned previously, some common chronic health problems are associated with stress. You or someone you know may have irritable bowel syndrome, fibromyalgia, intestinal ulcers, or severe headaches, including migraines. Unwanted weight gain is also associated with stress. The following sections take a closer look at these conditions.

**Irritable Bowel Syndrome (IBS)** Anxiety and stress worsen the signs and symptoms of irritable bowel syndrome (IBS). People with IBS have recurrent bouts of intestinal cramps, constipation, diarrhea, and mucus in bowel movements. Medical testing and physical examination, however, fail to find a physical cause for the condition. IBS is a common health problem in the United States; as many as one in five adults experience signs and symptoms of this disorder.[17]

Irritable bowel syndrome often occurs with *fibromyalgia syndrome* (*FMS*), a condition characterized by extreme fatigue, muscle and joint pain, headaches, and sleep disturbances for which no physical cause can be found. In some instances, a stressful event seems to trigger FMS.[18] People suffering from FMS tend to be depressed and anxious; however, these negative psychological states may be the result of the symptoms of the disorder, rather than the cause.

**Intestinal Ulcers** You probably know someone who has a stomach or other intestinal ulcer—each year, about a half million Americans develop **intestinal ulcers**.[19] Such ulcers are sores in the lining

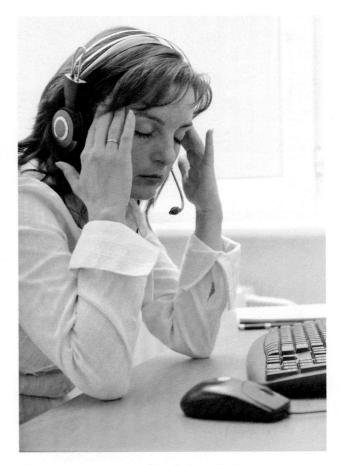

The most common type of headache is the "tension" headache.

of the esophagus (the "food tube"), stomach, or *duodenum*, which is the first part of the small intestine that leads from the stomach (see Figure 9.3). Ulcers form in the stomach ("peptic" or "gastric" ulcers) when its protective lining and overlying mucous layers do not resist the normal amount of *hydrochloric acid* that is secreted by the stomach. Ulcers of the esophagus develop when the acidic contents of the stomach chronically enter the structure and damage it. This action, *acid reflux*, often occurs when the ring muscle that serves as the "doorway" to the stomach from the esophagus relaxes. Cigarette smoking, alcohol, chocolate, fats, and peppermints can relax this muscle. In addition, lying down immediately after eating or overeating promotes acid reflux. People with intestinal ulcers usually experience burning or aching sensations in the middle of their abdomens from 30 minutes to 2 hours after eating. They may also feel bloated and nauseated after meals.

In many cases, the protective lining of the stomach may be chronically infected with the bacterium *Helicobacter pylori* (*H. pylori*). This microscopic organism is thought to weaken the stomach lining and make the person more susceptible to ulcers. However, not all individuals who are infected with *H. pylori* develop ulcers. Chronic cigarette smoking, alcohol ingestion, and aspirin and ibuprofen use also make the stomach lining susceptible to developing an ulcer.[15]

Unavoidable risk factors associated with ulcers are age and family history. As you age, your risk for ulcers increases; most ulcers are diagnosed in persons older than 40 years of age. Infection with *H. pylori* is an additional risk factor, although most people do not know if they are infected. The avoidable risk factors are cigarette smoking, chronic alcohol use, and regular use of anti-inflammatory drugs such as aspirin and ibuprofen.

Many people think that the "typical" individual who develops an ulcer has a hard-driving personality and endures a great deal of stress. Although stress does not cause ulcers, it seems to make them worse when they occur.[19] Furthermore, distressed people may smoke, drink too much alcohol, and not get enough sleep. Such unhealthy behaviors can negatively affect the immune system, reducing the body's ability to control *H. pylori* infection and making ulcers more likely.

Ulcers can be serious, especially if they bleed. Signs and symptoms of a bleeding intestinal ulcer include dark, tarry stools; a bloated sensation; and weakness. If you think you have a bleeding ulcer, seek medical attention immediately.

**Headaches** Nearly everyone has had a headache at one time or another. People who drink caffeinated beverages regularly may get headaches when they do not consume them, and physical ailments such as sinus infections often cause headaches. The most common type of headache is the *tension-type* ("tension") *headache*. People suffering from tension headaches report that the pain feels like a tight band has been placed around their forehead. The mechanisms that result in tension headaches are unknown, but stress can trigger tension headaches.[20] The typical tension headache is *not* accompanied by visual problems, stiff neck, nausea, vomiting, or fever.

Over-the-counter painkillers are usually effective for relieving tension-type headaches. For some people, simply applying hot packs to the head or neck and relaxing by having a massage are helpful. It is important to note that "rebound headaches" can occur when remedies that contain caffeine are used regularly to treat headaches.

*Migraines* are another type of recurring headache. About 12% of Americans suffer from migraine headaches, which are characterized by throbbing, intense pain that often affects one side of the head.[20] The cause of migraine headaches is unclear but thought to be related to genetic factors that affect the brain. Sometimes a migraine attack is preceded by *aura*, a nerve-related symptom that usually lasts for less than an hour. In most cases, the aura includes visual disturbances such as flashing lights or zigzag lines, but "pins and needles" sensations, numbness, and speech problems may occur as well (**Figure 3.3**). In addition to being disabled by the headache, people with migraines often experience nausea and vomiting. Be-

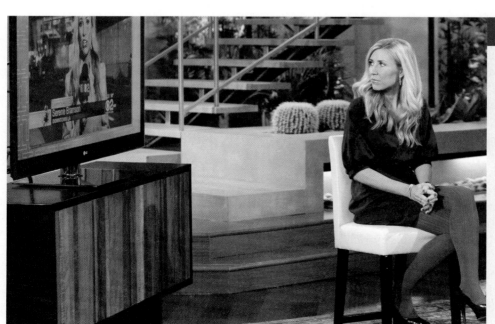

### Figure 3.3

**Migraines.** In 2011, Los Angeles TV news reporter Serene Branson (shown here) was broadcasting "live" when she began to garble her words. Although she appeared to have had a stroke, doctors later determined she had a severe migraine headache. Difficulty speaking is a sign of severe migraines as well as strokes.

cause their headaches are aggravated by light, sound, and routine physical activity, people with a migraine headache usually retreat to a darkened, quiet room to rest and recover. Migraine headaches often persist for several hours and are quite debilitating.

The first line of defense against migraines is identifying and avoiding their triggers. Some people develop migraines when they are anxious or under a lot of emotional stress. Others report having migraines when they do not get enough sleep or they have disrupted sleep patterns. In these cases, maintaining a regular, sufficient sleep schedule is crucial to avoiding attacks. Other persons have migraines that are triggered by consuming certain foods, including chocolate, aged cheeses, and red wines; and foods containing aspartame and monosodium glutamate (MSG). Keeping a food diary to determine which foods bring on headaches and then avoiding those foods are important.

In addition to managing or avoiding triggers, many people who have recurrent migraine headaches can take prescription medications to prevent the attacks.

The Consumer Health feature in this chapter discusses the usefulness of the herb feverfew as a natural means to prevent migraines.

If you suffer from frequent tension or migraine headaches, seek help from your physician. Headaches rarely signal life-threatening conditions. **Table 3.4** describes circumstances under which you should seek *immediate* medical attention for a headache.

**Overweight and Obesity** Do you lose your appetite or look for something sweet and creamy to eat when you are experiencing a lot of stress? About 80% of people alter their eating habits when they feel stressed out.[24] About half of the people who change their eating practices consume less food; the other half eats more food than usual and is referred to as *emotional eaters*. When under stress, emotional eaters usually choose tasty foods to eat. Such "comfort foods" tend to be high in sugar and/or fat, such as cookies, cake, and ice cream.[24]

As mentioned earlier in this chapter, stress increases the level of the stress hormone cortisol in the bloodstream. In response to increased blood cortisol levels, the pancreas releases the hormone *insulin*. The combined effect of cortisol and insulin is an increased desire to consume pleasurable, energy-rich foods—fatty and/or sweet foods. These hormonal adaptations are beneficial because the body needs a source of energy to fuel an immediate fight-or-flight response to threatening situations. In today's world, however, threats to well-being are usually chronic

| Table 3.4 |
| --- |
| **Serious Headache Signs and Symptoms** |

**Consult a physician if a headache:**

| | |
| --- | --- |
| • Is accompanied by stiff neck, confusion, weakness, double vision, unconsciousness, or convulsions | • Occurs after a blow to the head |
| • Is persistent in someone who has been free of headaches previously | • Worsens over days or weeks |
| • Is accompanied by fever, shortness of breath, nausea, or vomiting | • Is recurrent, especially in children |

*Source:* National Institutes of Health, National Institute of Neurological Disorders and Stroke. *Headache: Hope through research*. Retrieved on April 4, 2011, from http://www.ninds.nih.gov/disorders/headache/detail_headache.htm

and not life threatening, such as stressors generated by going to school, working, and dealing with family relationships and responsibilities. Furthermore, stressed-out Americans usually do not have to spend a lot of time hunting or searching for something tasty to eat, as their ancestors did hundreds of years ago. Adults can simply stop at a convenience store to buy a large sugar-sweetened drink, donuts, and candy bars as they drive to work, school, or home. When

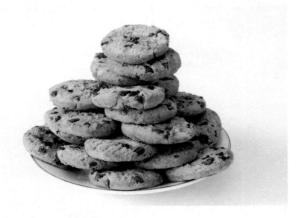

Are you an emotional eater?

# Consumer Health

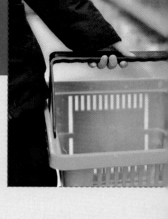

## Herbal Remedies for Stress Symptoms

Since ancient times, people have treated their stress symptoms with herbs and other plants. Many plants contain chemicals that have medicinal properties. Recently, many Americans have tried kava, valerian, and feverfew to relax or treat their stress-related symptoms. Does kava induce relaxation? Is valerian effective for treating insomnia? Can feverfew prevent migraines? Are these alternative therapies safe?

For hundreds of years, a ceremonial beverage made from the roots of the kava plant (*Piper methysticum*) has been used by South Pacific Islanders to reduce anxiety, relax muscles, and induce sleep. Although kava may relieve anxiety, its use cannot be recommended. Kava can cause serious liver damage, including liver failure, which can be deadly.[21] Furthermore, kava may interact with other drugs and intensify the effects of depressant drugs, including alcohol. Therefore, check with your physician before consuming products made from this herb.

Ancient Romans were aware of the medicinal value of the heliotrope plant, commonly known as valerian (*Valeriana officinalis*). Roots of the plant are dried, and then brewed into a tea that is used to induce sleep. Valerian is available in pills or mixed with alcohol to make a tincture. Valerian may have usefulness as a mild antianxiety

drug and produce few mild side effects when taken for 4 to 6 weeks.[22] Such side effects may include headaches, dizziness, upset stomach, and tiredness the morning following its use. The safety of taking valerian for longer than 6-week periods is unknown. It is a good idea to consult your physician before taking valerian.

Feverfew has been used for centuries to treat headaches, menstrual problems, and fever. Before supplements were available, people would chew the leaves of the plant, but this practice caused sores in the mouth and loss of taste. Feverfew may reduce the risk of migraines, but more research is needed to confirm this finding. There is not enough scientific evidence to support the use of feverfew for other health problems.

Feverfew does not seem to be toxic when consumed in recommended amounts.[23] Pregnant women, however, should not take the herb because it may cause the uterus to contract, increasing the risk of miscarriage or premature delivery. People who are allergic to ragweed and chrysanthemums are likely to be allergic to feverfew as well, so they should be careful when using the herb. Stop taking feverfew (or any herbal product) if you have adverse reactions. As in the case of all herbal treatments, check with your physician before trying feverfew.

the extra energy is not needed to cope physically with a stressful situation, it is stored as fat in the body for future energy needs. This adaptation often results in undesirable weight gain. Chapter 10 discusses overweight and obesity in detail.

**Heart Disease and Cancer** Chronic stress increases the risk of cardiovascular disease.[25] Some people's minds overreact to stressors, and their bodies respond by releasing excessive amounts of stress hormones into the bloodstream. This response may lead to inflammatory processes that cause high blood pressure and other physical changes that damage the inside walls of certain blood vessels. Additionally, scientists have found that platelets, cell fragments that participate in the blood clotting process, become stickier when a person is distressed.[25] When a blood vessel is damaged and bleeding occurs, platelets clump together and form a plug that may stop blood loss. If a person is injured during a fight for survival, the ease with which the platelets form blood clots can be lifesaving. Many stressful experiences, however,

do not include the risk of bleeding, yet the enhanced ability for blood clotting still occurs. In these instances, blood clots can be life threatening, particularly when a clot forms and blocks the blood flow to the heart muscle or the brain. A heart attack results when blood flow to the heart is blocked; a stroke can occur when blood cannot circulate through the brain.

Are there specific personality types that increase a person's risk of heart disease? For years, the popular belief is that people who have a *type A personality* (ambitious, restless, competitive, impatient, and hostile) are more likely to develop heart disease than people who do not have these characteristics. During the 1980s, medical researchers recognized that many people with type A personalities did not develop heart disease. More recently, scientists have associated a specific personality trait, *hostility*, with the development of heart and blood vessel diseases (cardiovascular disease). Hostile people harbor negative feelings, such as anger, hostility, and mistrust. A hostile person's immune system may respond to negative

**coping strategies** Behavioral responses and thought processes that people use to deal with stressors.

feelings by producing chronic inflammation, increasing the risk of heart disease.[26]

The stress response can reduce the effectiveness of the immune system, possibly interfering with its ability to detect and destroy cells that become cancerous. Most scientific studies, however, do not show an association between stress and cancer onset.[27] However, the effects of stress on the immune, nervous, and endocrine systems may lead to biochemical changes in the body that aid the growth of cancerous tumors. More research is needed to determine whether stress has tumor-promoting effects. Chapter 12 presents more information concerning the development of cardiovascular disease; Chapter 13 discusses the development of cancer.

## Healthy Living Practices

- To reduce the risk of intestinal ulcers, avoid cigarette smoking, chronic alcohol use, lying down after eating, overeating, and chronic use of anti-inflammatory drugs.

- If you experience a burning or aching sensation in the middle of your abdomen after eating, or feel bloated and nauseated after meals, you may have an intestinal ulcer. See your personal physician for diagnosis and treatment.

- To reduce the risk of tension headaches, learn to relax. Consult a physician if you have severe headaches.

## Coping with Stress

Stress is a consequence of living. In today's world, many people cannot fight or escape some of their stressors because the sources of this stress are difficult to pinpoint and control. In other instances, distressed individuals can identify their stressors, but they lack the resources to improve their situations. By learning ways to lessen the overall impact of everyday stressors on their health, many persons can live with their stress. To become more stress-resistant, for example, one can adopt a lifestyle that may reduce the negative effects of stress on the immune system, such as getting enough rest, exercising regularly, or becoming involved with spiritually uplifting activities.

**Coping strategies** are behavioral responses and thought processes that individuals use to deal actively with sources of stress. Coping strategies can be problem-focused, emotion-focused, or social support methods of managing stressful situations. Although many coping strategies are useful, some can be harmful to health.

According to the results of the Mental Health America Attitudinal Survey (2006), the major ways adults coped with stress were watching television, reading, listening to music, and talking to family members or friends.[1] Participants in the survey also cited prayer, meditation, and exercise as positive coping methods. However, many survey participants admitted using unhealthy practices to reduce stress, including eating (37%); smoking cigarettes, drinking alcohol, and using other drugs (26%); and hurting themselves (1%).

## Problem-Focused Strategies

*Problem-focused strategies*, such as planning, confronting, and problem-solving activities, are behaviors that can directly reduce or eliminate the negative effects of stressors. For example, setting priorities, managing money and time, planning for retirement, and retraining for a career change are strategies that can make people feel more in control of stressful situations. When individuals identify the sources of their stress and think that they have some control over their stressors, they feel less distress and experience fewer health problems. The "Changing Health Habits" activity in the Student Workbook at the end of the book can help you identify and change a distressing health-related habit.

**Managing Your Time** One of the most useful stress-reduction skills that you can learn is effective time management. Begin by making a list of all work, school, family, and leisure activities that you perform in a day. Then, analyze the list so that you can rank the activities according to level of priority. High-priority activities are those that must be accomplished if you are to meet your most important goals. Are some activities, such as watching television, chatting online, texting, or talking on the phone, relatively unimportant or "time wasters"? If so, these activities have low priority. To allocate and use time well, you may decide to eliminate some low-priority activities from your daily schedule.

After analyzing and ranking the high-priority activities, determine the amount of time that is needed

# Analyzing Health-Related Information

The following article about sleep appeared in *FDA Consumer*. Read the article and explain why you think it is a reliable or an unreliable source of information. Use the model for analyzing health information to guide your thinking; the main points of the model are noted here. You can find a full explanation of the model in Chapter 1.

1. Which statements are verifiable facts, and which are unverified statements or value claims?
2. What are the credentials of the person who wrote the article? Does this person have the appropriate background and education in the topic area? What can you do to check the person's credentials?
3. What might be the motives and biases of the person who wrote the article?
4. What is the main point of the article? Which information is relevant to the main point? Which information is irrelevant?
5. Is the source reliable? What evidence supports your conclusion that the source is reliable or unreliable?
6. Does the author attack the credibility of conventional scientists or medical authorities?

Based on your analysis, do you think that this article is a reliable source of health-related information? Summarize your reasons for coming to this conclusion.

## Sleepless Society

Tamar Nordenberg, staff writer for *FDA Consumer*

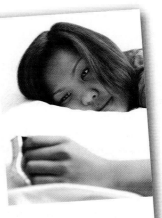

Millions of Americans undersleep by choice, burning the candle at both ends because of hectic work and family schedules. Americans sleep 7 hours each night on average, down from 9 hours in 1910 when people generally went to sleep as darkness fell.

"People don't respect sleep enough," says Daniel O'Hearn, a sleep disorders specialist at Johns Hopkins University. "They feel they can do more—have more time for work and family—by allowing themselves less time for sleep. But they do sleep; they sleep at work, or driving to work."

Like drunk driving, drowsy driving can kill. The National Highway Traffic Safety Administration estimates that more than 200,000 crashes each year involve drivers falling asleep at the wheel, and that thousands of Americans die in such accidents annually.

"Besides being an unpleasant sensation, when we're tired, we're less alert and less able to respond," says FDA drug reviewer Bob Rappaport, M.D. Lack of sleep can cause memory and mood problems, too, Rappaport says, and may affect immune function, which could lead to an increased incidence of infection and other illnesses. In studies performed on rats, prolonged sleep deprivation resulted in death.

Beyond the observable consequences of sleep deprivation, why humans—or any animal, for that matter—need sleep remains largely a mystery. "What we do know is that sleep is an important biological need, like food and drink, and that the brain is very active while we're sleeping," says James Kiley, director of the National Center for Sleep Disorders Research of the National Institutes of Health.

So just how much sleep does a person need? That can change throughout one's life based on age and other factors. For most people, though, 7.5 to 8.5 hours of sleep each night fulfills the basic physical need, but this is "very individual" and can range from as few as 4 or 5 hours to as many as 9 or 10. The Mayo Clinic of Rochester, Minnesota, defines an adequate amount of sleep as whatever produces daytime alertness and a feeling of well-being. People should not need an alarm clock to wake them, if they are getting enough sleep.

Source: Nordenberg, T. (1998). Sleepless society. *FDA Consumer*, 32(4):11.

to carry them out. Allow more time to complete the highest priority tasks than for those of lesser importance. Perform the high-priority tasks first. Putting off an important task (*procrastination*) often results from fear—fear of failure or doing a less-than-perfect job. If the task appears overwhelming, break it into smaller jobs that can be checked off as they are completed. Additionally, consider when your "best time" of the day is; plan to do the most challenging tasks during that period. To be successful in college, for example, you should allow time to attend all classes and prepare for each class, which includes setting some time aside for reviewing notes daily.

To manage time, using a calendar or personal computer to record appointments or when papers are due or exams are given can be helpful. Many people also make daily lists of "things to do," especially on very busy days. Allow some time for unexpected situations; it is not necessary to lock yourself into a rigid work schedule.

Of course, you also need time to relax, eat, exercise, socialize, and sleep. Arrange your schedule so that you can obtain 7 to 8 hours of sleep each night. Many college students are sleep deprived, and to stay alert, they often drink caffeinated beverages. Because excess caffeine can interfere with relaxation, you may need to reduce your consumption of these drinks.

If you work or have family responsibilities while you are in school, planning your time carefully is even more crucial. Individuals who balance the time that they spend performing task-centered responsibilities with that spent engaging in pleasurable activities are often able to improve their performance and feel a sense of accomplishment.

### Journal Writing

*In the past, I have seen a psychiatrist. There were times when I didn't want to go, either because I didn't have anything to say or I was in a good mood. But, I learned that no matter how I felt, it made me feel better just to talk about my life. Journaling acts somewhat like a psychiatrist or even a friend. It allows you to "get it off your chest" ... by writing down your feelings, you receive feedback from yourself.*

Coping with daily stressors may be easier if you keep a written record of personal events, thoughts, and feelings. Entering your thoughts in a journal regularly can help you focus on your emotional responses to situations. There are no rules to writing effective therapeutic journals. You do not have to write the passages in prose; some people express their feelings in poetry or as letters that are not to be mailed. Identify distressing problems or situations, and then write your thoughts concerning them, including ways to resolve these problems or manage the troublesome situations (see the Reflecting on Your Health activity at the end of this chapter).

## Emotion-Focused Strategies

Instead of directly dealing with stressors, many individuals use *emotion-focused strategies* to alter their appraisal of stressful situations. Such alterations can improve mood and reduce anxiety by making the events seem less threatening. Chapter 2 describes various defense mechanisms, such as denial and projection, that serve as emotion-focused coping strategies to defend one's mind against threats. Some people overeat or abuse alcohol to feel better during stressful periods. These unhealthy lifestyles generally relieve stress for the short term, but the consequences of overeating and drinking often create even more stress for the individual.

Emotion-focused strategies can have harmful impacts for individuals and those who must live or work with them. People need to recognize that stress is a part of life. Trying to avoid stressors and denying the need to manage stress usually do not reduce the long-term outcomes of stress on health.

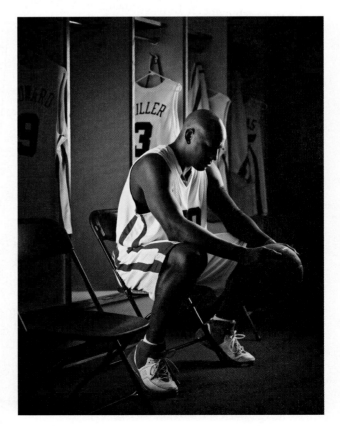

Not all emotion-focused strategies are counterproductive; some are helpful, especially if the strategy aids in mental relaxation or encourages more positive thinking. Humor can serve as a "stress buffer," lessening the negative health effects of both daily hassles and major life events.[28] For example, the homeowners who posted a "For Sale" sign in front of their hurricane-damaged house were using humor to relieve some of their distress. Additionally, forming constructive rather than destructive appraisals of stressful situations is a useful emotion-focused strategy. Many successful athletes cope with the stress of competition by appraising each competitive event as an opportunity to challenge themselves and achieve excellence in their sport. By viewing the competition as a challenge rather than a threat, athletes are less likely to experience the emotionally and physically destructive effects of stress on their performance.

## Social Support Strategies

Many individuals use *social support strategies* to cope with stressful situations. Social support strategies include seeking the advice, assistance, or consolation of close friends and relatives; participating in support groups; and obtaining spiritual help from members of the clergy or religious congregations.

When a major disaster occurs in a community, relief organizations such as the Red Cross provide valuable social and financial support services that reduce the impact of the catastrophe on peoples' lives. The knowledge that other people, even strangers, are willing to provide assistance is comforting and reassuring for many distressed individuals. Humans are not the sole providers of social support; lonely people who love animals often find comfort in the companionship of their pets (**Figure 3.4**).

### Healthy Living Practices

- [ ] Accepting stress as a part of life can reduce the negative or harmful impact of stress on your health.
- [ ] Planning for the future, setting priorities, and managing time can help you feel more in control of your life.
- [ ] Recording your thoughts and feelings in a journal can help you manage stress.
- [ ] Viewing challenging situations as opportunities to experience psychological growth can help you manage your stress.
- [ ] Seeking the companionship and social support of others can reduce your stress.

## Relaxation Techniques

Although no one can eliminate stress, you can use a variety of relaxation techniques to reduce its impact on your health. Furthermore, relaxation techniques help redirect your attention away from stressors and toward more pleasant thoughts.

As you relax, your intestinal functioning becomes normal, your breathing and heart rate slow, and your blood pressure declines. Practicing relaxation techniques when you feel stressed can help restore many body processes to normal, which reduces the potentially damaging effects that stress can have on your body. Relaxation activities often involve learning how to identify and relax your tense skeletal muscles while remaining mentally alert.

Most relaxation methods are relatively easy to learn, but to be effective, the individual needs a high degree of motivation, self-control, and willingness to practice the skills for about 10 to 20 minutes daily. Learn each technique to determine which ones are effective. At first, learning

### Figure 3.4

**Pets as Friends.** People who love animals often find comfort in the companionship of their pets.

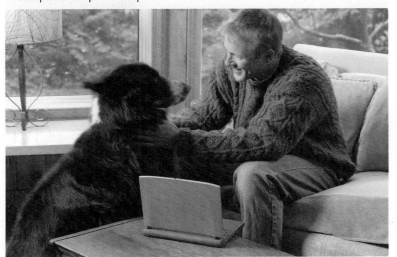

**temporomandibular (TEM-pe-row-man-DIB-you-ler)** joint The place where the lower jaw bone (mandible) attaches to the temporal bone of the skull.

**meditation** An activity in which one relaxes by mentally focusing on a single word, object, or thought.

to relax may be difficult, but by practicing at least one of these techniques every day, you should be able to master the activity within a couple of weeks.

## Deep Breathing

While having panic attacks, people often *hyperventilate* (pant for air) and feel as though they are suffocating. Hyperventilation alters the chemistry of the blood, which increases the heart rate and causes dizziness. By deliberately breathing more slowly and deeply, distressed people can feel more relaxed as their blood chemistry values return to normal. Concentrating on breathing more deeply allows people to shift their attention away from stressors and toward the breathing activity.

Under normal conditions, you breathe an average of 12 to 18 times per minute, but to relax, you need to breathe only 8 to 10 times per minute. The key is to take several deep breaths, using your abdominal muscles, and recognize how deep breathing feels different from your usual breathing pattern. Results from studies show that deep breathing is a quick and simple method to reduce the impact of stress on your health. You can use this breathing technique whenever you begin to feel excited or stressed; so, before your next exam, speech, or job interview, relax by simply breathing deeply.

*Of all the relaxation techniques we learned this semester, the deep breathing method was the most helpful. I can remember many situations when I've had to use it. While driving home from school, somebody pulled out in front of me and I had to make a ridiculous move to avoid hitting him head on. I didn't turn my car around and try to find him, which I would have done 6 months ago; I simply took some deep breaths and was thankful that no one, including myself, was injured.*

## Progressive Muscular Relaxation

Although some degree of skeletal muscular tension is necessary to maintain a comfortable body posture, excess tension in forehead, scalp, jaw, and neck muscles may contribute to the development of tension headaches. Distressed individuals often look tense because of their tightened facial muscles or clenched fists. Even when they are resting, stressed people still report feeling excess muscle tension. Teeth grinding is a common sign of stress that often occurs during sleep and may lead to headaches and pain in the **temporomandibular joint**, the joint where the lower jaw attaches to the skull in front of the ear (**Figure 3.5**).

The *progressive muscular relaxation technique* teaches people how to recognize the differences between a tensed muscle and a relaxed one. Individuals learn how to release muscle tension voluntarily, becoming aware of the relaxed sensations. When a person's skeletal muscles are completely relaxed, the individual is limp and feels calm. People often use the technique to fall asleep. The Managing Your Health feature titled "A Technique for Progressive Muscular Relaxation" highlights the steps of this particular stress reduction method.

## Meditation and the Relaxation Response

For some people, praying or meditating reduces stress. **Meditation** is an activity in which a person relaxes by mentally focusing on a single word, object,

### Figure 3.5

**The Temporomandibular Joint.** The temporomandibular joint is the point at which the lower jaw attaches to the skull in front of the ear. Pain in the temporomandibular joint may result from grinding teeth during sleep, a common sign of stress.

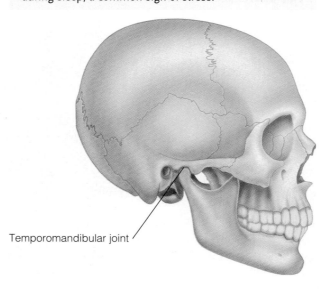

Temporomandibular joint

# Managing Your Health

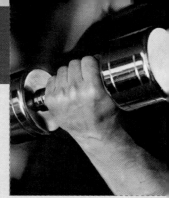

## A Technique for Progressive Muscular Relaxation

1. Choose a quiet location and sit in a comfortable position, hands down at your sides, and both feet flat on the floor.
2. Close your eyes and take a few deep breaths; concentrate on becoming as relaxed as possible.
3. With your arms at your sides, make a fist with one of your hands. Hold your clenched fist for about 5 seconds, release your hand from this position, and concentrate on the feeling as the muscular tension "drains" out of your hand.

This basic exercise is repeated as you tense muscles, hold the tensed position for 5 seconds, and then relax the major muscle groups in your body. It is important to focus on recognizing the difference between muscular tension and relaxation sensations. Continue breathing normally as the activity progresses. Begin with your head.

1. Tense your forehead and scalp muscles; feel the tight muscular sensations as you hold this position for 5 seconds; relax these muscles.

2. Tense your facial muscles; hold this position for 5 seconds; relax.
3. Tense the muscles of your neck and jaw; hold this position; relax.
4. Tense your back muscles—but not too tight; hold this position; relax.
5. Tense your right arm; hold; relax.
6. Tense your left arm; hold; relax.
7. Tense your chest muscles; hold; relax.
8. Tense your stomach muscles; hold; relax.
9. Tense your buttocks; hold; relax.
10. Tense your right leg—but not too tight; hold; relax.
11. Tense your left leg—but not too tight; hold; relax.

Now, imagine traveling back through your body searching for muscles that are not relaxed. As you find tense muscles, relax them. Maintain this position for several minutes, concentrating on your breathing. In this relaxed state, you may practice tranquil imagery and positive self-talk. To regain your normal physical activity, open your eyes, stand, and stretch your muscles.

---

or thought. *Mindfulness meditation* involves a variety of relaxation methods that focus your attention completely and in a nonjudgmental way on what you are doing or experiencing at the moment. Instead of repeating one word or thinking about a single thing or object, you allow your thoughts to flow and experience as much as you can about what you are sensing and thinking. According to results of scientific studies, people who practice mindfulness meditation are better able to regulate their emotional responses, and they report lower levels of emotional stress, anxiety, depression, and anger than people who do not use meditation to relax.[29]

You can engage in mindfulness-based stress reduction while performing ordinary activities such as eating or walking, or by studying an interesting photograph, painting, or object such as a seashell. By practicing this relaxation technique regularly, you can learn to regulate your attention and reduce your negative reactions to stress.

Herbert Benson incorporated features of meditation into his relaxation response, claiming that this method is effective for reducing blood pressure and drug abuse.[30] To practice Benson's method, find a quiet place where you can sit comfortably for 10 to 20 minutes. Close your eyes, breathe normally, and concentrate on repeating a simple word or maintaining a pleasant thought. Progressively relax groups of muscles, starting at your feet and moving up your body to your face. After relaxing your muscles, maintain this pose for at least 10 minutes. When you are ready to regain your usual degree of alertness, open your eyes, stand up, and stretch.

## Imagery

Imagery is a mental activity that is often combined with progressive muscular relaxation exercises to enhance physical relaxation. The technique is simple. After relaxing his or her muscles, the person thinks of a peaceful, pleasurable scene, using imagination or past experiences as a guide. While relaxed, the person "sees" the scene in his or her mind, and imagines other sensations as well. For example, someone who enjoys outdoor activities might recall floating down a small stream in a canoe. This individual would imagine the peaceful feeling of floating gently on the water as well as the sound of birds singing and water flowing. Imagery, or visualization, can be a creative and enjoyable way to relax as it disengages the mind from thinking about problems. Relaxation tapes or CDs often incorporate nature sounds with slow tempo music to facilitate imagery.

Athletes, actors, and other performers often use imagery to reduce their stress and enhance their performance. Before an event, for example, a pole vaulter often visualizes the entire sequence of events that takes place when approaching and vaulting over the pole. Although imagery is not a substitute for actually practicing the required skills, the technique is a useful training activity for many competitive athletes.

You do not have to be an athlete or an actor to use imagery to reduce your stress levels. Before facing a stressful situation, such as giving a speech or interviewing for a job, imagine the setting. Also imagine the other people's responses and your own behavior. Mentally rehearsing the situation can reduce your anxiety by making you feel better prepared. Then, immediately before the stressful event, breathe deeply to relax.

## Self-Talk

At times, people may have irrational or negative thoughts concerning their abilities to deal effectively with their stressors. Individuals can reduce their stress levels by identifying these self-defeating thoughts and replacing them with positive self-talk statements. Positive self-talk reflects a person's attributes and boosts self-confidence. However, thinking about oneself in a positive manner may be difficult for individuals who have low self-esteem. People with poor self-esteem often have self-degrading or self-critical thoughts, and they are unaccustomed to acknowledging their positive characteristics.

To practice positive self-talk, think of at least three affirmative statements to say about yourself, including your feelings, accomplishments, skills, and characteristics. Self-talk can be personal compliments ("I look great today"), statements of encouragement ("I can handle this problem"), or statements that reflect personal strengths ("I know I can ace that test"). Write these positive statements on a small card and place the card where you will see it daily. Repeat these statements to yourself every day and when you are feeling "stressed out." You can begin your daily relaxation sessions with progressive muscular relaxation followed by imagery, and then complete the stress management activity by repeating your positive self-statements.

## Physical Exercise

Whether it is gardening or ballroom dancing, physical activity can reduce stress by shifting one's attention away from stressors and toward the enjoyable aspects of the activity. Besides this psychological benefit, physical activity can metabolize the extra energy released during the stress response, lessening the impact of stress on the body. Additionally, engaging in physical activity with others can enhance social and spiritual well-being. Nearly everyone can think of at least one physical activity that they can enjoy on a regular basis.

Regular exercise improves mood and self-image, while reducing anxiety and stress.[31] Exercising regularly enhances the functioning of the immune system and may reduce symptoms of depression and anxiety.[32] Too much physical activity, however, can cause exhaustion or muscle damage, creating emotional stress. Athletes who engage in endurance activities and extensive physical training may have less effective immune systems, while they are in active training.

During strenuous physical activity, such as running, the nervous system releases endorphins that may be responsible for creating the "runner's high," the heightened sense of well-being that long-distance runners often experience. As mentioned earlier in this chapter, endorphins can relieve pain, but they also can reduce the activity of certain components of the immune system. Chapter 11 describes how most people can gain far more health benefits than harmful effects from regular, moderate exercise.

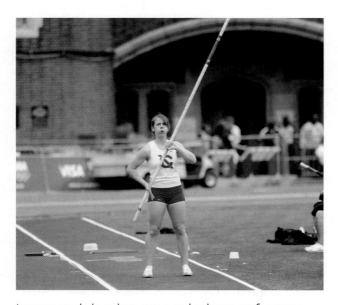

Imagery can help reduce stress and enhance performance.

**Figure 3.6**

**Managing Stress with Yoga.** Yoga includes specific physical exercises, breathing techniques, meditation activities, and dietary restrictions to promote a healthier body. After practicing yoga, trained individuals usually report feeling relaxed and refreshed.

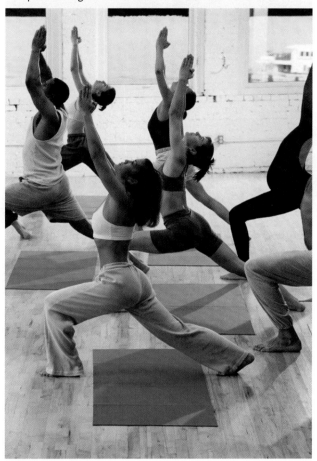

**Tai Chi and Yoga** Tai chi, a form of martial art that originated in China, emphasizes relaxation of the mind while the body is in motion. As people perform the gentle, gliding movements of tai chi, they focus their attention on this physical activity and disregard all other thoughts. In addition to tai chi, the other martial arts can be effective in reducing stress, increasing the body's flexibility, and boosting self-confidence. Tai chi, however, may be preferred by less physically active older adults because the exercises are less strenuous.

Yoga, a philosophy of living that originated in India thousands of years ago, includes specific physical exercises, breathing techniques, meditation activities, and dietary restrictions to promote a healthier body and manage stress (**Figure 3.6**). As individuals

practice the yoga exercises, they slowly move their bodies into positions that stretch their skeletal muscles. After maintaining these positions, trained individuals usually report feeling relaxed and refreshed. Although some of yoga's teachings concerning nutrition and the health benefits of stretching organs are not based on modern medical concepts, these exercises can enhance the body's muscular flexibility and reduce stress.[33]

Interest in tai chi and yoga is increasing in the United States. If you would like to learn the activities, check with the physical education department on your campus or the local fitness club to determine if they offer tai chi and yoga classes. Before beginning any new physical activity program, especially the martial arts and yoga, it is advisable to receive approval from your personal physician.

## Healthy Living Practices

- ☐ If dwelling on negative self-thoughts creates stress for you, think about your strengths and develop a list of affirmative self-statements to repeat regularly.
- ☐ Consider setting aside some time to relax every day, perhaps by using the techniques discussed in this chapter.
- ☐ Try breathing slowly and deeply before or during a stressful situation as a simple but effective way to relax.
- ☐ Engaging in tai chi, yoga, and moderate exercise and physical activity on a regular basis can reduce your stress.

## Across THE LIFE SPAN

### STRESS

Distressed adults may recall images of a carefree childhood, but children also experience stress. Common stressors for children include separation from a parent through divorce or death, moving to a new neighborhood and changing schools, and illness of a close family member.

When children are distressed, they often exhibit regressive behaviors, like clinging to and acting more

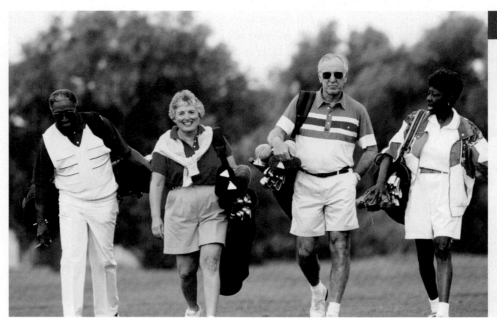

**Figure 3.7**

**Social Interaction Among Older Adults.** Many communities offer social and physical activities for older adults that can combat the stress of isolation.

dependent on their parents. In addition to acting immature, distressed youngsters may become depressed and withdrawn; suffer sleep disturbances, headaches, and stomachaches; or experience problems at school. Parents can help their children learn healthy ways to cope with stressful situations by teaching them problem-solving skills and relaxation exercises.

As mentioned in Chapter 2, the adolescent years are stressful because individuals undergo numerous physical and social changes during this time. Distressed youth who do not have effective and healthy coping mechanisms are likely to suffer from depression, abuse drugs, have serious traffic accidents, and experience problems with parents and school authorities. If an adolescent's stress response persists or is severe, professional counseling is necessary.

For many people, the older adult years can be very stressful. Aging individuals often feel bored or useless, especially if they have retired from the responsibilities of a job or raising a family. On the other

hand, many older adults are distressed because they must work to supply an income, or they must raise their grandchildren because their own children are unable, unwilling, or unavailable to do so. Older adults frequently experience distress when they must care for spouses with debilitating mental or physical illnesses.

Coping with loneliness and the deaths of friends or close family members is especially difficult for aging individuals as they face the reality of their own mortality. Suffering from disabling illnesses creates additional distress for many older adults. The inability to cope with stress can have serious results; rates of depression and suicide are high among the isolated elderly. To enhance the well-being of older adults, communities often have programs that encourage social interaction among aged members of the population (**Figure 3.7**). Additionally, elderly residents of most long-term care facilities can participate in social and physical activities that combat the stress of isolation.

# CHAPTER REVIEW

## Summary

*Stress* can refer to a threatening or demanding situation, a person's responses to a situation, or the interactions that take place between a person and a situation. Various situations or conditions, referred to as stressors, create stress. Individuals, however, can appraise the same situation differently. Situations with unwanted or negative outcomes produce distress, those with positive outcomes produce eustress. Stress can make life more challenging and interesting, but too much can make life miserable.

In a combined response, the nervous, endocrine, and immune systems prepare the body to confront or leave dangerous situations. Hans Selye proposed the general adaptation syndrome to describe the three stages of the body's adaptive physical responses to stressors. The stress response produces physical changes that include altering the activity and effectiveness of the immune system. As a result, enduring too many stressful life events can increase one's susceptibility to disease.

People often use either problem-focused, emotion-focused, or social support coping strategies to deal actively with stressful situations. Although these strategies can be effective methods of helping people take control over their stressors, some coping methods can be harmful to health. For example, emotional eating and avoiding and denying stressors are coping mechanisms that usually do not eliminate the sources of stress. Adopting healthy lifestyles can help one manage stress effectively.

Many stress management activities involve learning skills that enable one to relax. Relaxation can reverse many of the normal but damaging physical responses to stress. Relaxation techniques include deep breathing exercises, progressive muscular relaxation, meditation, and mental imagery. Journal writing, effective time management, positive self-talk, and moderate physical activity can also reduce stress.

Common childhood stressors include separation from a parent through divorce or death, moving to a new neighborhood and changing schools, and the illness of a close family member. Older distressed youths are often depressed, abuse drugs, and experience problems with parents and school authorities. Aging people often find that coping with loneliness, disability, and the deaths of friends or close family members is especially stressful.

## Applying What You Have Learned

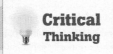
**Critical Thinking**

1. Using the techniques described in this chapter, develop a personal stress-reduction program that you can incorporate into your daily schedule. **Application**
2. You have two final exams scheduled for the same day. Describe how you could use a negative coping strategy to reduce your stress. Describe how you could use a positive coping method to deal with the same situation. **Application**
3. Plan a program that uses social support as a coping strategy to help distressed older adults who live in your community. **Synthesis**
4. Evaluate your present situation. Identify and list the sources of distress in your life. **Evaluation**

**Application**
using information in a new situation.

**Synthesis**
putting together information from different sources.

**Evaluation**
making informed decisions.

**Key**

# Reflecting on Your Health

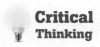

**Critical Thinking**

1. Review the physical adaptations to stress that are listed in Table 3.1. The last time you were faced with a stressful situation, did you experience these changes? How did you feel?
2. Recall that stress can have positive outcomes. Reflect on a stressful experience that made you feel happy, challenged, or successful. Why did the experience make you feel this way?
3. Each person can appraise a situation differently; what is distressing to one can be thrilling to another. Choose a situation that distresses you.

Why do you think it affects you in this manner? Do you think other people would find this situation distressing? Why or why not?
4. Chronic stress can have negative effects on health. What was the most stressful situation that you had to endure in the past year? How did this experience affect your health and well-being?
5. How do you usually react when faced with stressful situations? Are your responses positive or negative? How do you think you could reduce the impact of stress on your health?

# References

1. Mental Health America. (2006). Americans reveal top stressors: How they cope. Retrieved from http://www.mentalhealthamerica.net/index.cfm?objectid=ABD3DC4E-1372-4D20-C8274399C9476E26

2. Selye, H. (1976). *The stress of life* (2nd ed.). New York, NY: McGraw-Hill.

3. Black, P. H. (2006). The inflammatory consequences of psychologic stress: Relationship to insulin resistance, obesity, atherosclerosis, and diabetes mellitus, type II. *Medical Hypotheses, 67*(4):879–891.

4. Ayers, J. W., et al. (2009). Sorting out the competing effects of acculturation, immigrant stress, and social support on depression: A report on Korean women in California. *Journal of Nervous and Mental Disease, 197*(10):742–747.

5. Ibrahim, F. A., & Ohnishi, H. (2001). Posttraumatic stress disorder and the minority experience. In D. B. Pope-Davis & H. L. K. Coleman (Eds.), *The intersection of race, class, and gender in multicultural counseling* (pp. 89–126). Thousand Oaks, CA: Sage Publications.

6. Ro, M. (2002). Moving forward: Addressing the health of Asian American and Pacific Islander women. *American Journal of Public Health, 92*:516–519.

7. Heron, M. (2010). Deaths: Leading cause for 2006. *National Vital Statistics Reports, 58*(14): 1–100.

8. Blonna, R. (2005). *Coping with stress in a changing world* (3rd ed.). Boston, MA: McGraw-Hill.

9. Holmes, T. H., & Rahe, R. H. (1967). The social readjustment rating scale. *Journal of Psychosomatic Research, 11*:213–218.

10. Marx, M. B., Garrity, T. F., & Bowers, F. R. (1975). The influence of recent life experiences on the health of college students. *Journal of Psychosomatic Research, 19*:87–98.

11. Holmes, C., et al. (2009). Systemic inflammation and disease progression in Alzheimer disease. *Neurology, 73*(10):768–774.

12. Kiecolt-Glaser, J. K., et al. (2003). Chronic stress and age-related increases in the proinflammatory cytokine IL-6. *Proceedings of the National Academy of Sciences, 100*(15):9090–9095.

13. Wong, C. M. (2002). Post-traumatic stress disorder: Advances in psychoneuroimmunology. *Psychiatric Clinics of North America, 25*(2):369–383.

14. Levenson, J. L. (2003). Psychological factors affecting medical conditions. In R. E. Hales et al. (Eds.), *Textbook of psychiatry* (3rd ed., pp. 635–661). Washington, DC: American Psychiatric Press.

15. Orth-Gomér, K., et al. (2009). Stress reduction prolongs life in women with coronary artery disease: The Stockholm Women's Intervention Trial for Coronary Heart Disease. *Circulation, Cardiovascular Quality and Outcomes, 2*:25–32.

16. Ong, A. D., et al. (2009). Resilience comes of age: Defining features in later adulthood. *Journal of Personality, 77*(6):1777–1804.

17. National Institutes of Health, National Institute of Diabetes and Digestive and Kidney Diseases. (2007). *Irritable bowel syndrome.* Retrieved from http://digestive.niddk.nih.gov/ddiseases/pubs/ibs/

18. National Institutes of Health, National Institute of Arthritis and Neuromuscular and Skin Diseases. (2009). *Fibromyalgia.* Retrieved from http://www.niams.nih.gov/Health_Info/Fibromyalgia/default.asp

19. National Institutes of Health, National Institute of Diabetes and Digestive and Kidney Diseases. (2007). *H. pylori and peptic ulcers.* Retrieved from http://digestive.niddk.nih.gov/ddiseases/pubs/hpylori/index.htm

20. National Institutes of Health, National Institute of Neurological Disorders and Stroke. (2011, February). *Headache: Hope through research.* Retrieved from http://www.ninds.nih.gov/disorders/headache/detail_headache.htm

21. National Institutes of Health, National Center for Complementary and Alternative Medicine. (2010). *Herbs at a glance. Kava.* Retrieved from http://nccam.nih.gov/health/kava/

22. National Institutes of Health, National Center for Complementary and Alternative Medicine. (2010, July). *Herbs at a glance. Valerian.* Retrieved from http://nccam.nih.gov/health/valerian/

23. National Institutes of Health, National Center for Complementary and Alternative Medicine. (2010, July). *Herbs at a glance. Feverfew.* Retrieved from http://nccam.nih.gov/health/feverfew

24. Dallman, M. R. (2010). Stress-induced obesity and the emotional nervous system. *Trends in Endocrinology & Metabolism, 21*(3):159–165.

25. Ho, R. C. M., et al. (2010). Research on psychoneuroimmunology: Does stress influence immunity and cause coronary artery disease? *Annals of the Academy of Medicine of Singapore, 39*(3):191–196.

26. Brydon, L., et al. (2010). Hostility and physiological responses to laboratory stress in acute coronary syndrome patients. *Journal of Psychosomatic Research, 68*(2):109–116.

27. Ross, K. (2008). Mapping pathways from stress to cancer progression. *Journal of the National Cancer Institute, 100*(13):914–115, 917.

28. Taylor, M., et al. (2010). Psychosocial stress and strategies for managing adversity: Measuring population resilience in New South Wales, Australia. *Population Health Metrics, 8*:28. doi:10.1186/1478-7954-8-28

29. Greeson, J. M. (2009). Mindfulness research update: 2008. *Complementary Health Practice Review, 14*(1):10–18.

30. Benson, H. (1975). *The relaxation response.* New York, NY: William Morrow.

31. Kruk, J. (2009). Physical activity and health. *Asian Pacific Journal of Cancer Prevention, 10*(5):721–728.

32. Tsatsoulis, A., & Fountoulakis, S. (2006). The protective role of exercise on stress, stress system dysregulation, and comorbidities. *Annals of the New York Academy of Science, 1083*:196–213.

33. Kiecolt-Glaser, J. K., et al. (2010). Stress, inflammation, and yoga practice. *Psychosomatic Medicine, 72*(2):113. doi:10.1097/PSY.0b013e3181cb9377

go.jblearning.com/alters6e

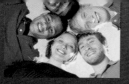

## Diversity in Health
Spouse Abuse: An International Problem

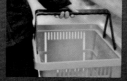

## Consumer Health
Natural Defense: Pepper Spray

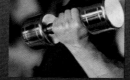

## Managing Your Health
Sexual Assault: Reducing Your Risk and Responding to an Attack

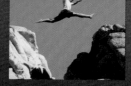

## Across the Life Span
Violence and Abuse

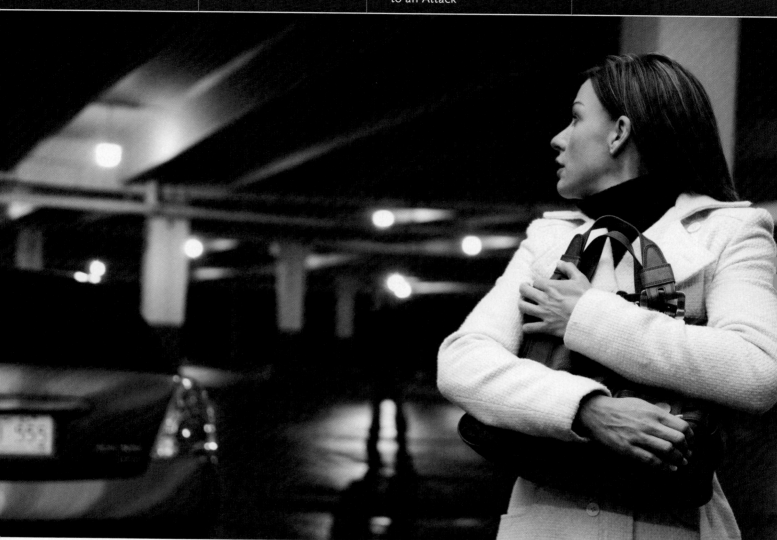

## Chapter Overview

How violence affects your health

Factors that contribute to violence

Major types of violence and abuse

How to assess your risk of becoming a victim of violence

What you can do to prevent and avoid violence

## Student Workbook

Self-Assessment: Am I in an Abusive Intimate Relationship?

Changing Health Habits: Can You Reduce Your Risk of Violence?

## Do You Know?

If watching violent television shows can make the viewer violent?

How to tell if your partner is likely to become physically abusive?

What to do if you are sexually harassed?

## CHAPTER 4

# Violence and Abuse

*Most of the campus security notices seemed to be for women, and I had a high school letter in wrestling, so I wasn't worried. Late one night, I was walking across campus, hardly watching where I was going, when a guy with a gun jumped out of some bushes and demanded my money. I gave him my watch and wallet, but he still hit me in the face with the gun barrel. I needed several stitches to close the wound.*

**A**ccording to the Federal Bureau of Investigation (FBI), in 2009 one violent crime happened about every 24 seconds in the United States.[1] Of these crimes, one aggravated assault occurred about every 39 seconds, one forcible rape took place almost every 6 minutes, and one murder happened nearly every 35 minutes.

In 2009, an estimated 702,000 children were abused or neglected in the United States, and an estimated 1,770 children died as a result.[2] Partner-against-partner violence is common in the United States. During their lifetimes, 1 in every 4 American women and 1 in every 14 American men suffer sexual and/or physical abuse at the hands of their intimate partners.[3] For many Americans, violence is a way of life.

> *"...one aggravated assault occurred about every 39 seconds..."*

**violence** Interpersonal uses of force that are not socially sanctioned.

**assault** The intentional use of force to injure another person physically.

**abuse** Taking advantage of a relationship to mistreat a person.

Every society tolerates certain controlled uses of force, for example, spanking a misbehaving child or playing contact sports. In this chapter, **violence** refers to interpersonal uses of force that are not socially sanctioned. Such violence occurs when at least one person intentionally applies or threatens physical force against one or more people. These incidents are usually one-sided—for example, a perpetrator attacking a victim—but they are sometimes mutual, such as in a barroom brawl, a schoolyard scuffle, or a fight between a husband and wife.

No one is exempt from violence; it may be directed against infants, children, adolescents, and older adults. Certain groups of people, such as African Americans, homosexuals, and Jews, are often targets of violence (*hate crimes*). Over the past 20 years, American citizens have become victims of violence as domestic and foreign terrorists waged deadly attacks in the United States.

Most physical violence in the United States could be regarded as nonsexual crimes against persons, primarily assault, robbery, and homicide. **Assault** is the intentional use of force to injure someone physically. **Abuse** occurs when one takes advantage of a relationship to mistreat a person, often by using frequent threats of force. Examples of abuse include spouse abuse, child abuse, elder abuse, and sexual harassment.

At some time in your life, you may have been a victim of abuse or violence, or you may have been indirectly involved in violent incidents. As a child, you may have been verbally abused by a parent or punched or kicked by a playground bully. As a teenager, you may have been slapped, shoved, or forced to have sex by someone you dated. As an adult, you may have been threatened or assaulted by a person with a weapon, as was the male college student in the chapter opener. How likely are you to become a victim of abuse or violence in the days to come?

Many Americans feel that their lives are more dangerous than in the past, but national rates of violent crime have declined dramatically since 2000. In 2009, the estimated number of murders, rapes, and aggravated assaults decreased by about 7.5% from the 2000

estimate.[4] Nevertheless, males, blacks, American Indians, teens, and young adults experienced higher rates of violent crime than did others.[5] This chapter explores the causes of violence and describes its effects on health. Additionally, this chapter provides practical steps you can take to reduce your risk of being a victim.

## How Violence Affects Health

Many patients who seek treatment in hospital emergency rooms are victims of violence. Although some victims just need medical attention for minor cuts or bruises, others have more serious injuries such as lost teeth, broken bones, and firearm or knife wounds that may require hospitalization (**Figure 4.1**). Additionally, victims of rape or attempted rape may need immediate treatment to reduce the risk of sexually transmitted infections (STIs) and unintentional pregnancies.

In some cases, victims of violence suffer serious permanent physical disabilities such as blindness, brain damage, and loss of body movement (*paralysis*). Additionally, the stress of fighting or living in an abusive situation alters the functioning of the immune system, which can lower one's resistance against infectious illnesses. Death is, of course, the most serious consequence of violence. Homicide is the second leading cause of death for Americans 15 to 24 years of age.[6]

### Figure 4.1

**The Aftermath of Violence.** Injuries resulting from violence often require medical treatment.

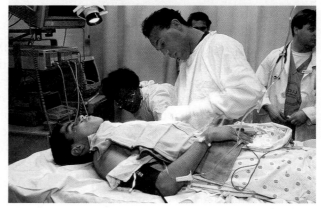

Even if they do not have physical injuries, victims of violence or abuse usually experience some degree of psychological damage that often includes anxiety and depression. Anxious or depressed people have a high risk of abusing drugs, developing eating disorders, and having suicidal thoughts. When people encounter violence outside their homes, the experience can create serious problems for the victims' family life. Family relationships may become strained, suspended, or even ended as a consequence. Violence that occurs within a family setting is very harmful. Cases of marital separation or divorce often involve violence against a spouse or child. To recover from the psychological effects of violence, people should seek help from qualified mental healthcare professionals.

A possible social effect is the *intergenerational* transmission of violence, in which abused children mature and become abusive parents, perpetuating family violence.[7] This particular effect, however, occurs with only some abused children; others have personality factors that buffer them from the long-term effects of child abuse. Overall, the financial costs of violence on physical, psychological, and social health are staggering; the cost in human misery is immeasurable.

## What Causes Violent Behavior?

Violence is complex; there is no single cause of violence, nor is violent behavior limited to a particular group of people. Nevertheless, several factors contribute to violence, including poverty, substance abuse, availability of guns, psychological problems, and poor self-esteem. In many instances, however, violence is learned behavior. As mentioned earlier, children who are exposed to violence in their homes are more likely to be abusive or violent as adults than children who do not witness violence.

Does exposure to violent screen media, particularly movies, video games, and television programs, contribute to violent behavior? The average American third to twelfth grader spends more than 6 hours per day using various forms of screen media.[8] In general, children who watch acts of violence in screen media are more likely to exhibit aggressive and violent behavior than children who do not view violence in such media.[8] How do television shows and other forms of screen media contribute to violence in the United States?

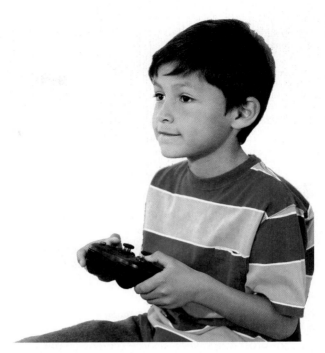

Violent video games offer opportunities for children to learn violent behavior.

Screen media, including violent computer games and movies, offer opportunities for young people to learn violent behavior. Watching violent movies, for example, provides indirect ways to participate in the violence, experience emotional states associated with being violent, and observe the outcomes of violence. Television programs and movies often glamorize violent and abusive people, and the perpetrators may avoid punishment. If violence is portrayed as an effective way of getting what one wants, an impressionable young observer may resort to violence when he or she is in similar situations. Another concern is that young people who often use violent forms of screen media for entertainment may become "desensitized" to real cases of violence and tolerate such behavior as a result.

Televisions are equipped with "V-chips" that enable adults to block certain programs from being viewed by children, but only 20% of parents use this control.[8] The screen media industry provides various rating systems to help parents select software and programs with acceptable content for children. Many parents find the ratings confusing, and some children misuse the ratings to find violent programs. Thus, parents should exercise good judgment concerning which media are appropriate for their children as well as monitor their offsprings' use of screen media as a form of entertainment.

# Major Types of Violence and Abuse

## Sexual Violence

*My first sexual experience was very unpleasant. It happened on San Padre Island over Spring Break when I was a freshman. I was 18, and he was 25 years old. He took me to an area where no one could see him or hear me. I was naive and thought I could stop him, but I couldn't. I had wanted to wait until I was married, or at least in love with the person.*

**Sexual violence** involves some type of sexual activity gained through force, threat of force, or coercion. **Rape** is sexual intercourse by force or with a person who is not able to give legal consent, such as a 12-year-old child. Both men and women can be the perpetrators or targets of rape and sexual assault. Nevertheless, females are the targets of most attempted or completed rapes. One of 6 American women and 1 of 33 American men have been victims of an attempted or completed rape at some time in their lives.[9]

College campuses are not safe havens for women. According to one major research report, about 1 in 36 female college students are victims of a completed or attempted rape during an academic year.[10] Most of the completed rapes occur in campus residential housing; the remainder of these assaults took place in fraternity houses.

In most cases, a woman is raped by someone she knows, particularly a current or former husband, current or ex-boyfriend, a date, classmate, or live-in (*cohabiting*) partner. Although men are not as likely to be raped as women, they are usually raped by male strangers and acquaintances.[9] *Marital rape* generally refers to the use or threat of violence against one's spouse to force sexual activity. *Acquaintance rape* is forced sexual activity that occurs between unmarried adults who know each other. If the couple is involved in a dating relationship, it is called *date rape*. In acquaintance rape, the rapist has a need to demonstrate his dominance over women, but he is sexually motivated as well. He intends to have sex with a woman he has met, not sexually assault her. When she de-

clines his sexual advances, however, he rapes her. In other instances, a man may expect sex as repayment for money spent for dinner or entertainment. He may think it is acceptable to insist on having sex, even if his date says "no" and physically resists. Survey data suggest that many men who rape do not think of themselves as rapists, especially if the victim is someone they know.

The use of alcohol or other drugs may weaken a person's inhibitions and alter his or her usual behavior. While intoxicated, a man may act more sexually aggressive toward his partner, and an intoxicated woman may be less able to prevent forced sex. The deliberate use of Rohypnol and other so-called date-rape drugs to sexually assault unsuspecting women is a growing problem in the United States. Rohypnol causes not only loss of consciousness but also loss of memory concerning events that occurred when the drug was taken. Chapter 7 includes information concerning date-rape drugs.

**Reporting Sexual Assault** Data from crime surveys suggest that sexual crimes occur more often than previously suspected. Rape victims frequently feel ashamed and embarrassed and are often reluctant to report their experiences to the authorities. Moreover, they may fear further victimization by the assailant or negative reactions from family, friends, and coworkers. Some victims, however, fail to report the assault because they simply do not want to become involved in the criminal justice system. Many victims of acquaintance rape are often unwilling to report the incidents because they feel partially to blame. For example, a female college student may feel that if she had consumed less alcohol or smoked less marijuana

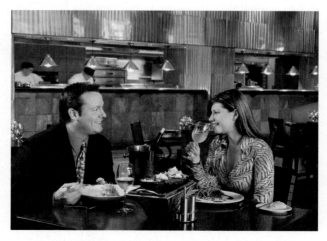

When intoxicated, a man may act more sexually aggressive toward his date or partner, and an intoxicated woman may be less able to prevent forced sex.

# Managing Your Health

## Sexual Assault: Reducing Your Risk and Responding to an Attack

### To avoid stranger rape:

- Avoid high-risk situations such as being alone in isolated areas or using drugs that affect your physical responses to a threat or your decision-making abilities.
- Walk with your head up, looking alert and confident.
- Consider carrying pepper spray. (See the Consumer Health box later in this chapter.)
- Have your keys or remote carlock device in your hand as you approach your parked vehicle so that you do not have to stand outside your car looking for them. Check the area around your parked car and in the back seat before you enter it.
- If your car becomes disabled, do not accept a stranger's help. Place a "Help, call police" sign in the window. Stay inside of the car until police arrive. Do not hitchhike. Carry a cell phone and keep it on for quick use in an emergency.
- Keep the doors and windows of your car and home locked. Install deadbolt locks and peepholes on all outside doors of your home.
- Be wary of strangers who want you to open your door to them; they may intend to harm you. If they ask to use your phone, tell them you will make the call for them. Even if they appear to be from a business, do not open the door.

### If you are attacked:

- Yell or scream "Fire" instead of "Help" to get people's attention. Do not stop screaming; making a loud commotion may scare your attacker away.
- Do not allow yourself to be moved to another location. Resist being forced into a car. If you leave the original scene of the assault, it becomes more likely that you will be seriously injured or murdered.
- *Avoid* kicking a man's groin area; men are wary of this maneuver and guard their genitals. Instead, making a swift, hard kick across the attacker's kneecap can disable the person, allowing you to escape.
- If your attacker has a weapon, he may intend to kill you regardless of whether you comply with his demands. In this instance, rape prevention experts often recommend that you use extreme actions to confuse or intimidate the criminal such as throwing up, acting psychotic, or pretending to have AIDS, a heart attack, or other life-threatening condition. In other instances, you may pretend to cooperate with your attacker, perhaps even acting as though you are attracted to him. By waiting until his guard is down, you may be able to make a surprise move in your defense.

### To avoid date rape:

- Agree to meet a "blind date" at a crowded location, or agree only to a group dating situation until you feel comfortable going out with the individual.
- Be wary of dates who show unreasonable or inappropriate behaviors in public, such as aggressiveness, rudeness, dominance, or hostility in social situations that do not involve sex. These individuals may display the same behaviors when alone with you.
- Do not send mixed verbal and/or nonverbal messages about your feelings that can confuse your date. Clearly say "no" to unwanted sexual advances.

---

at a party, she would have been able to resist the sexual advances of others.

Sexual assault victims should obtain immediate medical attention for their injuries. Hospital emergency rooms often have staff who are trained to manage rape cases. In addition to receiving treatment for physical injuries, many rape victims need testing for sexually transmitted infections, medication to prevent pregnancy, and counseling to cope with the situation.

If the victim chooses to prosecute the rapist, she should preserve all physical evidence because it might assist the police. For example, she should not wash any part of her body or change clothes. Semen and pubic hair from the attacker can be used to identify this individual. Victims who are unsure if they want to take legal action against their assailant can contact a rape crisis center for free advice from trained counselors. Most major metropolitan areas have rape crisis centers; their phone numbers may be listed un-

**family (domestic) violence** Violence or abuse between family members, people who are involved in intimate relationships, or unrelated individuals who live together.

der "Rape Hotline" or "Women Self-Help" in phone books. The following Managing Your Health feature provides some suggestions to lower your risk of becoming a sexual assault victim as well as what to do in case you are attacked.

# Family Violence

**Family (domestic) violence** is a pattern of behavior characterized by physical assaults, including sexual violence; psychological/emotional abuse; and threats to cause harm that occur among family members, couples in intimate relationships, or unrelated individuals who live together. Such violence includes assaults and murders of spouses, children, and older family members. Between 1998 and 2002, family violence accounted for 11% of all violence.[11] In 2009, family members were responsible for almost one-fourth of all murders.[12] Child and elder abuse are often classified as forms of family violence; the Across the Life Span feature of this chapter provides information concerning these forms of family violence.

**Intimate Partner Violence** *Intimate partner violence (IPV)* involves actual or threatened physical or sexual violence, as well as emotional abuse, by a spouse, ex-spouse, lover, former lover, or date. In 2009, about 1 in 4 women who experienced nondeadly acts of violence were victimized by an intimate partner.[12] About 1 in 20 men who experienced nonfatal violence was a victim of an intimate partner.

In many instances, perpetrators of IPV emotionally abuse their partners for a period before they become overtly violent toward them.[13] Violent acts may range from slapping, shoving, and punching to beating and murder. Typically, verbal and emotional abuse accompany the physical violence. *Dating violence*, the threat or use of force against one's partner during courtship, is quite common. About 10% of high school students reported that they had been hit, slapped, or physically hurt (on purpose) by their boyfriend or girlfriend in 2009.[14] Furthermore, 10% of the female students and about 5% of the male high school students reported that they had been forced to have sex, at some point in their lives.

Intimate partner violence also occurs in homosexual relationships. In a survey of more than 800 urban men who have sex with men, almost one-third of

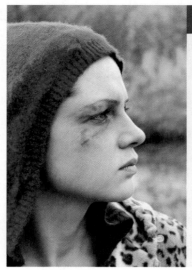

the subjects reported they had experienced abuse in a past or current relationship.[15] IPV between lesbian couples is quite high; according to various surveys, 17% to 52% of lesbians reported they had been physically abused by their partners.[16]

Compared to women, men are more likely to injure seriously or murder their female intimate partners (**Figure 4.2**).[13] In 2009, of the female murder victims for whom their relationships to the offenders were known, about 35% were murdered by their husbands or boyfriends.[17] Although both sexes commit violent acts against their dates or partners, women usually engage in violence against their male partners as acts of self-defense.

What factors contribute to violence between intimate partners? Such violence exists within every racial, ethnic, socioeconomic, and religious group. The rates of intimate partner violence, however, are higher among the poor, the unemployed, and those with low-status occupations. Additionally, children who are exposed to violence between their parents have a greater risk of abusing their lovers later in life.[18] As a result of witnessing violence between their parents, these children may grow up thinking such abuse is a "normal" aspect of intimate relationships.

Another major factor that contributes to intimate partner violence is drug use. Often, one or both partners have consumed alcohol or used other mind-altering drugs when the violence between them erupts. Both perpetrators and victims tend to have low self-esteem and be highly dependent on their partners. Some men and women have difficulty asserting themselves without becoming angry and resort to aggressive behavior to control and intimidate

## Table 4.1

### Signs of Danger in a Relationship

**A partner who is likely to become physically abusive:**

- Insists that you do things that you do not want to do and prevents you from doing things that you would like to do
- Argues with you over any issue
- Does not accept responsibility for his or her mistakes and blames you or other persons for his or her problems
- Prevents you from associating with your family and friends and threatens to end the relationship if you do not stop interacting with others
- Displays excessive jealousy or is too possessive
- Attempts to control your behavior, for example, tells you how to dress or wear your hair
- Is verbally abusive, for example, criticizes you or says degrading things to you either in private or in public
- Expects you to do everything perfectly and according to his or her wishes, and expects you to know what they are, even without being told
- Pushes, slaps, or shoves you during disagreements
- Reacts violently ("loses control" over his or her behavior) toward you or others when things go wrong or not according to his or her wishes
- Exhibits cruelty to other persons or animals, usually without remorse

*Source:* Adapted from Mariani, C. (1996). *Domestic violence survival guide.* Flushing, NY: Looseleaf Law Publications.

their partners. The activity "Am I in an Abusive Relationship?" in the Student Workbook at the end of the book can help you determine if your partner is abusive. Furthermore, **Table 4.1** lists certain behaviors and attitudes that often characterize physically abusive individuals. Because dating violence is often a precursor of marital violence, you should leave a relationship if your partner displays any of these characteristics.

Why do men and women stay in abusive relationships, sometimes for decades? Women often remain in these situations because of their emotional attachment to and economic dependency on the abuser. They often feel trapped and isolated.[19] Furthermore, an abusive partner may be apologetic and loving after episodes of violence, raising the victim's hopes that the violence has ended. Spouse abuse is not just an American phenomenon; the Diversity in Health feature "Spouse Abuse: An International Problem" discusses the nature of this behavior in non-Western societies.

## Sexual Harassment

**Sexual harassment** is the intentional use of annoying and offensive sexually related comments or behaviors to intimidate people or coerce them into unwanted sexual activity. Such abusive behavior can include unwelcome requests for dates, sexually offensive jokes, lewd comments, or touching and fondling. It is difficult to determine the scope of the problem because surveys often use different definitions of *sexual harassment.* Furthermore, sexual harassment is not always easy to recognize. For example, if someone tells a sexually offensive joke, under what circumstances would you consider this sexual harassment?

Sexual harassment can happen anywhere. College instructors, for example, engage in sexual harassment if they provide special treatment, such as awarding a passing grade, to students who submit to their sexual advances. In addition to schools, sexual harassment frequently occurs in the workplace, where it creates stress and reduces employees' job satisfaction, performance, and loyalty. It is especially devastating for individuals who feel that their grade, job, or career depends on enduring the harassment or submitting to the intimidating person.

How can one handle a person who engages in sexual harassment? Some people simply avoid or ignore harassing persons; others choose to confront their tormentors by telling them, verbally or in writing, to stop the annoying and unprofessional comments or behaviors. If the harassment persists, victims can pursue more aggressive steps, including reporting the behavior to management or taking legal action. Many educational institutions and businesses have policies concerning sexual harassment that follow guidelines established by the federal government's *Equal Employment Opportunity Commission (EEOC).* These policies usually identify steps that people can take to file harassment-related complaints. Before initiating such action, a person should document episodes of sexual intimidation, recording the date and nature of the unwanted comments or behaviors. In many in-

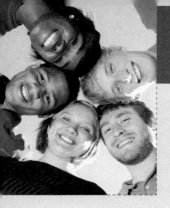

# Diversity in Health

## Spouse Abuse: An International Problem

Throughout the world, women of all cultural, religious, ethnic, and socioeconomic groups are abused by their intimate partners. Throughout the world, at least one-third of all women have experienced violence or abuse on one or more occasions during their lifetimes.[20] According to results of a study conducted by the World Health Organization, rates of IPV ranged from 15% in Japan to about 70% in Peru and Ethiopia.[21] In many societies, husbands are not punished for acting out violently against their wives, and the female victims often accept blame for their mistreatment.

Why does spouse abuse persist? Certain non-Western cultures ascribe low status to women. Many men living in these societies do not consider wife battering and other forms of mistreatment of their spouses as violence or abuse. Additionally, certain practices in such cultures increase the financial dependence of women on their spouses, which makes it difficult for them to leave their abusive husbands. For example, women living in some countries lose their inheritance or the opportunity to earn an income outside of the home when they marry. The economic power in these countries is unequally distributed in favor of men, and as a result, husbands feel entitled to control their wives and families. Male domination continues at community and state levels as women are often denied access to education and government positions. Thus, they lack the knowledge and political power necessary to change public policy. To eliminate violence against women, people from around the world must work to change the attitudes, behaviors, and laws that negatively affect the status of women.

---

stances, the abusive person has harassed other workers or students; therefore, a victim may be able to strengthen his or her case against this person by asking other victims to serve as witnesses.

## Stalking

Sensational stories about celebrities who are pursued relentlessly by overly aggressive, obsessive fans have led to interest and research into *stalking* behavior. Anyone, however, can be the victim of a stalker. The term "stalker" generally refers to a person who willfully and repeatedly harasses or threatens another person. Stalking behavior typically includes following the targeted individual, hanging around this person's home, making harassing or threatening phone calls, leaving threatening voicemail messages, or vandalizing his or her property. Other examples of harassment include sending unwanted text messages or gifts and making unwelcome visits to the targeted person's workplace (see **Table 4.2**).

According to a report by the U.S. Department of Justice, an estimated 3.4 million Americans were victimized by stalkers in a 12-month period that spanned 2005 and 2006.[22] In only about 10% of the cases, the stalker was a stranger to his or her victim. According to victims, most of the stalkers were a former intimate partner or a friend, roommate, or neighbor.[22]

### Table 4.2

### Typical Stalking Behaviors

**A stalker:**

- Repeatedly makes unwanted, intrusive, and frightening communications to the victim by phone, mail, and/or email
- Repeatedly leaves or sends unwanted items, presents, or flowers to the victim
- Follows or waits for the victim at places such as home, school, or work
- Makes direct or indirect threats to harm the victim or the victim's children, relatives, friends, or pets
- Damages or threatens to damage the victim's property
- Posts information or spreads rumors about the victim at social websites, in public places, or by word of mouth
- Obtains personal information about the victim by accessing public records, using Internet search services, going through the victim's garbage, or contacting the victim's friends, coworkers, or neighbors

*Source:* Adapted from Stalking Resource Center, National Center for Victims of Crime (n.d.). Retrieved June 22, 2007, from http://usdoj.gov.ovw/aboutstalking.htm.

The majority of stalkers are males; the largest group of stalkers is composed of lonely, emotionally disturbed men who have been rejected by their partners.[23] Despite his ex-partner's efforts to avoid him, the stalker often hopes he can convince her to rekindle the relationship. When she ignores or rebuffs his efforts, he becomes angry with her and wants to harm her emotionally or physically.

Stalking can lead to violence, including homicide. Stalkers physically attack an estimated one-fourth to about one-third of their victims.[24] Warning signs of a violent stalker include the use of verbal threats and prior involvement in an intimate relationship with the victim. Even if the victim is not physically threatened or harmed, he or she usually experiences extreme emotional distress and often seeks legal means to make the stalker stop the harassing behavior. Victims often continue to suffer severe emotional effects long after the stalking ends, and they may need treatment for depression and post-traumatic stress disorder.

If you are being stalked, what can you do to discourage the stalker and end his or her terrifying behavior? If the stalker is a former intimate partner, experts advise that either you or a family member

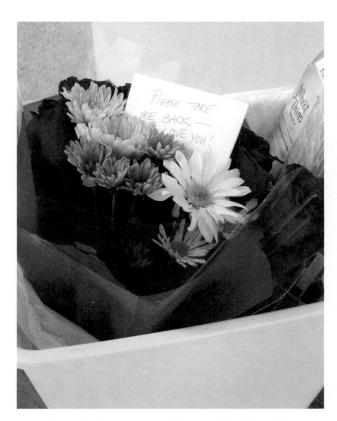

Men who stalk women may send unwanted gifts, such as bouquets of flowers, to their victims.

confront the stalker to tell him or her that the relationship is over and you have no interest in renewing it. After that, avoid all communication with the person but keep records of his or her harassing behavior. If the stalker persistently telephones you, have an answering machine record calls on that line and get a separate, unlisted phone number for other callers. If the stalker uses email messages or text messages to annoy you (*cyberstalking*), contact your Internet service (ISP) or cell phone service provider for help. Additionally, seek support and help from family, friends, neighbors, and coworkers by telling them about the stalking incidents. Finally, make sure your home is secure, and if you feel threatened by the stalker, notify the police.

## Community Violence

**Community violence** refers to violence that happens in public settings such as street corners, bars, and public places. Among youths, community violence often occurs as *gang violence*. Typical members of a gang are males between 8 and 24 years of age who share similar racial or ethnic backgrounds. Such gangs are prevalent in certain neighborhoods of U.S. cities and are becoming more common in many suburbs. Between 2002 and 2008, the number of gangs increased by almost 30%.[25] According to one government estimate, approximately 1 million gang members were involved in criminal activity throughout the United States during 2008.[26] Gang-related criminal activities include armed robberies, drug trafficking, car theft, identity theft, and murder.[26]

Violence is a characteristic of gang activities—gang members often resort to violence to defend their territory. Violent gang activities are more likely to occur on city streets during weekend evenings. The late-night drive-by shooting, for example, has come to be associated with gang violence.

Why are some youths attracted to gangs, placing themselves at high risk for serious injury and even death? Adolescents may join gangs for social reasons, especially if their communities offer few opportunities for safe social activities. Additionally, gang membership provides an opportunity for some youths to belong to a group and find self-identity, that is, to "be someone." Involvement with gangs, however, dramatically increases one's risk of being murdered. In 2006, homicide was the number one cause of death for African American males between 15 and 34 years

**institutional violence** Violence that occurs mainly in institutional settings such as college campuses or workplaces.

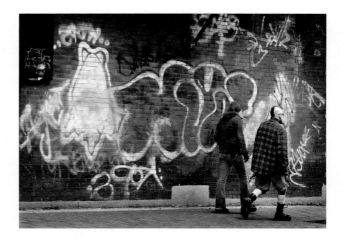

of age and the second leading cause of death for Hispanic males between 10 and 34 years of age.[27]

## Institutional Violence

**School Violence** Most acts of **institutional violence** occur in schools, where students attack their peers or even their teachers and school administrators. Earlier generations of students may have shoved and punched to settle arguments; today's students may use guns and knives.

In the past few years, several incidents in which students used guns to kill their classmates and teachers made headline news. Such terrible events, however, are rare. Less than 1% of murders involving youth take place on school property. In 2009, American youth were much less likely to carry weapons to school and engage in fighting than in 1993.[14]

What can be done to reduce the risk of violence at school? Many urban schools now resort to using metal detectors and hiring uniformed police in an attempt to curb school violence. Other steps to manage the problem include training elementary school teachers and administrators to identify potential troublemakers in their classrooms. Children who are prone to become violent often model the aggressive behaviors of their parents. Such high-risk children have dif-

ficulty controlling their anger; tend to poke, shove, or annoy other people; act impulsively; bully other children; and defy authorities, including parents and teachers. In many communities, schools now offer conflict resolution classes for children that emphasize socially acceptable ways of settling disputes.

**Violence on College Campuses** On April 16, 2007, Cho Seung-Hui, a 23-year-old psychologically disturbed college student, shot 32 students and faculty to death on the Virginia Polytechnic Institute (Virginia Tech) campus before taking his own life (**Figure 4.3**). The violent incident raised serious questions about the safety of American university students and sparked efforts to improve campus security and identify troubled college students before they react

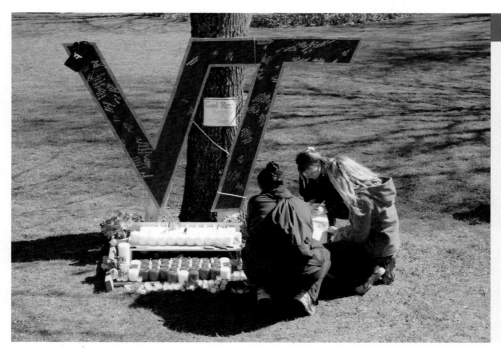

### Figure 4.3

**College Violence.** On April 16, 2007, a psychologically disturbed college student shot 32 students and faculty to death on the Virginia Polytechnic Institute campus before taking his own life.

violently. Prior to the Virginia Tech shootings, the results of nationwide surveys conducted between 1995 and 2002 indicate college students were less likely to be victims of violent crime than nonstudents of the same age.[28] According to these surveys, the majority of violent crimes against college students occurred off campus and during the evening or at night (6 P.M. to 6 A.M.). Only about one-third of the violent crimes committed against college students were reported to the police.

The *Student Right to Know and Campus Security Act* requires administrators of colleges and universities that receive federal funds to report information concerning the number of murders, assaults, rapes, and other specific crimes that take place on their campuses. Additionally, the administrators must develop programs that are designed to educate students about personal safety and campus security. To reduce the violence on their campuses, many college administrators have adopted security measures such as restricting access to campus buildings, setting up emergency call boxes on campus, improving lighting near walkways and parking lots, limiting visitation hours in residence halls, and initiating escort services for female students. For information about the types and extent of crime at your college or university, visit the Department of Education's Office of Postsecondary Education website http://ope.ed.gov/security/GetOneInstitutionData.aspx for an interactive tool that provides data concerning numbers of reported crimes on college campuses. You can also contact staff at the campus police department.

## Workplace Violence

Workplace violence is any act of violence or abuse directed toward an individual who is performing his or her job. Although most people will never experience the most dangerous types of workplaces, such as psychiatric hospitals and prisons, any workplace can be a setting for violence. In 2009, homicide was the third leading cause of death for American workers.[29] The stereotype of workplace violence as vengeful acts committed by disgruntled former workers is misleading. Work-related homicides are most likely to occur during armed robberies of retail businesses such as grocery stores, restaurants, bars, and gas stations. Employees with the highest risk of being murdered while working are cab drivers, convenience store attendants, police, and security guards.

Certain workers have a high risk of becoming violent, particularly when they are laid off, fired, or not promoted. Persons most likely to resort to workplace violence are men between the ages of 25 and 40 who are loners, have marital and other family problems, appear angry and paranoid, abuse alcohol and/or other drugs, and blame others for their problems. Women are less likely to commit violent acts in workplaces, but they are more likely to be victims.

## Terrorism

Terrorism is intentional violent acts against civilians to produce extreme fear, severe property damage, and numerous deaths. Terrorists may attack specific cultural or political symbols, such as places of worship or government buildings; or more random targets, such as restaurants, subway stations, and airplanes (**Figure 4.4**). Regardless of whether terrorists are citizens of the country they attack or foreigners, a major purpose of terrorism is to frighten the general population and make them feel vulnerable and helpless.

### Figure 4.4

**New York City, September 11, 2001.** On this day, foreign terrorists used commercial jets to attack the World Trade Centers and the Pentagon.

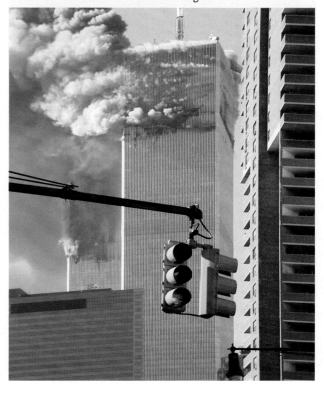

The use of conventional bombs by terrorists is not new, but recently, terrorists have adopted more sinister methods of killing civilians and destroying property. The arsenal of terrorist weapons now includes poisonous chemicals, life-threatening infectious agents such as the bacterium that causes anthrax, and explosives strapped to suicidal individuals who intentionally blow themselves up in crowded places.

In addition to physical injuries, survivors of a terrorist attack often experience long-term psychological consequences such as post-traumatic stress disorder (PTSD) and depression. Extensive media reporting of the disastrous event, however, indirectly affects the psychological health of those outside the zone of destruction. National surveys conducted after the September 11, 2001, attacks on the World Trade Centers and Pentagon indicate many Americans who were not directly affected by the attacks suffered from extreme psychological stress symptoms as a result of the terrorism.[30,31] After September 11, 2001, U.S. government officials took steps to reduce the risk of terrorism by, for example, erecting video surveillance cameras in public places and increasing airport security. Nevertheless, many Americans think additional terrorist attacks in the United States are likely. Living with such fear increases the risk of stress-related health problems such as those discussed in Chapter 3.

## Assessing Your Risk of Violence

What are the chances that you, or some of the people you care about deeply, are at risk for violence? The risk is difficult to determine because many violent incidents, especially rapes and spouse battering, are never reported to the police. Nevertheless, some people are more likely to suffer serious or fatal injury than others. The likelihood of a particular person experiencing such harm depends on specific risk factors, including his or her family situation, living conditions, personality, and activities.

Family disruption is a major risk factor for family and community violence. Parental conflict that leads to separation, divorce, or desertion contributes to family disruption, as does the presence of criminal or drug-addicted parents. Neighborhood conditions, such as high rates of unemployment, can lead to high rates of family disruption. Other risk factors

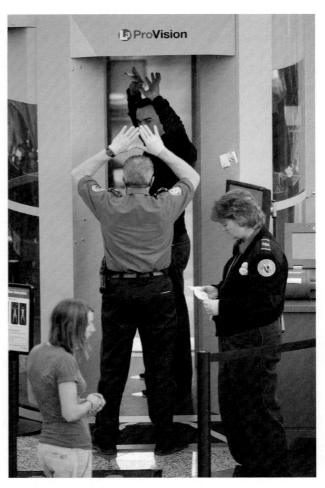

Increased airport security measures were an outcome of the September 11, 2001 terrorist attacks.

for family violence are social isolation, the presence of children with special needs, and a large number of children in the family. Conditions that contribute to school violence are poor discipline in the classroom, weak administrators, poor enforcement of rules, and low levels of student and parent interest in academic achievement.

As mentioned earlier in this chapter, the availability of alcohol, other drugs, and guns dramatically escalates the likelihood of serious injury or death in violent situations. A significant percentage of people who commit violent crimes test positive for alcohol, marijuana, cocaine, or combinations of mind-altering drugs at the time of their arrest. In 2009, firearms were used in about 67% of the nation's murders, 43% of robberies, and 21% of aggravated assaults.[32]

Certain individuals are more likely than others to find themselves in places and situations in which violence is likely to occur. Age is a major risk factor. Americans younger than 25 years old are more likely to become involved in violence than are older persons. Americans between 12 and 24 years of age experience the highest rates of violent crimes; in 2009, almost one in four murder victims were younger than 22 years of age.[33] Another key risk factor is sex. While in their homes, women are as likely as men to use force, but in community settings they are far less likely to do so. Men are more likely than women to be arrested for perpetrating crimes of violence, and they are more likely to be the victims of such crimes. Women, however, have a greater risk of being killed by their spouses than men do.

Race and ethnicity are two other characteristics strongly associated with involvement in violent incidents. In 2009, African Americans were more likely than whites to be victims of sexual assault and aggravated assault.[34] In that year, however, almost half of the murder victims were white and half of the victims were African Americans.

An objective of *Healthy People 2020* is to reduce the homicide rate from 6.1 per 100,000 (the rate in 2007) to 5.5 per 100,000 Americans by 2020.[35] This is one national health indicator in which progress has been made; the homicide rate decreased to 5.1 murders per 100,000 Americans in 2009.[36]

## Preventing and Avoiding Violence

Although many Americans doubt that violence can be prevented, they do think it can be controlled. To reduce violent crime, communities are turning increasingly to environmental measures such as improved street lighting, neighborhood watch organizations, and surveillance by closed-circuit cameras. Many large companies have taken specific steps to reduce workplace violence, such as hiring security staff, controlling access to offices, requiring employees to wear identification badges, and offering employee assistance programs that provide referrals for counseling services.

You can take numerous practical steps to reduce your personal risk of victimization. Many avoidance measures are simple and inexpensive, and they work. To be effective, however, these measures must become part of your routine. The most effective action is staying away from high-risk situations and people. For example, a woman who does not attend a binge drinking party cannot be raped by a male at the party; a man who stays out of a high-crime district is unlikely to be a victim of a drive-by shooting. Simply put, people should avoid high-risk places and dangerous persons.

Another violence preventive measure is to avoid using destructive responses such as angry verbal exchanges, including insults and name calling, to manage interpersonal conflicts. Arguments are the most frequently cited circumstances that result in murder. In 2009, for example, arguments were involved in about 4 of 10 murders in which the circumstances were known.[37] If you become involved in a heated dispute or threatening situation, keeping calm may prevent the situation from escalating into a violent one. For example, breathe deeply, count to 10, "bite your tongue," or make some excuse and quickly leave the scene. The relaxation techniques described in Chapter 3 can help you maintain your composure in such situations. If you have a "short fuse" and get angry easily, counseling can help you learn conflict management strategies such as impulse control, anger management, and negotiation techniques.

## Home Security Measures

Improving your home's security can discourage and prevent criminals from victimizing you. In many break-ins, the intruder simply came through an unlocked door or window. Before you leave your residence, check to see if it is secure. The most important safety measure is to have and always use good deadbolt locks on doors. If your entry door does not have windows, consider having a peephole installed in the door. When someone knocks at your door, do not open it until you have peered through the peephole and are certain that you can safely welcome the visitor into your home. Also, keep windows securely locked, especially when you are not home. Contact your police department or the campus security center to see if they will perform a free safety inspection of your residence. If you can keep a pet at your residence, consider getting a large dog for a companion and "bodyguard."

Following are other helpful safety measures:

- When you go out of your home, leave some lights and a radio on to give the impression that someone is there.

- When you return to your home, do not enter if you see signs of a break-in or suspicious persons in the area. Go instead to a neighbor's or public place and call the police. If surprised, burglars often become assailants and attack the robbery victims.

- Lock the door immediately after entering your home or dorm room.

## Community Security Measures

If you live in a dangerous neighborhood, consider moving to a safer one if you can. This is the most effective measure you can take to avoid violence. If you cannot leave the neighborhood, look for a place to live that is farther away from the most dangerous streets. If the new area looks safer, ask a few residents, and even local police, if they would prefer to live elsewhere. The police may have local crime statistics, so you can compare crime rates of various neighborhoods.

Daily life is filled with people and situations that cannot be avoided, but you can use certain tactics to reduce your chances of victimization. If your usual routine requires traveling through dangerous neighborhoods, remove yourself from these high-risk areas by taking safer routes, even if they are out of your way. Avoid isolated places, especially when you are alone. Jogging trails in parks, deserted buildings, infrequently used sections of libraries, and nearly empty parking lots and garages are places where violent incidents are likely to occur.

A considerable percentage of violent crimes, especially sexual assaults, happen between 6 P.M. and midnight. Thus, if you must go out at night, do not go alone. Additionally, stay in places where you can see other people. Being in the presence of others greatly reduces your risk of violence. If you are alone at night and on campus, use the college's escort service or use the "buddy system" when walking to and from buildings.

Following are other community safety measures:

- Do not walk, jog, or bike alone, especially at night.
- Wear a whistle to signal an alarm or carry a can of pepper spray to use if threatened (see the Consumer Health feature).
- Look alert.
- Park in a well-lit busy area. Check inside and underneath the car before entering. If you need to use public transportation, choose well-populated stops.
- If violence erupts anywhere near you, run away if you can.

## Reducing the Risk of Violence While in a Car

Regardless of the time of day, as soon as you enter your car, lock the doors. Keep your car doors locked, and take the keys with you, even when you leave the car for a minute. Do not give rides to strangers or stop to help others. If you spend a lot of time in your car, keep a charged cell phone with you to call for assistance in any emergency. If you are involved in a minor accident, stay in your car; call the police, and keep the doors locked and the windows rolled up until they arrive.

If someone demands that you surrender your car, do not argue with or resist the person: Get out of the car and quickly move away from the area. Then, contact the police. If you are driving and someone in a nearby vehicle drives aggressively and irresponsibly, avoid getting angry with the person. If a driver tailgates your car, flashes high beams at you, or makes angry gestures, do not stop to discuss the matter. Avoid making eye contact with this individual. In this situation, *do not* drive to your home because he or she is likely to follow you and confront you when you get out of your car. You can discourage this person from continuing to follow you by driving to a busy highway or other high-traffic area. If you still feel threatened, drive to a well-lit public place; obviously, police stations or fire stations are the best choices.

## Workplace Safety Measures

In the workplace, learn your company's security measures, for example, the locations of fire alarms, so that you can activate one in case of any trouble. Keep your cell phone with you at all times. Perhaps most important, strive to get along with coworkers and the public. Help create a positive working environment and relationships by displaying a friendly attitude, good manners, tact, and diplomacy. The "Changing Health Habits" activity in the Student Workbook at the end of the book can help you identify and change habits that may increase your risk of becoming a victim of violence.

## Self-Protection

When faced with the threat of force, your actions can influence the outcome of the situation. For example, you may obtain help from others by calling the police, pressing an alarm button, blowing a whistle, or screaming "Fire" to attract attention. When cornered and facing a threatening person alone, you can try to defuse the situation verbally by reasoning with your assailant. If you become overwhelmed by fear or con-

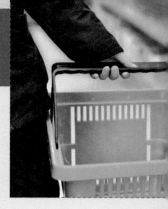

# Consumer Health

## Natural Defense: Pepper Spray

One way to protect yourself against an aggressor is to use pepper spray. Pepper spray contains capsaicin, a compound that is found in hot chili peppers. When sprayed in an assailant's eyes, pepper spray produces a painful burning sensation. Almost immediately, the person's eyelids swell shut and tears begin to flow. The spray also causes the attacker to experience difficulty breathing and lose control over body movements. These effects last about 20 to 30 minutes, which gives you time to escape the situation and call police. Pepper spray is an effective and safe way to subdue an attacker, but it may take a few seconds to work on enraged or drugged individuals.

Hardware or variety stores often sell pepper spray in small canisters that can be carried on a key chain or in a coat pocket or purse. Some states may impose age or other restrictions concerning the use of pepper spray. Therefore, before buying the product, check with local law enforcement agencies to determine if it is legal to use pepper spray. Always follow the package directions when using it as a defense and keep the canister out of the reach of children and irresponsible persons.

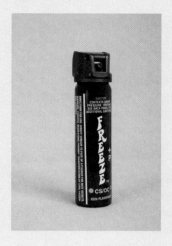

clude that you cannot escape, your response may be to offer no resistance. However, the gut responses to danger are the fight-or-flight reactions described in Chapter 3. Sometimes flight—simply running away—is the best means of escaping threatening situations. The opposite response is to defend yourself by fighting. Many Americans carry with them, or keep handy in their homes, a weapon for self-defense such as a gun, knife, or chemical defense spray. When danger threatens, other people may rely on improvised weapons such as car keys, scissors, or a flashlight. Some people seek training in personal defense or in firearm use to enhance their ability to defend themselves (**Figure 4.5**).

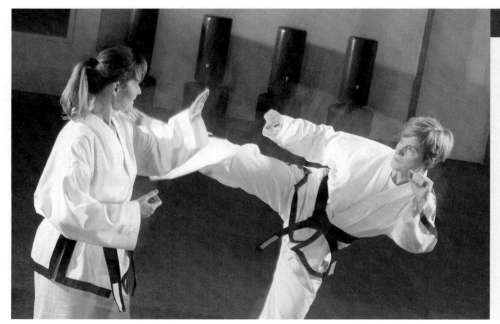

### Figure 4.5

**In Self-Defense.** Fighting back is one way of responding to violent situations.

Should victims always resist their attackers? No uniform answer can be given. Each potential victim must assess each situation quickly to decide how to respond under the circumstances. In situations involving intimate partner abuse or stalking, civil protection orders that separate and prohibit contact between the abuser or stalker and the victim can be effective in preventing further abuse.

## Reporting Violence

If you are attacked, you must decide whether to report the incident. You should report any attempted or completed crime of violence by strangers or acquaintances to the police. Most large police departments include specially trained family violence and sexual assault units that provide sympathetic and appropriate responses. A 9-1-1 call usually gains access to the appropriate emergency services.

In certain instances, you may feel reluctant to inform police about what happened to you. Consider reporting the incident to an agency, such as a rape crisis center or a women's self-help service, that can assist you in dealing with legal authorities and medical establishments. Nationwide, a 24-hour, toll-free family violence hotline can be reached at 1-800-799-7233.

Seeking help is beneficial to the victim's recovery from violence. Managing the short- and long-term effects of the violent incident on the victim's family and friends also is important. Useful services include marital counseling, couple therapy, financial and legal aid, and family therapy. Access to such services and information concerning local self-help groups can usually be arranged through your campus student health center or through social service agencies in your community.

**Child Maltreatment 2009**

U.S. Department of Health & Human Services
Administration for Children and Families
Administration on Children, Youth and Families
Children's Bureau

*Source:* U.S. Department of Health and Human Services, Administration on Children, Youth, and Families. (2010). *Child maltreatment 2009.* Retrieved from http://www.acf.hhs.gov /programs/cb/pubs/cm09/index.htm

### Healthy Living Practices

- To reduce your risk of violence, avoid high-risk places and dangerous people. Take steps to make your environment safe.
- If a dispute turns into a heated argument, try to keep calm to prevent the threatening situation from escalating into a violent one.
- Conflict-management skills can help defuse tense, angry situations. Some college campuses offer courses in conflict management; consider taking a class to learn these techniques.
- There is no single way to react whenever someone threatens your safety; therefore, assess each situation to decide how to respond under the circumstances.
- If you are a victim of violence, report the attack to police. In addition, obtain prompt treatment of your physical injuries and emotional distress.

### Across THE LIFE SPAN

### VIOLENCE AND ABUSE

**Child physical abuse** includes beating, squeezing, burning, cutting, suffocating, binding, and poisoning a child who is younger than 18 years of age. Although child physical abuse takes place in institutional settings, such as day care centers and schools, homes are by far the most common setting. Most physical violence against children is not committed by strangers or casual acquaintances but by parents and other adults known to the victims, such as neighbors, baby-sitters, and family friends. Abused children younger than 2 years of age are at greatest risk of fatalities, primarily from head injuries. Many children, however, receive less severe injuries on a regular basis. Such violence is not confined to impoverished families or to any particular racial or ethnic group.

Studies show that abused children behave more aggressively at every stage of the life span. As adults, they are more likely to be violent against dates, spouses, their children, and, later, their elderly parents.

Why do some parents abuse their children? Parents who are physically abusive to each other have a high risk of abusing their own children. Additionally, abusive parents generally lack effective parenting skills and frequently have faulty or unrealistic expectations about their children's behavior. For example, a parent may shake a 3-month-old infant to make it stop crying or kick a 2-year-old child for not using the toilet. Abusive parents tend to be under tremendous psychological stress and often are isolated from people who could provide helpful advice and social support. Regardless of the parents' situation, suspected or observed cases of child neglect or abuse can be reported anonymously by calling the *Childhelp National Child Abuse* hotline (1-800-422-4453). In some states, a person must report suspected cases of child abuse or neglect to authorities.

Data from various studies indicate that many adults were victims of sexual abuse during childhood. **Child sexual abuse** refers to sexual activity with a child that takes place as a result of force or threat, or by taking advantage of an age difference or a caretaking relationship. A *pedophile* is an individual who is sexually attracted to children and fantasizes about having physical contact with them. A *child molester* acts on his or her urges by having sexual activity with vulnerable children. Most molesters are heterosexual males who generally target girls between 8 and 10 years old. The abuse usually involves fondling a child's body, but it may include completed or attempted vaginal, anal, or oral sex. According to a survey of more than 17,300 adult Americans, 16% of men and

**child physical abuse** Physical violence against a child who is under 18 years of age.

**child sexual abuse** Sexual activity involving a child that takes place as a result of force or threat.

**pedophile** (**PE-doe-file**) An individual who is sexually attracted to children.

**incest** Sexual relations between family members who are not spouses.

about 25% of women experienced sexual abuse as children.[38] Such abuse often causes long-term serious psychological problems.[39]

Many people think that child molesters are strangers who are mentally ill, looking for children to kidnap, rape, and murder. In fact, most cases involve adults whom the children know and trust, such as baby-sitters, family friends, relatives, teachers, camp counselors, coaches, and clergy. Only 3% of murdered children younger than 5 years of age were killed by strangers.[40] However, children who have unsupervised access to personal computers provide a way for sophisticated child abusers to communicate with and befriend vulnerable children through Internet chat rooms, social networking sites, or electronic bulletin boards. Adult caregivers must teach their children about child abusers who prowl the Web, posing as children to gain actual children's confidence.

**Incest** refers to sexual experiences between family members who are not married to each other. In many instances, incest involves an adult and his or her young children, step-children, or grandchildren. Vic-

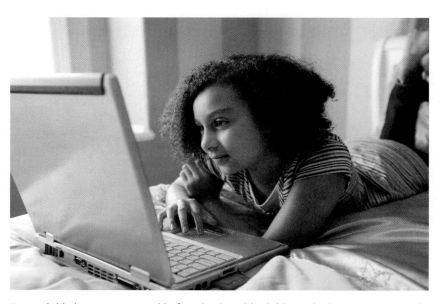

Some child abusers target and befriend vulnerable children who have unsupervised access to personal computers.

The following article promotes an herbal tea formulated to reduce a person's level of anger. Read the article and evaluate it using the model for analyzing health-related information. The main points of the model are noted here; the model is fully explained in Chapter 1.

1. Which statements are verifiable facts, and which are unverified statements or value claims?
2. What are the credentials of the person who wrote the article? Does this person have the appropriate background and education in the topic area? What can you do to check the person's credentials?
3. What might be the motives and biases of the person making the claims?

4. What is the main point of the article? Which information is relevant to the main point of the article? Which information is irrelevant?
5. Is the source reliable? What evidence supports your conclusion that the source is reliable or unreliable? Does the source of information present the pros and cons of the topic or the benefits and risks of the tea?
6. Does the source of information attack the credibility of conventional scientists or medical authorities?

Based on your analysis, do you think that this article is a reliable source of health-related information? Summarize your reasons for coming to this conclusion.

## Aunt Annie's Tranquillity Tea

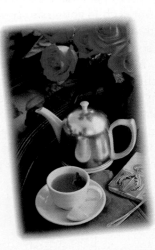

As you know, I've been using herbs all my life to treat everything from acne to zinc deficiency. Most of my knowledge about herbs didn't come from books or the Internet, it was passed down to me in my Great Aunt Annie's diary. Annie had a fabulous herb garden in the back of her house. One afternoon in 1914 she made the most amazing discovery, which she later recorded in her diary. She had dug up some comfrey root and picked a bunch of pennyroyal and lobelia leaves from the garden. Since coltsfoot was blooming, she thought it might be a nice change to add some of its leaves to her usual tea recipe. She brewed a pot of tea from the mixture and drank about 2 cups of it. The tea was delicious. Very soothing.

Less than an hour later, Great Uncle Jeb came in from the barn, tracking dirt all over Aunt Annie's new carpet. Now I need to tell you that Annie had a terrible temper—she was only 4' 8" tall, but she used to push big old Jeb around a lot. Needless to say, Uncle Jeb was expecting the worst from his wife. But this time, instead of flying off the handle and kicking Jeb, as she was prone to do, Aunt Annie laughed and hugged him. Happy as a kitten rolling in catnip, Annie cleaned up the mess. Uncle Jeb suspected Annie had added something different to her usual tea recipe, so he had her sit down and recall the herb mixture. Using her recipe, Jeb made a pot of that tea for Annie to drink every day for the rest of her life. When Uncle Jeb began making whiskey in the barn and staying out late with his friends, Annie never raised a fuss. She just sat in the bent oak rocking chair, sipping her tea.

If you want to try Aunt Annie's Tranquillity Tea on someone you know who's got a bad temper, I'll send the recipe to you. I'm the editor of this magazine, so just send $10 for shipping and handling to my address, which is on the inside of the front cover. I'd love to hear about your experiences with the tea; be sure and let me know how it worked for you.

Your friend,

**Herb**

Herb Z. Gardenia

tims may be boys, although girls are at much greater risk. Incest is often nonviolent, but forced, and it typically escalates over time. Ignorance or fear may keep the child from disclosing the abuse to others. Because of its psychological and physical impact on the youthful victim, incest is a serious form of sexual abuse. The risk factors for incest are similar to those of nonsexual abuse: childhood sexual victimization of the perpetrator and high levels of stress within the family.

To prevent child sexual abuse, parents should teach their young children how to recognize and report sexual abuse, regardless of their relationships with perpetrators. Because most cases involve people the youngsters know, simply telling children "Don't talk to strangers" is not sufficient advice. Very young children need to learn which parts of their bodies are private. Additionally, children need to learn that if anyone touches them in ways that make them feel uncomfortable, they should report the incidents to parents, teachers, or other responsible adults.

**Elder abuse** is the use of physical or sexual violence against an older adult; some researchers include verbal threats and neglect in their definitions. Physical and psychological abuse of older persons takes place not only in institutional settings such as hospitals and nursing homes, but especially in family settings. Such abuse occurs in all racial and ethnic groups and at all socioeconomic levels. An estimated 3% of older Americans experience abuse.[41] As the average age of the American population increases, many experts expect that the prevalence of elder abuse will increase as well.

The causes of elder abuse are complex. Older adults with chronic health conditions are most likely to be victimized by their spouses or adult children who must care for them. Caring for frail, aged relatives can be frustrating and stressful. Furthermore, the caregiver may depend on the older adult relative for his or her housing and income. In such situations, resentful caregivers may resort to abusive behavior. In severe cases, violence against older adults is associated with certain mental illnesses and drug (usually alcohol) abuse. If you observe an older adult being abused or neglected, report the situation to a local adult protective services agency.

# CHAPTER REVIEW

## Summary

*Violence* refers to interpersonal uses of force that are not socially sanctioned. A violent social incident occurs when at least one person intentionally applies or threatens physical force on others. Violence is a major public health problem because it produces staggering physical, psychological, and social consequences. For many Americans, violence is a way of life; no one is exempt from violence.

Assault is the intentional use of force to injure someone physically; abuse occurs when one takes advantage of a relationship to mistreat a person. Examples of abuse include spouse abuse, child abuse, and sexual harassment.

Regardless of whether physical harm occurs, violent victimization always damages psychological health. Psychological effects of violence include anxiety, depression, and suicidal thinking. Anxious or depressed people have a high risk of drug abuse and eating disorders. Family relationships may become strained or end as a result of violence. Furthermore, intergenerational transmission of violence occurs when abused children mature and abuse their own children. To recover from the psychological effects of violence, one should seek help from mental healthcare professionals.

Violence is complex; there is no single cause of violence, and neither is violent behavior limited to a particular group of persons. Factors that contribute to violence include poverty, substance abuse, certain psychological disorders, and poor self-esteem. In many instances, violence is learned behavior. Watching violent media, for example, may contribute to violent behavior.

Sexual violence involves areas of the body that are sensitive to sexual arousal. Such violence involves sexual activity gained through force, threat of force, or coercion. The majority of sexual assaults are committed not by strangers but by acquaintances, friends, family members, and spouses. Family (domestic) violence encompasses both friends and family members and usually takes place in homes. Community violence includes acts that occur between strangers or acquaintances, usually in public places. Institutional violence occurs mainly within institutional environments such as schools, workplaces, or prisons. Terrorism involves violent acts against civilians to produce extreme fear, severe property damage, and numerous deaths.

To reduce the likelihood of becoming a victim of violence, individuals should limit their exposure to risky situations and take steps to make their residences secure. When faced with a violent situation, a person can obtain help from others by attracting attention, defuse the situation by reasoning with an assailant, or simply run away. In some instances, the threatened individual may need to defend himself or herself physically.

Most physical violence against children is committed by adults known to the victims, such as relatives, neighbors, or baby-sitters. Most violence against children occurs in their homes. Girls, especially those between the ages of 8 and 10 years, are more likely to be targets of sexual abuse than are boys. Parents should teach their young children how to recognize and report sexual abuse. Children who experience violence often suffer emotional and social injuries that remain long after physical injuries have healed.

Elder abuse occurs in all racial and ethnic groups and at all socioeconomic levels. Family members are responsible for the vast majority of abuse directed toward older adults. As the average age of the American population increases, many experts predict that the incidence of elder abuse will also increase.

# CHAPTER REVIEW

## Applying What You Have Learned

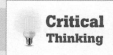 **Critical Thinking**

1. If your friend reports being sexually harassed by a college professor, what advice could you give to him or her? **Application**
2. You have to attend classes or work at a job in the evenings. Determine at least two steps you can take to reduce your risk of violence on campus or at work. **Analysis**
3. Plan a program to increase security in your dorm or on your campus. Consider forwarding it to an official at the university who might be interested in your plan, such as the Dean of Student Affairs. **Synthesis**
4. Evaluate your present security situation. Determine situations in your life that provide some risk of violence and describe ways in which you can reduce these risks. **Evaluation**

go.jblearning.com/alters6e

**Application**
using information in a new situation.

**Analysis**
breaking down information into component parts.

**Synthesis**
putting together information from different sources.

**Evaluation**
making informed decisions.

**Key**

## Reflecting on Your Health

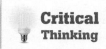 **Critical Thinking**

1. As mentioned in this chapter, visual media can influence a person's attitudes toward violence. Choose a violent movie or television show that you watched recently. What impact, if any, did it have on your feelings about violence?
2. Do you like to play violent computer games? If so, how does this activity affect your attitudes toward violence?
3. What could you do to avoid getting into an abusive relationship with an intimate partner? If you are already in an abusive relationship, what are your feelings about your partner? What would make you change your current situation?
4. How safe do you feel at home or in the dorm? What worries you most about the safety of your environment? What steps could you take to make your residence more secure?
5. If you were out walking alone at night and realized someone was following you, describe what you would do to reduce your risk of being attacked. Do you think that it is safe for you to walk alone at night? Why or why not?

# References

1. U.S. Department of Justice, Federal Bureau of Investigation. (2010). *Crime clock statistics*. Retrieved on March 23, 2011, from http://www2.fbi.gov/ucr/cius2009/about/crime_clock.html

2. U.S. Department of Health and Human Services, Administration on Children, Youth, and Families. (2010). *Child maltreatment 2009*. Retrieved on March 23, 2011, from http://www.acf.hhs.gov/programs/cb/pubs/cm09/index.htm

3. Tjaden, P., & Thoennes, N. (2000). *Extent, nature, and consequences of intimate partner violence: Findings from the National Violence Against Women Survey* (Publication NCJ 181867). Washington, DC: U.S. Department of Justice, Office of Justice Programs.

4. U.S. Department of Justice, Federal Bureau of Investigation. (2010). Crime in the United States, 2009. Retrieved on March 23, 2011, from http://www2.fbi.gov/ucr/cius2009/index.html

5. U.S. Department of Justice, Bureau of Justice Statistics. (2010, March 1). *Key facts: Violent crime*. Retrieved on March 30, 2011, from http://bjs.gov/index.cfm?ty=kftp&tid=31

6. Miniño, A. M., et al. (2010). Deaths: Preliminary data for 2008. *National Vital Statistics Reports, 59*(2):1–72. Retrieved on March 24, 2011, from http://www.cdc.gov/nchs/data/nvsr/nvsr59/nvsr59_02.pdf

7. Tremblay, R. E., et al. (2005). Physical aggression during early childhood: Trajectories and predictors. *Canadian Child and Adolescent Psychiatry Review, 14*(1):3–9.

8. American Academy of Pediatrics. (2009). Policy statement—media violence. *Pediatrics, 124*(5):1495–1503.

9. Tjaden, P., & Thoennes, N. (2006). *Extent, nature, and consequences of rape victimization: Findings from the National Violence Against Women Survey*. Atlanta, GA: National Institute of Justice and the Centers for Disease Control and Prevention.

10. Fisher, B. S., et al. (2000). *The sexual victimization of college women* (Publication NCJ 182369). Washington, DC: National Institute of Justice, Bureau of Justice Statistics, U.S. Department of Justice.

11. Durose, M. R., et al. (2005). *Family violence statistics: Including statistics on strangers and acquaintances* (Publication NCJ-207846). Retrieved on March 30, 2011, from http://bjs.gov/index.cfm?ty=pbdetail&iid=828

12. U.S. Department of Justice, Office of Justice Programs, Bureau of Justice Statistics. (2010). *National Crime Victimization Survey: Criminal victimization, 2009*. Retrieved on March 30, 2011, from http://bjs.gov/content/pub/pdf/cv09.pdf

13. U.S. Centers for Disease Control and Prevention, National Center for Injury Prevention and Control, Division of Violence Prevention. (2011). *Understanding intimate partner violence*. Retrieved on March 25, 2011, from http://www.cdc.gov/violenceprevention/pdf/IPV_factsheet-a.pdf

14. Eaton, D. K., et al. (2010). Youth risk behavior surveillance—United States, 2009. *Morbidity and Mortality Weekly Report, Surveillance Summaries, 59*(SS5):1–148.

15. Houston, E., & McKirnan, D. J. (2007). Intimate partner abuse among gay and bisexual men: Risk correlates and health outcomes. *Journal of Urban Health: Bulletin of the New York Academy of Medicine, 84*(5):681–690.

16. Ristock, J. L. (2003). Exploring dynamics of abusive lesbian relationships: Preliminary analysis of a multisite, qualitative study. *American Journal of Community Psychology, 31*(3–4):329–341.

17. U.S. Department of Justice, Federal Bureau of Investigation. (2010). *Crime in the United States: Expanded homicide data*. Retrieved on March 30, 2011, from http://www2.fbi.gov/ucr/cius2009/offenses/expanded_information/homicide.html

18. McKinney, C. M., et al. (2009). Childhood family violence and perpetration and victimization of intimate partner violence: Findings from a national population-based study of couples. *Annals of Epidemiology, 19*(1):25–32.

19. Frank, J. B., & Rodowski, M. F. (1999). Review of psychological issues in victims of domestic violence seen in emergency settings. *Emergency Medical Clinics of North America, 17*(3):657–677.

20. World Health Organization. (2010). International day for elimination of violence against women. Retrieved on March 25, 2011, from http://www.who.int/violence_injury_prevention/media/news/2010/25_11/en/index.html

21. World Health Organization/London School of Hygiene and Tropical Medicine. (2010). *Preventing intimate partner and sexual violence against women: Taking action and generating evidence*. Geneva, Switzerland: Author.

22. U.S. Bureau of Justice Statistics. (2009). 3.4 million people report being stalked in the United States. Retrieved on March 30, 2011, from http://www.bjs.gov/content/pub/press/svuspr.cfm

23. Lamberg, L. (2001). Stalking disrupts lives, leaves emotional scars. *Journal of the American Medical Association, 286*(5):519, 522–523.

24. U.S. Centers for Disease Control and Prevention. (2008). Notice to readers: National Stalking Awareness Month—January 2008. *Morbidity and Mortality Monthly Report, 57*(3):72.

25. Egley, A., et al. (2010, March). Highlights of the 2008 National Youth Gang Survey. *OJDP Fact Sheet*. Retrieved on March 29, 2011, from http://www.ncjrs.gov/pdffiles1/ojjdp/229249.pdf

26. U.S. Department of Justice, National Drug Intelligence Center. (2009). *National gang threat assessment 2009* (Document ID: 2009-M0335-001). Retrieved on March 29, 2011, from http://www.justice.gov/ndic/pubs32/32146/index.htm#Contents

27. Heron, M. (2010). Deaths: Leading causes for 2006. *National Vital Statistics Reports, 58*(14):1–100.

28. Baum, K., & Klaus, P. (2005). *Violent victimization of college students, 1995–2002* (Publication NCJ 206836). Washington, DC: U.S. Department of Justice, Bureau of Justice Statistics, Office of Justice Programs. Retrieved on March 26, 2011, from http://www.bjs.gov/index.cfm?ty=pbdetail&iid=593

29. U.S. Department of Labor, Bureau of Labor Statistics. (2010). *2009 census of fatal occupational injuries, CFOI charts*. Retrieved on March 29, 2011, from http://www.bls.gov/iif/oshwc/cfoi/cfch0008.pdf

30. Holman, E. A., et al. (2008). Terrorism, acute stress, and cardiovascular health: A three-year national study following the September 11th attacks. *Archives of General Psychiatry, 65*(1):73–80.

31. Galea, S., et al. (2005). Posttraumatic stress disorder in the general population after mass terrorist incidents: Considerations about the nature of exposure. *CNS Spectrums, 10*(2):107–115.

32. U.S. Department of Justice, Federal Bureau of Investigation. (2010). *Crime in the United States, 2009.* Retrieved on March 29, 2011, from http://www2.fbi.gov/ucr/cius2009/offenses/violent_crime/index.html

33. U.S. Department of Justice, Bureau of Justice Statistics. (2011, March 30). Key facts at a glance: Violent crime rates by age of victim. Retrieved on March 30, 2011, from http://www.bjs.gov/content/glance/vage.cfm

34. U.S. Department of Justice, Bureau of Justice Statistics. (2011, March 30). Victim characteristics. *National Crime Victimization Survey.* Retrieved on March 30, 2011, from http://www.bjs.gov/index.cfm?ty=tp&tid=92

35. U.S. Department of Health and Human Services, Public Health Service. (n.d.). 2020 topics and objectives, injury and violence prevention. *Healthy People 2020.* Retrieved on March 31, 2011, from http://healthypeople.gov/2020/topicsobjectives2020/objectiveslist.aspx?topicid=24

36. U.S. Department of Justice, Federal Bureau of Investigation. (2010). Rate: Number of crimes per 100,000 inhabitants by population group, 2009. Table 16. *Crime in the United States, 2009.* Retrieved on March 31, 2011, from http://www2.fbi.gov/ucr/cius2009/data/table_16.html

37. U.S. Department of Justice, Federal Bureau of Investigation. (2010). Expanded homicide data table 10: Murder circumstances by relationship, 2009. *Crime in the United States, 2009.* Retrieved on March 29, 2011, from http://www2.fbi.gov/ucr/cius2009/offenses/expanded_information/data/shrtable_10.html

38. Middlebrooks, J. S., & Audage, N. C. (2008). *Effects of childhood stress on health across the lifespan.* Atlanta, GA: Centers for Disease Control and Prevention, National Center for Injury Prevention and Control.

39. Huyer, D. (2005). Childhood sexual abuse and family physicians. *Canadian Family Physician, 51*:1317–1319.

40. U.S. Department of Justice, Bureau of Justice Statistics. (2011, March 30). *Homicide trends in the United States: Infanticide.* Retrieved on March 30, 2011, from http://www.bjs.gov/content/homicide/children.cfm

41. Gibbs, L. M., & Mosqueda, L. (2007). The importance of reporting mistreatment of the elderly. *American Family Physician, 75*(5):628.

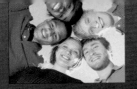

## Diversity in Health
Menopause

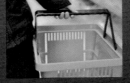

## Consumer Health
Home Pregnancy Tests

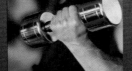

## Managing Your Health
Genetic Counseling and
Prenatal Diagnosis |
Enlargement of the Prostate

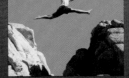

## Across the Life Span
Sexual Development

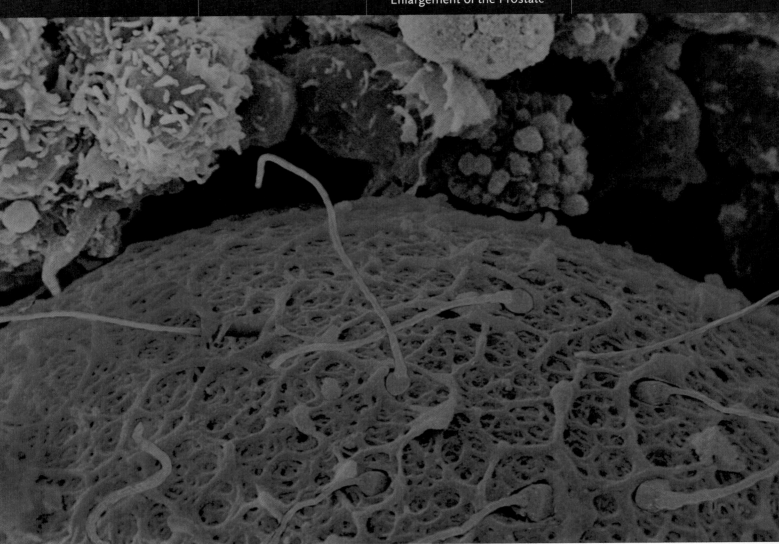

# Chapter Overview

The functions and structures of the male and female
  reproductive systems

What happens throughout the menstrual cycle

How a woman can prepare her body for pregnancy

How a fetus develops

The changes in a pregnant woman from conception
  through the postpartum period

The causes of and treatments for infertility

The benefits and drawbacks of contraceptive methods

# Student Workbook

Self-Assessment: Contraceptive Comfort and Confidence
  Scale | Attitudes Toward Timing of Parenthood Scale

Changing Health Habits: Do You Want to Improve Your
  Reproductive Health?

# Do You Know?

How well your contraceptive method works compared to
  others?

What causes birth defects?

When a woman is most likely to get pregnant?

## CHAPTER 5

# Reproductive Health

T his striking photograph depicts the essence of **sexual reproduction**: the fertilization of an egg (ovum) by a sperm, a process also called conception. The photograph is color enhanced; the outside of the egg is shown as orange and the sperm as blue. A layer of cells that extend from the egg covers its surface. During the maturation of the egg, these outer cells secrete a thick gel-like material that covers the egg beneath. Together, the gel and the outer cells form a protective covering, which sperm must penetrate by means of digestive enzymes in their heads. Although it is difficult to see in this photograph, the head of only one sperm is making its way through these outer layers to ultimately fertilize this egg.

When the sperm enters the egg, it triggers the egg's final maturation. Following this process, the hereditary material from the sperm and the mature egg unite, forming a new cell—the zygote. This single cell has the potential to develop into a new individual.

Fertility is the ability to conceive a child, while infertility is the inability of a couple to conceive a child after 1 year of unprotected sex. Couples may have reduced fertility for a variety of reasons; it is not necessarily be-

> *"This striking photograph depicts the essence of sexual reproduction: the fertilization of an egg (ovum) by a sperm..."*

cause of "a problem" with one partner or the other. Factors that slig'.tly impair the fertility of both sexual partners may interact to render a couple infertile. These factors include a low sperm count, a high percentage of abnormally shaped sperm, scarring in the female genital tract, structural defects of the uterus, and hormonal imbalances. Treatments for infertility are specific to the causes and include surgical procedures, hormone therapy, medication, and lifestyle changes. In addition to these therapies, physicians can harvest eggs and sperm to assist fertilization and implantation.

Whether physician-assisted or accomplished with no intervention at all, fertilization is preceded by a variety of physiologic processes that make it all possible, and that is where we begin this chapter.

# The Male Reproductive System

The male reproductive system is structured for the development and maturation of sperm and for delivering sperm to the vagina. **Figure 5.1** is a diagram of a posterior view (a) and a lengthwise section of the male reproductive tract (b).

## The Internal Organs of Sexual Reproduction

**Sperm Development** Sperm are produced in the **testes** (singular, *testis*), which hang outside the body (in the angle formed between the legs) encased in a sac of skin called the **scrotum**. The testes have two

## Figure 5.1

**The Male Reproductive System.** (a) Posterior view of the internal organs, and (b) lengthwise section (side view) of the internal organs.

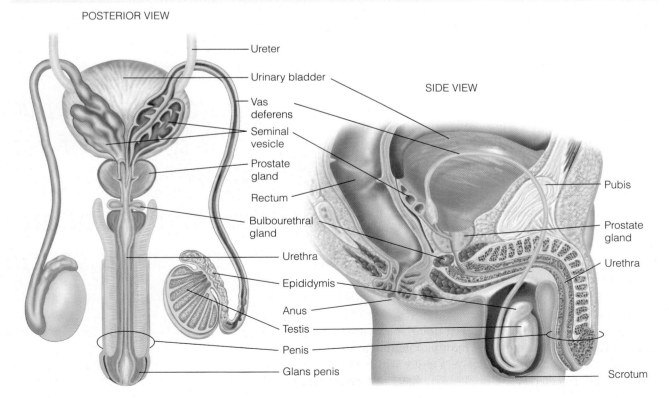

POSTERIOR VIEW

- Ureter
- Urinary bladder
- Vas deferens
- Seminal vesicle
- Prostate gland
- Rectum
- Bulbourethral gland
- Urethra
- Epididymis
- Anus
- Testis
- Penis
- Glans penis

SIDE VIEW

- Pubis
- Prostate gland
- Urethra
- Scrotum

major functions: production of the sex hormone testosterone and production of sperm cells. The testes are packed with hundreds of feet of tubes (called *seminiferous tubules*) in which sperm are made. Each day, the testes of an adult male produce hundreds of millions of sperm. Various conditions are necessary for proper sperm production.

In a review of environmental and lifestyle effects on the development of sperm, Richard Sharpe notes that factors that result in a rise in scrotal temperature have a negative effect on sperm development. The testes must be cooler than body temperature to produce normal sperm; the position of the scrotum keeps the temperature of the testes below that of the rest of the body. However, behaviors that result in the scrotum not being able to dissipate heat can result in increased temperature of the testes. Such behaviors include taking long, hot baths and staying seated for long periods, especially when wearing tight pants. Obesity in men has also been shown to adversely affect sperm development.[1]

**Semen Formation**  After sperm are manufactured in the seminiferous tubules, they are gently moved along by the fluid in which they are suspended. The sperm move through a network of ducts to the **epididymis** (plural, *epididymides*). The epididymis is a coiled tube that lies on the back of each testis. Here is where the sperm mature, developing the ability to swim and to fertilize an egg.

Rhythmic contractions of the muscular walls of the epididymis slowly move the sperm to the **vas deferens** when maturation is complete. The vas deferens is a tube that links the epididymis and the urethra, the passageway through which sperm exit the body. Sperm are stored in the vas deferens until they are released from the body during **ejaculation**, their emission from the penis during **orgasm**, the peak of sexual excitement. Sperm can be stored for a few days in these ducts. If not ejaculated within that time, the sperm die and are ingested by the body's white blood cells. Newly synthesized sperm take their place. For this reason, men who have had vasectomies should not be concerned that sperm are accumulating in their bodies.

The sperm are suspended in relatively little fluid while stored in the vas deferens. A variety of organs referred to as accessory sex glands add fluid to the sperm as they exit the body during ejaculation. This fluid contains nutrients to fuel the sperm as they journey up the female reproductive tract, alkaline substances to neutralize the acidity of the vagina, and other chemicals to aid sperm movement. The

**epididymis** (EP-ih-DID-ih-mis) A coiled tube that lies on the back of each testis and in which sperm mature.

**vas deferens** (VAS DEF-er-enz) A tube that links the epididymis and the urethra, the passageway through which sperm exit the body.

**ejaculation** The emission of semen from the penis during orgasm.

**orgasm** The peak of sexual excitement.

**semen** The ejaculate; the secretions of the accessory sex glands (called seminal fluid) and sperm.

**seminal vesicles** (SEM-ih-nal VES-ih-klz) Paired male sex organs located near the junction of the two vasa deferentia, which produce thick fructose-containing secretions that are added to the ejaculate.

**prostate gland** A single, walnut-sized gland that lies just below the bladder, surrounding the urethra. The prostate produces a milky alkaline fluid that is added to the ejaculate.

secretions of the accessory sex glands (called seminal fluid) and the sperm make up the **semen**, or *ejaculate*.

During ejaculation, sperm are swiftly propelled through the vas deferens by the rhythmic contractions of its muscular walls. Just prior to the merging of the two vasa deferentia where they meet the urethra, the secretions of the paired seminal vesicles flow into the ejaculate. The thick secretions of the **seminal vesicles** add much of the volume to the ejaculate (approximately 60%) and contain the sugar fructose, which provides nutrition for the sperm.

As the ejaculate continues traveling through the male reproductive tract, the **prostate gland** adds its secretion. This single, walnut-sized gland lies just below the bladder. It surrounds the urethra and produces a milky fluid that protects sperm from the acidic environment of the woman's vagina.

During sexual arousal, the bulbourethral glands produce a mucuslike fluid that precedes the ejaculate. The bulbourethral glands (also called Cowper's glands), paired glands about the size of peas, are located on either side of the urethra just below the prostate. The secretions of these glands help neutralize the acidity of the male urethra and the vagina. These glands also contribute a small amount of lubrication for sexual intercourse. However, this fluid may contain sperm. For this reason (and others), the withdrawal method of birth control is not highly reliable.

**penis** A cylindrical external organ of sexual reproduction in males, which hangs in front of the scrotum.

**ovaries** Internal organs of female sexual reproduction within which eggs (ova) develop.

**follicles** Masses of cells in the ovaries that contain immature ova (eggs) in various stages of development. Each follicle contains one ovum.

**puberty** (PEW-ber-tea) A stage of sexual development during which the endocrine (hormone) and reproductive systems mature.

**ovulation** The maturation and release of an egg from an ovary, usually each month from puberty to menopause.

**uterine tubes** Passageways that extend from each ovary to the uterus.

## The External Organs of Sexual Reproduction

The scrotum and the **penis** are the external organs of sexual reproduction (external genitals) in males (see Figure 5.1). Three columns of spongy tissue in the inner structure of the penis (**Figure 5.2**) become filled

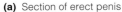

### Figure 5.2

**The Erect and Flaccid Penis.** (a) During an erection, blood fills the spongy erectile tissue of the penis. (b) When the blood drains from this tissue, as it does after orgasm, the penis becomes flaccid.

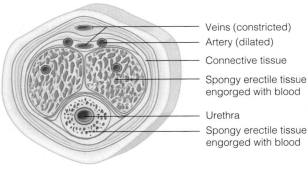

Veins (constricted)
Artery (dilated)
Connective tissue
Spongy erectile tissue engorged with blood
Urethra
Spongy erectile tissue engorged with blood

**(a)** Section of erect penis

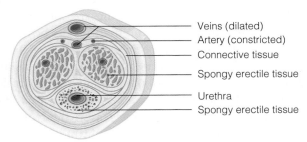

Veins (dilated)
Artery (constricted)
Connective tissue
Spongy erectile tissue
Urethra
Spongy erectile tissue

**(b)** Section of flaccid penis

with blood during sexual arousal, which causes the penis to enlarge and become firm so that it can be inserted into the vagina. During sexual intercourse, the penis can become stimulated enough to result in orgasm, during which ejaculation occurs.

## The Female Reproductive System

The female reproductive system is structured for the development and maturation of ova, for receiving sperm, for providing an environment in which a fertilized ovum can develop and mature, and for giving birth to the developed fetus. **Figure 5.3** is a diagram of a lengthwise section of the female reproductive tract (a) and a posterior view (b).

## The Internal Organs of Sexual Reproduction

**Egg Development** Ova are produced in the **ovaries**, which are two oval organs suspended by ligaments (a type of connective tissue) in the pelvic cavity. The almond-sized ovaries contain **follicles**, which are masses of cells that contain immature ova in various stages of development (**Figure 5.4**). Each follicle contains one ovum.

Unlike male sex cells, *all* female sex cells begin to develop before birth. This process stops before birth, and the potential eggs remain dormant throughout childhood. Each month after the onset of sexual maturity, or **puberty**, but prior to menopause, a few ova continue their development. Most of the time one ovum matures and bursts from an ovary each month; this process is **ovulation**. The ovulation of two ova can lead to the development of fraternal twins, if both are fertilized. Identical twins result when the two cells formed from the fertilized ovum's first division continue development as independent organisms. A woman's reproductive life span lasts from puberty to age 50 years (on average); only about 400 ova mature during this period.

**Where Eggs Are Fertilized and Then Develop** During ovulation, the egg is released into the pelvic cavity. Lying close to the ovaries are the fimbriae, the fringed edges of the **uterine tubes** (see Figure 5.3), also called *fallopian tubes* or *oviducts*. The uterine tubes are shaped somewhat like trumpets, with their wider ends near the ovaries and their narrower ends connected to the uterus. As the fimbriae move, they create a current of fluid that gently sweeps the

**Figure 5.3**

**The Female Reproductive System.** (a) Side view (lengthwise section) of the internal organs, and (b) posterior view of the internal organs.

**(a)**

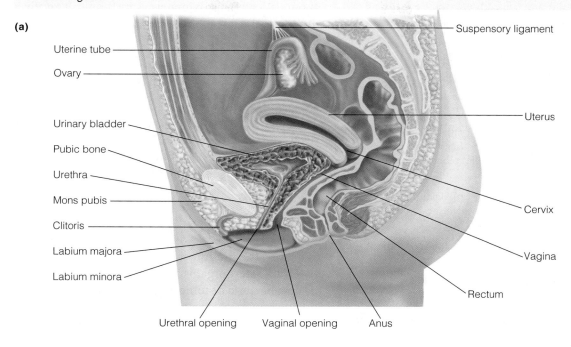

Suspensory ligament

Uterine tube

Ovary

Uterus

Urinary bladder

Pubic bone

Urethra

Mons pubis

Clitoris

Cervix

Labium majora

Labium minora

Vagina

Rectum

Urethral opening  Vaginal opening  Anus

**(b)**

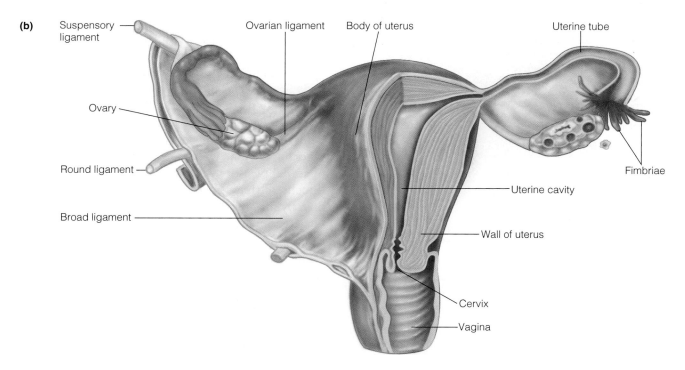

Suspensory ligament

Ovarian ligament

Body of uterus

Uterine tube

Ovary

Round ligament

Fimbriae

Uterine cavity

Broad ligament

Wall of uterus

Cervix

Vagina

The Female Reproductive System    **125**

**uterus** A hollow, muscular, pear-shaped organ that protects and nourishes the embryo/fetus during development.

**cervix** The narrow neck of the uterus.

**vagina** A tube about 10 cm (approximately 4 in.) long that receives the penis during intercourse, allows the passage of the menstrual flow, and is a birth canal.

**vulva** The collective term for the external female genitals. The vulva surrounds the vaginal opening.

**clitoris** (KLIT-oh-ris) A female organ of sexual arousal. Located under a protective hood of tissue, the clitoris lies in front of the urethra.

**labia minora** (LAY-bee-ah my NOR-ah) Two thin, hairless folds of skin that extend from over the clitoris to an area behind the vagina. The labia minor cover and protect the vaginal opening ad urethra.

**labia majora** (LAY-bee-ah mah-JOR-ah) Hairy, rounded, and thick folds of skin that lie adjacent to the labia minora and extend forward to unite at the mons pubis.

**mons pubis** A mound of fatty tissue that lies over the pubic bone, cushioning it.

## Figure 5.4

**The Developing Ovum.** A highly magnified, colorized photograph of a developing ovarian follicle with developing egg (ovum).

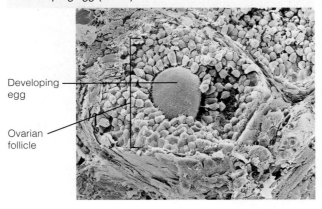

Developing egg

Ovarian follicle

ovum into the tube. If sperm are present, the uterine tube is also the site of fertilization. The fertilized ovum moves through the uterine tube as it journeys to the uterus.

The **uterus** is a hollow, muscular, pear-shaped organ that protects and nourishes the developing organism. The fertilized egg implants in the wall of the uterus and grows and develops during pregnancy, which is discussed shortly.

The uterus opens into the vagina at the **cervix**, the narrow neck of the uterus. The cervix produces mu-

cus. At certain times of the month, the consistency of the cervical mucus changes, facilitating sperm movement into the uterus around the time of ovulation and hindering it at other times. The **vagina** is a tube about 10 cm (approximately 4 in.) long. It receives the penis during intercourse, allows the passage of the menstrual flow, and is a birth canal.

## The External Organs of Sexual Reproduction

The female external genitals (see Figure 5.3a) collectively are called the **vulva**. The vulva surrounds the vaginal opening. The urethra, the tube that carries urine from the bladder to the outside, lies anterior to the vagina.

Although the urethra is shared by the urinary and reproductive systems in men, it has no reproductive or sexual function in women. Because it is close to the anal area, the urethra can become infected by digestive tract microorganisms during sexual intercourse if these bacteria become lodged in this tube. If microorganisms are not washed from the urethra by urine, they may multiply and cause urethritis (also commonly known as cystitis, a urinary tract infection, or a bladder infection). Healthcare providers recommend that women who often develop such infections urinate after sexual intercourse and drink plenty of fluids to keep the urethra washed free of bacteria.

Located under a protective hood of tissue, the **clitoris** lies anterior to the urethra. This tiny structure has spongy tissue like that of the penis and becomes engorged with blood during sexual arousal. Like the penis, it has numerous nerve endings that send messages to the brain, which are interpreted as sensations of sexual pleasure when this organ is stimulated indirectly during sexual activity. (Rubbing the clitoris directly may result in discomfort.)

Extending from over the clitoris to an area behind the vagina, two thin, hairless folds of skin called the **labia minora** (meaning "small lips") cover and protect the vaginal opening and urethra. Within the area bounded by the labia minora, lying near the vaginal and urethral openings and the clitoris, are various glands that secrete lubricating substances during sexual activity. Next to these skin folds are the hairy, more rounded, and thicker **labia majora** ("large lips"). The labia majora extend forward to unite in a mound of fatty tissue called the **mons pubis**. The mons pubis provides a cushion over the pubic bone, a portion of the pelvic bones that is in front of the genitals.

The breasts are also external organs of sex and reproduction in women. Breasts primarily consist of fat and glandular tissue (**Figure 5.5**). Exercise will not increase breast size; it can develop only the underlying pectoral muscles. Although their major purpose is the production of milk to sustain an infant after birth, the breasts are also sensitive to sexual stimulation. The nipples contain nerve endings that are sensitive to touch; smooth muscles in the nipples contract during sexual arousal, causing the nipples to become erect.

## The Menstrual Cycle

Women, unlike men, experience a cyclic waxing and waning of their sex hormones each month. These hormonal changes orchestrate physiologic changes in the ovaries and uterus. These changes are collectively called the **menstrual cycle**, which literally means "monthly cycle." The average length of a cycle is 28

**menstrual (MEN-strool-al) cycle** The monthly changes in the levels of the female sex hormones that orchestrate physiological changes in the ovaries and uterus.

**menses** (MEN-seez) The menstrual period; the sloughing of the endometrium.

**endometrium** (EN-doe-ME-tree-um) The inner lining of the uterus.

days, but menstrual cycles generally vary from 21 to 35 days in length.[2]

The menstrual cycle is usually described as beginning on the first day of the **menses** (menstrual period; **Figure 5.6**). The menses are the sloughing of the inner lining of the uterus, which is the **endometrium**. This lining develops gradually during the month, preparing for the implantation of a fertilized egg. If fertilization and implantation do not occur, the ovum dissolves and hormonal changes result in the lining

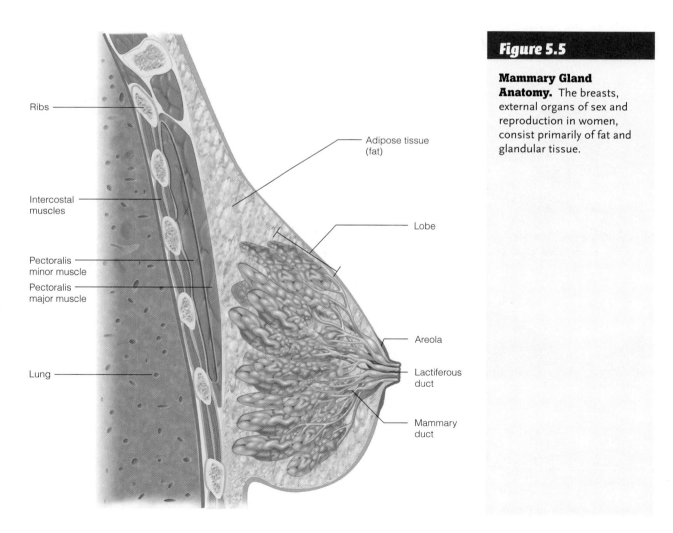

Ribs

Intercostal muscles

Pectoralis minor muscle

Pectoralis major muscle

Lung

Adipose tissue (fat)

Lobe

Areola

Lactiferous duct

Mammary duct

### Figure 5.5

**Mammary Gland Anatomy.** The breasts, external organs of sex and reproduction in women, consist primarily of fat and glandular tissue.

**estrogen** (ES-tro-jen) A hormone secreted by ovarian follicles, the groups of cells within which ova mature. With progesterone, estrogen stimulates the continued development and thickening of the uterine lining.

**progesterone** (pro-JES-te-rone) A hormone secreted by the corpus luteum. With estrogen, progesterone stimulates the continued development and thickening of the uterine lining.

**corpus luteum** (KOR-pus LOO-tea-um) The ruptured follicle left behind after ovulation.

**placenta** (plah-SEN-tah) A structure that develops after implantation of a fertilized ovum in the uterine wall and consists of maternal and fetal tissues that secrete hormones that help maintain the pregnancy.

Each month during her childbearing years, a woman's body prepares for a pregnancy. Usually only one ovarian follicle reaches the final stage of development in any particular cycle. About midcycle, hormonal changes trigger ovulation, the release of the egg from the ovary. The corpus luteum (meaning "yellow body") secretes high amounts of progesterone and lesser amounts of estrogen, which cause the uterine lining to grow, thicken, and develop a rich blood supply in preparation for the implantation of a fertilized ovum. If fertilization does not occur, the corpus luteum degenerates and stops producing hormones. Without hormonal stimulation, the uterine lining degenerates and is passed out of the body through the vagina during the menses.

If fertilization occurs, the corpus luteum does not degenerate. It produces estrogen and progesterone throughout pregnancy, maintaining the lining of the uterus. As the pregnancy develops, so does the **placenta**, a structure consisting of maternal and fetal tissues that also secretes hormones that help maintain the pregnancy. In addition, oxygen, nutrients, and wastes move between mother and fetus across the placenta, which is connected to the fetus by the umbilical cord.

being cast from the body. Each month a new lining develops.

What happens to the uterine lining is controlled by the hormones estrogen and progesterone. **Estrogen** is a hormone secreted by ovarian follicles, the groups of cells within which ova mature (see Figure 5.4); **progesterone** is secreted by the **corpus luteum**, the remnant of a follicle that has released its ovum.

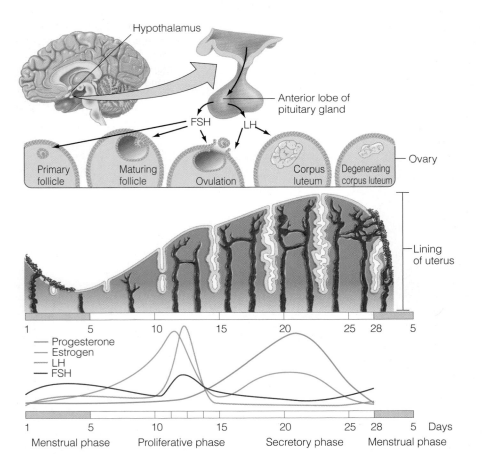

**Figure 5.6**

**The Menstrual Cycle.** The cycle begins on the first day of the menses. Hormones from the hypothalamus control the release of the hormones follicle-stimulating hormone (FSH) and luteinizing hormone (LH) from the anterior pituitary. Estrogen is secreted by the ovarian follicles, and progesterone is secreted by the corpus luteum. The rise and fall of hormone levels are related to ovulation and to the building up and sloughing off of the uterine lining.

## Premenstrual Syndrome

Approximately 70% to 90% of American women in their reproductive years report mild to moderate discomfort during the week prior to menstruation as their hormonal levels drop. More than 20% report that premenstrual symptoms such as anxiety/tension, mood swings, decreased interest in activities, appetite changes/food cravings, aches, and cramps interfere with their relationships and their daily activities.[3] This condition, originally termed *premenstrual tension syndrome* because most women experiencing it reported tension and anxiety among their symptoms, is now simply referred to as **premenstrual syndrome**, or **PMS**. A range of 5% to 8% of women report severe impairment of their daily activities because of PMS symptoms.[3] This debilitating condition is called *premenstrual dysphoric disorder* (PMDD). Research results provide some evidence that both PMS and PMDD may be partly the result of interactions between sex hormone levels and certain brain neurotransmitters.[4]

Most women with mild to moderate PMS are helped by one or more of the following treatments: counseling, lifestyle modification such as including exercise in their daily regimen, or medications prescribed for specific symptoms. Fluoxetine (Prozac) has shown usefulness in the treatment of PMS, acting to reduce symptoms of depression and anxiety that are linked to problems with the proper regulation of serotonin, a brain neurotransmitter. Additionally, many women are helped by using low-dose, combined oral contraceptives. Nutritional treatments include a diet low in salt, alcohol, caffeine, and sugar. Taking calcium supplements may reduce the severity of symptoms of PMS. Women with more severe symptoms of PMS and with PMDD may benefit from medications prescribed for their specific situation and symptoms.[4]

## Toxic Shock Syndrome

A disease called *toxic shock syndrome (TSS)* is associated with the menses. This disease became well known in the 1980s, when hundreds of women who used certain high-absorbency tampons during their menstrual periods were stricken. In TSS, staphylococcal (STAFF-ih-low-KAH-kul) bacteria grow in the blood-soaked tampon and in vaginal tissues, producing toxins that can enter the woman's bloodstream. Although TSS is associated with a wide variety of surgical conditions unrelated to the menses

**premenstrual syndrome (PMS)** Symptoms such as anxiety, mood swings, aches, and cramps that occur prior to the menses and that significantly interfere with daily life.

**pregnancy** The gestational process; the process of development of a new individual from fertilization until birth.

**teratogens** Various environmental influences such as drugs, alcohol, viruses, and dietary deficiencies that can damage the embryo or fetus early in pregnancy.

(such as skin, bone, and soft-tissue infections), about two-thirds of all cases are related to tampon use during the menses. Additionally, TSS can occur from use of contraceptive diaphragms and sponges, but such occurrences are rare. Although TSS is an uncommon disease, women from 15 to 34 years old are at the highest risk. Approximately 5% of all persons who contract TSS die from the infection.[5]

The most common symptoms of TSS are fever, muscle pain, headache, dizziness, diarrhea, vomiting, and a sunburn-like rash. One to two weeks after the onset of the disease, the skin of the palms, fingers, toes, and soles of the feet begins to peel. Generally, TSS patients are hospitalized and treated with fluids and antibiotics.

To avoid contracting TSS from tampon use, women who use tampons should change them often and alternate their use with pads throughout the menses. Women should use only the level of absorbency they require. If during tampon use a woman experiences fever, rash, dizziness, or diarrhea, she should remove the tampon and seek medical attention immediately.

## Pregnancy and Human Development

**Pregnancy** is the gestational process, that is, the process of development of a new individual from fertilization until birth. What can a woman do to prepare her body for pregnancy? What can she do during the *prenatal* period, the time during which she is pregnant, to increase her chances of delivering a healthy baby?

## Prepregnancy and Prenatal Care

Various **teratogens**, environmental influences such as drugs, alcohol, viruses, cigarette smoking, and

**amniocentesis** A prenatal test performed generally between the 15th and 18th weeks of gestation, in which some of the amniotic fluid that surrounds the fetus is removed and studied to determine whether the fetus has a genetic abnormality.

dietary deficiencies, can damage the embryo or fetus. The most highly sensitive periods of the developing structures of the embryo and fetus to teratogens oc-

cur primarily during the first 8 weeks after conception, possibly before a woman knows that she's pregnant. Therefore, if you are trying to become pregnant, to avoid birth defects you should take care of your body as if you were pregnant. The Analyzing Health-Related Information feature found later in this chapter discusses folic acid (folate), a B vitamin critical to proper neural tube development of the embryo. **Table 5.1**

## Table 5.1

### Selected Teratogens Known to Cause Birth Defects

| Teratogen | Explanation |
|---|---|
| *Maternal Infectious or Noninfectious Disease* | |
| Cytomegalovirus | A herpes-type virus that can cross the placenta and infect the embryo. Found in about 1% of newborns. Most defects affect the nervous system. Risk of brain damage is 50% after infection early in pregnancy. One in 10 affected fetuses die. |
| Diabetes mellitus | Risk of major malformations is about 18%. Heart malformations and neural tube defects are most frequent. Risk is greatest in uncontrolled or poorly controlled diabetes. |
| Phenylketonuria (PKU), untreated | Excess phenylalanine, not the defective gene, causes birth defects such as intellectual disability and malformations of the heart. |
| Rubella | The German measles virus can cross the placenta and infect the embryo. Infection during the first 3 months of pregnancy is likely to result in abnormalities such as deafness, heart defects, and intellectual disability. |
| *Drugs, Other Chemicals, and Radiation* | |
| Alcohol | Main characteristics of the birth defects caused by maternal alcohol consumption are growth deficiency, hyperactivity, distractibility, small head, under-development of the brain, and intellectual disability. No safe level of alcohol consumption during pregnancy is known. |
| Anticonvulsant medication | Probability of birth defects varies with medications, dosage, and stage of pregnancy. |
| Chemotherapeutic agents | Drugs used to treat cancer can also harm the embryo or fetus. |
| Cocaine | Some possible birth defects from cocaine use during pregnancy are bleeding in the brain, death of part of the brain tissue, underdeveloped head and brain, prematurity, and seizures. |
| Diethylstilbestrol (DES) | A drug formerly prescribed for women who were in danger of having a miscarriage. This drug affected some of their female offspring, causing unusual vaginal, cervical, and uterine changes beginning in adolescence. Increased risk for developing a certain type of vaginal and cervical cancer. |
| Ionizing radiation | Extremely high exposure to x-rays or exposure to radiation used in cancer therapy can affect the embryo or fetus and result in an underdeveloped head and brain. |
| Accutane | This synthetic form of vitamin A is used to treat certain types of acne. Birth defects that may result from use during pregnancy (when taken by mouth) include malformations of the ear, brain, and heart. Healthcare providers also suggest avoiding megadoses (more than 10,000 I.U.) of vitamin A during pregnancy. |
| Thalidomide | A drug taken for morning sickness in the 1960s. Taking this drug between 20 days and 36 days after conception resulted in major anatomic deformities of the limbs and heart. |

# Managing Your Health

## Genetic Counseling and Prenatal Diagnosis

You and your spouse have decided it's time to have a baby. You are both worried that a genetic disease may run in one of your families. (A genetic disease is caused by problems with the hereditary, or genetic, material.) Also, you're worried about the risk of birth defects because "mom" will be far past age 35 when she gives birth, and the likelihood of genetic diseases is higher then than at younger ages. What can you both do to ensure the genetic health of your baby?

Your first step might be to discuss your concerns with an obstetrician/gynecologist. Your healthcare practitioner may send both of you to a genetic counselor to explore the incidence of genetic disease in your families and to determine the probability of you and your spouse having a child with a genetic disorder.

There are many reasons to seek genetic counseling. Parents with a child who has a genetic disease often choose genetic counseling to determine the probability that future children will be affected. In populations at high risk for certain genetic diseases, such as African Americans and sickle cell anemia, or Ashkenazi Jews and Tay-Sachs disease, families or prospective parents may visit genetics centers to undergo screening tests. Once screening has been done and the carriers and noncarriers of the disease have been identified, the genetic counselor can advise them of their probability of passing on problem genes to children.

After the baby is conceived and prior to birth, various techniques are available to tell for sure if the baby is affected with any of a wide variety of disorders. Tests performed on the fetus (or related tissues) to determine its health are called prenatal diagnoses. Methods that are frequently used are ultrasound, **amniocentesis**, and chorionic villus sampling (CVS). These methods can detect many, but not all, fetal abnormalities.

Ultrasound scanning, or sonography, is a common, painless, safe, and relatively inexpensive procedure for prenatal diagnosis that has been used since the 1960s. Ultrasound uses high-frequency sound waves to visualize the fetus, which can be seen as early as 7 weeks of development. The ultrasound probe is moved over the woman's abdomen. Sound waves enter the uterus and bounce off fetal structures in ways that reflect their density and makeup. The reflected waves are projected on a monitor screen (**Figure 5.A**), and their patterns are interpreted by a healthcare provider. Using this technique, a healthcare provider can detect many structural abnormalities, estimate the age of the fetus, confirm if multiple fetuses are present, and confirm fetal position. In addition, ultrasound is often used to help guide needle placement in amniocentesis, fetal blood sampling, and chorionic villus sampling.

Another common type of prenatal diagnosis is amniocentesis, which was developed in the 1960s and was widely used by the 1970s. Amniocentesis involves the removal of some of the amniotic fluid that surrounds the fetus. This watery fluid protects the baby from jarring movements and contains waste products and some cells from the fetus. Geneticists observe these cells to determine whether the fetus will be born with a genetic abnormality. In addition, medical technicians can perform tests on the fluid to determine the presence of substances that are indicators of various conditions, such as certain neural tube defects and Rh disease (a blood incompatibility problem between mother and fetus).

To extract some amniotic fluid and cells from around the fetus, the physician inserts a thin, long needle through the abdominal and uterine walls of the mother until the needle pierces the amniotic sac (**Figure 5.B**). (The physician guides the needle using ultrasound so that it will not injure the fetus, and anesthetizes the abdominal wall with a local anesthetic.) After the fluid is withdrawn, the cells must be grown, or cultured, which takes approximately 4 weeks. This technique is now performed as early as 11 weeks of gestation but is routinely

### Figure 5.A

**Ultrasound in Pregnancy.** The ultrasound probe produces sound waves that bounce off fetal tissues. As the probe is moved across a pregnant woman's abdomen, images that provide information about the position, size, and physical condition of the fetus are visualized on a screen.

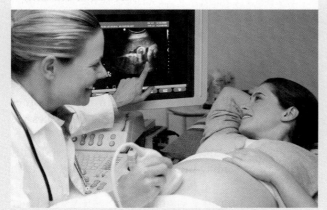

*(Continues)*

## Figure 5.B

**Amniocentesis.** In the amniocentesis procedure, a long, thin needle is used to pierce the mother's abdominal wall and uterus and withdraw amniotic fluid. Free fetal cells are found in this fluid and can be analyzed for the fetus's gender, age, and indications of chromosomal abnormalities.

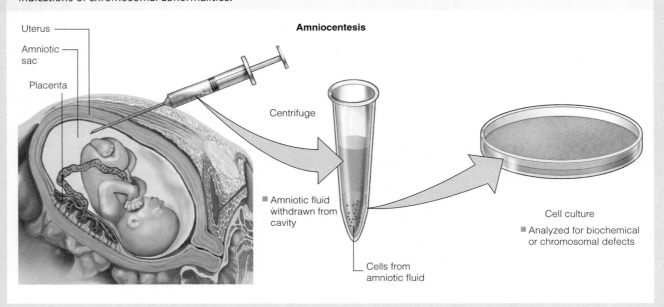

performed between 15 and 18 weeks, so diagnosis is generally completed by the 19th to 22nd week. This procedure is considered safe; the risk of miscarriage resulting from amniocentesis is 0.2% to 0.3% (1 in 300 to 500).

Fetal blood sampling was developed in the 1970s. Extracting blood from the fetus is risky; however, blood can be withdrawn safely from the umbilical vein. With this technique, physicians can screen infants for various blood disorders such as sickle cell anemia and hemophilia and check for fetal oxygen levels or infection. The risk of miscarriage with this technique is up to 2% (2 in 100). This technique is least risky when performed between weeks 18 and 21 of pregnancy but can be done as early as week 17.

lists various teratogens and their detrimental effects on the embryo/fetus.

A woman preparing for pregnancy should have a medical checkup to determine if her level of antibodies against rubella (German measles) is sufficient. She should also be screened for sexually transmitted infections (STIs), especially AIDS, and should avoid changing the cat's litter box to protect herself from contracting toxoplasmosis (infection with a microscopic parasite found in cat feces). Additionally, a woman preparing for pregnancy should seek her healthcare provider's advice regarding the use of medications.

It is important that a woman contemplating pregnancy eat a well-balanced and nutritious diet to enter this critical period with sufficient nutrient stores and blood levels to meet the needs of the pre-embryo and embryo before the placenta is established. (The body has both short-term and long-term nutrient storage capabilities.) Chapter 9 describes some nutritional recommendations for a prepregnancy diet; a woman should also consult her healthcare practitioner regarding proper nutrition during pregnancy. A pregnant woman should not assume that she is "eating for two" in the sense that she should double her food intake. Her need for calories, protein, and calcium are only somewhat greater than her prepregnancy needs. Excessive weight gain during pregnancy may mean excess body fat retained long after pregnancy. Although certain nutrients are extremely important (such as folate, which helps prevent neural tube defects), a pregnant woman should take only the vitamin supplements that her

**Chorionic villus sampling (CVS)** was also developed around 1970 but came into wide use in the 1980s. The chorion is the outermost of the fetal membranes (**Figure 5.C**) that facilitate the exchange of nutrients, gases, and other materials such as waste products between the fetus and the mother. The umbilical cord extends from the fetus to the chorion. Finger-like projections called villi (singular, *villus*) extend from the chorion into maternal tissues at the placenta, the part of the chorion that joins mother and fetus. In this way, the blood of the fetus, circulating through blood vessels in the chorion and its villi, comes into close contact (but does not mix) with maternal blood vessels. To perform CVS, a physician inserts a thin tube or a needle into the vagina and up into the uterus or can enter the uterus by puncturing the abdomen. The instrument vacuums up a tiny sample of villi. Although this technique has the advantages of early testing (weeks 10 to 12) and quick analysis of cells (no culturing is needed), the risk of miscarriage is approximately 1% (1 in 100). CVS was previously thought to cause birth defects of the limbs in some pregnancies, but it has been determined that such defects occur at the same rate as in pregnancies without CVS.

Today, using ultrasound to guide them, physicians are able to sample fetal skin and certain other tissues. In addition, some conditions can be treated before birth with a blood transfusion or one of the forms of fetal surgery currently available. The choices that remain are terminating the pregnancy or carrying the fetus to term. If the second choice is made, prenatal diagnosis is extremely helpful to ensure that the baby receives the best possible medical care for its condition, beginning from its first breath.

## Figure 5.C

**Chorionic Villus Sampling.** One way to perform CVS is to insert a tube, or catheter, into the vagina, up through the cervix, and into the uterus. This tube is used to collect pieces of chorionic villi, which are part of the outer fetal tissue called the chorion (not part of the fetus). These cells are analyzed for chromosomal abnormalities.

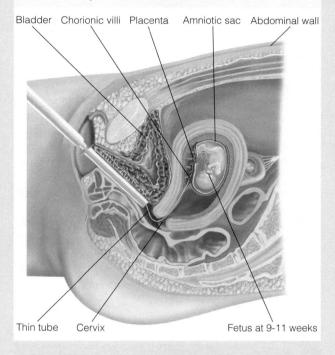

Bladder   Chorionic villi   Placenta   Amniotic sac   Abdominal wall

Thin tube   Cervix   Fetus at 9-11 weeks

healthcare provider prescribes. Some nutrients, such as vitamin A, are teratogens in certain quantities.

It is critical that a woman avoid drinking alcohol, smoking cigarettes, and taking any drugs (unless they have been prescribed) when preparing for pregnancy and during pregnancy. Alcohol consumption can cause a fetal alcohol spectrum disorder, which can result in a variety of birth defects, including intellectual disability, growth deficiency, and hyperactivity. Smoking a pack or more of cigarettes per day can result in a low-birth-weight baby who is weak, has a reduced brain size, and is vulnerable to illness. If a pregnant woman is addicted to drugs, her baby will be born addicted as well. In addition, she is more likely to experience complications during pregnancy and have a baby with severe birth defects. Taking drugs and drinking alcohol occasionally can also damage the embryo or fetus. No safe level of these teratogens has been determined.

Women older than 35 years of age have a higher risk of having babies with Down syndrome (a genetic abnormality resulting in intellectual disability) than younger women. Older women may choose to have diagnostic tests such as amniocentesis and chorionic villus sampling during pregnancy to detect possible genetic disease or other abnormalities in the fetus. In addition, couples often seek genetic counseling before becoming pregnant. If anyone in a couple's family has a genetic disease, seeking genetic counseling may be prudent. (The Managing Your Health essay "Genetic Counseling and Prenatal Diagnosis" discusses prenatal tests and counseling.)

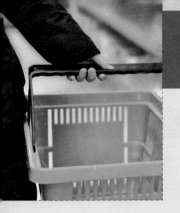

# Consumer Health

## Home Pregnancy Tests

Most pregnancy tests rely on the detection of the hormone **human chorionic gonadotropin (hCG)**. This hormone is produced by embryonic tissues destined to become the placenta, the organ that allows the exchange of nutrients, gases, and wastes between the fetus and a pregnant woman. Pregnancy tests to detect hCG can be conducted on either blood or urine. Urine tests are most frequently used to detect hCG because urine is easier to collect than blood. This is the type of test in home test kits.

The way pregnancy tests work is that hCG binds with specific antibodies in the test kit. If a woman is not pregnant, hCG will not be present in her urine, binding will not occur, and the test will be negative. If a woman is pregnant, hCG will be present in her urine, binding will occur, and the test will be positive.

Home pregnancy tests are easy to use. These tests contain either a plastic stick with an absorbent part that is placed in the urine flow or immersed in a container of collected urine, or a plastic device with an opening containing absorbent material into which drops of urine are placed. While a woman waits, the urine moves through the absorbent material inside either type of device, and the hCG (if present) attaches to an antibody that has a color label such as blue or red. The hCG-antibody complex then moves to another window where it binds to a second antibody attached to the absorbent material in either a line, symbol, color, or the word *pregnant*. If hCG is not present in a woman's urine, the line, symbol, color, or the word *pregnant* will not appear.

It is important to follow the directions of a home test carefully and wait the prescribed length of time to "read" the result. Testing the first urine of the day is best because hCG is most concentrated in the first urine. The manufacturers of home pregnancy tests claim that a woman can test her urine on the first day of her missed period or before, and that she will obtain results that are 99% accurate. However, hCG levels are usually quite low this early in pregnancy. It may be advisable to obtain a blood test from your healthcare practitioner for a reliable early result or to wait at least a week after your missed period to use a home pregnancy test, using the first urine of the day. Be sure to check the expiration date on the package and only use tests that have not expired. You may also decide to repeat the test in a few days no matter what the result.

Ask your pharmacist for help if you are unsure which test to choose. A woman who has a positive test should see her healthcare provider immediately for a confirmatory test and appropriate prenatal care.

## Healthy Living Practices

- ☐ Women preparing for pregnancy should have a medical checkup, eat a well-balanced and nutritious diet, and avoid drinking alcohol, smoking cigarettes, or using other drugs.
- ☐ Women and men concerned about the possibility of passing a genetic condition on to their offspring can seek genetic counseling when considering pregnancy.

Many women want to know if exercising during pregnancy will hurt the fetus. Generally, if a woman was exercising before she became pregnant, she can continue exercising while she is pregnant. However, a healthcare provider may suggest modifications in a pregnant woman's workout regimen. Also, some healthcare providers recommend that their previously sedentary patients start a mild exercise program to help them become stronger and develop stamina for the birth process. Chapter 11 discusses exercising and pregnancy in more detail in its Across the Life Span section.

## Determining If You or Your Partner Is Pregnant

How do you know if you or your partner is pregnant? By noticing certain physical signs, you may become aware of this condition. A pregnant woman will not menstruate, so a missed menstrual period may be the first sign. However, a pregnant woman may experience *implantation bleeding* about a week before the expected time of the menstrual period. This small amount of blood flow from the uterus occurs when the fertilized ovum nestles into the uterine wall. Additionally, the breasts may feel sore, she may feel nauseated at certain times during the day or all day, and she may feel tired, moody, or both. These signs are bodily reactions to changes in hormone levels during pregnancy.

If a woman suspects that she is pregnant, she may choose to conduct a home pregnancy test or visit her gynecologist/obstetrician for such a test. The Consumer Health feature "Home Pregnancy Tests" discusses how pregnancy tests work and provides guidelines for conducting such a test.

If a woman has missed more than one menstrual period and is certain that she is not pregnant, she should see her healthcare provider. *Amenorrhea* (ah-MEN-oh-REE-ah), or abnormal stoppage of the menses, is most often caused by stress, weight loss, or strenuous exercise regimens. However, it can have more serious causes, such as hormonal imbalances or tumorous growths.

## Pregnancy and Fetal Development

Pregnancy usually lasts 38 weeks, or approximately 9 months. The delivery date is calculated to be 40 weeks from a woman's last menstrual period because *conception* (fertilization) usually occurs in the middle of the cycle. Typically pregnancy is described in terms of trimesters, or 3-month periods, during which certain

**chorionic villus sampling (CVS)** A prenatal test performed generally between the 10th and 12th weeks of gestation, in which some of the fetal extraembryonic tissue is removed and analyzed to determine whether the fetus has a genetic abnormality.

**human chorionic gonadotropin (hCG)** In a pregnant woman, a hormone produced by embryonic tissues destined to become the placenta. Pregnancy tests rely on the detection of this hormone in the blood.

developmental events take place. (Because months are more than 4 weeks, the month-to-week correlations given here are approximate.)

The first trimester is a crucial time of development when all the organ systems of the body are forming and becoming functional. Cells in the embryo migrate to key developmental positions, shaping the individual as it takes on a human form. In contrast, the second and third trimesters are periods of growth and refinement of the organ systems. **Figure 5.7** through **Figure 5.11** depict the development

---

### Figure 5.7

**Fertilization and Implantation.** The first event in human development is fertilization, which takes place in the uterine (fallopian) tube. The fertilized ovum begins to divide as it moves along the tube to the uterus and is now referred to as a pre-embryo. At 4 days after fertilization, the developing ball of cells begins to fill with fluid, a stage of pre-embryonic development termed the blastocyst. Approximately 6 days after fertilization, the blastocyst implants in the back wall of the uterus. During implantation, the embryo attaches firmly to the inner lining of the uterus. This illustration shows the journey of the fertilized ovum from the fallopian tube to the uterus. Occasionally, implantation takes place outside of the uterus, a condition known as ectopic pregnancy. Pre-embryos may implant on an ovary, on the intestine, or in a fallopian tube. All ectopic pregnancies endanger the mother's life.

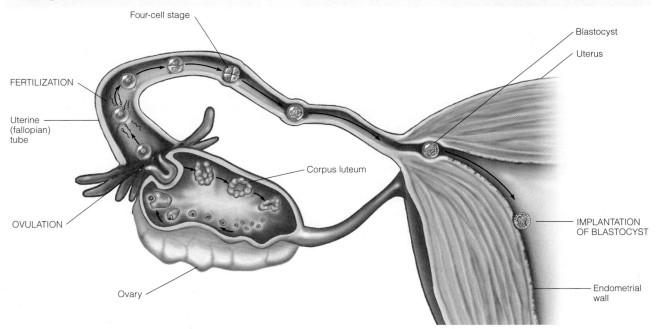

**Figure 5.8**

**Human Embryo Between 4 and 5 Weeks of Development.** As the pregnancy moves into the 3rd week, the pre-embryo is only 0.10 in. long. The flattened pre-embryo develops into a cylindrical embryo. Some of the organs, such as the heart, begin to develop. This 4.5-week-old embryo has established the beginnings of most of the major organ systems of the body. Its C-shaped body has a featureless head, a middle with the heart and liver bulging from the body, and a tail. During the 5th week, the embryo doubles in length from 4 mm (0.18 in.) to 8 mm (0.38 in.). The brain grows rapidly. Wrists, fingers, and ears begin to form during the 6th week of development. Although development has been rapid, growth has not. By the end of the 6th week, the embryo is a mere half-inch long.

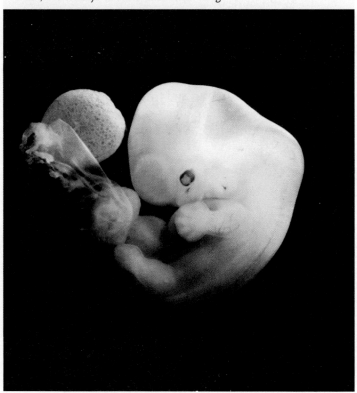

**Figure 5.9**

**Human Fetus About 11 to 12 Weeks of Development.** During the 7th week, eyelids begin to cover the eyes, and the face begins to look somewhat human. By the 8th week, the last week in the embryonic period, the embryo grows to about an inch. Most of the body systems are functional by this time. The fetal period begins at week 9, lasts throughout the rest of the pregnancy, and is characterized by growth and functional maturation of the organs. During weeks 9 through 13 (the 3rd month), facial features become more well developed, with eyelids completely covering the eyes and then fusing shut. (The eyes can be seen through the thin eyelids.) The genitals begin to develop, and the heart is now a four-chambered structure.

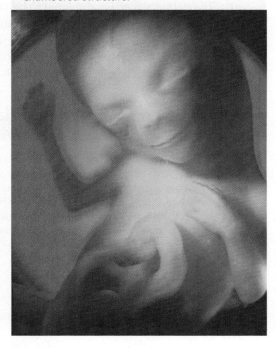

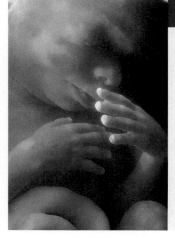

**Figure 5.10**

**Human Fetus About 5 Months (20 Weeks) of Development.** The second trimester comprises the 4th, 5th, and 6th months of development, or weeks 14 through 26. The organs that developed during the first trimester mature and grow during this trimester. As the 4th month passes, the genitals become fully formed. The sensory organs nearly finish their development and refinements of body structures occur. The mother becomes aware of fetal movements around the 5th month of pregnancy, the stage of development of the fetus in the photo. By the end of the 5th month, as fat deposits are laid down, the fetus begins to look more like a baby. Only 12 inches long and weighing 1 pound, it probably could not survive on its own. However, if born by the end of the 6th month, the fetus has a chance of surviving with special medical care.

of the **pre-embryo** (the first 2 weeks of development), the **embryo** (weeks 3 through 8), and the **fetus** (weeks 9 through 38). Figure 5.7 also describes ectopic pregnancy, implantation of the embryo outside of the uterus.

While the fetus is developing, changing, and growing over 9 months, changes also take place in the mother's body. **Figure 5.12** summarizes these changes. In addition, the pregnant woman may experience nausea, vomiting, frequent urination, leg cramps, vaginal discharge, fatigue, and constipation

during the first trimester. Nausea, vomiting, and leg cramps (if present) usually subside by the second trimester. At that time, additional changes may take place. In her last two trimesters, a pregnant woman

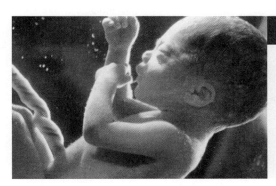

### Figure 5.11

**Human Fetus Nearly Full Term—8 to 9 Months.** During the third trimester, months 7 through 9 or weeks 27 through 38, the fetus primarily gains weight. Its lungs develop more fully, eyelids open, and the nervous system undergoes further development. However, the nervous system is not fully developed and its maturation continues after birth. At the end of the third trimester, the average fetus weighs about 7.5 pounds and is 20 inches long.

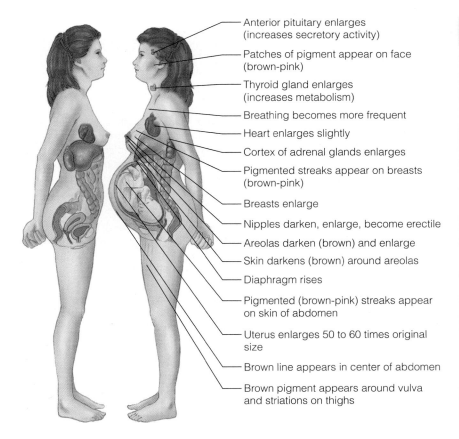

Anterior pituitary enlarges (increases secretory activity)

Patches of pigment appear on face (brown-pink)

Thyroid gland enlarges (increases metabolism)

Breathing becomes more frequent

Heart enlarges slightly

Cortex of adrenal glands enlarges

Pigmented streaks appear on breasts (brown-pink)

Breasts enlarge

Nipples darken, enlarge, become erectile

Areolas darken (brown) and enlarge

Skin darkens (brown) around areolas

Diaphragm rises

Pigmented (brown-pink) streaks appear on skin of abdomen

Uterus enlarges 50 to 60 times original size

Brown line appears in center of abdomen

Brown pigment appears around vulva and striations on thighs

### Figure 5.12

**A Summary of the Physical Changes That Take Place During Pregnancy.** (*Left*) The unpregnant female body; (*Right*) Changes that appear by 30 weeks of fetal development.

may experience swelling of the legs and feet, varicose veins, backache, heartburn, and shortness of breath, in addition to continuing vaginal discharge, frequent urination, fatigue, and constipation. **Table 5.2** lists various problem conditions that may occur during pregnancy. As women of childbearing age get older, their risks for pregnancy complications and adverse outcomes increase.[6]

## Table 5.2

### Pregnancy Problems and Symptoms

| Name of Condition (Alternative or former names) | Definition | Cause | Symptoms | Treatment |
|---|---|---|---|---|
| Ectopic pregnancy | Fertilized egg implants outside the uterus. Majority occur in the uterine tube. | Problems with anatomy of uterine tubes, possibly resulting from pelvic inflammatory disease, uterine surgery, or use of IUD. | Loss of menses, pelvic or abdominal pain, abnormal vaginal bleeding. | Surgery to remove embryo. Nonsurgical treatments may be used in certain situations. |
| Pregnancy-induced hypertension [PIH] (Preeclampsia) (Toxemia of pregnancy) | A group of metabolic disturbances. | Unknown. | High blood pressure, water retention, and an excess of protein in the urine, occurring in the third trimester. Primarily a disease of first pregnancy. Occurs with higher frequency in adolescent women and those older than 35 years. | Bed rest. Medication to reduce blood pressure and prevent seizures. Delivery usually cures the condition. |
| Eclampsia | An extension of PIH to the point of seizure, coma, or both. | Unknown. | Increase in blood pressure from that in PIH, abdominal pain, blurry vision, headache, shakiness. May occur in third trimester or postpartum. | Convulsions and high blood pressure are treated with medication. Delivery takes place as soon as patient is stabilized. |
| Diabetes mellitus associated with pregnancy (Gestational diabetes mellitus [GDM]) | A metabolic disorder that leads to high glucose levels in the blood (see Chapter 9). In pregnancy, poor control of blood glucose levels can lead to fetal abnormalities. | Hormonal changes of pregnancy often result in a display of diabetes in women with risk factors for the disease. | See Table 9.5. Women with risk factors for diabetes (obesity and family history) should be screened prior to and during pregnancy for this disease. | Control of blood glucose level with diet and/or insulin injections. |

*Sources:* Adapted from Rivlin, M. E., & Martin, R. W. (Eds.). (2000). *Manual of clinical problems in obstetrics and gynecology* (5th ed). Philadelphia: Lippincott, Williams & Wilkins; and Zuspan, F. P., & Quilligan, E. J. (1998). *Handbook of obstetrics, gynecology, and primary care.* St. Louis, MO: Mosby.

# The Birth Process

**labor (parturition)** (PAR-too-RISH-un) The process of childbirth.

No one is certain what events signal the beginning of **labor**, the process of childbirth. Labor is also called **parturition** and takes place in three stages: cervical dilation, fetal delivery, and placental delivery. The birth process normally takes about 13 hours for the woman who is giving birth for the first time. In women who have previously given birth, the time shortens considerably and is about 8 hours.

Two main events occur during dilation: rhythmic contractions of the uterine muscles cause the cervix (the opening of the uterus) to dilate (widen) and to efface (thin out). In the nonpregnant state, the cervix is hard and tubelike with an extremely narrow opening. During the first stage of labor, the cervix becomes soft. The opening widens and the tissue stretches so that by the end of the first stage of labor the cervical opening is 3.5 in. to 4 in. wide and the tubular cervix

no longer exists as such—it flattens and becomes continuous with the lower portion of the uterus (**Figure 5.13**). During this time—or prior to labor in some cases—the amniotic sac ruptures (the water breaks), releasing the amniotic fluid. This fluid cushions the fetus during development. The baby must be born within 24 hours of the rupture, or serious infection could occur.

In the beginning of her labor, a woman's uterine contractions may last for 30 seconds and be 15 to 20 minutes apart. As labor progresses, the contractions become stronger, longer, and more closely spaced. By the end of the first stage of labor, during a period called transition, contractions occur every 1 to 2 minutes and last up to a minute each.

## Figure 5.13

**The Stages of Labor.** (a) The position of the fetus at the beginning of labor. (b) Dilation, the cervix (the opening to the uterus) widens and thins. (c) Expulsion, the baby is born. (d) Placental delivery.

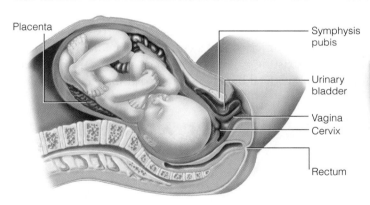

**(a) Early first-stage labor**

Placenta
Symphysis pubis
Urinary bladder
Vagina
Cervix
Rectum

**(b) Later first-stage labor: the transition**

Ruptured amniotic sac

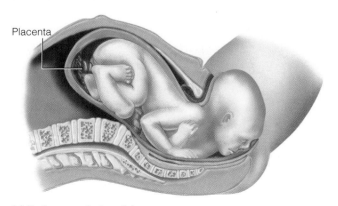

**(c) Early second-stage labor**

Placenta

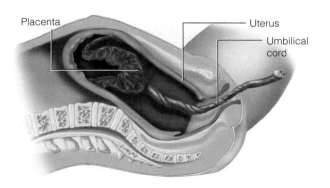

**(d) Third-stage labor: delivery of placenta**

Placenta
Uterus
Umbilical cord

Some women experience preparatory contractions that are not a part of labor, which are called **Braxton-Hicks contractions**, or false labor. False labor contractions can be distinguished from the contractions of true labor in that they occur irregularly, the intervals between contractions do not shorten, and the contractions do not increase in strength. A woman experiencing these contractions should consult her physician to confirm that she is not in labor.

During the second stage of labor, the baby is born. The average time for this stage is 30 to 60 minutes. Uterine contractions continue and move the baby into the birth canal (vagina). The woman pushes and bears down, aiding this process. The head usually appears first, but some babies are born in the breech position, feet or buttocks first. A **breech birth** is a more complicated delivery than a head-first delivery and may require surgical removal of the baby through the abdominal wall—a cesarean section. During a vaginal delivery, the physician may perform an **episiotomy**, making a cut in the tissue surrounding the vaginal opening to widen the opening. This cut is usually made in the direction of the anus. Without this procedure, the skin and surrounding tissues may sustain more damage and heal with more difficulty than surgically cut tissue does.

After the baby is born, its nose and mouth are cleared of mucus by suctioning. The umbilical cord is clamped in two places and cut between the clamps to prevent bleeding. Healthcare practitioners assess the baby's ability to adjust to life outside the uterus at 1 minute and then 5 minutes after birth.

Within 15 to 30 minutes after delivery of the baby, the uterus continues to contract, separating the fetal placental tissues from maternal tissues. During this third stage of labor, the placenta is expelled from the uterus. Figure 5.13 summarizes the birth process, showing the three stages of labor (a–d).

## Circumcision

Although few data are available, they show that from about 61% to 79% of male newborns are circumcised in the United States.[7] In some groups, such as followers of the Jewish and Islamic faiths, circumcision rates approximate 100% because the procedure is practiced for religious and cultural reasons. *Circumcision* is a surgical procedure to remove the foreskin of the penis, which is a fold of skin covering the end of the penis. The photos in **Figure 5.14** show both an uncircumcised and a circumcised penis.

Existing scientific evidence demonstrates potential medical benefits of newborn male circumcision,

### Figure 5.14

**Circumcision.** (a) Uncircumcised penis. (b) Circumcised penis.

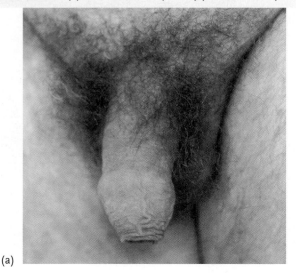

(a)

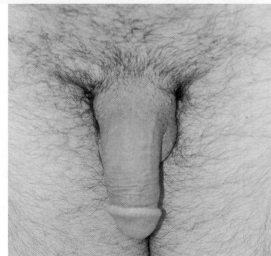

(b)

such as lowered risk of urinary tract infections, especially in infants younger than 1 year of age, lowered risk of penile cancer, and lowered risk of STIs, especially herpes (HSV-2) and HIV infection. Circumcision also reduces the prevalence and transmission of human papillomavirus, which is linked to the development of cervical cancer.[8] However, the policy statement of the American Academy of Pediatrics,[9] which was reaffirmed in 2005,[10] notes that, in general, the differences in risk are small and the data are not sufficient to recommend routine circumcision of male newborns at this time. Additionally, circumcision has some risks as does any surgical procedure, though complications are rare and usually minor. Therefore, the AAP suggests that parents, in conjunction with their pediatricians, decide what is in the best interest of the child. If the decision is made for circumcision, the Academy strongly recommends giving the infant pain relief medication.

## The Postpartum Period

The *postpartum period* is the 6 weeks after childbirth during which a mother's body returns to its prepregnant state. One of the areas of the body affected greatly, of course, is the reproductive system. The uterus returns nearly to its original size. Within 2 weeks, the cervical opening closes to a slit, and tissue damage that occurred to it during the birth process heals. The vagina, bruised and swollen from the newborn traveling through it, returns to normal after about 3 weeks. The episiotomy and any torn tissues surrounding the vaginal opening heal within 1 week.

A variety of other organ systems and tissues in the mother's body change during pregnancy and return to their prepregnant state during the postpartum period and beyond. For example, muscles in the pelvic region gradually regain their original tone, but this process may take up to 6 months. During the first few days after delivery, a woman may have trouble urinating due to bruising of the bladder, the effects of anesthetics, and swelling of the ureters, tubes that lead from the kidneys to the bladder. The ureters may remain swollen for up to 3 months, although problems with urination usually last only a few days. During the birth process and the expulsion of the placenta, a woman loses blood. Her blood plasma and red blood cell volumes usually return to the normal nonpregnant state by the end of the postpartum period, but may take a few additional weeks. Hormonal changes are comparatively rapid after delivery; some return to normal levels by the end of the first postpartum day, but others take 1 to 2 weeks to normalize.

Many women experience *postpartum depression*, especially in the week after delivery. Approximately 40% to 85% of women experience mild depression, often referred to as "the baby blues." This mild form of depression, often accompanied by mood swings, is thought to be a result of the physical and mental stresses of childbirth, as well as the variety of physical (including hormonal) changes that take place during that time. Symptoms include periods of crying, sleep disturbances, loss of appetite, and confusion. Whereas the baby blues do not require medical attention, more serious postpartum depression does. This disorder can occur up to 1 year after giving birth and affects 10% to 15% of mothers.[11]

At the beginning of the postpartum period, many women also start breastfeeding their infants. The benefits of breastfeeding are discussed in the Across the Life Span section of Chapter 9.

### Healthy Living Practices

- If you are female and in your reproductive years, have missed a period, are nauseated at times, feel tired often, and are experiencing moodiness, check with a healthcare practitioner; you may be pregnant.

- Manufacturers claim that home pregnancy tests can be used prior to or on the day of a missed period or thereafter to determine pregnancy. However, early results may be unreliable. A healthcare practitioner can provide laboratory testing to confirm pregnancy.

# Infertility

**Infertility** is the inability of a couple to conceive a child after 1 year of unprotected sex and affects 7.4% of married women in the United States.[12] Some infertility experts suggest that couples wait for 2 years before seeking help for infertility. Infertility is not necessarily the result of "a problem" with one partner or the other. Factors that slightly impair the fertility of both sexual partners may interact to render a couple infertile.

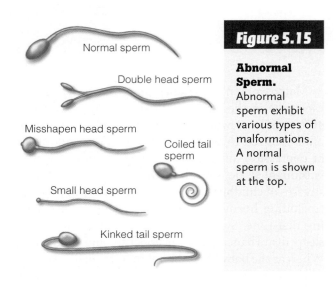

Normal sperm

Double head sperm

Misshapen head sperm

Coiled tail sperm

Small head sperm

Kinked tail sperm

**Figure 5.15**

**Abnormal Sperm.** Abnormal sperm exhibit various types of malformations. A normal sperm is shown at the top.

## Factors That Affect Fertility

One reason for male infertility is faulty sperm production. In normal sperm production, the semen contains approximately 80 million to 120 million sperm per milliliter (mL). Because the ejaculate volume ranges from 2 to 8 mL, slightly less than a teaspoon to nearly 2 teaspoons, the total sperm ejaculated ranges from about 200 million to 800 million. A sperm count lower than 20 million sperm per mL, 40 million to 160 million total in the ejaculate, may impair fertility.

In addition to a low sperm count, a high percentage (usually more than 40%) of abnormally shaped sperm can affect male fertility. Abnormally shaped sperm such as those with two heads or abnormally shaped heads or tails (**Figure 5.15**) may not be able to swim well. These defects may reduce their chances of reaching the egg.

Male infertility is often related to a variety of environmental factors or diseases. Cigarette smoking, chronic alcoholism, various medications, and prolonged illnesses with accompanying fever all affect sperm production. Infection with the mumps virus can render a man sterile.

A man can also have a problem with sperm transport, which can cause infertility even if the sperm count is adequate for conception. Infections caused by certain STIs can block the vas deferens and injure these tubes. Erectile dysfunction is also a common cause of infertility if a man is unable to ejaculate.

There is a variety of causes of infertility in women. In some instances, the vagina cannot be penetrated because of an intact hymen (a membrane that partially covers the vagina and that is usually ruptured at the first intercourse) or to vaginismus (involuntary, painful contractions of the vagina). Some abnormalities in the structure of the vagina, which may be present at birth or caused by scarring from STIs or trauma, allow only partial penetration. Unknowingly complicating the problem, couples having trouble with penetration often use lubricants that kill sperm. For example, one type of the popular K-Y Jelly has spermicidal properties.

Once sperm travel up the vagina, they must pass through the cervix to reach the uterus and the fallopian tubes. Secretion of mucus by the cervix is important for sperm motility. Infection can damage the glands that secrete mucus or result in the presence of white blood cells. The properties of this mucus also change if a woman has an estrogen deficiency. Such changes in the quality and quantity of mucus can impair the sperm's ability to reach an egg.

Structural defects of the uterus do not usually cause infertility; usually such problems result in repeated miscarriage. However, the uterine (fallopian) tubes can be another fertility trouble spot. Infection with *Neisseria gonorrhoeae* or *Chlamydia trachomatis* (see Chapter 14) can result in severe tissue destruction, completely blocking the tubes and causing sterility. Infections of other origins, such as from appendicitis or IUD complications, may result in less severe blockage. Pregnancy may occur, but the risk is increased for ectopic pregnancy. Endometriosis, the growth of abnormal tissue in the abdomen, is another cause of sterility, ectopic pregnancy, or both.

The ovaries can be the source of impaired fertility. Hormonal imbalances can interfere with ovulation, and a mumps infection, radiation, and chemotherapy can damage the ovaries. Additionally, function of the ovaries declines as a woman ages, reducing her ability to conceive. Occasionally, because of an unknown cause, a young woman can experience a decline in the function of the ovaries known as primary ovarian insufficiency, in which she prematurely "runs out" of cells destined to become eggs.[13] Dietary deficiencies, frequent strenuous exercise, smoking, and obesity have also been shown to negatively affect ovary function and the ability to conceive.[14-16]

## Treating Infertility

To treat infertility, a physician skilled in this practice begins with extensive histories of the couple's health. This may be followed by a series of relatively simple tests such as a sperm count to rule out common causes of infertility. Other, more extensive, physical examinations may be necessary to determine the cause. In some instances, the cause cannot be determined. Treatments are specific to the known causes of the infertility and include surgical procedures, hormone therapy, medication, and lifestyle changes. In addition, nutritional treatment is currently being investigated. Research results reveal that either sperm quality or pregnancy rate rose in men after treatment with oral antioxidants, such as vitamins C and E, zinc, and folate.[17]

In addition to these therapies, physicians can harvest ova and obtain semen to assist fertilization and implantation. For example, if a couple has problems with sperm reaching the cervix, cervical conditions that are hostile to sperm, or the health of the sperm themselves, a physician may suggest artificial insemination, which has been practiced in the United States for more than 50 years. During this procedure, semen is placed in the cervical opening during the time of ovulation. With intrauterine insemination, concentrated sperm are placed in the uterus.

Women who have no uterine tubes or blocked tubes that do not respond to surgery often choose in vitro fertilization (IVF) to conceive. *In vitro* means "in a test tube" or "in the laboratory." In vitro fertilization involves fertilization of ova with sperm in laboratory glassware, with subsequent implantation of zygotes (fertilized eggs) in the woman's uterus. The birth of the first baby conceived through in vitro fertilization took place in 1978.

In 1992, a new IVF technique called intracytoplasmic sperm injection, or ICSI, was developed to fertilize eggs directly. Early IVF techniques involved putting eggs and sperm together and allowing sperm to swim to and fertilize the eggs. In the late 1980s, a technique was developed in which a few sperm were injected into the space between the egg and its barrier, increasing the chance of fertilization. The ICSI technique involves injecting a single sperm directly into the egg. It is used when men have a very low sperm count, nonmotile sperm, or sperm unable to penetrate the chemical barrier that protects the egg.

Any treatment of infertility in which the sperm and eggs are both handled outside of the body is called assisted reproductive technology. Although assisted reproductive technology has been helpful, studies urge some caution. The use of assisted reproductive technology increases the risk of multiple births and infants born with low birth weights (under 5.5 pounds) for both multiple births and single births. These risks increase the chances of long-term neurological problems such as cerebral palsy.[18]

# Contraception

Most of the time, people engage in sexual intercourse for nonreproductive reasons. The timing may not be right for a pregnancy, or their family may be complete. Therefore, couples usually use some form of **birth control**, or **contraception**, which are methods to avoid pregnancy. You can assess your attitude toward the timing of parenthood by using the self-assessment scale in the Student Workbook pages at the end of the book.

Couples and individuals have many factors to consider when choosing a birth control method. They might consider its cost, effectiveness, reversibility, side effects, ease of use, convenience, and effectiveness against STIs. They must also consider their age and whether they need contraception on a regular basis or if they have only infrequent contraceptive needs. Many people are also concerned about the ways in which a contraceptive interferes with or fits in with their lovemaking. Some people have religious considerations to think about when making this choice.

Because a woman has a long reproductive life lasting some 30 to 35 years (from her teenage years until age 50 on average), the form of contraception she chooses may vary to meet her needs throughout the stages of her life. A variety of contraceptive methods is available, each with its own risks, benefits, and level of effectiveness. Most methods are based on the female reproductive cycle and rely on a woman's taking action. However, many methods can rely on the action of both partners and be incorporated into lovemaking.

The effectiveness of a contraceptive method is an important factor to consider. The *theoretical effectiveness* of a contraceptive refers to the number of women who will *not* become pregnant out of 100 couples using a method consistently and properly as their only means of birth control for 1 year. For example, if a method is 80% effective, 80 of 100 women using this method will not become pregnant over a year; 20 women will become pregnant. *Actual effectiveness* refers to the number of women who will *not* become pregnant of 100 couples using a method under usual conditions. Many people forget to use the method or use it improperly, lowering its effectiveness. (Unprotected sex has an effectiveness rate of 15%; 85 out of 100 women will become pregnant over a year.) **Table 5.3** lists the effectiveness of the various forms of birth control.

## Table 5.3

### Effectiveness of Various Birth Control Methods

| Method | Actual Effectiveness (%) | Theoretical Effectiveness (%) |
| --- | --- | --- |
| Abstinence | — | 100 |
| Fertility awareness | 75 | 91–99 |
| Coitus interruptus (withdrawal) | 73 | 96 |
| Spermicides | 71 | 82 |
| Diaphragm | 86 | 94 |
| Contraceptive sponge (women who have not given birth) | 84 | 91 |
| Contraceptive sponge (women who have given birth) | 68 | 80 |
| Lea's Shield | 85 | Not available |
| FemCap | 86 | Not available |
| Male condom | 85 | 98 |
| Female condom | 79 | 95 |
| Combined oral contraceptives (the pill) | 92 | 99.7 |
| Progestin-only pill (the mini-pill) | 97 | 99.5 |
| Contraceptive patch (Ortho Evra) | 92 | 99.7 |
| Contraceptive vaginal ring (NuvaRing) | 92 | 99.7 |
| Contraceptive implant (Implanon) | 99.95 | 99.95 |
| Depo-Provera | 97 | 99.7 |
| IUDs (across types) | 99.2–99.9 | 99.4–99.9 |
| Female sterilization | 99.5 | 99.5 |
| Male sterilization | 99.85 | 99.9 |

The "Contraceptive Comfort and Confidence Scale" in the Student Workbook pages at the end of the book can help you assess whether the method of contraception that you are using or considering is, or will be, effective for you.

## Abstinence and Natural Methods

With respect to contraception, **abstinence** means refraining from vaginal intercourse. Without this act, a woman cannot get pregnant (unless sperm are introduced artificially into her reproductive tract by a physician or possibly if sperm are deposited at the opening to the vagina and are able to travel into the vagina and then into the uterus). Abstinence is 100% effective and is an excellent alternative for young men and women who feel they are not ready to have sex. Also, people choose to abstain from sex during various periods of their lives for varied reasons.

**Natural family planning**, or **fertility awareness** (formerly called the *rhythm method*), is a group of birth control techniques in which a couple abstains from sexual intercourse during the time of the month when a woman is most likely to conceive. Although the theoretical effectiveness of natural family planning/ fertility awareness is high—91% to 99% depending on the method—the actual effectiveness of these methods is about 75% because it is often difficult to determine when ovulation has occurred and fertilization can take place. However, when couples consistently use two indicators of fertility, mucus inspection and temperature (the mucothermal method), and strictly adhere to the guidelines of using these methods together, the methods have been shown to be more than 98% effective.[19]

Ovulation usually (but not always) takes place about 14 days before the woman's next menstrual period. If she has sex up to 72 hours before ovulation, she can become pregnant because sperm live approximately this long. The egg survives for 24 hours, so fertilization can occur for 1 day after ovulation also. In summary, fertilization can take place up to 3 days before and 1 day after ovulation.

The time of ovulation varies with the length of a woman's cycle and may vary within cycles of a consistent length. In fact, a woman can ovulate anytime during her cycle and can even become pregnant during her menstrual period. The following are four ways to determine (but without 100% certainty) when ovulation takes place: the temperature method, the calendar method, mucus inspection, and the mucothermal method. All but the calendar method are based on changes that take place in a woman's body around the time of ovulation.

To use the *temperature method*, a woman takes her temperature with a special basal thermometer before she gets out of bed every day for a few months. Because the body temperature usually dips just before and rises just after ovulation (**Figure 5.16**), charting body temperature for a few months can help a woman determine when she ovulates and if ovulation is regular.

To use *mucus inspection*, a woman notes when her cervical mucus changes consistency. Four days before ovulation, cervical mucus (which flows to the vagina) becomes clearer and thinner. She should avoid intercourse from this time until the mucus changes back to its cloudier, thicker appearance. The *mucothermal method* combines this method with the temperature method described in the previous paragraph.

To use the *calendar method*, the woman records the length of her menstrual cycles for a year, beginning on day 1 of menstrual bleeding. After determining the length of her shortest and longest cycles, she uses a chart or formula provided by her healthcare practitioner to determine which days of the month she could become pregnant. This method works best when a woman has cycles that are consistently the

**abstinence** A method of birth control that involves refraining from vaginal intercourse.

**natural family planning (fertility awareness)** Formerly called the rhythm method; a group of birth control techniques in which a couple abstains from sexual intercourse during the time of the month when a woman is most likely to conceive.

**coitus interruptus (withdrawal)** (KO-ih-tus in-ter-RUP-tus) A form of birth control in which the man removes his penis from his partner's vagina and genital area, interrupting intercourse before ejaculation.

**spermicides** Chemicals that kill sperm.

same length. If a woman's cycle varies greatly, "safe" times within her cycle will be shorter than if her cycles are more regular.

**Coitus interruptus**, or **withdrawal**, is another natural form of birth control. To use this method, the man senses when he is close to ejaculation, and then removes his penis from his partner's vagina and genital area, interrupting intercourse. There are many problems with this method, however. A man must exercise a great deal of self-control, removing his penis from the vagina at a time when his desire may be to thrust more deeply. Also, he must be able to sense when he has enough time to remove himself before ejaculation. Additionally, sperm from a recent ejaculation may be present in the urethra and may be carried to the tip of the penis with drops of pre-ejaculatory fluid and result in pregnancy. To reduce the possibility of sperm in the pre-ejaculate, a man should urinate after ejaculation and carefully clean all semen from the penis. With perfect use, coitus interruptus is 96% effective. However, during actual use this form of contraception is only 73% effective. None of the natural methods of birth control protects against the transmission of STIs.

## Chemical Methods

**Spermicides** are chemicals that kill sperm. The most common active ingredient in spermicides marketed in the United States is nonoxynol-9. The inactive ingredients make up the carrier, or base, of the spermicides,

## Figure 5.16

**Basal Body Temperature Variations During the Menstrual Cycle.** In this graph, basal body temperature is shown to vary during this "model" menstrual cycle. The time of ovulation is determined by noting the fall in temperature just before ovulation and the rise over 3 days just after. Remember, most menstrual cycles are not as regular as this model cycle. Safe days vary widely among women and may vary widely among an individual's cycles. The days prior to ovulation are considered "unsafe" because a woman does not yet know whether ovulation has occurred.

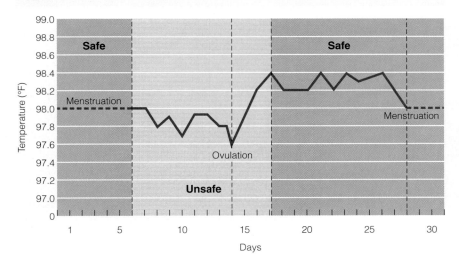

which are sold as foams, creams, jellies, films, suppositories, and tablets. (Spermicides are also added to many brands of condoms.) The carrier distributes the spermicide in the vaginal canal. Shortly before vaginal sex, foams, creams, and jellies are placed high in the vagina near the cervix using an applicator, as shown in **Figure 5.17** (a and b). Spermicidal films are placed near the cervix. Suppositories and tablets are placed in the vagina and given time to dissolve. Correct placement of the spermicide and timing of insertion are critical to the spermicide's effectiveness, which is 82% if these products are used correctly and consistently.

Advantages to using spermicides are that the side effects (such as allergy and vaginal irritation or infection) are minimal, they are used only when birth control is needed, and they are easy products to obtain over the counter. Disadvantages are a low rate of effectiveness and an increase in the frequency of genital irritation and lesions caused by nonoxynol-9. The presence of genital lesions and irritated membranes increase the risk of contracting a sexually transmit-

## Figure 5.17

**Contraceptive Foam and Jelly, Diaphragm, FemCap, and Lea's Shield.** (a) Contraceptive foam or jelly is placed high up in the vagina, covering the cervix, using a plunger-type applicator. (b) Contraceptive jelly and applicator. (c) The diaphragm is ringed with contraceptive spermicide prior to insertion. The diaphragm is pinched to narrow it and is then placed high in the vagina, covering the cervix. (d) Diaphragm.

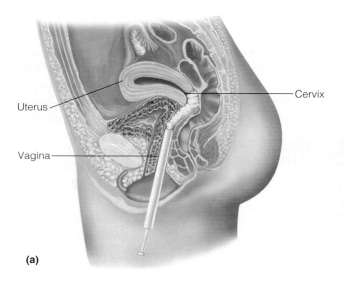

(a)

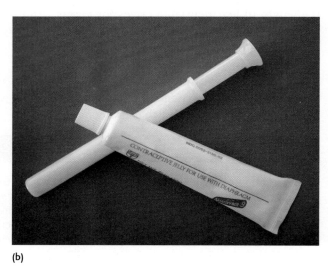

(b)

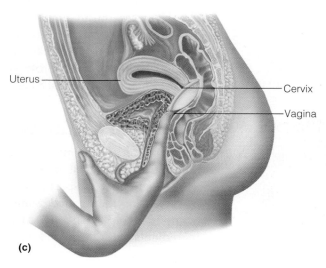

(c)

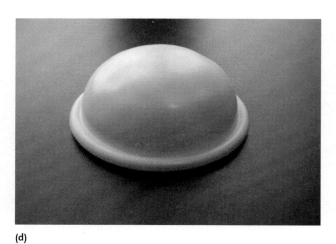

(d)

ted infection such as HIV during intercourse with an infected partner.[20]

Some women use **douching** as a contraceptive method. Douching is the use of specially prepared solutions to cleanse the vagina. Douching is *not* effective for contraception. By the time a woman can douche after sexual intercourse, sperm have already reached the cervix and uterus and cannot be washed away. Additionally, if a woman has used a contraceptive product containing spermicide, or has used spermicide alone as a contraceptive, douching may wash away the chemical and render it inactive.

**douching** (DOOSH-ing) The use of specially prepared solutions to cleanse the vagina; not an effective birth control method.

**barrier methods** Types of birth control that block the path that sperm must take to reach the ovum; these forms of contraception include male condoms, female condoms, diaphragms, and cervical caps.

## Barrier Methods

**Barrier methods** of contraception block the path that sperm must take to reach the ovum. These forms

### Figure 5.17 (Continued)

(e) A small amount of spermicide is spread on the rim and brim of the side of the FemCap that will face outward, away from the cervix. A larger amount of spermicide is spread in the groove on the side of the FemCap that will face inward, toward the cervix. The FemCap is pinched to narrow it and is then placed high in the vagina with the bowl facing upward and the long brim entering first. The FemCap is placed to cover the cervix completely. (f) FemCap. (g) Lea's Shield. This contraceptive device is also pinched for insertion and pushed up into the vagina as far as it can go. It is used in conjunction with spermicide.

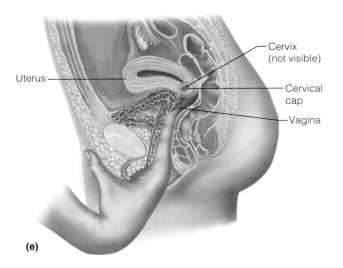

**(e)**

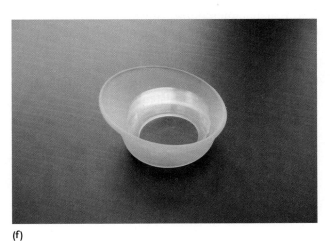

**(f)**

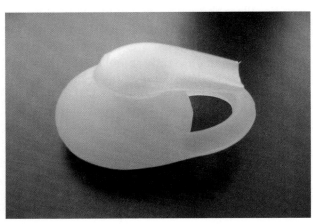

**(g)**

**condom** A sheath used to cover the penis during sexual intercourse to help prevent pregnancy or sexually transmitted infections.

of contraception include diaphragms, cervical caps, male condoms, and female condoms.

**Diaphragms and Diaphragm-like Products** The diaphragm has been in use in the United States longer than 60 years. Shown in Figure 5.17c and Figure 5.17d, a *diaphragm* is a dome-shaped rubber cup bordered by a flexible spring that is designed to cover the cervix and surrounding area. This prescription item must be fitted by a healthcare practitioner.

Before inserting a diaphragm, place spermicide on both its sides and around its rim. Compress the spring, collapsing the diaphragm so that it can be inserted into the vagina. When the diaphragm reaches the cervical area, its spring pops open, causing the diaphragm to assume its dome shape and to be held firmly in place over the cervix.

After insertion, a diaphragm is effective for 6 hours, so a woman could insert the diaphragm well before sexual intercourse. However, spermicide must be added before each additional act of intercourse. After the last intercourse, the diaphragm must be left in place for at least 6 hours but must not be worn for more than 24 hours because of risk of infection. Used properly and consistently, the diaphragm is 94% effective.

The Today Vaginal Contraceptive Sponge, an over-the-counter single-use, disposable *sponge* that contains spermicide and is used like a diaphragm, was taken off the market in the United States in 1995. The Food and Drug Administration (FDA) discovered that the water system used in the manufacture of the product was contaminated with bacteria that cause diarrhea, although the sponges were never shown to be contaminated with this pathogen. A New Jersey pharmaceutical company purchased the Today sponge from its original manufacturer in 1999. The FDA approved U.S. sales of the Today sponge in April 2005.

In 2002, the FDA approved *Lea's Shield*, a diaphragm-like vaginal barrier contraceptive. The shield, shown in Figure 5.17g, is composed of three parts: a bowl, a one-way valve, and a loop. After coating the inside of the bowl around the hole, the front of the rim, and the outer part of the valve with spermicide, pinch the rim of the shield and slide the device high up in the vagina. The bowl of the shield covers the cervix. The valve vents air during insertion, which creates a suction that helps hold the shield in place.

The loop is used to remove the device and to prevent its rotation during use. Lea's Shield can be inserted up to 24 hours prior to intercourse and should remain in place for 8 hours afterward but for no longer than 48 hours total. The actual effectiveness of the shield is 85%.

The *cervical cap* works much the same way as the diaphragm, but it is smaller and covers only the cervix. In 2003, the FDA approved the FemCap (Figure 5.17f). Like Lea's Shield, the FemCap can be inserted up to 24 hours prior to intercourse and should remain in place for 8 hours afterward but for no longer than 48 hours total. Before inserting, put a small amount of spermicide in the dome of the FemCap, spread a thin layer on the brim, and put a small amount in the folded area between the brim and the dome. The FemCap is inserted with the long brim entering first and the dome-side down. The actual effectiveness of the FemCap is 86%.

**Condoms** A **condom** is a sheath, usually made of thin latex or polyurethane, that covers the erect penis (male condom) or lines the vagina and covers the labia (female condom) to provide a barrier against fertilization or sexually transmitted infections.

*Male condoms*, the only form of birth control presently available for men other than vasectomy, are one of the most popular forms of birth control in the United States. The use of male condoms is also described in Chapter 14. Used for the prevention of pregnancy, condoms are 85% effective with actual use and 98% effective with consistent and proper use.

*Figure 5.18* illustrates the correct procedure for putting on a male condom: Put the condom on after the penis has become erect but before there is genital contact with a partner. Hold the top half-inch of the condom, squeezing the air out. This space will form a reservoir for semen. If air is not removed from this space, the semen cannot collect at the condom tip. Place the rolled-up condom over the head of the penis (Figure 5.18a). While still holding the tip, unroll the condom to cover the penis to its base (Figure 5.18b and c). Gently smooth out any air that may have been trapped between the condom and the penis. After ejaculation, hold the condom firmly at its base to prevent slippage while you withdraw the still-erect penis from your partner's body. Remove the condom from the penis (Figure 5.18d), being careful not to spill semen on your partner and not to touch the exterior of the condom to your genital area. The outside of the condom may have become contaminated from an infected partner. Discard the used condom.

Approved by the FDA in 1993, the Reality female condom, a polyurethane sheath with a ring at each end, lines the vagina. Its use is also described in Chapter 14. Female condoms, used consistently and properly as a form of birth control, are approximately 95% effective. Their actual effectiveness, however, is 79%.

**Figure 5.19** shows a female condom and the correct procedure for inserting one: Holding the closed end of the condom, squeeze the ring inside the condom so that it flattens and can be inserted into the vagina (Figure 5.19a). Insert the flattened ring and condom into the vagina (Figure 5.19b), gently pushing it up to the cervix as shown in Figure 5.19c. You should be able to feel the ring positioned past the pubic bone. Straighten out the part of the condom lining the vagina if it is twisted. The outside ring should cover the labia, as shown in Figure 5.19d. After intercourse, first twist the condom to close it at the vaginal opening, which will prevent sperm and pathogens from

touching your genital area. Remove the condom with gentle pulling and discard. Female and male condoms are intended for one-time use.

## Hormonal Methods

There are two basic types of hormonal contraception: combined estrogen and progestin contraceptives, and progestin-only contraceptives. With the exception of progesterone-only mini-pills, hormonal methods of birth control prevent pregnancy by suppressing ovulation.

**Combined Estrogen and Progestin Contraceptives Combined oral contraceptives** (COCs; "the pill") suppress ovulation through the combined actions of estrogen and progestin (a synthetic form of

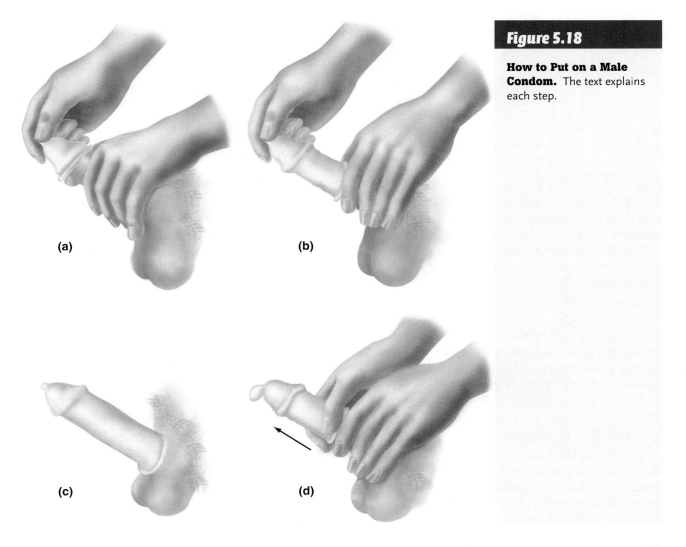

(a)

(b)

(c)

(d)

**Figure 5.18**

**How to Put on a Male Condom.** The text explains each step.

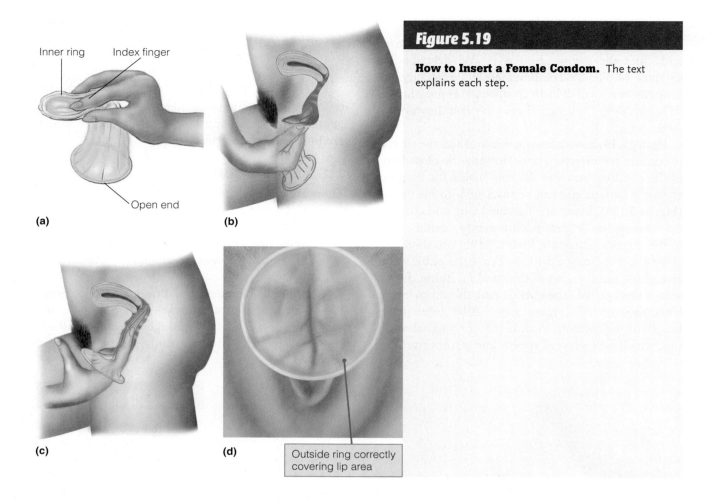

**Inner ring** **Index finger**

**Open end**

**(a)**

**(b)**

**(c)**

**(d)**

Outside ring correctly covering lip area

**Figure 5.19**

**How to Insert a Female Condom.** The text explains each step.

progesterone). With the exception of extended-cycle oral contraceptives (Seasonale and Seasonique) and Lybrel, which are described later in this section, menstruation occurs monthly.

The Guttmacher Institute notes that the pill is the most common method of birth control reported by women who use birth control methods.[21] The pill has numerous advantages. It is highly effective, decreases menstrual cramps, decreases the length of the menses and the amount of blood lost, has a protective effect against pelvic inflammatory disease, reduces the risk for ovarian and endometrial cancer (cancer of the uterine lining), reduces the risk for benign (noncancerous) breast disease, and helps prevent osteoporosis (thinning of the bones). The pill is a readily reversible form of contraception.

COCs have been available for nearly 50 years and are some of the best-studied prescription medications. The amount of estrogen and progestin in pills has decreased over the years, so today's pills are much safer than pills of the past. Cardiovascular disease is

the most serious complication of the pill. Women at high risk for developing this complication of COC use are those who are older than 50 years of age or who are older than 35 years of age and smoke cigarettes. Women who are sedentary, overweight, and have high blood pressure, diabetes mellitus, or an elevated serum cholesterol level are also at high risk. **Table 5.4** lists symptoms that may warn of a potential health complication when using the pill. The mnemonic (memory aid) ACHES can help you remember these symptoms.

A review of studies on the risk of cervical cancer in women taking COCs reveals that risk increases with increasing duration of use.[22] The studies included women on combined oral contraceptives and some on progestin-only preparations, which are discussed shortly. Risk was shown to decline after use stopped. After 10 years, the risk was the same as that for women who never used oral contraceptives.

*Extended-cycle oral contraceptives* contain lower doses of hormones than conventional birth control

## Table 5.4

### Warning Signs and Symptoms of a Potential Health Complication When Using "The Pill" or an IUD

| | Pill | | | IUD |
|---|---|---|---|---|
| A | Abdominal pain (severe) | | P | Period is late; abnormal spotting or bleeding |
| C | Chest pain (severe), shortness of breath | | A | Abdominal pain or pain wth intercourse |
| H | Headache (severe), may include dizziness, weakness, numbness | | I | Infection (sexually transmitted) exposure, abnormal discharge |
| E | Eye problems: vision loss, blurring, double vision, flashing lights | | N | Not feeling well, fever, chills |
| S | Sudden, severe leg or arm pain; leg or arm numbness | | S | String is missing or is shorter or longer |

pills and are taken for 84 days instead of the usual 21 before menstruation occurs. With this pill, a woman has only four menstrual periods per year, one each season, instead of the usual 13. In addition to suppressing ovulation, this pill prevents buildup of the lining of the uterus. Therefore, the menses are light. Seasonale was approved by the FDA in 2003 and Seasonique in 2006. With Seasonale, a woman takes an inactive pill during the days of her period, and with Seasonique, she takes a low-dose estrogen pill. The low-dose estrogen appears to reduce breakthrough bleeding during the time between menses.

Lybrel was approved by the FDA in 2007. Like Seasonale and Seasonique it is a low-dose pill, but it is taken 365 days per year. Over time menstruation stops, but a woman may experience some breakthrough bleeding and spotting, especially during the first few months of use. Thus, a woman choosing to use this form of COC should weigh the convenience of not menstruating with the uncertainty of breakthrough bleeding and spotting. The health benefits, health risks, and theoretical effectiveness of Lybrel, Seasonale, and Seasonique are comparable to other COCs.

The *contraceptive patch* (Ortho Evra) was approved by the FDA in 2001 and became available in late April 2002. The patch delivers hormones through the skin for 1 week. A woman uses three patches over 3 weeks, and then "goes off" the patch, during which time menstruation occurs. A primary advantage of the patch over conventional birth control pills is convenience: A woman needs to remember to change the patch only once a week rather than remembering to take a pill every day. Results of research show that women who used the patch were more satisfied with this contraceptive method than with contraceptive pills.[23]

In 2001, the FDA approved the *contraceptive vaginal ring* (NuvaRing), which became available in mid-2002. This doughnut-shaped device fits in the vagina much like a diaphragm but works by releasing progestin and estrogen. Instead of taking a pill every day, a woman keeps the ring in place for 3 weeks, and then removes it for 1 week, during which time she menstruates. Like the patch, the vaginal ring offers convenience: A woman only needs to remember to remove the ring after 3 weeks and insert a new one after a week without it.

**Progestin-Only Contraceptives** Implanon, Depo-Provera, and mini-pills are all forms of progestin-only contraceptives. Progestin works to suppress ovulation in much the same way as combined oral contraceptives.

Implanon, approved by the FDA in 2006, is a matchstick-sized *contraceptive implant*. It is surgically inserted under the skin of the upper arm. While there, it releases progestin slowly and can inhibit ovulation for 3 years.

*Depo-Provera*, which has been used in the United States since 1992, is an injection of progestin that inhibits ovulation for 3 months. *Mini-pills* are progestin-only pills that are taken continually. Introduced in 1970, they have been in use for approximately 40 years.

Although highly effective, progestin-only contraceptives have a few serious disadvantages. These con-

**intrauterine device (IUD)** A small contraceptive device that either is covered with copper or contains a reservoir of progestin and is inserted into the uterus.

**emergency contraception (EC)** Birth control methods that help prevent pregnancy after sexual intercourse, rather than before or during sex.

traceptives change a woman's menstrual cycle. In addition to amenorrhea (no periods), these changes can include opposite effects: an increased number of days of menstruation with light bleeding or an increased number of days with heavy bleeding. Women find some of these changes unacceptable. Another disadvantage is that long-term use of progestin-only contraceptives may cause thinning of the bones because of low estrogen.

## Intrauterine Devices

An **intrauterine device (IUD)** is a small apparatus that a healthcare practitioner inserts into the uterus (**Figure 5.20**). A string hangs from the base of the IUD and extends into the vagina; the presence of the string is an indication that the IUD is still in place. The active ingredient of the IUD is either copper, which covers the IUD, or progestin, which is contained in a reservoir within the IUD.

IUDs are among the safest, most effective, and least expensive reversible contraceptives available. Although their modes of action aren't precisely understood, IUDs seem to work primarily by inhibit-

ing the ability of sperm to reach and fertilize the egg. IUDs also appear to thin the uterine lining and sometimes may prevent ovulation. Table 5.4 lists signs and symptoms that may warn of a potential health complication when using an IUD. The mnemonic PAINS can help you remember these symptoms.

## Emergency Contraception

**Emergency contraception (EC)** helps prevent pregnancy *after* sexual intercourse, rather than before or during sex. Therefore, some types of EC are called "the morning-after pill." Despite the nickname, EC does not have to be used right away but can be used up to 3 to 5 days after sex, depending on the method. Women often choose EC if they did not use another form of contraception or if they think their method did not work. EC is also used in cases of rape.

Emergency contraception methods are not 100% effective, but they reduce the likelihood that a woman will become pregnant by about 75% after unprotected sex or after sex with a method that has failed. Because of the lower level of effectiveness of EC compared to other birth control methods, it is not a wise choice for use as a woman's primary method. Like most forms of birth control, EC does not protect against sexually transmitted infections.

Three types of emergency contraception are currently available in the United States: a progestin-only pill (Plan B), various brands of combined oral contraceptives, and insertion of the copper IUD. Both types of emergency contraceptive pills do one of three

### Figure 5.20

**The Intrauterine Device.** An IUD is a small apparatus that is inserted into the uterus. The active ingredient of an IUD is either copper or progestin. The far right photo shows two typical IUDs.

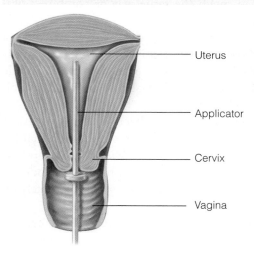
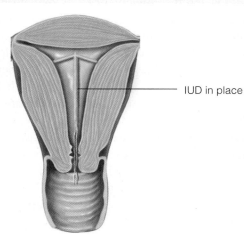
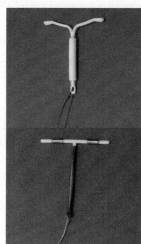

Uterus

Applicator

Cervix

Vagina

IUD in place

things, depending when in the cycle they are taken and whether fertilization has already taken place: They temporarily stop the release of an egg from the ovary, they prevent fertilization, or they prevent a fertilized egg from implanting in the uterine wall. Emergency contraception will not abort an embryo already implanted. Insertion of the copper IUD works in the latter two ways as emergency contraception.

## Sterilization

**Sterilization** is a permanent form of birth control. In the past, sterilization was only available as a surgical procedure, but in 2002 the FDA approved a nonsurgical, irreversible method of female sterilization called Essure. Using a local anesthetic, a physician inserts a tiny spring into each fallopian tube by passing it through the vagina and then the uterus. Over 3 months, the spring irritates the tube, causing it to produce scar tissue that blocks the tube. After the 3-month period, a physician injects dye into the uterus and up into the tubes. An x-ray of the dye-injected area shows whether the tubes are fully blocked.

The surgical form of female sterilization is a **tubal ligation** and involves cutting and tying off the uterine tubes by means of clips, rings, or burning so that

the sperm and egg cannot unite. Male sterilization is a **vasectomy** and involves cutting and tying off the vas deferens to prevent sperm from becoming part of the ejaculate. Tubal ligation is a medically more complicated and more costly procedure than vasectomy, but both are highly effective. Failure is most often the result of surgical error or the spontaneous rejoining of the tubes. **Figure 5.21** illustrates tubal ligation and vasectomy.

The surgical forms of sterilization can be reversed, but subsequent pregnancy rates vary depending on factors such as the type of procedure that was performed, the health of the tubes being rejoined, and the health and age of the patient. Microsurgical techniques provide excellent success rates.

**sterilization** A permanent form of birth control that requires a surgical procedure.

**tubal ligation** Female sterilization that is performed by cutting and tying off the uterine tubes so that the sperm and egg cannot unite.

**vasectomy** Male sterilization that is performed by cutting and tying off the vas deferens to prevent sperm from becoming part of the ejaculate.

### Figure 5.21

**Sterilization Methods.** Female sterilization (a), or tubal ligation, involves cutting and tying off the fallopian tubes. Male sterilization (b), or vasectomy, involves cutting and tying off the vas deferens.

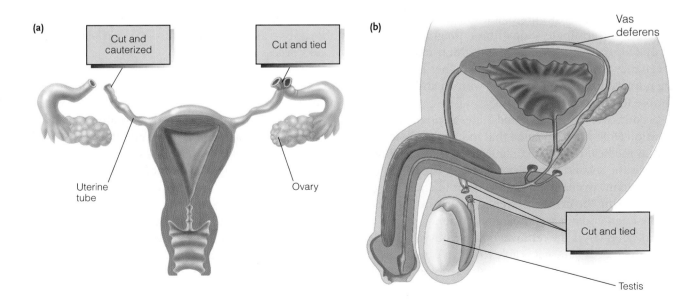

(a)

Cut and cauterized

Cut and tied

Uterine tube

Ovary

(b)

Vas deferens

Cut and tied

Testis

**abortion** Removal of the embryo or fetus from the uterus before it is able to survive on its own.

**medical abortion** A method of drug-induced abortion performed within 9 weeks of the first day of the last period.

**surgical abortion** Includes various methods of induced abortion in which the contents of the uterus are physically removed.

## Healthy Living Practices

- The most effective means to prevent an unwanted pregnancy are sexual abstinence, the use of an IUD, and sterilization, followed closely by hormonal methods.

- If you are using a hormonal method of birth control, consult your healthcare provider when you are taking antibiotics to determine if you should use a backup method of contraception while taking this medication.

- To reduce the risk of contracting or transmitting sexually transmitted infections, use a condom during sexual intercourse. The best way to protect yourself against STIs is to practice sexual abstinence.

## Abortion

Sometimes contraceptive methods fail and an unplanned pregnancy occurs that a woman or a couple chooses to terminate. Sometimes pregnancy seriously jeopardizes a woman's health and ending the pregnancy is the only means of saving her life. There are numerous other reasons why women and couples choose to terminate a pregnancy.

A controversial 1973 United States Supreme Court decision (*Roe v. Wade*) ruled that induced abortion is a legal medical procedure. States may regulate abortions in the second trimester to protect the health of the pregnant woman, but the decision to end a pregnancy during the first trimester is the private concern of a woman and her healthcare practitioner.

An **abortion** is the removal of the embryo or fetus from the uterus before it is able to survive on its own. During a *spontaneous abortion*, the body expels the embryo, usually because of serious genetic defects, although there may be other causes. Spontaneous

abortions (miscarriages) generally occur during the first trimester. Ten percent to 20% of pregnancies end in spontaneous abortion.

An *induced abortion* is one that does not happen on its own. It is caused by taking certain drugs (a medical abortion) or by having certain physical procedures performed (a surgical abortion). During the first trimester, both types of abortions can be performed.

A **medical abortion** can be performed within 9 weeks of the first day of the last period and uses a combination of the drugs mifepristone and misoprostol. Mifepristone causes changes in the pregnant woman's body so that it cannot sustain the pregnancy and the embryo/fetus detaches from the uterine wall. Misoprostol causes the uterus to contract and expel its contents. According to the Centers for Disease Control and Prevention (CDC), about 13% of abortions are performed this way.[24]

In a **surgical abortion**, a physician physically removes the contents of the uterus. *Vacuum (suction) aspiration* is used from 3 to 12 weeks of gestation. It can be performed in the physician's office in approximately 10 to 20 minutes with the use of a local anesthetic. To perform a vacuum aspiration, the physician dilates (widens) the cervix slightly and inserts a slender, hollow plastic tube through the vagina and cervix into the uterus. The tube is connected to a suction aspirator, which draws the tissue out of the uterus and into a container (**Figure 5.22**).

Vacuum aspiration is used for 78% of abortions;[24] the embryo is less than an inch long at this time. Thus, 91–92% of abortions are performed either medically (using drugs) or with vacuum aspiration early in pregnancy. According to CDC data, most abortions—almost two-thirds—are performed at 8 weeks or less of gestation.[24]

If the abortion is performed between 12 and 15 weeks of gestation, the uterus is often scraped with a tool called a curette after the vacuum aspiration is completed. This procedure is commonly called a *D&C*, which means dilation and curettage.

Abortions that are performed during 15 to 21 weeks of development are performed somewhat like a D&C, but forceps are also used to remove larger pieces of tissue. Therefore, the cervix must be dilated to a greater extent to allow the entry of the forceps. This procedure is called a dilation and evacuation, or *D&E*. General anesthesia is often used for this procedure. According to the CDC, only about 7% of abortions are performed between 14 and 20 weeks of gestation.[24]

## Figure 5.22

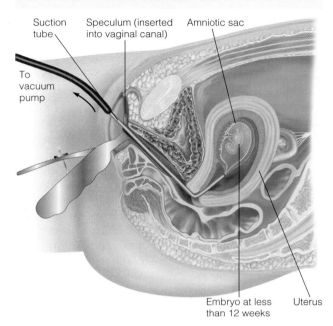

**Vacuum (Suction) Aspiration.** During this procedure, a thin, hollow tube is inserted through the vagina and cervix to the uterus. A suction aspirator (vacuum pump) draws tissue out of the uterus and into a container.

Suction tube

Speculum (inserted into vaginal canal)

Amniotic sac

To vacuum pump

Embryo at less than 12 weeks

Uterus

There are two basic methods of abortion for the 1% that is performed at 21 weeks of gestation or more: induction, and intact dilation and extraction. *Induction* is a form of abortion in which labor is artificially induced (started). Saline abortions are one method of induction: A physician inserts a long needle through the abdominal wall and into the amniotic sac. A salt solution is injected into the sac, which causes the quick death of the fetus. The uterus begins contractions within 12 to 24 hours, and the woman delivers a dead fetus. This procedure is performed using a local anesthetic. Other types of solutions and prostaglandins (hormone-like substances that cause the uterus to contract) are also used for induction.

A special type of D&E procedure called an *intact dilation and extraction* (IDX or intact D&X) is the so-called partial birth abortion procedure. President George W. Bush signed the Partial-Birth Abortion Ban Act in November 2003, which criminalizes the procedure. Physicians from many states challenged the constitutionality of the law. Three federal judges from California, New York, and Nebraska ruled that the legislation had many constitutional defects and rejected the ban. The question of the constitutionality of the law went to the Supreme Court, and on April 18, 2007, the high court ruled in a 5–4 decision that the federal Partial-Birth Abortion Ban Act of 2003 was constitutional.

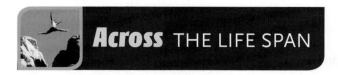

**Across** THE LIFE SPAN

## SEXUAL DEVELOPMENT

The gender of an individual is set at the time of fertilization and is determined by the type of sex chromosomes (genes) it receives from its parents. Females have two X chromosomes; males have an X and a Y.

During the 7th week of development, the embryo with a Y chromosome begins to develop testes. The developing testes secrete male hormones collectively called androgens. These hormones direct the development of a male reproductive system. Embryos and fetuses without a Y chromosome begin to develop ovaries during the 9th week. The absence of androgens results in the development of a female reproductive system.

After birth, the secretion of the androgen testosterone in male babies nearly ceases and does not resume until puberty, the time of sexual maturation. The female reproductive system does not become active until that time as well.

Puberty is a stage of development during which the endocrine (hormone) and reproductive systems mature. Puberty begins at approximately 10 to 11 years of age and concludes about 5 or 6 years later. Girls usually enter puberty about 2 years earlier than boys do. Scientists do not know what triggers this developmental process.

During childhood, the production of a hormone that stimulates the release of male and female sex hormones is suppressed. At the onset of puberty, the suppression ceases and the brain begins releasing the hormone that regulates the production of testosterone in males and estrogen in females. As puberty proceeds, the brain secretes greater and greater amounts of this hormone; thus more and more testosterone or estrogen is secreted. These hormones stimulate the physical changes of puberty. These changes include growth spurts resulting from the growth of the skeleton (especially the long bones), the development of pubic and underarm hair, and the growth and maturation of the reproductive tract.

In males, building levels of testosterone result in an enlarging of the testes and penis, deepening of the voice as a result of an enlargement of the voice

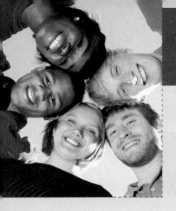

# Diversity in Health

## Menopause

Menopause is a time of transition for every woman who reaches her 50s, but transition is about the only thing women universally experience during this time. The symptoms of menopause and attitudes regarding this process vary extensively among women across cultures. Why do these differences exist?

One hypothesis is that if a society regards menopause as a positive time, the symptoms of menopause reported by its women will decrease in number and severity. Certain evidence seems to support this hypothesis. For example, during their childbearing years, the Rajput women of Northern India are socially constrained and cannot move about freely in their villages. Those who no longer menstruate are freed of this constraint. Interestingly, these women report no symptoms of menopause. Similarly, Mayan women look upon menopause as a lifting of the burden of childbearing. They, too, report no symptoms of hot flashes or cold sweats such as are typically reported by North American women. Additionally, Yanomamo women (forest-dwellers who live near the border between Brazil and Venezuela) eagerly await menopause, which is considered the time of "older age," for this time of life brings increased status and decision-making power in their society.

In a multiethnic study of U.S. women, Green and Santoro found that most menopausal symptoms varied by ethnicity and culture as well. Night sweats and hot flashes were reported more often by African American and Hispanic women, while vaginal dryness was reported most often by Hispanic women. And even though other menopausal symptoms varied among Hispanic women, the symptoms correlated with their country of origin.

Nevertheless, the diversity of the symptoms and experiences of women of various cultures regarding menopause cannot be attributed solely to differences in culture. Ayers, Forshaw, and Hunter took a broader look at the correlation between menopausal symptoms and attitudes toward menopause, conducting a review of cross-cultural studies on the subject. The researchers determined that women with more negative attitudes toward menopause reported more symptoms of menopause when experiencing this life transition, and those with less negative attitudes experienced fewer symptoms.

Menopausal symptoms and experiences must also be evaluated in the context of risk factors for death and disease. But just as it affects attitudes, culture affects lifestyle, and lifestyle affects health. Thus, culturally influenced lifestyles affect susceptibility to disease, the aging process, and the quality of life and, in turn, may account for some of the differences in the perception of menopausal symptoms among women. Cultural differences in the experience of menopause exist but appear to be so intertwined with the various facets of a woman's life that the effect of culture alone may be difficult to assess.

*Sources:* Ayers, B., et al. (2010). The impact of attitudes towards the menopause on women's symptom experience: A systematic review. *Maturitas,* 65(1):28–36; Green, R., & Santoro, N. (2009). Menopausal symptoms and ethnicity: The Study of Women's Health Across the Nation. *Women's Health,* 5(2):127–133; and Melby, M. K., et al. (2005). Culture and symptom reporting at menopause. *Human Reproduction Update,* 11:495–512.

box, development of facial hair, broadening of the shoulders, and enlargement of the arm, chest, and leg muscles. Under the direction of testosterone, the seminiferous tubules begin manufacturing sperm. A significant developmental event in pubertal boys is semen emission during sleep, called nocturnal emissions or wet dreams. Initially, sperm are not present in the semen.

In females, estrogen results in the development of the breasts and the rounding of the hips. Females experience **menarche**, the first menstruation, at around 12 years of age. The normal range for menarche is 8 to 15 years of age. A delay of the menarche may occur in girls with chronic diseases, such as diabetes mellitus, those with disorders that affect their nutritional status, such as anorexia nervosa, and those undergoing strenuous training, such as Olympic hopefuls.

When a woman reaches 45 to 55 years of age, most of her ovarian follicles (eggs) have matured, and the remaining follicles are old. During some months, these aging follicles do not reach maturity and ovulation does not take place. Without mature egg follicles, the normal cyclic secretion of estrogen and progesterone does not occur, and the menses become irregular. Eventually, all follicles stop maturing, estrogen and progesterone are no longer secreted, and the menses cease. The cessation of the menses is called menopause. This term means the final menstrual period, but it is widely used to refer to the few years of transition when a woman passes from her reproductive years to her nonreproductive years. The Diversity in Health essay discusses menopausal symptoms and attitudes across cultures.

As the hormonal changes of menopause take place, women usually experience symptoms such as hot flashes and physiologic changes such as thinning of the vaginal walls and vaginal dryness. In addition, the loss of estrogen results in an increased risk of osteoporosis and heart disease.

In a 2007 report, the International Menopause Society (IMS) updated recommendations on postmenopausal hormone therapy (HT), clarifying the sometimes confusing and conflicting information that became available beginning in 2002.[25] These recommendations were the most recent as of late 2011. In 2002, data from the Women's Health Initiative (WHI) trial were published and showed that HT did not protect postmenopausal women against heart attacks as previously thought.[26] Since the initial 2002 report more information has become available, and more importance has been placed on the fact that the study population for the WHI trial was women with a mean age of recruitment of 63 years.

The IMS recommends that "hormone therapy should be part of an overall strategy including lifestyle recommendations regarding diet, exercise, smoking and alcohol for maintaining the health of postmenopausal women. The risks and benefits of HT differ for women around the time of menopause compared to those for older women." The IMS notes that, if used, HT and its dosage should be tailored to each patient by her physician, and that menopausal women should become knowledgeable of the risks

and benefits of the therapy. The IMS concludes that HT is "effective in preventing the bone loss associated with the menopause," "may be cardioprotective if started around the time of menopause and continued long-term," "has benefits for connective tissue, skin, joints and intervertebral disks," "may reduce the risk of colon cancer," and "is associated with a reduced risk of Alzheimer's disease." Combined estrogen–progestin regimens rather than estrogen alone provide a reduced risk of endometrial cancer. Regarding potential serious adverse effects of HT, the IMS concludes that the possible risk of breast cancer is less than 0.1% per year and that the risk of blood clots and stroke increases with age but is minimal until age 60 years.[25]

Men also undergo changes in their reproductive systems during middle age. Men are fertile throughout their lives, although the number of healthy, active sperm they produce decreases as they grow older. Middle-aged men experience a decline in testosterone, ejaculate with less force and less volume, and take longer to regain an erection after orgasm. In addition, the prostate gland usually enlarges. See the Managing Your Health essay "Enlargement of the Prostate."

Although both men and women undergo changes in their reproductive systems beginning at middle age, these changes do not have to impair their ability to have a healthy, enjoyable sex life extending into their elderly years.

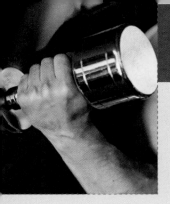

# Managing Your Health

## Enlargement of the Prostate

If you are male and older than 45 years, your prostate may be enlarging slowly. If you are not yet 45 years old, prostate enlargement may be in your future. This process of enlargement is common for middle-aged and older men; it is part of the aging process and may never be a cause for concern. However, about 50% of men in their 60s and about 90% of men in their 70s and 80s complain of problems caused by an enlarged prostate gland, also known as prostatic hyperplasia, or benign prostatic hypertrophy (BPH).

How can an enlarged prostate affect your health? Notice in Figure 5.1 that the prostate gland surrounds the urethra beneath the urinary bladder. As the prostate enlarges, it may squeeze the urethra, hampering the flow of urine through this tube. Therefore, the symptoms that may appear first as a result of BPH are difficulty in beginning to urinate, a decrease in the force of the urine stream, a dribbling of urine after urinating, a sensation of a full bladder after urinating, and a need to urinate 5 or 10 minutes after urinating.

As the prostate squeezes the urethra more and more, the muscles of the bladder wall respond by thickening as they forcefully push urine through the constricted urethra. This thickened bladder is irritated easily, however, and contracts more readily. Therefore, the following symptoms develop: an urgency to urinate and/or leaking of urine; more frequent urination, especially at night; and painful urination. Eventually, urine flow can be blocked to the point that emergency treatment is necessary.

There are several treatments for BPH. Surgery is usually undertaken when symptoms are severe. During the surgery, the portion of the prostate squeezing the urethra is removed. Laser therapy, radio frequency therapy, or microwave therapy can be used to destroy the enlarged prostate tissue as well. These procedures are less invasive than traditional surgical techniques are and usually have fewer long-term side effects and complications.

Another treatment is balloon dilatation. During this procedure, an inflatable device is inserted into the urethra through the opening at the tip of the penis. The device is inflated at the area of constriction and is then removed. This procedure widens the urethra to alleviate symptoms. Various medications also ease the symptoms of BPH.

Enlargement of the prostate may also be caused by prostate cancer. This cancer is the second most common cause of cancer deaths in men (lung cancer being the first). However, it usually does not appear in men younger than 55 years, and it is generally a slow-growing

form of cancer. Its symptoms overlap with those of BPH and include difficult, frequent, and painful urination and blood in the urine.

The symptoms of BPH and prostate cancer are more than just a nuisance. The restriction or blockage of urine flow can damage the kidneys; prostate cancer can spread, resulting in death. To avoid the discomforts and possible serious consequences of these conditions, therefore, the prostate should be examined regularly. The American Cancer Society recommends that men older than 50 years have a digital rectal examination every year. During this examination, the physician inserts a gloved, lubricated finger into the rectum. Because the prostate lies next to the rectum (**Figure 5.D**), the physician can palpate (feel by pressing lightly) the size of the prostate.

Newer diagnostic techniques include transrectal ultrasound, in which the physician inserts an ultrasound probe into the rectum that results in an image of the prostate on a monitor.

A blood test has been developed to help detect prostate cancer. This test is known as prostate-specific antigen (PSA) and helps find many prostate cancers years before they would otherwise be detected. See Chapter 13 for a discussion of current recommendations for using the PSA test.

### Figure 5.D

**Digital Examination of the Prostate.** The physician can feel an enlargement of the prostate gland by inserting a gloved finger into the rectum.

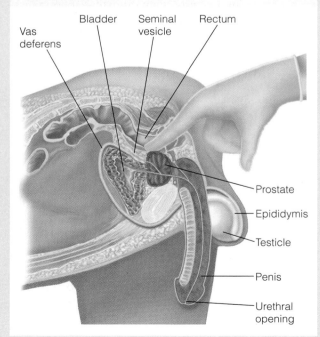

# Analyzing Health-Related Information

Explain why you think this web page about folic acid is a reliable or an unreliable source of information. Use the "Assessing Information on the Internet" portion of the model for analyzing health-related information to guide your thinking; the main points of the model are noted here. The model is fully explained in Chapter 1. If you wish to visit this site, the web address is www.cdc.gov/ncbddd/folicacid.

- What is the source of the information?
- Is the site sponsored by a nationally known health or medical organization or affiliated with a well-known medical research institution or major university? If not, is the site staffed by well-respected and credentialed experts in the field?
- Does the site include up-to-date references from a well-known, respected medical or scientific journal or links to reputable websites, such as nationally recognized medical organizations?
- Is the information at the website current?

Based on your analysis, do you think that this web page is a reliable source of health-related information? Summarize your reasons for coming to this conclusion.

If you are unsure of the credibility of the site after answering the preceding questions, continue with the following six Analyzing Health-Related Information questions.

1. Which statements on the website are verifiable facts, and which are unverified statements or value claims?
2. Does the person, organization, or institution that developed the website have the appropriate background and credentials in the topic area? What can you do to check credentials?
3. What might be the motives and biases inherent to the website?
4. What is the main point of the article, ad, or claim made on the site? Which information is relevant to the issue, main point, product, or service? Which information is irrelevant?
5. Does the source of information present the pros and cons of the topic or the benefits and risks of the product?
6. Does the source of information attack the credibility of conventional scientists or medical authorities?

Based on your additional analysis, do you think that this web page is a reliable source of health-related information? Summarize your reasons for coming to this conclusion.

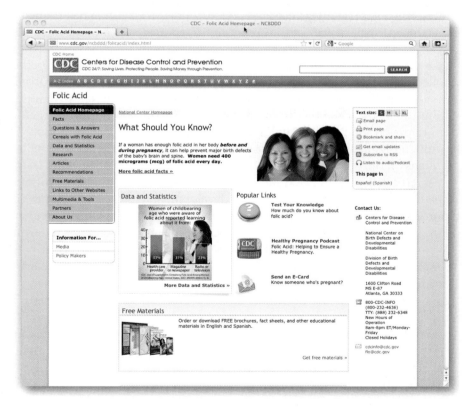

# CHAPTER REVIEW

## Summary

Sexual reproduction involves the fertilization of an egg by a sperm, forming the first cell of a new individual. The male reproductive system produces sperm (male sex cells) and delivers them to the vagina of the female. Sperm are produced in the testes and are moved along the male reproductive tract with the seminal fluid secreted by accessory sex glands during ejaculation.

Eggs (ova; female sex cells) develop and mature in the female reproductive system, which also receives sperm and provides an environment in which a fertilized ovum can develop. Eggs mature in the ovaries, are fertilized in the uterine tubes, and develop in the uterus during pregnancy.

Women experience cyclic monthly hormonal changes that orchestrate physiologic changes that take place in the ovaries and uterus. The changes are collectively called the menstrual cycle. During the menstrual cycle, an ovum matures and is released from the ovary while the lining of the uterus thickens in preparation for the implantation of a fertilized ovum. If pregnancy does not occur, the uterine lining sloughs off during the menses.

If fertilization takes place, the embryo/fetus develops in the uterus of the female. This developmental process is termed pregnancy, or gestation. Various environmental influences (teratogens) such as drugs, alcohol, viruses, and dietary deficiencies can damage the embryo or fetus early in pregnancy. A woman preparing for pregnancy should have a medical checkup; eat a well-balanced and nutritious diet; avoid drinking alcohol, smoking cigarettes, and taking drugs; and possibly seek genetic counseling.

Women who become pregnant may notice physical signs of this condition such as a missed period, nausea, fatigue, and moodiness. A woman can conduct a home pregnancy test or have a laboratory test performed to determine if she is pregnant.

Pregnancy lasts about 38 weeks and is typically described in terms of trimesters, or 3-month periods. During the first trimester, all the organ systems of the body form and become functional. The second and third trimesters are periods of growth and refinement of the organ systems.

The process of childbirth (labor) takes place in three stages: dilation, expulsion, and placental delivery. During dilation, the uterine muscles contract, causing the cervix to widen (dilate) and thin out (efface). During the second stage of labor the baby is born. Within 15 to 30 minutes after delivery of the baby, the placenta is expelled from the uterus.

Couples often want to avoid pregnancy for various reasons, so they choose some form of birth control, or contraception. Contraceptive methods are varied and can be grouped into seven categories: abstinence and natural methods, chemical methods, barrier methods, hormonal methods, intrauterine devices, sterilization, and emergency contraception. Each method has different advantages, disadvantages, and levels of effectiveness. Abstinence, sterilization, IUDs, and hormonal methods are the most effective means of contraception. Using condoms and practicing abstinence are the best ways to prevent the transmission of sexually transmitted infections while at the same time preventing pregnancy.

Sometimes contraceptive methods fail and an unplanned pregnancy occurs that a woman or a couple chooses to terminate. Women and couples choose to terminate a pregnancy for other reasons, including health concerns of the mother. Terminating a pregnancy involves the removal of the embryo or fetus from the uterus before it is able to survive on its own. This process is called an induced abortion. In the United States today, there is great controversy over a woman's right to choose induced abortion. More than 90% of abortions are performed either medically (using drugs) or with vacuum aspiration early in pregnancy; almost two-thirds are performed at 8 weeks or less of gestation.

The sex of an individual is set at the time of fertilization and is determined by the type of sex chromosomes (genes) that the embryo receives from its parents. The male and female reproductive tracts develop during gestation. Further maturation does not continue until puberty, the time of sexual maturation, which begins at approximately 10 to 11 years of age and concludes about 5 or 6 years later. Men and women both undergo changes to their reproductive function during middle age. Women have a cessation of the menses as a result of physiologic and hormonal changes and can no longer reproduce. Men can reproduce throughout their lives but at middle age experience a decline in testosterone and sexual functioning.

# Applying What You Have Learned

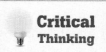
**Critical Thinking**

1. A woman is 42 years old, unmarried, and has sex regularly with a single sexual partner. She has been using an intrauterine device but has developed an infection with the insertion of her most recent IUD. She must change to another method of birth control. If you were this woman, which method would you choose? Provide evidence that your choice is prudent. **Application**

2. In this chapter, much attention is given to the theoretical and actual effectiveness of various types of birth control. When you look at Table 5.3, which column should carry more weight in your decision making—the theoretical or the actual effectiveness? Give reasons for your answer. **Analysis**

3. You have been asked to lead a discussion in your health class about maximizing maternal and fetal health during pregnancy. You may discuss any information in this chapter relevant to this issue. (You may add topics not mentioned in this chapter as well.) List the topics you will discuss and briefly describe the importance of each. **Synthesis**

4. Devise an assessment that will help people evaluate their attitudes toward abortion. Explain why you think that your assessment tool will accurately evaluate these attitudes. **Evaluation**

| **Application** | **Analysis** | **Synthesis** | **Evaluation** | |
|---|---|---|---|---|
| using information in a new situation. | breaking down information into component parts. | putting together information from different sources. | making informed decisions. | **Key** |

# Reflecting on Your Health

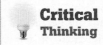
**Critical Thinking**

1. Contracting sexually transmitted infections can endanger your health and your ability to have children. What is the relationship between responsible sexual behavior and reproductive health in your life?

2. If you are a man, what did you learn in this chapter about female reproductive health that was new to you? If you are a woman, what did you learn in this chapter about male reproductive health that was new to you? How will this new knowledge affect your behavior toward the opposite sex? How might it affect your attitudes?

3. Most contraceptive methods focus on the female reproductive system. Because of this focus, should women have the primary responsibility for contraception? Why or why not?

4. In the United States, a woman's right to choose to have an abortion (other than a "partial-birth" abortion) is protected by law. Do you think that the law should be changed to criminalize abortion in general? If so, why? Should abortion be legal only in certain circumstances? If so, when?

5. Table 5.1 lists selected teratogens. If a woman knowingly exposes her embryo or fetus to teratogenic drugs such as alcohol, should she be prosecuted in the criminal justice system? Why or why not?

# References

1. Sharpe, R. M. (2010). Environmental/lifestyle effects on spermatogenesis. *Philosophical Transactions of The Royal Society B, 365*:1697–1712.

2. The National Women's Health Information Center. (2009). *Menstruation and the menstrual cycle fact sheet.* Retrieved on February 22, 2011, from http://www.womenshealth.gov/faq/menstruation.cfm#d

3. Freeman, E. W., et al. (2011). Core symptoms that discriminate premenstrual syndrome. *Journal of Women's Health, 20*(1):29–35.

4. Shulman, L. P. (2010). Gynecological management of premenstrual symptoms. *Current Pain and Headache Reports, 14*(5):367–375.

5. Centers for Disease Control and Prevention. (2005). Toxic shock syndrome. Retrieved on February 23, 2011, from http://www.cdc.gov/ncidod/dbmd/diseaseinfo/toxicshock_t.htm

6. Luke, B., & Brown, M. B. (2007). Elevated risks of pregnancy complication and adverse outcomes with increasing maternal age. *Human Reproduction, 22*:1264–1272.

7. Centers for Disease Control and Prevention. (2008). Male circumcision and risk for HIV transmission and other health conditions: Implications for the United States. Retrieved on February 23, 2011, from http://www.cdc.gov/hiv/resources/factsheets/circumcision.htm

8. Tobian, A. A. R., et al. (2009). Male circumcision for the prevention of HSV-2 and HPV infections and syphilis. *New England Journal of Medicine, 360*:1298–1309.

9. American Academy of Pediatrics. (1999). Circumcision policy statement. *Pediatrics, 103*:686–693.

10. American Academy of Pediatrics. (2005). AAP publications retired and reaffirmed. *Pediatrics, 116*:796.

11. Brett, K., & Barfield, W. (2008). Prevalence of self-reported postpartum depressive dymptoms—17 states, 2004–2005. *Morbidity and Mortality Weekly Report, 57*:361–366.

12. Centers for Disease Control and Prevention. (2009). Infertility. Retrieved on February 24, 2011, from http://www.cdc.gov/nchs/fastats/fertile.htm

13. De Vos, M., et al. (2010). Primary ovarian insufficiency. *Lancet, 376*(9744):911–921.

14. Olive, D. L. (2010). Exercise and fertility: An update. *Current Opinions in Obstetrics and Gynecology, 22*(4):259–263.

15. Brewer, C. J., & Balen, A. H. (2010). The adverse effects of obesity on conception and implantation. *Reproduction, 140*(3):347–364.

16. Anderson, K., et al. (2010). Lifestyle factors in people seeking infertility treatment—A review. *Australian and New Zealand Journal of Obstetrics and Gynaecology, 50*(1):8–20.

17. Ross, C., et al. (2010). A systematic review of the effect of oral antioxidants on male infertility. *Reproductive Biomedicine Online, 20*(6):711–723.

18. Basatemur, E., & Sutcliffe, A. (2008). Follow-up of children born after ART. *Placenta, 29*:S135–S140.

19. Frank-Herrmann, P., et al. (2007). The effectiveness of a fertility awareness based method to avoid pregnancy in relation to a couple's sexual behavior during the fertile time: A prospective longitudinal study. *Human Reproduction, 22*:1310–1319.

20. Herold, B. C., et al. (2011). Female genital tract secretions and semen impact the development of microbicides for the prevention of HIV and other sexually transmitted infections. *American Journal of Reproductive Immunology, 65*:325–333.

21. Guttmacher Institute. (2010). Facts on contraceptive use in the United States. Retrieved on February 24, 2011, from http://www.guttmacher.org/pubs/fb_contr_use.html

22. International Collaboration of Epidemiological Studies of Cervical Cancer, Appleby, P., Beral, V., Berrington de González, A., Colin, D., Franceschi, S., et al. (2007). Cervical cancer and hormonal contraceptives: collaborative reanalysis of individual data for 16,573 women with cervical cancer and 35,509 women without cervical cancer from 24 epidemiological studies. *Lancet, 370*:1609–1621.

23. Wan, G. J., et al. (2007). Treatment satisfaction with a transdermal contraceptive patch or oral contraceptives. *Contraception, 75*:281–284.

24. Pazol, K., et al. (2011). Abortion surveillance—United States, 2007. *Morbidity and Mortality Weekly Update, 60*(1):1–39. Retrieved on February 25, 2011, from http://www.cdc.gov/mmwr/pdf/ss/ss6001.pdf

25. Pines, A., Sturdee, D. W., Birkhäuser, M. H., Schneider, H. P. G., Gambacciani, M., & Panay, N., on behalf of the Board of the International Menopause Society. (2007). IMS updated recommendations on postmenopausal hormone therapy. *Climacteric, 10*:181–194.

26. Women's Health Initiative Memory Study Investigators. (2004). Conjugated equine estrogens and global cognitive function in postmenopausal women: Women's Health Initiative Memory Study. *Journal of the American Medical Association, 291*(24):2959–2968.

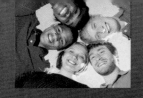
**Diversity in Health**
The Virtue of Virginity

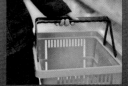
**Consumer Health**
Ginseng and Sexual Prowess

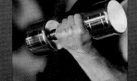
**Managing Your Health**
Minding Your Sexual Manners

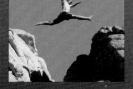
**Across the Life Span**
Sexuality

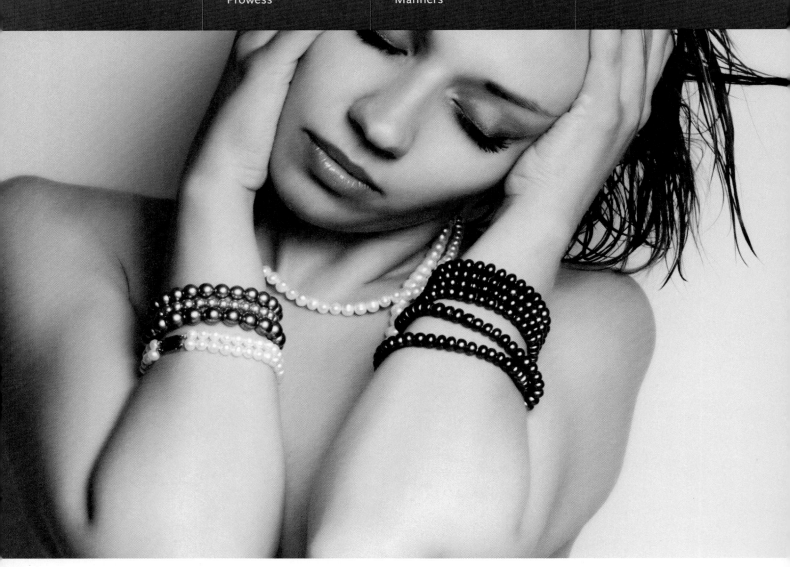

# Chapter Overview

How biological and psychological factors influence sexual behavior

The phases of sexual response cycles

Symptoms of and treatments for sexual dysfunctions

How culture affects sexuality

Nature versus nurture and sexual orientation

The diversity of sexual behavior

Definitions and theories of love and commitment

# Student Workbook

Self-Assessment: Male Sexual Quotient Self-Assessment Questionnaire | The Love Attitudes Scale

Changing Health Habits: Would a Behavior Change Improve Your Relationship?

# Do You Know?

What are common sexual practices?

How living together affects future marriage?

How to communicate effectively?

# Relationships and Sexuality

**"...promoters and advertisers know that 'sex sells.'"**

Sex is everywhere in our society. You can find sexually explicit images and information in movies, books, and TV shows, on the Web, and in the lyrics of popular music. If you browse through magazines or scan billboards, you are likely to see pictures of attractive young men and women in advertisements for clothes, perfumes, and cars. Whether their product is a movie, jewelry, or pair of jeans, promoters and advertisers know that "sex sells." What does sex mean to you?

The term *sex* refers to one's gender, male or female, as well as to sexual intercourse and other intimate physical activities that involve the genitals. **Sexuality**, however, is more than gender or reproductive organs. Sexuality is the aspect of personality that encompasses an individual's sexual thoughts, feelings, attitudes, and actions. Each person has a unique collection of private and public sexual experiences that shapes his or her sexuality.

**sexuality** The aspect of personality that encompasses a person's sexual thoughts, feelings, attitudes, and actions.

Numerous biological, psychological, social, and cultural forces interact to influence a person's sexual development, sexual health, and interpersonal relationships (**Figure 6.1**). Sexuality is woven into every aspect of human life; sex affects a person's identity, self-esteem, emotions, personality, relationships, lifestyle, and overall health.

Being knowledgeable about sexuality is important for maintaining good health and optimal well-being. Misinformation can lead to serious consequences, such as unintentional pregnancies or sexually transmitted infections. Additionally, people who are well informed about sexuality can communicate effectively with their medical practitioners and sexual partners regarding reproductive or sexual concerns.

Throughout life, you make various sexually related decisions, such as deciding with whom to have an intimate sexual relationship. Such decisions can have serious effects on your health and well-being, as well as those of others. By considering how your actions may affect yourself and your sexual partners, you can become a more sexually responsible person.

### Figure 6.1

**Sexuality Model.** Numerous biological, psychological, social, and cultural forces interact to influence sexual development, sexual health, and interpersonal relationships.

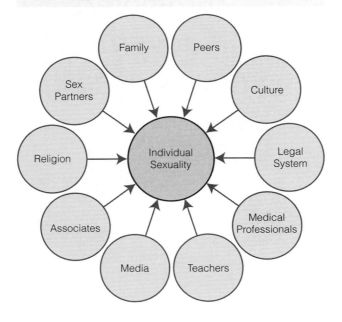

## Human Sexual Behavior

The reproductive activity of most complex animals includes behaviors commonly referred to as courtship and mating. Unlike other animals, humans exhibit a variety of complex sexual behaviors that do not necessarily result in reproduction. People often engage in sexual activity for pleasure and relaxation or to help maintain the emotional bonds of their intimate relationships. Some individuals, however, use their sexuality to dominate, exploit, or harm others. What factors influence human sexual behavior?

### The Biology of Sexual Behavior

The motivation to pursue sexual activity—the sex drive, or *libido*—is an instinctual behavior moderated by the sex hormones. The ovaries and the testes, glands that make up part of the hormonal (endocrine) system, secrete these chemical messengers. The endocrine system is so named because of the endocrine glands, such as the ovaries and the testes, which secrete the hormones. Glands are individual cells or groups of cells that secrete substances. They are called *endocrine* because they release substances within (*endo-*) the body, rather than secreting substances that exit the body, such as sweat.

The endocrine system plays an important role in sexual functioning. The pituitary, located in the brain, and the ovaries and testes produce hormones that affect sexual functioning (**Figure 6.2**). Additionally, the hypothalamus, located above the pituitary, produces hormones that trigger the secretion of pituitary hormones. During puberty in males, pituitary hormones activate the maturation of the male reproductive structures and the release of increased levels of the male sex hormone, testosterone. Testosterone plays a role in the maturation of the male reproductive structures, stimulates the development of sperm, and triggers and maintains the development of the secondary sexual characteristics such as the growth of a beard and the deepening of the voice. During puberty in females, pituitary hormones cause maturation of the ovaries, which then begin secreting the female sex hormones estrogen and progesterone. Estrogen stimulates maturation of the uterus and vagina, development of the female secondary sexual characteristics such as the development of breasts, and a change in the distribution of body fat.

During middle age, the production of sex hormones declines. After 40 years of age, men produce less testosterone and fewer sperm, although accelerated declines appear to be slowed by practicing healthy behaviors, such as avoiding overweight and obesity.[1] Despite this reduction, elderly men can still father children. When women reach menopause, usually between 45 and 55 years of age, their estrogen and progesterone levels decrease dramatically. As a result, menopausal women are no longer fertile. However, most healthy elderly men and women continue to have an interest in sex, and they engage in sexual activity. Research conducted for the 2010 AARP Survey of Midlife and Older Adults reveals that among those older than 70 years of age, 80% of men and 39% of women believed that a satisfying sexual relationship was important to the overall quality of life. In addition, 15% of men and 5% of women older than 70 years reported engaging in sexual intercourse at least once a week.[2]

## The Psychology of Sexual Behavior

Certain thoughts, sensations, and emotions modulate sexual behavior, as do the sex hormones. Included in this psychological mix are factors that can influence sexual behavior positively, such as satisfaction with one's body, good physical and emotional health, absence of beliefs that can hinder sexual responsiveness or enjoyment, previous positive sexual experiences, and high self-esteem.

Many **sexologists**, scientists who study human sexuality, think that people who have high self-esteem are more likely to have positive attitudes concerning their sexuality than persons with poor self-concepts. However, people frequently judge their bodies and sexual prowess against unrealistic standards of physical attractiveness and sexual ability that are presented in the media. As a result, some individuals develop feelings of sexual inadequacy and low self-esteem because they feel sexually unattractive or inept. People who have these feelings may be unable to enjoy their sexuality and may be unable to form fulfilling intimate relationships.

If you are male, you may want to assess your level of sexual function and satisfaction by taking the "Male Sexual Quotient Self-Assessment Questionnaire" in the Student Workbook pages at the end of this book.

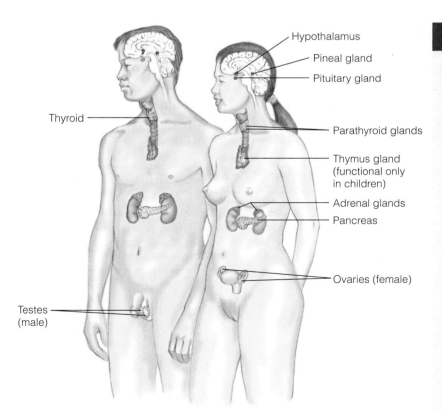

Thyroid

Testes (male)

Hypothalamus
Pineal gland
Pituitary gland
Parathyroid glands
Thymus gland (functional only in children)
Adrenal glands
Pancreas
Ovaries (female)

### Figure 6.2

**Endocrine Glands.** The pituitary, ovaries, and testes produce hormones that affect sexual functioning. The hypothalamus produces hormones that trigger the secretion of pituitary hormones.

**testosterone** A male sex hormone (androgen) that plays a role in the development of functionally mature sperm and is responsible for the development and maintenance of male secondary sexual characteristics such as the deepening of the voice and the growth of facial hair.

**vasocongestion** A condition in which the spongy tissue of the penis and clitoris expands with blood during sexual arousal.

**myotonia** An increase in muscle tension throughout the body during sexual arousal.

# The Sexual Response

The sexual response in both males and females is governed primarily by the nervous system rather than by hormones. Hormones are chemicals secreted in one part of the body that have an effect in another. **Testosterone**, the "male" hormone (women also secrete testosterone), helps maintain the sex drive, or libido.

The two major physical changes that occur during sexual arousal are vasocongestion and myotonia. **Vasocongestion** occurs as blood flow away from the sexual organs is reduced. The spongy tissue of the penis and clitoris expands with blood and these structures become erect. **Myotonia**, an increase in muscle tension, occurs throughout the body.

**The Masters and Johnson Model** Both sexes have broader responses than just these events. This pattern of responses is termed the *sexual response cycle*. First defined by Masters and Johnson, it is usually thought of as having four phases: excitement, plateau, orgasm, and resolution (**Figure 6.3**).

During the *excitement phase* of the sexual response cycle, both men and women have a heightened sexual awareness. Certain thoughts, sights, touches, and even sounds or odors lead to a rush of blood to the clitoris and vaginal opening in women and to the penis in men.

In men, the penis expands as blood fills spaces in its columns of spongy tissue. As a result, the penis becomes erect, and the expansion of the tissue compresses the veins that take blood away from this organ (see Figure 5.2). Consequently, as blood flow into the penis increases, blood flow out of the penis decreases. This decrease in outward blood flow maintains the erection.

In women, glands in the vulvar area secrete mucus-like fluid. The congestion of blood in the vulvar area and in the vagina swells the labia and pushes fluid through the vaginal wall. These fluids are lubricants for sexual intercourse. Blood also rushes to the breasts. In response, the breasts swell. The nipples become erect as smooth muscles contract. Many women also exhibit a sex flush at this time, a reddening of the skin as blood flow through it increases.

As sexual excitement continues, the *plateau phase* begins. The heart rate, blood pressure, respiration rate, and level of muscle tension all increase. During the plateau phase, the erection of the male intensifies as the penis is massaged rhythmically by intercourse (anal or vaginal), manual stimulation, or oral stimulation. Sensory impulses from tactile sensations in both sexes reinforce their sexual sensations. In women, the lower third of the vagina constricts around the penis. The upper two-thirds of the vagina widens as the uterus and cervix lift up, creating a space for the semen. Continued stimulation of the clitoris and penis leads to the next phase of the sexual response—the orgasmic phase.

In men, ejaculation occurs during the *orgasmic phase*. This involuntary response (over which men can exert some voluntary control) results when the nervous system sends messages to muscles in the walls of the vas deferens and urethra to contract. At the same time, the seminal vesicles and prostate receive messages to release their secretions. The pelvic muscles also rhythmically contract. Orgasm in women is characterized by rhythmic contractions of the pelvic muscles and vaginal walls. Both sexes experience a peak of sexual pleasure at orgasm. Erection and ejaculation are the two primary components of the male sex act. The clitoris of the female becomes erect during sexual activity and she achieves orgasm, but women do not ejaculate like men.

## Figure 6.3

**The Masters and Johnson Model of the Female and Male Human Orgasmic Responses.** The female response is much more variable than is the male response, as shown by the three female patterns and one male pattern illustrated here.

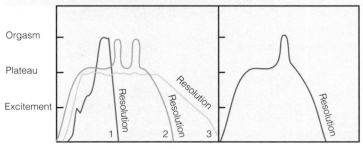

Female response          Male response

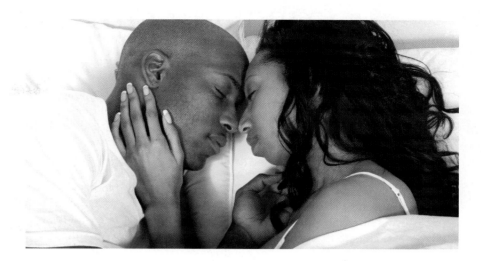

During the *resolution phase* the body returns to its prearousal state. The heart rate, blood pressure, and respiration slow; the muscles relax. In males, the erection subsides (the penis becomes flaccid) and sometimes fatigue sets in. Depending on the man and his age, he will not be able to develop another erection for a few minutes to a few hours. This time is the *refractory period*. Unlike men, women have the capacity to reach the orgasmic phase again (have multiple orgasms) in sequence or rather quickly after dropping to the plateau phase.

**Other Sexual Response Models** The Masters and Johnson model is considered a biological and linear model of sexual response. It is considered biological because it encompasses only physiologic aspects of the sexual response and not emotional or psychological aspects. It is considered linear because it has a beginning, middle, and end, starting at one place and ending at another. Although this model may reflect the male sexual response well, it may not be as reflective of the female sexual response.

Whipple and Brash-McGreer developed a circular model of female sexual response based on a previous linear four-stage model developed by Reed. The circular model shows that a woman's reflection on a sexual encounter affects her desire for the next sexual encounter. Satisfying sexual experiences reinforce her desire for another, whereas negative sexual experiences detract from her desire. This circular model recognizes that the pleasure and emotional satisfaction

derived from one sexual experience can lead to desire for the next sexual experience.[3]

Basson also developed a cyclical model of the female sexual response, which is shown in **Figure 6.4**.[4] This model heavily incorporates emotional and psychosocial aspects. Sexual stimuli act on the sex drive

## Figure 6.4

**Basson's Blended Intimacy-Based and Sexual Drive-Based Circular Model of the Female Sexual Response.** Women seek sexual intimacy for reasons beyond the physiologic sex drive, such as a desire to increase emotional closeness. This model shows that both the sex drive and the desire for emotional intimacy may motivate a woman to be responsive to sexual stimuli. In addition, biological and psychological factors combine to determine whether she becomes sexually aroused. For example, past sexual abuse may interfere with arousal even if she desires intimacy with her partner. Positive past experiences, however, will promote arousal. Her emotional and physical satisfaction from the sexual experience will then increase her desire for emotional intimacy, continuing the cycle of response.

*Source:* Reprinted from Basson, R. (2001). Female sexual response: The role of drugs in the management of sexual dysfunction. *Obstetrics and Gynecology, 98*(2):350–353.

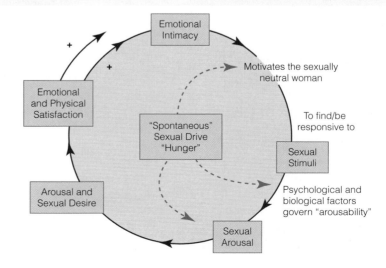

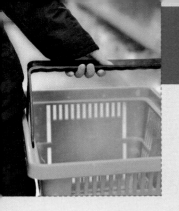

# Consumer Health

## Ginseng and Sexual Prowess

You've probably seen ads for ginseng in magazines, on television, or on the Web. The ads often make claims such as "Ginseng will boost your energy and sexual stamina," or "Ginseng has been used for centuries in maintaining overall health and vitality," or "Ginseng will reduce stress and the effects of aging." "Can it do that?" you wonder.

Ginseng is an herb that grows wild or is cultivated in eastern Asia and North America. For hundreds of years, the root of the plant has been used in Asia for medicinal purposes and as an aphrodisiac because it often looks like a human body (**Figure 6.A**). But what do we know about ginseng? Will it make you more sexually "potent"? Can it harm you or, alternatively, enhance your health?

On the positive side, sperm motility and ability to fertilize an egg (capacitation) are enhanced after sperm are incubated with extracts of ginseng. Are sperm motility and capacitation enhanced in men who take ginseng? There is still no answer to that question. Does ginseng affect sexual arousal or performance? Ginseng has been shown to significantly enhance libido and copulatory behavior in male rats and mice. This herb appears to have a direct effect on penile tissue, which could be respon-

sible for its copulatory performance-enhancing actions and has been used to treat erectile dysfunction.

On the negative side, medical researchers know that drug interactions occur with many herbals. Ginseng, in particular, may alter bleeding (or clotting) time, the time it takes for blood to stop flowing from a tiny wound. Ginseng also interacts with anticoagulant drugs, which "thin" the blood; that is, they decrease the ability of the blood to clot. Therefore, anticoagulants and ginseng should not be taken together. Ginseng also may interfere with the heart medication digoxin (digitalis), which affects the force and rate at which the heart beats.

In addition to its interaction with anticoagulants and digoxin, ginseng should not be used if a person is taking estrogens or corticosteroid drugs such as cortisone because of possible additive effects. Ginseng may also affect blood glucose levels, so it should not be taken by persons with diabetes mellitus. For those on the antidepressant drug phenelzine sulfate (Nardil), ginseng could provoke a manic episode (an extreme excited state). Its general side effects may include headache and involuntary muscular contractions.

Should you take ginseng to boost your sexual prowess? This herb is commonly used in Asia to treat sexual dysfunction in humans. In addition, animal studies provide evidence that ginseng may be useful in such treatment, and it may enhance libido and copulatory behavior in males. Results of one small Asian study show that Korean red ginseng improved sexual arousal in menopausal women. However, a review published in the *Journal of Sexual Medicine* in 2010 states that "although there's a positive trend towards recommending ginseng as an effective aphrodisiac, however, more in depth studies involving [a] large number of subjects and its mechanism of action are needed before definite conclusions could be reached." With all this evidence in mind, you might not want to rely on ginseng for better bedroom calisthenics just yet.

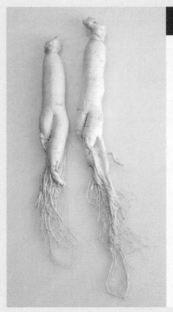

### Figure 6.A

**Ginseng Root.** The use of the ginseng root as an aphrodisiac presumably began as a result of its human-like shape.

Sources: De Andrade, E., et al. (2007). Study of the efficacy of Korean red ginseng in the treatment of erectile dysfunction. *Asian Journal of Andrology,* 9:241–244; Oh, K. J. (2010). Effects of Korean red ginseng on sexual arousal in menopausal women: Placebo-controlled, double-blind crossover clinical study. *Journal of Sexual Medicine,* 7:1469–1477; Shamloul, R. (2010). Natural aphrodisiacs. *Journal of Sexual Medicine,* 7:39–49; Zhang, H., et al. (2007). Ginsenoside Re promotes human sperm capacitation through nitric oxide-dependent pathway. *Molecular Reproduction and Development,* 74:497–501.

as biologic and psychological factors come into play, such as satisfaction with her sex partner, her self-image, and previous sexual experiences. A positive psychological state can lead to sexual arousal and then sexual desire. The resulting emotional and physical satisfaction she experiences from sexual activity leads to emotional intimacy with her partner and reinforces her being receptive to the next sexual encounter.

## Sexual Dysfunctions

A *dysfunction* is an impaired bodily process or a behavior that hinders the development or maintenance of healthy relationships. *Sexual dysfunctions* relate to the psychological and physical conditions that interfere with the sexual response.

## Erectile Dysfunction (Impotence)

A common problem with the sexual response that occurs in men, particularly middle-aged and older men, is *impotence*. More properly called **erectile dysfunction (ED)**, impotence is the inability of a man to develop and/or sustain an erection firm enough for penetration. The incidence of ED rises as men age: 5% in men aged 20 to 39 years, 15% in men aged 40 to 59 years, 44% in men aged 60 to 69 years, and 70% in men 70 years or older.[5] Some men with various degrees of erectile dysfunction are able, with proper stimulation, to reach orgasm and ejaculate.

Until the last 15 years or so, impotence was thought to be primarily a psychological problem, a conclusion based on research studies conducted by well-known sex therapists Masters and Johnson. However, medical researchers have discovered that approximately 70% to 80% of cases of impotence are caused by physical problems. The most common cause of physically based impotence is blood vessel disease. Lifestyle factors that affect ED are smoking, alcohol consumption, and physical activity. Smoking increases the risk of ED and is associated with its progression. Physical activity decreases the risk of ED, while moderate alcohol consumption (two drinks per day for men) decreases the risk of ED compared to no alcohol consumption or heavier consumption.[6]

To develop and maintain an erection, blood must fill the spongy tissue of the penis and compress the veins that bring blood away from the penis. If a man has fatty deposits clogging his penile arteries, blood flow to the penis may be insufficient to develop and

**erectile dysfunction (ED)** A sexual dysfunction in which a man is unable to develop and/or sustain an erection firm enough for penetration of the vagina. Also called impotence.

**premature (rapid) ejaculation** A common male sexual dysfunction in which a man consistently attains orgasm either before or shortly after intercourse and before he wishes it to occur.

maintain an erection. The drugs Viagra (sildenafil), Levitra (vardenafil), and Cialis (tadalafil) work by widening blood vessels in the penis, thus increasing blood flow.

Erectile dysfunction can also be caused by a variety of other conditions, such as diabetes mellitus;[5] damage to the spinal nerves or other nerves involved in erection; damage to the arteries that bring blood to the penis; certain medications used to control high blood pressure, anxiety, or depression; illness or injury that damages the penis; and hormonal imbalances. Research results show that use of a testosterone patch improves sexual function in men aged 50 to 70 years who exhibit symptoms of hormonal imbalance.[7]

Alcohol and illegal drugs such as marijuana, heroin, and cocaine have also been shown to affect penile function negatively. In addition, stress can be a cause of erectile difficulties. Epinephrine (adrenaline), a chemical released by the body during the stress reaction, impedes a man's ability to have an erection.

Physicians warn that minor physical problems can cause erectile difficulties that can worry a man and lead to psychological problems with erection. A significant finding to help distinguish between a physical and psychological cause for impotence is whether the man has a normal pattern of erections while asleep but not while engaged in sex with his partner. Men are encouraged to seek medical help for impotence immediately so that underlying, and possibly serious, physical problems can be diagnosed and treated promptly. If physical problems are not the cause, the psychological health of the patient as well as the health of his relationships should be explored.

## Premature (Rapid) Ejaculation

**Premature ejaculation (PE)**, also called **rapid ejaculation**, is the most common male sexual dysfunction, affecting from 3% to 30% of men of all ages, cultures, and ethnicities.[8] The wide range is due to a previous lack of definition, so studies often defined premature ejaculation in differing ways. However, the term was finally defined in 2008 by the Ad Hoc Committee of the International Society for Sexual Medicine. PE means that a man consistently attains orgasm either before or shortly after intercourse begins (generally in less than 1 minute all or nearly all of the time) and before he wishes it to occur, resulting in distress for a man and also for his partner.[7] Using this definition, the International Society for Sexual Medicine expects that the proportion of men affected by PE may be less than 3%.[8]

The cause of PE is a controversial topic among medical researchers and psychologists who study sex-related disorders. One hypothesis suggests that PE is related to anxiety. Another hypothesis is that men who exhibit premature ejaculation may be physically more sensitive to sexual stimulation. In the past decade, however, the focus has shifted from psychological factors to biological factors that may underlie PE, such as genetically based differences in ejaculation or neurotransmitter problems. (Neurotransmitters are chemical messengers that allow nerve cells to communicate with one another.) Consequently, treatment focus is shifting from behavioral techniques to drugs.[9] Nonetheless, specialists in sexual dysfunction advise that a variety of therapies may be useful in helping men with PE and suggest that a man or couple with this problem see a sex therapist as well as a physician.

Dapoxetine is a drug that is currently being considered for approval by the FDA for the treatment of PE, although the drug was rejected initially by the FDA in 2005. Dapoxetine is a short-acting antidepressant that allows the neurotransmitter serotonin to be used more effectively by the brain. (Serotonin is a brain chemical that affects emotions, behavior, and thought.) If approved, dapoxetine would be the first drug approved to treat PE. Although the drug appears to be effective and generally well tolerated by patients, it has serious side effects with long-term use, which include psychiatric problems, weight gain, skin reactions, lowered sex drive, nausea, and headache. These side effects have been one stumbling block in the FDA approval process. Another similar drug called Escitalopram is also in development. Topical anesthetic creams are available, but they are messy, must be applied prior to sex and then thoroughly washed off, and may numb the partner's tissues if not removed completely.[9]

## Hypoactive Sexual Desire Disorder

*Hypoactive sexual desire disorder* (HSDD) refers to a persistent low interest in sex with personal distress resulting from this low desire.[10] This disorder affects both men and women, although HSDD occurs more often in women. Interest in sex declines with age in both men and women as hormone levels drop. Thus, older women and men may not be as distressed as younger persons by a lowered sex drive and may consider it part of the normal aging process. Consequently, HSDD may have a lower frequency in older persons than in younger persons.

A study of a large national sample of U.S. women using the Women's International Study of Health and Sexuality (WISHeS) questionnaire supports this hypothesis.[11] Results of the study reveal that 24% to 36% of women between the ages of 20 and 70 years had low sexual desire. Nonetheless, not all of these women had HSDD because not all of them experienced personal distress as a result of their low desire. In premenopausal women aged 20 to 49 years, 24% had low sexual desire. In naturally postmenopausal women aged 50 to 70 years (those who had not had menopause induced surgically by removal of the ovaries), 29% had low sexual desire—a 5% increase with age. However, a much larger percentage of the younger women were distressed by their low desire: 59% of the younger age group who experienced low sexual desire versus 33% of the older age group. Thus, in calculating HSDD in these two groups of women, the researchers determined that the younger women had a higher rate of HSDD (14%) than the older women (9%).

Hypoactive sexual desire disorder has a variety of psychological and physical causes, such as restrictive views regarding sex, a history of sexual abuse, relationship problems, certain chronic diseases such as rheumatoid arthritis, fatigue, stress, illness, and abnormal hormone levels. Stahl suggests that HSDD may be the result of a dysfunction of certain "reward pathway" neurotransmitters in the brain.[10]

Treatment of HSDD includes the identification and elimination of the cause. Problems within the relationship or those rooted in long-held, deep-seated feelings and beliefs require counseling and therapy for resolution. Other treatments include relaxation techniques, hormone treatments, and changes in medications that a patient may be taking. Drugs that act on the dysfunctional "reward" pathways in the brain may hold promise for the future treatment of HSDD as well.[12]

## Female Sexual Arousal Disorder

When a woman becomes sexually excited, the blood vessels in the pelvic area widen, tissues expand, and fluid seeps through the walls of the blood vessels in the vaginal area, providing lubrication for sexual intercourse. *Female sexual arousal disorder* (FSAD) is a condition in which a woman is continually unable, over an extended period of time, to attain or maintain adequate lubrication along with the swelling response during sexual activity. If the absence of this response is the result of a physiologic cause, such as the changes of menopause, injuries to the genital area, damage to nerves, the side effect of medications, or illness, the condition is considered a sexual dysfunction resulting from a medical condition, and it is not considered FSAD. The causes of FSAD include depression, stress, relationship problems, past sexual or emotional abuse, and self-image problems.

Treatments for the absence of adequate lubrication during sexual activity vary depending on the cause. Treatments for sexual dysfunction caused by a medical condition include hormone replacement therapy, prescription intravaginal hormone creams, and nonprescription lubricants. The EROS clinical therapy device, which is a small vacuum pump designed to increase blood flow to the area, helps some women. In addition, research results show sildenafil citrate (Viagra) to be a moderately useful treatment.[13] Treatments for FSAD include sex therapy and psychological therapy.

## Vaginismus

**Vaginismus** is a sexual dysfunction of women in which the muscles of the lower third of the vaginal canal contract involuntarily (and often painfully) at the anticipation of sexual intercourse, the insertion of tampons, or a pelvic examination, and cause distress. The muscular contractions are strong enough to prevent penetration. Women with vaginismus do not usually have other sexual dysfunctions and can achieve orgasm by stimulating the clitoris.

Vaginismus appears to have both physical and psychological causes. A variety of physical conditions can cause pain during intercourse (*dyspareunia*; dis-pah-ROO-nee-ah) and result in vaginismus. Causes of dyspareunia include a poorly healed episiotomy (an incision made to widen the vaginal opening during the birth process); infections, sores, or lesions of the vagina or vulva; estrogen deficiency; sexually transmitted infections (STIs); or inadequate lubrication during intercourse. If a woman experiences pain during intercourse because of one or more of these conditions, involuntary vaginal contractions may occur as the body attempts to protect itself from penetration and subsequent pain. If the cause of the pain

eventually subsides, the contractions may still occur as a conditioned response. Recent research suggests that vaginismus and dispareunia should be considered as one "genito-pelvic penetration/pain disorder" because the two conditions generally occur together, and reliable diagnosis of vaginal spasm is difficult.[14]

*Psychogenic vaginismus* usually begins without a physical cause. The results of studies show that this type of vaginismus occurs as a protective response to perceived pain or violation of the body, with common causes being child sexual abuse, early traumatic sexual experiences, early traumatic gynecological examinations, inadequate sex information, and cultural and religious taboos.

Treatments for vaginismus are usually tailored to the individual and are multidimensional. Education helps correct misconceptions a woman may have about the genitals in general and the vagina in particular. (For example, a woman may believe that the vagina is particularly narrow and delicate, and therefore easily harmed by penetration.) Psychiatric or psychological therapy may be useful for a woman alone or for her and her partner. Physical treatment generally includes using vaginal inserts of graded sizes to slowly help a woman overcome her fear of penetration, but this step can be taken only when a woman feels ready.

## Culture and Sexuality

Society strongly influences the sexual attitudes and behaviors of a population by identifying acceptable sexual activities and placing restrictions on others. For example, some cultures value sexual abstinence before marriage; others value sexual experimentation during childhood. A **value** is a belief that an idea, object, or action has worth. The Diversity in Health essay "The Virtue of Virginity" provides a cross-cultural perspective concerning the value of sexual abstinence before marriage.

An individual usually formulates a personal value system before adulthood. A *value system* is a collection of beliefs that helps a person identify and classify things as being good or bad, or neither good nor

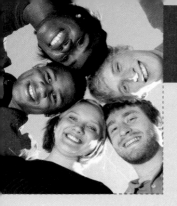

# Diversity in Health

## The Virtue of Virginity

In many cultures and to many people, virginity is a virtue that is presented on the wedding night to one's spouse. Since ancient times, people from various cultures have used the condition of a bride's hymen to determine if this virtue is intact. Although the hymen has no known biological function, this thin membranous tissue usually covers part of the outer entrance to the vagina. Most hymens have at least one opening that is wide enough to permit the discharge of menstrual blood. In many instances, this opening is too narrow for a penis to penetrate without tearing the surrounding tissue, but the hymen can also be torn while engaging in nonsexual activities, such as riding a bicycle, exercising, or using tampons.

According to the Old Testament of the Bible, a man who thought that his bride was not a virgin on their wedding night was entitled to have his townspeople stone her to death. In some ancient societies, a newly wed woman who could not prove her virginity might be banished from her hometown, tortured, or killed. Her lover, if known, often received the same treatment. Today, virginity is still an important criterion for selecting a mate, especially in India, Indonesia, China, Taiwan, Iran, Turkey, and Arab nations. In most of these places, however, a new bride with sexual experience usually receives less harsh treatment than in the past. She may be rejected by her husband and returned to her family as "used goods."

Facing embarrassment and ridicule from neighbors, the woman's family may disown her.

According to Islamic tradition, a woman's virginity is the basis for her honor and that of her family, her future groom, and his family. Muslims, followers of Islam, would arrange early marriages for their female children to ensure that these girls entered puberty as virgin brides. Fatima Mernissi, a sociologist in the African country of Morocco, thinks that Muslim men maintain their respect and pride by controlling the sexuality of their wives, daughters, and sisters. In many Muslim communities, young women are required to be heavily veiled in the presence of strange men and in public (see **Figure 6.B**). If they do not wear veils, young women may be punished severely.

Marriage and social customs in rural parts of Africa, Asia, and the Mediterranean often include some ritual that "proves" the bride has lost her virginity on her wedding night. In parts of Greece, the groom's friends gather outside the window of the newly married couple on the morning after the wedding to receive the news that the bride is no longer a virgin. After the groom makes the expected announcement, the gathering of friends celebrates by firing guns into the air. In many Middle Eastern villages it is customary for the groom to display bloodstained sheets as evidence of wedding night virginity loss. In some societies with such traditions, new brides keep a small amount of chicken blood handy to drip on sheets during the wedding night, or they make a small cut near the vaginal opening that will bleed during sexual intercourse. The social value of virginity is

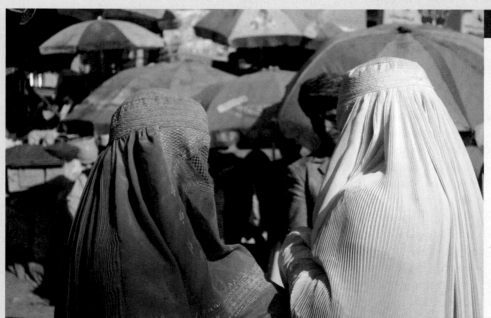

### Figure 6.B

**Culturally Appropriate Clothing.** In some Islamic traditions women wear the body-covering burka in public. A mesh screen covers the eyes. These women are at a bazaar in Afghanistan.

so powerful that cosmetic surgeons in Japan and Italy routinely reconstruct hymens so that their unmarried female patients who have been sexually active or have torn hymens for reasons unrelated to sex can present themselves with the needed tissues intact.

Economic factors also play a major role in perpetuating the value of premarital virginity. In many cultures, property is handed down from fathers to sons. Therefore, families strive to protect their financial interests and lines of inheritance by seeking virgin brides for male relatives. An unmarried woman who is not a virgin could be pregnant with a male child whose father is from another family. Without DNA testing to confirm a child's paternity, rural people in underdeveloped regions rely on an intact hymen as a sign of virginity. Along with this view of women as property, cultural norms of sexual chastity, female virginity, pure bloodlines, and family honor may also serve to control women's behavior.

In some societies, virginity tests, which usually involve inspection of the hymen, are used to document premarital virginity. For example, virginity testing existed in Turkey until 2002 when laws were changed that had previously allowed school administrators to require virginity testing for female students. In 2010, the Indonesian government was urged by Amnesty International to block attempts to institute virginity and pregnancy testing for high school girls. In some areas of South Africa, virginity "tests" that are born of ancient tribal customs and that have no relationship to whether a young woman is really a virgin are still practiced alongside public genital inspection for an intact hymen (**Figure 6.C**). In addition, virginity testing of boys was reported in areas of South Africa in 2009. The "test" is based on the tightness of the foreskin and the manner of urination; however, South African urologist Barney Hattingh notes that it is impossible to tell whether a boy or a man had previously engaged in sexual intercourse. South Africans who support virginity testing explain that this tradition is important not only to retain long-held customs but also to promote sexual abstinence in a country with a high rate of HIV/AIDS.

Is disease prevention the "new" virtue of virginity? It may be, but promoting virginity by means of virginity testing is viewed by its opponents as nothing more than degrading abuse. Virginity testing is placing ancient cultures and human rights on a collision course and makes virginity look less like a virtue and more like a condition to endure.

*Sources:* Amnesty International. (2010, November 11). Indonesia urged to block discriminatory pregnancy tests for school girls. Retrieved on March 7, 2011, from http://www.amnesty.org/en/news-and-updates/indonesia-urged-block-discriminatory-pregnancy-tests-schoolgirls-2010-11-11; Brulliard, K. (2008, September 26). Zulus eagerly defy ban on virginity test; S. Africa's progressive constitution collides with tribal customs. *Washington Post*. Retrieved on March 7, 2011, from http://www.washingtonpost.com/wp-dyn/content/article/2008/09/25/AR2008092504625.html; Mernissi, F. (2003). Beyond the veil: Male–female dynamics in Muslim society. London, England: Saqi Books; Mthethwa, B. (2009, December 12). Virginity testing keeps boys pure. Retrieved on March 7, 2011, from http://www.timeslive.co.za/sundaytimes/article231102.ece

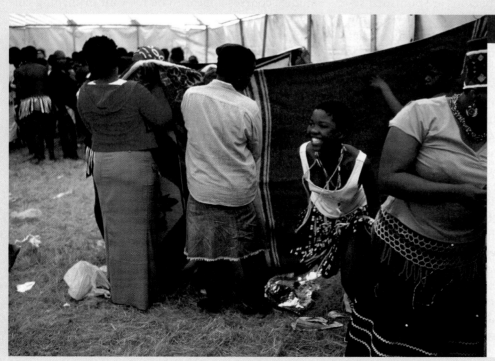

### Figure 6.C

This smiling girl has just completed her virginity testing in rural Natal, South Africa.

**gender** The classification of a person's sex based on many criteria, among them anatomic and chromosomal characteristics.

**gender identity** An individual's perception of himself or herself as male or female.

**gender role** Patterns of behavior, attitudes, and personality attributes that are traditionally considered in a particular culture to be feminine or masculine.

**sexual stereotype** The widespread association of certain perceptions with one gender.

**sexism** Discrimination and bias against one sex.

bad. This value system guides the reasoning and behavior of the individual, especially in sexual decision making.

Many Americans derive their sexual values from Judeo-Christian religious teachings. However, people in the culturally diverse U.S. population adhere to a variety of sexual values, some of which conflict with traditional Judeo-Christian teachings. No universally accepted set of sexual values applies to Americans.

Widely accepted values can help people determine behavioral norms, but these norms often change over time and across cultures. Before World War I, for example, it was socially unacceptable for "proper" American men or women to expose much of their bodies in public. Today, most Americans think that it is acceptable for people to wear clothing that exposes much of their bodies, especially in warm weather. However, in some cultures, persons are punished severely if they appear in public dressed in revealing outfits; the only acceptable style of clothing is that which has been worn for centuries (Figure 6.B).

## Gender Identity and Roles

**Gender** is the classification of a person's sex based on many criteria, among them anatomic and chromosomal characteristics. **Gender identity** is an individual's perception of himself or herself as male or female. Various biological, social, and environmental forces mold a child's gender identity.

Before birth, genetic and hormonal factors influence the sexual development of the embryonic brain. After birth, social factors have a major impact on gender identity. As children interact with people, they observe and learn gender roles and sexual stereotypes. A **gender role** refers to patterns of behavior, attitudes, and personality attributes that are traditionally considered in a particular culture to be feminine or masculine. A **sexual stereotype** is the widespread association of certain perceptions with

one gender. Examples of sexual stereotypes are associating the color blue with boys and pink with girls or associating passiveness with females and aggressiveness with males.

Throughout the world, obvious biological differences between the sexes form the basis for traditional gender roles. In many cultures, for example, women are responsible for routine child-rearing and household management. This traditional gender role assignment likely developed for a variety of reasons, such as a woman's biological role in giving birth and nursing infants. It is also likely that because men, in general, are physically stronger than women are, their customary roles have been protecting and providing for their families, especially in hunter-gatherer or agrarian societies.

In addition to biological factors, culture (often determined by race and ethnicity) and religion heavily influence sexual attitudes and behaviors. In many cultures, men learn to be sexually aggressive and women learn to be sexually passive. According to these sexual stereotypes, men are always eager for sex, and they are expected to demonstrate their interest and aggressiveness by initiating sexual encounters. Women are expected to be less interested in sex than men are but to accept the sexual advances of men (such as their partners) willingly.

In the United States, parents, friends, teachers, and the media influence children's perceptions of gender roles. Academic engagement, peers, and women's studies courses appear to be relevant in shaping college students' perceptions of gender roles.[15]

Some Americans reject traditional gender stereotypes because these attitudes and practices can create and foster sexism. **Sexism**, discrimination and bias against one sex, is common in many societies. For many women in the United States and other countries, sexist practices affect their status and health at work, school, and home. Sexual harassment and violence against women are forms of sexism. Men can experience sexism as well; white American males often feel the object of sexist practices in the workplace when hiring guidelines favor females.

Over the past two decades, societal norms in the United States have moved to a more liberal interpretation of appropriate role behaviors for women. Women are now more comfortable asking men out on dates. Men and women may feel free to initiate or refuse sexual activity. Additionally, a growing number of Americans feel free to choose nontraditional careers and adopt flexible gender roles. In a few families, traditional sex roles are reversed. For example, a woman may decide to work outside of the home while her male partner chooses to stay at home to care for their children and manage household tasks.

## Transgender

**Transgender** is an umbrella term for various groups of people who do not conform to traditional gender roles and includes transsexuals, crossdressers, intersex persons, drag performers, and androgynes. According to data released in 2011 from the Williams Institute at the University of California, Los Angeles (UCLA), 0.3% of the U.S. adult population is transgender.[16]

*Transsexuals* are persons whose gender identity conflicts with his or her biological sex, a condition known as *gender dysphoria*. Such an individual feels trapped in the body of the opposite sex. Transsexuals frequently undergo psychotherapy and hormonal treatments to help them deal with their gender identity conflicts; others choose to have sex reassignment surgery to change their sexual appearances. Physicians who perform sex reassignment surgeries usually remove certain reproductive organs and reconstruct the genitals of the patient to make them resemble those of the opposite sex. After transsexual surgery, however, the newly fashioned reproductive organs do not function like the organs of people who were born with them. **Figure 6.5** is a before and after photo

of Chastity Bono—actor, writer, musician, transgender activist, and daughter of Sonny Bono and Cher. Chastity Bono is now Chaz Bono, a male.

Unlike transsexuals, *crossdressers* are comfortable with their gender, but they occasionally dress and act like the opposite sex. Most crossdressers are heterosexual men. *Drag performers* dress like the opposite sex as well, but they do it as a job or as play; it is not an identity for them.

*Intersex* persons have disorders of sex development (DSD) resulting in some combination of male and female internal and external sexual organs. These characteristics are the result of the action of genes and are present at birth. In 2010, a gene that influences the activity of other genes involved in human sex determination was discovered.[17] With 1 in 1,000 individuals affected by DSD, research is ongoing to better understand the genes involved in the development of a person's sex and how they work.

Androgynous persons, or *androgynes*, have traits with no gender value—they do not fit easily into male or female categories—or they have traits attributed to the opposite sex. These characteristics may be physical or behavioral.

## Sexual Orientation

One of the most emotionally charged aspects of human sexuality is **sexual orientation**, that is, the direction of a person's romantic thoughts, feelings, and attractions. Results of one study reveal that of a nationally representative sample of 9,400 U.S. college and university students, 93.9% identified themselves as **heterosexual** (sexually attracted to members of the opposite sex).[18] Of the remainder, 2.4% identified themselves as **homosexual**, and 3.7% as **bisexual**. Homosexuals are sexually attracted to members of

### Figure 6.5

**Chastity Bono to Chaz Bono.** Born the daughter of Sonny Bono and Cher, Bono's transition from female to male began in 2008, was physically completed in 2009 with gender reassignment surgery, and was legally completed in 2010 when a California court agreed to change Bono's gender and name. (a) Chastity Bono in 1998. (b) Chaz Bono in 2011.

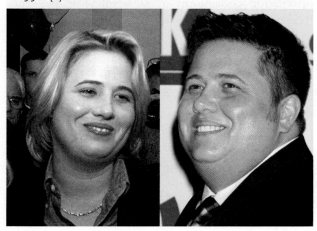

(a)                        (b)

**Figure 6.6**

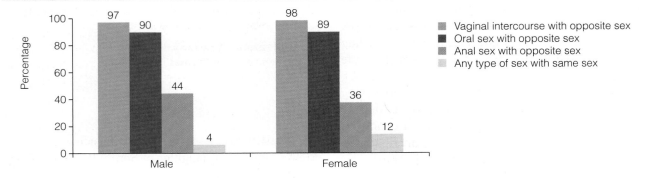

**Sexual Behavior.** Sexual behavior in lifetime among males and females 25–44 years of age: United States.
*Source:* Chandra, A., et al. (2011, March 3). Sexual behavior, sexual attraction, and sexual identity in the United States: Data from the 2006–2008 National Survey of Family Growth. *National Health Statistics Reports*, no. 36. Retrieved on March 14, 2011, from http://www.cdc.gov/nchs/data/nhsr/nhsr036.pdf

their own sex; bisexuals engage in sexual activity with both sexes. Results from the National Survey of Family Growth (NSFG), conducted by researchers at the Centers for Disease Control and Prevention (CDC) and published in 2011, show that 6% of men and 12% of women aged 25 to 44 years engaged in sex with a same-sex partner at least once over their lifetime (**Figure 6.6**).

Of the homosexual population in the study, 55% were males and 45% were females. Of the bisexual population in the study, 29% were males and 71% were females. These percentages of sexual orientation are similar to the results of many other studies.[19]

Homosexual men and women are commonly referred to as *gay* people; homosexual women are also called *lesbians*. Sexologist Alfred Kinsey proposed that sexual orientation is a continuum with exclusively heterosexual and homosexual designations at opposite ends and degrees of bisexuality within this continuum (**Figure 6.7**).[20] Sexual orientation does not vary much across sociodemographic groups.[19]

## Nature or Nurture?

Do people, particularly homosexuals, choose their sexual orientation? Formerly, there was widespread belief that homosexuality was learned behavior, and that children became homosexual by having early social and sexual experiences with gay individuals. At present, researchers cannot find a common childhood characteristic that predicts adult sexual orientation. Children may have same-sex experiences with other children, but most of them develop heterosexual orientations as they mature. Some gays and lesbians report that they knew they were different at an early age, but they did not recognize their homosexuality until they were in their teens or early 20s.

Today, researchers and mental health experts generally agree that people do not decide their sexual orientation and cannot alter their sexual preferences, whether they are at either end of the sexual orientation continuum or somewhere in-between. Researchers have been studying the biological basis of homosexuality, and results of studies of the early

**Figure 6.7**

**Kinsey's Continuum of Sexual Orientation.** Sexuality researcher Alfred Kinsey thought that sexual orientation is a continuum with exclusively heterosexual and homosexual designations on the ends and degrees of bisexuality between them.

| 100% Heterosexual | A few homosexual fantasies or experiences | More heterosexual than homosexual | Bisexual | More homosexual than heterosexual | A few heterosexual fantasies or experiences | 100% Homosexual |
|---|---|---|---|---|---|---|

**homophobia** An intense fear of or hostility toward homosexuals.

1990s show physical differences in small groups of cells in the hypothalamus of the brains of heterosexual and homosexual men.[21] In 1993, molecular geneticist Dean Hamer and his colleagues announced that a particular region of the X chromosome in homosexual males was involved in male sexual orientation in some, but not all, gay men.[22] Males inherit this sex chromosome (condensed piece of hereditary material) from their mothers. The particular region of the X chromosome was dubbed the "gay gene." However, the results of more recent research suggest that homosexuality is under the control of more than a single gene. Scientists are now studying how genes that control homosexuality are maintained in the population.[23]

## Sexual Orientation and Society

Since ancient times, homosexuality has existed in most societies. Homosexuals are members of every racial, ethnic, socioeconomic, religious, and occupational group. Although many homosexuals choose to conceal their sexual orientation, especially from their coworkers and neighbors, others have decided to express their sexual preferences openly.

**Homophobia** is an intense fear of or hostility toward homosexuals. However, not every person who objects to homosexuality is afraid of gay people or is hostile toward them. Therefore, *antihomosexual* may be a more descriptive term than *homophobic* to describe people who harbor such fears and hostilities.

Many heterosexuals do not accept homosexuality because they think gay sexual behavior is unnatural or it contradicts their religious beliefs. Other people are afraid of contact with gays because they associate acquired immune deficiency syndrome (AIDS) with homosexuality. Results of a May 2010 Gallup poll on tolerance for gay rights revealed that 57% of respondents thought that homosexuality was an acceptable alternative lifestyle, up from 44% in 1996, while 40% thought it was unacceptable, down from 50% in 1996.[24]

U.S. President Bill Clinton signed the "Defense of Marriage" bill in 1996, which does not recognize marriages between homosexuals and allows states to ignore same-sex marriages that have been performed in other states. Gay couples, however, often cohabit and form lifetime commitments, commonly called domestic partnerships. Because domestic partners often contribute to the economic survival of their households, share property, and raise children, they want the same legal rights and protections that heterosexual married couples have, such as the right to claim insurance benefits when their partners die. When asked in 2010 whether marriages between same-sex couples should or should not be recognized by the law as valid, with the same rights as traditional marriages, 44% of Gallup poll respondents said they should be valid, up from 27% in 1996, while 53% said they should not be valid, down from 68% in 1996.[24]

There are very few places in the world where gay couples can legally marry. As of September 2011, the countries allowing same-sex marriage were Argentina, Belgium, Canada, Iceland, The Netherlands, Norway, Portugal, South Africa, Spain, and Sweden. In the United States, Connecticut, Iowa, Massachusetts, New Hampshire, New York, Vermont, and the District of Columbia allowed same-sex marriage, but most states in the United States banned same-sex marriage or referred to marriage as being between a man and a woman. The state of California allowed same-sex marriage from June 16, 2008, through November 5, 2008.

Many countries allowed same-sex registered partnerships or civil unions as of July 2011, including Austria, Croatia, Denmark, Finland, France, Germany, Great Britain, Hungary, Ireland, Luxembourg, New Zealand, and Switzerland. In the United States, same-sex civil unions were allowed in Delaware, Hawaii, Illinois, New Jersey, and Rhode Island. Civil unions allow various benefits depending on the state or country, such as recognition of the relationship, family leave benefits, and group insurance. In the United States, civil unions provide state-level spousal rights. Some states allow registered domestic partnerships: California, Oregon, Nevada, Washington, Hawaii, Maine, Wisconsin, and the District of Columbia. Domestic partnerships grant nearly all or some state-level spousal rights to unmarried couples.

**Healthy Living Practices**

☐ Consider seeking professional counseling if you are confused or troubled by your sexual orientation.

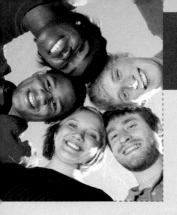

# Diversity in Health

## Common Sexual Practices Between Partners

Most heterosexuals are familiar with the notion of "having sex" or **sexual intercourse** as vaginal sex, the insertion of a penis into a vagina. Vaginal sex, or **coitus**, is the most common and popular form of intimate sexual activity between partners. According to findings from the National Survey of Sexual Health and Behavior (NSSHB) conducted by researchers from the Center for Sexual Health Promotion at Indiana University, about three-fourths of men and women aged 25 to 39 years and more than half aged 20–24 and 40–49 years engaged in vaginal intercourse in the month prior to taking the survey.[25] Results from the NSFG show that 97% of men and 98% of women aged 25–44 years had vaginal intercourse at least once over their lifetime (see Figure 6.6).

The report *American Sexual Behavior: Trends, Sociodemographic Differences, and Risk Behavior* from the University of Chicago's National Opinion Research Center states that, on average, adult Americans say that they engage in vaginal intercourse about once a week. Married individuals report having vaginal sex more frequently than never-married, divorced, or widowed persons. The results of various surveys indicate that the longer a couple has been married, the less frequently they engage in coitus.[19]

Men engaging in *anal intercourse*—whether with other men or with women—was reported much less frequently than vaginal intercourse was. The highest incidence of past-month homosexual/heterosexual "insertive" anal intercourse (inserted penis into anus) was among men aged 25–29 years at 10.3%.[25] Lifetime heterosexual anal sex for men aged 25–44 years was reported as 44% on the NSFG (see Figure 6.8). The highest incidence of homosexual past-month "receptive" anal intercourse (received penis in anus) was among men aged 50–59 years at 2.9%.[25]

For women, the incidence of anal intercourse is low. The highest incidence of past-month anal intercourse reported on the NSSHB was among those aged 18–24 years at about 7% to 8%.[25] Lifetime anal sex for females aged 25–44 years was reported as 36% on the NSFG (see Figure 6.6).

Many women and men find receptive anal intercourse unappealing because the practice can be painful, it increases the risk of contracting sexually transmitted infections especially HIV, and it increases the risk of developing urinary tract infections. The lining of the rectum tears easily—much more easily than the vagina—elevating the risk of bacteria and viruses entering the bloodstream. Lubricants that are often used with anal sex may irritate the tissues, increasing the risk further. Using latex condoms during anal sex reduces but does not eliminate this risk. For women, if anal intercourse is followed by vaginal intercourse, bacteria can be spread from the rectum into the vagina or the *urethra*, the tube that carries urine from the bladder. After anal sex, one should wash the fingers and penis thoroughly before engaging in additional sexual activity, and a fresh condom should be used. Women should urinate after vaginal sex to help remove some of the bacteria that have entered the urethra, reducing the risk of a bladder infection.

People often engage in *petting*, more recently called *mutual masturbation*, as a pleasurable substitute for or a prelude to intercourse. During these activities, two or more people stimulate themselves or another sexually, often with the hands, without vaginal or anal intercourse. Mutual masturbation activities include a variety of sex acts that range from kissing and fondling breasts to performing oral sex. Additionally, people may rub their genital areas together, without penetration. For people who want to reduce their risk of pregnancy or sexually transmitted infections, mutual masturbation can be a safe alternative to vaginal or anal sex.

Although not as popular as vaginal intercourse, oral sex is a common sexual activity. **Cunnilingus** is the use of the mouth and tongue to stimulate a woman's genitals; **fellatio** refers to oral stimulation of a male's genitals. In the early part of this century, heterosexuals, even those who were married, rarely practiced oral sex. By the 1970s, sex manuals and sexuality textbooks had begun to suggest that couples incorporate oral sex into their sexual routines. Women who are unable to have orgasms during coitus are often able to have them while receiving oral sex.

In a study of more than 2,000 college students using an anonymous online survey, researcher Wendy Chambers of the University of Georgia found that 39.1% of virgins had given oral sex to someone in their lifetime and that 95.5% of nonvirgins had. Of the respondents, 53.5% considered oral sex to be an intimate act, compared to 91% who considered sexual intercourse to be an intimate act.[26]

Results of the NSSHB show that the percentage of males who gave oral sex to a female within the month before the survey peaks at ages 25–29 years at 40%, and the percentage of males who gave oral sex to a male within the month is highest at ages 20–24 years at 5.2% and at 50–59 years at 6.4%. The percentage at other ages is much lower for male-on-male oral sex within the month. Results of the NSSHB also show that the percentage of females who gave oral sex to a male within the month before the survey peaks at ages 25–29 years at 49.9%, and the percentage of females who gave oral sex to a female within the month peaks at ages 16–17 years at 4.2%. The percentage at other ages is much lower for female-on-female oral sex within the month.[25] On the NSFG, lifetime percentages for oral sex with the opposite sex were 90% for men aged 25–44 years and 89% for women of the same age group (see Figure 6.6).

## Solitary Sexual Behavior

In 1994, statements on masturbation by the U.S. Surgeon General M. Joycelyn Elders resulted in her being forced to resign her post. Her comments were in response to a question at a United Nations conference on AIDS and suggested that masturbation might be taught as a means to limit the spread of HIV/AIDS. Although masturbation was a taboo subject to speak about publicly at that time, Elders recognized in 2010 that "we have finally included masturbation in our national conversation" as she discussed the reports from the National Survey of Sexual Health and Behavior.[27]

Data from the NSSHB show that solo masturbation is a common sexual practice in the United States. From 28% to 69% of men report that they masturbated alone within the month prior to the survey and from 12% to 52% of women did as well. Percentages varied by age group, with the lowest percentages reported by the oldest age group (70+ years old) and the highest percentages reported by those aged 25 to 29 years. This was true for both men and women.[25] The results of a British survey released in 2008 show that 73% of men and nearly 37% of women aged 16 to 44 years reported masturbating within the month prior to the survey.[28]

## Celibacy

**Celibacy**, or **sexual abstinence**, is refrainment from sexual intercourse, usually by choice. Celibacy can be a way of life; the clergy of some religions practice sexual abstinence. Some celibate individuals engage in alternative sexual practices such as masturbation. Temporary sexual abstinence during the woman's peak period of fertility is a feature of natural family planning methods (see Chapter 5). Late

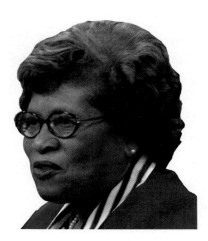

Former U.S. Surgeon General M. Jocelyn Elders.

> **sexual intercourse** Penetration of the vagina by a penis.
>
> **coitus** (KO-ih-tus) The act of a penis penetrating a vagina, often referred to as vaginal intercourse.
>
> **cunnilingus** Use of the mouth and tongue to stimulate a woman's genitals.
>
> **fellatio** Use of the mouth and tongue to stimulate a male's genitals.
>
> **celibacy (sexual abstinence)** Refrainment from sexual intercourse, usually by choice.

in pregnancy, couples may decide to avoid vaginal intercourse, especially if the activity is too awkward and uncomfortable.

Celibacy is not known to be harmful; indeed, it is the most effective measure for preventing pregnancies and sexually transmitted infections.

### Healthy Living Practices

- ☐ Wash after touching the anal area so as not to spread bacteria that live in the rectum to other parts of the body.
- ☐ To reduce the risk of transmitting the virus that causes AIDS, use latex condoms during vaginal or anal intercourse.
- ☐ Practicing sexual abstinence is the most reliable way to avoid pregnancy and sexually transmitted infections.

## Romantic Relationships

### Defining Love

Giving and receiving love are so important to a person's well-being that social scientists have speculated about love and studied its origins, characteristics, and stages. What is love? Why do people fall in love?

*Love* is difficult to define because the term has different meanings for different people. One definition is that love is a collection of behaviors, thoughts, and emotions that are associated with a psychological attraction toward other individuals. There are numerous kinds or degrees of love and a variety of feelings associated with love. Liking, fondness, affection, attraction, infatuation, and lust are feelings related to love. Also, the love of two friends can be quite dif-

**caring** The expression of concern for someone's well-being.

**intimacy** Disclosure of one's most personal thoughts and emotions to a trusted individual.

**attachment** The desire to spend time with someone to give and receive emotional support.

**commitment** The determination to maintain a relationship even when times are difficult.

**affection** Fondness.

**respect** The feeling that another has value and deserves attention.

ferent from the feelings between parent and child or husband and wife. According to sexologists William H. Masters and Virginia E. Johnson, all forms of love involve the element of **caring**, the expression of concern for someone's well-being.

Zick Rubin, one of the first psychologists to develop a questionnaire to measure the meanings of love, attempted to differentiate between loving and liking. He found that loving had characteristics of intimacy, attachment, caring, and commitment while liking had characteristics of affection and respect.[29] **Intimacy** is the disclosure of one's most personal thoughts and emotions to a trusted individual. **Attachment** is the desire to spend time with someone to give and receive emotional support. **Commitment** is the determination to maintain the relationship even when times are difficult. **Affection** is a feeling of fondness toward another. **Respect** is the feeling that another has value and deserves attention.

Most humans seek loving relationships with other individuals to meet their emotional needs. Love that

is fulfilling is reciprocal; that is, when one loves another, he or she is loved in return. Individuals who are in love feel free to achieve self-actualization (see Chapter 2) because their relationship fosters mutual independence as well as emotional, social, and spiritual growth.

# Psychologists' Theories About Love

Beginning with Sigmund Freud in 1922, psychologists have tried to explain the phenomenon of love. Early "love theorists" such as Freud were clinical psychologists, professionals who diagnose, treat, and study mental or emotional problems and disabilities. Most of their theories relied on ideas that people loved others as a remedy for their own problems or deficiencies, rather than loving others for themselves.

In recent decades, social psychologists have formulated theories on love. These professionals explore questions by examining the individual in a social context while taking into account personality, which is the distinctive pattern of behavior, thoughts, motives, and emotions that characterizes an individual.

In 1956, Eric Fromm presented his ideas about love in *The Art of Loving*.[30] A basic idea in Fromm's book, as noted in its title, is that loving is an art and, as such, must be learned and practiced. Fromm also distinguishes between types of love, such as motherly love and erotic love.

In 1973, John Alan Lee theorized that six styles of loving exist.[31] His ideas have since been upheld by results of studies of other researchers. *Table 6.1* lists these styles with their names (derived from the Greek), meanings, and characteristics. To see with

## Table 6.1

### Lee's Six Styles of Loving

| Name | Meaning | Characteristics |
|------|---------|-----------------|
| Ludus | Game-playing love | Enjoying "chasing" love interests but not "catching" them |
| Eros | Romantic, passionate love | Believing in "true" love and "instant" chemistry |
| Storge | Affectionate, friendly love | Believing that love grows out of friendship |
| Mania | Possessive, dependent love | Believing that your lover's attention is all that matters |
| Pragma | Logical, practical love | Thinking that the best lover for you will fit a predetermined set of criteria |
| Agape | Selfless love | Wanting to bear your lover's burdens so that he or she does not suffer |

which of Lee's style you most closely align, take "The Love Attitudes Scale" provided in the Student Workbook section at the end of this book.

In 1986, Robert Sternberg developed a triangular theory of love that incorporates three components—intimacy, commitment, and passion—as symbolized by the points of a triangle, as **Figure 6.8** shows.[32] His intimacy component includes behaviors that foster a feeling of warmth, while the commitment component refers to the decision to love as well as to make a relationship last. Passion, in the love triangle, refers not only to sexual passion but also to the fulfillment of needs that elicit a passionate response. The balance of these three components affects the shape of the triangle. Amount of love affects the area of the triangle.

People in a love relationship often have feelings of intimacy, commitment, and passion that differ from those of their partners. Although two people may be in love with each other, their "love triangles" will not match if one loves the other more than is reciprocated, and if one differs from the other in the balances of the three kinds of love. According to Sternberg, couples with similar love triangles are more likely to be satisfied with their relationships because they share more love-related feelings and attitudes, as Figure 6.10b shows, there are couples with mismatched triangles, as in Figure 6.10c. Sternberg has developed a questionnaire to measure love according to his love triangles theory.[33,34]

Finally, Sternberg asserts that although there are only three components of love, these three components combine in various ways to produce seven kinds of love.[34] For example, an absence of all three components (intimacy, commitment, and passion) results in nonlove. The presence of all three components results in consummate love. **Table 6.2** lists Sternberg's kinds of love and their components.

## Figure 6.8

**Sternberg's Love Triangle.** Psychologist Robert Sternberg created a model that incorporates three components of love—intimacy, commitment, and passion—at the points of a triangle. Couples with identical "love triangles" (a) are more likely to be satisfied with their relationships because they share more sexual feelings and attitudes than couples with similar (b) or highly mismatched triangles (c).

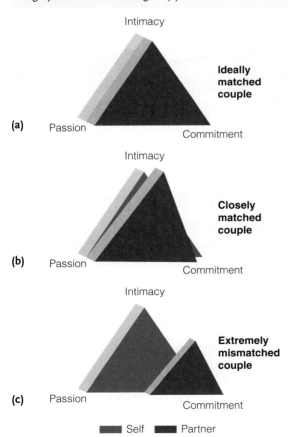

## Table 6.2

### Sternberg's Seven Kinds of Love

|  | Components of Love | | |
|---|---|---|---|
| **Kind of Love** | **Intimacy** | **Passion** | **Commitment** |
| Nonlove | 2 | 2 | 2 |
| Liking | 1 | 2 | 2 |
| Infatuated love | 2 | 1 | 2 |
| Empty love | 2 | 2 | 1 |
| Romantic love | 1 | 1 | 2 |
| Companionate love | 1 | 2 | 1 |
| Fatuous love | 2 | 1 | 1 |
| Consummate love | 1 | 1 | 1 |

*Source:* From *Cupid's arrow: The course of love through time* by Dr. Robert J. Sternberg, Cambridge University Press, 1998. Reprinted by permission of the author.

**compatible** Capable of existing together in harmony.

## Love Attachments

The early bonds, or attachments, that develop between parents and their offspring may influence the ability of the children to form close, secure relationships when they are adults. *Attachment* is a biological drive in which a child seeks nearness to or contact with a specific person, such as a parent, when he or she is frightened, tired, hungry, or ill. A child will exhibit attachment behavior, such as eye contact, smiling, crying, and clinging, to obtain or maintain desired proximity to this person. How the person responds to the child largely determines the type of attachment the child will form: secure, ambivalent, or avoidant.

For example, when an infant is hungry, he or she will exhibit attachment behavior, such as crying, which usually evokes a nurturing response from the attachment figure (e.g., mom or dad). A nurturing response to this need usually includes touching, eye contact, smiling, and providing milk. When the infant receives this nurturing response consistently, trust is built. When the infant does not receive this response consistently, the child may develop mistrust and may stop his or her attachment behavior. Over time, symptoms may emerge such as lack of eye contact, destructive behavior, and poor peer relationships. Some children who have poor attachments to their parents may avoid becoming emotionally close to people in adulthood.

Experts think that children who have emotionally distant and neglectful parents may mature into anxious lovers. *Anxious lovers* often have considerable doubts about the quality of their sexual relationships, are unable to trust their partners, and may be unable to form long-term commitments. However, if parents meet the emotional needs of their children and frequently display affection toward them, the children are likely to mature into secure lovers. Secure lovers are more likely to form trusting and committed relationships with other adults than are anxious lovers.

## Love Changes over Time

Early in a relationship, when physical attraction is greatest and partners know very little about one another, their passion is high. Preoccupied with their sexual desire for each other, passionate lovers think about their partners and want to be with them constantly.

Some people experience *infatuation*, a passionate but unrealistic attraction to someone. Infatuated individuals often exaggerate the positive characteristics of their partners while ignoring their faults. A relationship that is based on infatuation may not survive, especially when one or both lovers become aware of their partners' weaknesses and find these faults unacceptable.

Eventually, the intense sexual attraction that characterizes the initial stage of a romantic relationship subsides. The couple, if sexually active, usually engages in sex less frequently than in the earlier phase of their relationship. They enjoy being together, but they can endure separations. Other aspects of their relationship, such as companionship, often deepen. Although couples in this stage of love have conflicts, committed partners usually try to resolve their problems.

Not every couple experiences the stages of love in this order. Sometimes passionate love affairs evolve from companionate relationships, such as when friends become lovers. Whatever the course of a romantic relationship, however, it will have phases of growth and change.

The following Managing Your Health feature "Minding Your Sexual Manners" provides suggestions for socially responsible sexually related behaviors.

### Healthy Living Practices

☐ To help you make responsible decisions concerning your sexuality, consider how your sexual behavior affects yourself and others.

## Establishing Romantic Commitments

Have you ever been in love? Why did you fall in love with that person? Studies have shown that physical attraction is the most important factor that determines whether two individuals become romantically interested in one another. People often use other criteria as well, such as social status, occupation, and wealth, to select their sexual partners. Not surprisingly, Americans spend millions of dollars annually to enhance their "sex appeal" by purchasing makeup, jewelry, clothing, and expensive cars.

Initially, two people who are physically attracted to each other usually make and hold eye contact.

# Managing Your Health

## Minding Your Sexual Manners

The following guidelines can help you make socially responsible decisions regarding your sexual behavior.

1. Never force sex on another person, regardless of the situation.
2. Understand that at any time in a relationship, when a person says no, that means no, not yes or maybe.
3. Avoid situations that can impair your ability to make responsible sexual decisions, especially situations that involve alcohol and other drug use.
4. Be prepared to prevent pregnancies or sexually transmitted infections. Do not engage in risky sexual behaviors. Protect yourself and your partner by using a new latex condom with each act of sexual intercourse.
5. Communicate your concerns about the risks of pregnancy and sexually transmitted infections to your partner.
6. Share the responsibility of preventing pregnancies and sexually transmitted infections with your partner.
7. Respect the sexual privacy of your partner and your relationship.
8. Consider the feelings of others. Public displays of intimate behavior can offend or embarrass people.
9. Do not sexually harass others.
10. Treat your partner with care and respect.

*Source:* Adapted from Hatcher, R. A., Sanderson, C. A., & Smith, K. L. (1990). Sexual etiquette 101. *SIECUS Report,* 18:9.

Couples may describe this behavior as "falling in love at first sight." After two people find each other physically appealing, they need to determine if they are **compatible**; that is, if they are capable of existing together in harmony.

Which characteristics are important for establishing long-term satisfying and compatible relationships? Individuals in such relationships are usually close in age, and they usually share similar racial, ethnic, religious, and educational backgrounds (**Figure 6.9**). Members of couples who have extremely different backgrounds or many dissimilar characteristics can certainly form satisfying and lasting relationships, but these situations are less common than those described previously.

Sexual satisfaction is another characteristic related to the establishment of long-term satisfying and compatible relationships. Several studies show an

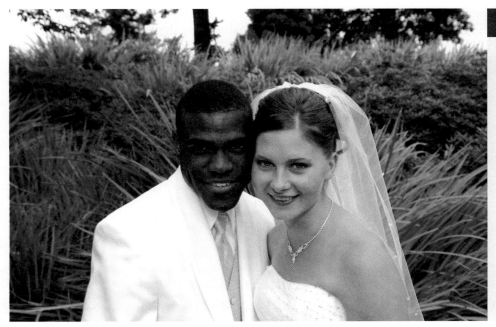

### Figure 6.9

**Many Personal Characteristics Contribute to Compatibility.** Although this man and woman do not share the same racial background, they are similar in age and may have other similarities that foster their compatibility as a couple.

association between sexual satisfaction and overall relationship satisfaction.[35] One study focused on the association between sexual satisfaction and relationship quality in premarital heterosexual couples.[36] Research results showed that over time, sexual satisfaction was positively associated with relationship satisfaction, love, and commitment for both men and women. When change occurred in sexual satisfaction over time, change also occurred in relationship satisfaction, love, and commitment. Overall, sexual satisfaction had stronger links with relationship quality for men than for women.

## Types of Romantic Commitments

**Cohabitation** In the second half of the twentieth century, a growing number of unmarried people decided to live with their heterosexual partners. In 1960, 439,000 adult heterosexual couples lived together; by 2008, the number had risen more than 15-fold to 6.8 million.[37] The practice of unmarried couples living together is called **cohabitation**.

Why do people live together rather than get married? Among young people, the widespread belief is that cohabitation is a way to find out if they and their partners really get along. Cohabitation is viewed as a way to avoid a bad marriage and eventual divorce. However, results of studies show that people who cohabit before marriage (with the exception of those who are engaged and have set a wedding date) are *not* more likely to enjoy longer and happier marriages than individuals who do not live together before

marrying. Studies conducted in the United States, Sweden, and Canada document higher divorce rates among couples who cohabited before marriage than among those who did not. Research results suggest that this increased risk of divorce may be due to the result of self-selection; that is, persons who are less able to sustain long-term relationships may choose to cohabit prior to marriage, rather than to marry without first living with their partners.[37] Additionally, research data show that multiple cohabiting experiences do not help people learn to have better relationships. In fact, persons with multiple cohabiting experiences are more likely to have failed future relationships than persons who do not cohabit. Although this negative correlation of cohabitation on later marriage stability is not totally understood, no positive contribution of cohabitation to marriage has been found.[38]

Despite a negative correlation between cohabitation and marriage stability, cohabitation is emerging as a significant experience for young adults and is replacing marriage as the first living-together union. Researchers estimate that 25% of unmarried women in the United States between the ages of 25 and 39 are currently living with a heterosexual partner. An additional 25% are estimated to have cohabited at one time.[37]

**Marriage** In the United States and in most other countries, marriage is a legally binding commitment between an adult man and an adult woman. Most Americans desire marriage as a lifelong and loving partnership, and expect sexual faithfulness, emotional support, mutual trust, and lasting commitment. However, research results show a moderate decline in marital quality since the 1970s (**Figure 6.10**).

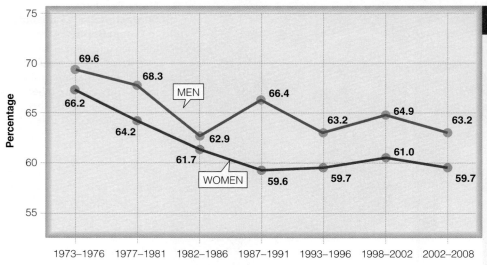

### Figure 6.10

**Percentage of Married Persons Age 18 Years and Older Who Said Their Marriages Were "Very Happy," by Period, United States.**

*Source:* Data from General Social Survey, conducted by the National Opinion Research Center of the University of Chicago. Sprecher, S. (2002). Sexual satisfaction in premarital relationships: Associations with satisfaction, love, commitment, and stability. *Journal of Sex Research*, 39(3):190–196.

Along with being less satisfied with their marriages, Americans are also marrying a bit later in life today than in recent decades. In 1960, the median age at first marriage was 20 years for women and 23 years for men. (The median is the point below which 50% of the scores fall.) By 2007, the median age of first marriage had increased to 26 years for women and 28 years for men. Americans have also become less likely to marry; from 1970 to 2008 the annual number of new marriages per 1,000 unmarried women aged 15 years and older declined 51%.[37]

What factors help make a marriage successful? Partners in successful marriages often demonstrate positive problem-solving and communication skills. When conflicts arise, couples with these skills can openly discuss their feelings, and they are willing to negotiate and compromise to find solutions. Additionally, partners in successful marriages share basic values, have mutual concerns, and exhibit high degrees of physical intimacy.

**Extrarelational Sex** Some people have sexual relationships with individuals who are not their spouses or primary sex partners. Although most Americans disapprove of such **extrarelational sex**, particularly when married couples are involved, results from the General Social Survey on American Sexual Behavior show that 21.7% of men and 12.6% of women had sexual relations with a person other than their spouse while married.[19] Rates are highest among persons who are "not too happy" with their marriage (30%), those who rarely attend church (22%), and those who are separated (39.4%). Having sex with someone other than one's spouse is commonly referred to as *extramarital sex* or *adultery*. The majority of married Americans report that they are faithful to their spouses.

**Separation and Divorce** Despite having high hopes for happiness and success during their wedding celebrations, many couples see their marriages end in separation or divorce. Nearly half of recent first marriages may end in divorce; the divorce rate for younger persons has risen in recent years. Accurate data concerning the number of married persons who separate permanently are unavailable. Teenage marriages are especially vulnerable to dissolution. Women who marry when they are younger than 20 years of age are much more likely to be in a failed marriage than women who marry

when they are at least 20 years of age. In addition, divorce rates are higher for high school dropouts than for college graduates, and for marriages in which there is conflict over money matters, an extramarital affair has taken place, or an alcohol/drug problem exists.[37]

Early in the twentieth century, divorce was uncommon in this country. In 1940, the U.S. divorce rate was 2 divorces per 1,000 persons. The divorce rate rose during World War II and peaked at more than 4 divorces per 1,000 at the war's end. The rate fell during the 1950s to nearly prewar rates, and rose again in the 1960s and 1970s. From 1979 through 1981, the U.S. divorce rate was at its highest level of the twentieth century, slightly more than 5 divorces per 1,000. The decline in the divorce rate has been relatively steady since that time, and in 2009 was at 3.4 for every 1,000 persons (**Figure 6.11**).

### Figure 6.11

**U.S. Divorce Rates: 1940 to 2009.** Since 1981, the divorce rate has declined in the United States.
*Sources:* U.S. Bureau of the Census, National Center for Health Statistics.

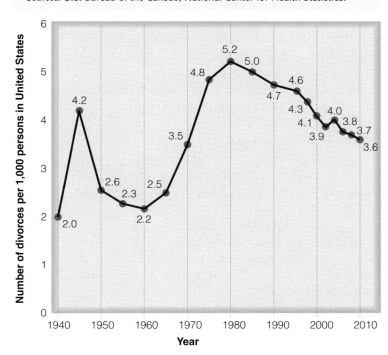

# Communication in Relationships

Effective communication is a cornerstone of interpersonal and sexual relationships. To communicate effectively, people must express themselves as accurately and as clearly as possible but also must listen with attentiveness, openness, and patience. To express yourself accurately and clearly, first say exactly what you mean. If you avoid being straightforward so that you will not hurt someone's feelings, for example, the person with whom you're communicating may not understand your message. Second, your statements must be specific, not vague. For example, telling your partner that you would like him to be more spontaneous will probably make him question what you really mean. Do you always want him to act in a spontaneous manner? Has he never been spontaneous? Or do you really mean that you had wanted him to accept yesterday's last-minute party invitation, and wished that he could have just dropped what he was doing, changed his clothes, and dashed out the door with you? Third, avoid sending mixed messages. For example, don't tell your partner that everything is fine when she can tell from your behavior and expression that you are really feeling "down." Or, don't say, "I don't want to worry you, but I think I have a sexually transmitted infection."

Another mechanism to foster effective communication is to express your feelings using "I" statements when discussing issues with a partner. Then, go on to say what you need to try to maintain (or change) the feeling. Statements that begin with "You" can hinder open communication between partners, particularly if the speaker is criticizing the listener's behavior or blaming this person for something. For example, instead of saying "You always spend too much time with your friends," you could say, "I feel lonely and miss you terribly when you are out with your friends." (Express the feeling.) "Could I join you on those occasions so that we could spend more time together?" (State the remedy.) Try not to fall into the trap of "false" I statements. "I feel like you spend too much time with your friends" is really a "you" statement.

Besides being able to express oneself clearly, an effective communicator has good listening skills. Failure to hear information accurately or completely can create misunderstandings that result in conflicts. In discussions, good listeners restate or paraphrase what they have heard their partners say. This practice allows speakers, if necessary, to correct or clarify what they have said. For example, if your partner says, "When we get together with your friends or your family, you always ignore me," you could respond by saying, "I didn't realize that you feel neglected in those situations. What can I do to make you feel more included?"

In addition to words, people use nonverbal forms of communication, such as body positioning (body language) and facial gestures, to express their thoughts (**Figure 6.12**). Touching is a form of nonverbal communication that can convey important information about intimate sexual feelings. Many people report that being held, kissed, massaged, or fondled by their partners is as sexually gratifying as sexual intercourse. Sensual touching does not have to involve the genitals; gently massaging your partner's back, for example, can convey your feelings of love to this individual.

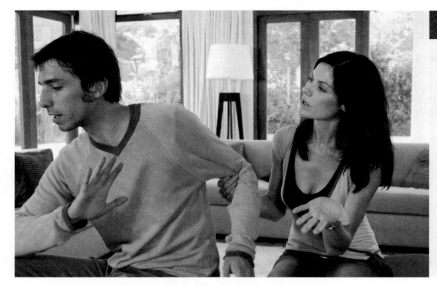

**Figure 6.12**

**Nonverbal Communication.** Nonverbal forms of communication, such as body postures and facial gestures, can convey thoughts. What do this couple's nonverbal signals communicate?

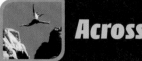

## Across THE LIFE SPAN

### SEXUALITY

Most preschoolers masturbate. Parents who think masturbation is a healthy and normal aspect of sexuality usually let their children know that the behavior is inappropriate in public but do not attempt to stop this behavior in private. Preschool children typically play games in which they act out adult gender roles. By this age, children have learned that there are differences between the sexes. Children are curious about sexuality; they may "play doctor" by examining each others' genitals. Additionally, young children often ask questions such as "Where did I come from?" If parents are uncertain how to answer this or other questions about sexual matters, they can usually find a collection of age-appropriate sexuality books at their libraries that they can read with their children after reading them themselves.

It is not unusual for elementary school-age children to engage in mutual sex play, activities that may include rehearsing adult sexual behaviors. Sex experts consider such sex play normal behavior when it is playful, occurs infrequently, and does not involve coercion.

The ability to reproduce begins during puberty. Many teens avoid sexual activity because they fear becoming pregnant, contracting sexually transmitted infections, and losing self-esteem or parental trust. The media, however, expose American youth to sexually explicit images that may conflict with parental values and encourage sexual experimentation. Additionally, peers or older persons can exert consider-

able pressure on teens to engage in sex. To help youth maintain their abstinence, parents and educators can teach teens how to use sexual assertiveness skills.

Despite efforts to promote teenage abstinence, only about half of American high school students refrain from having sex. By grade 10, about 40% of young girls in the United States have had sexual intercourse. By grade 12, about 65% have engaged in coitus.[39]

Results of the Youth Risk Behavior Surveillance, 2009, conducted by the CDC revealed that by age 13 years, more boys reported having engaged in sexual intercourse than girls. About 25% of male black students indicated that they had engaged in sexual intercourse before age 13; this percentage was well more than twice that of their Hispanic peers and more than five times that of their white peers. Overall, 15.2% of black students, 6.7% of Hispanic students, and 3.4% of white students initiated sexual intercourse before 13 years of age.[39]

In comparing behavior trends in youth from 1991 through 2007, the CDC has found that the percentage of high school students who have ever had sexual intercourse has decreased from about 54% in 1991 to about 46% in 2009. More students are using condoms; in 1991 about 46% of sexually active students used a condom during their last sexual intercourse, while in 2009, 61% reported having done so.[40]

The teenage birth rate in 2009 was the lowest it has ever been since the CDC began keeping track of birth rates for teenagers in 1960 (**Figure 6.13**). The preliminary 2009 birth rate for teenagers 18 to 19 years old was 66.2 births per 1,000 females of that age group. This rate was about 60% lower than in 1960 (166.7 per 1,000) and 30% lower than in 1991 (94.0 births per 1,000). For those in the 15- to 17-year-old age group,

## Figure 6.13

**Birth Rates for Teenagers by Age: United States, 1960–2009.**

Source: Ventura, S. J., & Hamilton, B. E. (2011). U.S. teenage birth rate resumes decline. *NCHS Data Brief*, no. 58. Retrieved March 14, 2011 from http://www.cdc.gov/nchs/data/databriefs/db58.pdf

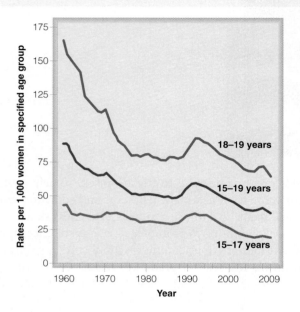

birth rates fell to 20.1 per 1,000 young women, which is 48% lower than in 1991 (38.6 births per 1,000) and 54% lower than in 1960 (43.9 births per 1,000).

Compared to women in their 20s, pregnant teenagers have a greater risk of experiencing serious complications during pregnancy and delivery as well as of giving birth to premature, underweight babies. Premature infants are born before the 37th week of pregnancy. The risk of giving birth to a premature, low-birth-weight infant is especially high for pregnant adolescents between 10 and 14 years of age. Underweight premature newborns have a greater risk of serious health and developmental problems than do normal-weight newborns who are born at term, that is, between the 37th and 41st weeks of pregnancy.

Most unmarried teenage girls who give birth to live infants keep their babies rather than give them up for adoption. Adolescent mothers are more likely to be unmarried, poor, and have less education than mothers who give birth when they are older. Many teenage mothers have difficulty improving their educational and socioeconomic levels when they become adults.

Teenaged fathers do not usually marry the teenaged mothers of their children, even though the relationship between the teens may have been ongoing for 6 months or longer. If the father is 20 years or older, he is more likely than his teenaged counterpart to marry the mother. As the child becomes older, the teenaged father typically becomes less and less involved with the child. When asked why they did not live with or marry their children's mothers, teenaged fathers cite financial concerns as one major issue.[41]

With respect to older adults, sex has enduring importance. Sexuality does not end because a person is older. According to findings from the National Survey of Sexual Health and Behavior, 20% of Americans who are 70 to 79 years of age engage in sexual intercourse a few times per year, 20% a few times per month, and 5% two or three times per week. Those aged 80 years and older enjoy sexual intercourse as well; almost 19% in this age group had sexual intercourse a few times per month. Twenty-one percent of those in their 70s received oral sex and 25% gave oral sex within the past year. Fifteen percent of those aged 80 years and older received oral sex and 22% gave oral sex within the past year.[41] Sexual inactivity in the later years of life is more often the result of medical disabilities or lack of a sexual partner rather than lack of desire.

Older adults experience a gradual decline in sexual functioning. Therefore, elderly individuals should recognize that their sexual responses are likely to be different from when they were young adults. For example, it usually takes longer for the older adult to become adequately sexually stimulated before sex, and orgasms are less intense. Chronic diseases such as diabetes and heart disease can further limit an aged person's sexual responses or interest in sex. Certain antihypertensive and antidepressant medications can produce side effects that impair sexual functioning; affected individuals should discuss their sexual problems with their physicians. Frequently, changing medications can be helpful. In some cases, medical treatments are available that can improve sexual functioning. Elderly individuals who have sexual impairments that do not respond to treatment can rely on noncoital forms of sexual expression such as kissing, caressing, cuddling, and oral sex to obtain pleasure and fulfillment. For some, affectionate behavior is more crucial to happiness than sex is.

Besides physical factors, significant social changes such as the loss of a spouse or moving into a nursing home can have negative impacts on the sexuality of aged individuals. Widows and widowers may have difficulty meeting sexual partners. Elderly nursing home residents may not feel free to express their sexuality because they lack privacy. As the number of elderly Americans rises, addressing sexual needs in this age group will become an increasingly important issue.

# Analyzing Health-Related Information

Search the word *impotence* using Google or another search engine. Choose a website that sells an impotence product. Explain why you think the website you chose is a reliable or an unreliable source of information. Use the "Assessing Information on the Internet" portion of the model for analyzing health-related information to guide your thinking; the main points of the model are noted here. The model is fully explained in Chapter 1.

- What is the source of the information?
- Is the site sponsored by a nationally known health or medical organization or affiliated with a well-known medical research institution or major university? If not, is the site staffed by well-respected and credentialed experts in the field?
- Does the site include up-to-date references from a well-known, respected medical or scientific journal or links to reputable websites, such as nationally recognized medical organizations?
- Is the information at the website current?

Based on your analysis, do you think that this web page is a reliable source of health-related information? Summarize your reasons for coming to this conclusion.

If you are unsure of the credibility of the site after answering the preceding questions, continue with the following six Analyzing Health-Related Information questions.

1. Which statements on the website are verifiable facts, and which are unverified statements or value claims?
2. Does the person, organization, or institution that developed the website have the appropriate background and credentials in the topic area? What can you do to check credentials?
3. What might be the motives and biases inherent to the website?
4. What is the main point of the article, ad, or claim made on the site? Which information is relevant to the issue, main point, product, or service? Which information is irrelevant?
5. Does the source of information present the pros and cons of the topic or the benefits and risks of the product?
6. Does the source of information attack the credibility of conventional scientists or medical authorities?

Based on your additional analysis, do you think that this web page is a reliable source of health-related information? Summarize your reasons for coming to this conclusion.

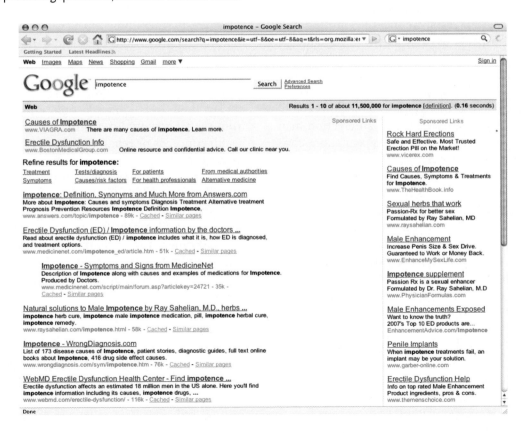

# CHAPTER REVIEW

## Summary

Human sexuality is a complex set of thoughts, feelings, attitudes, and behaviors that are related to reproduction as well as to being male or female. Numerous biological, psychological, social, and cultural forces interact to influence sexuality. Sexuality influences all aspects of an individual's life, including identity, self-esteem, emotions, personality, relationships, lifestyle, and health. Being knowledgeable about sexuality is important for maintaining good health and optimal well-being.

The sexual response of individuals engaging in sexual activity is usually described in phases. During the excitement phase, both men and women have a heightened sexual awareness. During the plateau phase, the heart rate, blood pressure, respiration rate, and level of muscle tension all increase and the erection of the male intensifies. During the orgasmic phase, men ejaculate, while women's vaginal walls contract rhythmically. During the resolution phase, the body returns to its prearousal state. Other models of the sexual response include emotional or psychological aspects as well as these physiologic aspects.

Some people have sexual dysfunctions that interfere with their sexual response. Common sexual dysfunctions include erectile dysfunction, the inability of a man to develop and/or sustain an erection firm enough for penetration; premature ejaculation, consistently attaining orgasm either before or shortly after intercourse begins and before he wishes it to occur; hypoactive sexual desire, a low interest in sex that causes distress, which occurs in both sexes but is more prevalent in women; and vaginismus, a sexual dysfunction of women in which the muscles of the lower third of the vaginal canal contract involuntarily at the anticipation of vaginal penetration.

Instincts, sensations, and hormones drive reproductive behavior, but social, cultural, and religious factors heavily influence a person's sexual attitudes, values, and behaviors. Sexually responsible people consider how their sexual behavior affects themselves and others.

Gender is the classification of the sex of a person based on many criteria, among them anatomic and chromosomal characteristics. Gender identity is an individual's perception of himself or herself as male or female. Various biological, social, and environmental forces mold a child's gender identity. A *gender role* refers to patterns of behavior, attitudes, and personality attributes that, in a particular culture, are traditionally considered feminine or masculine. In the United States today, gender roles are undergoing dramatic changes and are becoming more flexible than in the past.

Sexual orientation, the direction of one's romantic thoughts, feelings, and attractions, can be toward the same sex, the opposite sex, or both sexes. Today, researchers and mental health experts generally agree that people do not decide their sexual orientation and cannot alter their sexual preferences, whether they are at either end of the sexual orientation continuum or somewhere in-between.

Sexual partners may engage in a variety of intimate activities, including mutual masturbation as well as vaginal, oral, and anal sex. However, sex does not require a partner for it to be a pleasurable experience—most people solo masturbate at some point during their lives. Some people choose to refrain from sexual activity for a variety of reasons, such as health concerns or religious beliefs. Abstaining from sexual activity is not known to be harmful, and it is an effective measure for preventing pregnancies and sexually transmitted infections.

People need to establish and maintain satisfying attachments to others for optimal health and well-being. People who have high self-esteem, are satisfied with their bodies, are in good health, and have positive feelings about their sexuality are likely to form fulfilling intimate relationships. Although love is difficult to define, people in loving relationships share feelings of caring, respect, attachment, commitment, and intimacy.

Various psychologists have developed theories about love. However, experts generally agree that love changes over time. Early in a relationship, when physical attraction is greatest and partners know very little about one another, their passion is high. Eventually, the intense sexual attraction that characterizes a romantic relationship in its initial stages subsides. Other aspects of the relationship, such as companionship, often deepen. Compatibility, the ability to exist in harmony, is crucial in the development of a healthy emotional attraction between partners. Usually important for establishing a compatible relationship is the sharing of similar interests, attitudes, and values.

More couples are choosing to cohabit before marriage, but this practice results in a higher risk of divorce than not living together prior to marriage. Those who are married are less satisfied with their marriages and are marrying later in life than in recent decades. Effective communication is an essential ingredient for maintaining satisfying and successful marriages and intimate relationships.

Children are curious about sex; they frequently play sex games with other children and ask their par-

ents questions about sex. Children's sex play is normal behavior when it is playful, occurs infrequently, and does not involve coercion.

The teenage birth rate has declined dramatically since the 1960s. Compared with women in their 20s, pregnant teenagers have a greater risk of serious complications during pregnancy and delivery, as well as of giving birth to premature and underweight newborns. Additionally, adolescent mothers are more likely to be unmarried, poor, and have less education than mothers who give birth when they are older. Many teenage mothers have difficulty improving their educational and socioeconomic levels when they become adults.

Sexuality does not end at a particular age. Most healthy elderly men and women continue to be interested and participate in sexual activity. However, sexual functioning declines with aging; sexual responses in older persons are different from when they were young adults. As the number of elderly Americans rises, addressing sexuality needs in this age group will become an increasingly important issue.

## Applying What You Have Learned

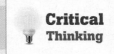
**Critical Thinking**

1. Develop a plan to improve the way you convey your feelings in relationships. **Application**
2. Analyze your present intimate relationship or a past one. Explain why you think it will be (or was) a short-term or long-term relationship. **Analysis**

3. Propose a checklist of characteristics that you could use to select a suitable partner. Explain why these characteristics are important. **Synthesis**
4. Develop a position concerning the promotion of masturbation as a safe sex alternative. How would you defend your position? **Evaluation**

| **Application** | **Analysis** | **Synthesis** | **Evaluation** | **Key** |
|---|---|---|---|---|
| using information in a new situation. | breaking down information into component parts. | putting together information from different sources. | making informed decisions. | |

## Reflecting on Your Health

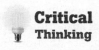

**Critical Thinking**

1. What is the source of your sexual values (e.g., your parents, your religious upbringing)? Do you feel comfortable with those values? Why or why not? Do you feel as though your peers share some or all of your values, or do you feel intimidated or pressured to change your values?

2. Do you think that "traditional" gender roles are appropriate in American society today? If you think that some are appropriate and some are not, pick one example from each category and explain your feelings about their appropriateness or inappropriateness.

3. Do you agree with former Surgeon General Jocelyn Elders's opinion that sex education in U.S. schools could include instruction about masturbation particularly for the purpose of reducing the spread of sexually transmitted infections, especially HIV/AIDS? Why or why not?

4. Think about a current or former intimate relationship you had. Do you think that your love relationship fits one of Lee's six styles of loving or one of Sternberg's kinds of love? How does it fit or not fit?

5. Think about the nature of your verbal interactions with someone important to you—a parent or spouse, for example. How could you communicate more effectively with that person using suggestions in this chapter?

## References

1. Travison, T. G., et al. (2007). The relative contributions of aging, health, and lifestyle factors to serum testosterone decline in men. *Journal of Clinical Endocrinology and Metabolism, 92*:549–555.

2. Fisher, L. L., et al. (2010). *Sex, romance, and relationships: AARP survey of midlife and older adults.* Retrieved on March 3, 2011, from http://assets.aarp.org/rgcenter/general/srr_09.pdf

3. Whipple, B. (2002). Women's sexual pleasure and satisfaction. A new view of female sexual function. *The Female Patient, 27*:39–44.

4. Basson, R. (2001). Female sexual response: The role of drugs in the management of sexual dysfunction. *Obstetrics and Gynecology, 98*:350–353.

5. Selvin, E., et al. (2007). Prevalence and risk factors for erectile dysfunction in the US. *American Journal of Medicine, 120*:151–157.

6. Kupelian, V., et al. (2010). Relative contributions of modifiable risk factors to erectile dysfunction: Results from the Boston Area Community Health (BACH) Survey. *Preventive Medicine, 50*(1–2):19–25.

7. Kazi, M., et al. (2007). Considerations for the diagnosis and treatment of testosterone deficiency in elderly men. *The American Journal of Medicine, 120*:835–840.

8. International Society for Sexual Medicine. (2010). Premature ejaculation: Advice for men from the International Society for Sexual Medicine [Patient information sheet]. Retrieved on March 6, 2011, from http://www.issm.info/v4/data/education/patient/patient.asp

9. Hellstrom, W. J. (2011). Update on treatments for premature ejaculation. *International Journal of Clinical Practice, 65*(1):16–26.

10. Stahl, S. M. (2010). Circuits of sexual desire in hypoactive sexual desire disorder. *Journal of Clinical Psychiatry, 71*(5):518–519.

11. Leiblum, S. R., Koochaki, P. E., Rodenberg, C. A., Barton, I. P., & Rosen, R. C. (2006). Hypoactive sexual desire disorder in postmenopausal women: US results from the Women's International Study of Health and Sexuality (WISHeS). *Menopause, 13*:46–56.

12. Stahl, S. M. (2010). Targeting circuits of sexual desire as a treatment strategy for hypoactive sexual desire disorder. *Journal of Clinical Psychiatry, 71*(7):821–822.

13. Schoen, C., & Bachmann, G. (2009). Sildenafil citrate for female sexual arousal disorder: A future possibility? *Nature Reviews Urology, 6*(4):216–222.

14. Binik, Y. M. (2010). The *DSM* diagnostic criteria for vaginismus. *Archives of Sexual Behavior, 39*:278–291.

15. Bryant, A. N. (2003). Changes in attitudes toward women's roles: Predicting gender-role traditionalism among college students. *Sex Roles, 48*(3/4):131–142.

16. Gates, G. J. (2011, April). *How many people are lesbian, gay, bisexual, and transgender?* The Williams Institute, School of Law, University of California Los Angeles. Retrieved on April 12, 2011, from http://www2.law.ucla.edu/williamsinstitute/pdf/How-many-people-are-LGBT-Final.pdf

17. Pearlman, A., et al. (2010). Mutations in MAP3K1 cause 46,XY disorders of sex development and implicate a common signal transduction pathway in human testis determination. *The American Journal of Human Genetics, 87*:898–904.

18. Ford, J. A., & Jasinski, J. L. (2005). Sexual orientation and substance use among college students. *Addictive Behaviors, 31*:404–413.

19. Smith, T. W. (2006). *American sexual behavior: Trends, sociodemographic differences, and risk behavior* (GSS Topical Report No. 25). Chicago, IL: University of Chicago, National Opinion Research Center.

20. Kinsey, A. C., Pomeroy, W. B., Martin, C. E., & Gebhard, P. H. (1953). *Sexual behavior in the human female.* Philadelphia, PA: W. B. Saunders.

21. LeVay, S. (1991). A difference in hypothalamic structure between heterosexual and homosexual men. *Science, 253*:1034–1037.

22. Hamer, D. H., Hu, S., Magnuson, V. L., Hu, N., & Pattatucci, A. M. (1993). A linkage between DNA markers on the X chromosome and male sexual orientation. *Science, 26*:321–327.

23. Iemmola, F., & Camperio Ciani, A. (2009). New evidence of genetic factors influencing sexual orientation in men: Female fecundity increase in the maternal line. *Archives of Sexual Behavior, 38*:393–399.

24. Gallup Poll. (2010). *Gay and lesbian rights.* Retrieved on March 9, 2011, from http://www.gallup.com/poll/1651/Gay-Lesbian-Rights.aspx

25. Herbenick, D., et al. (2010). Sexual behavior in the United States: Results from a national probability sample of men and women ages 14–94. *The Journal of Sexual Medicine, 7*(Suppl 5):255–265.

26. Chambers, W. C. (2007). Oral sex: Varied behaviors and perceptions in a college population. *Journal of Sex Research, 44*:28–42.

27. Elders, M. J. (2010). Sex for health and pleasure throughout a lifetime. *The Journal of Sexual Medicine, 7*(Suppl 5):248–249.

28. Gerressu, M., Mercer, C. H., Graham C. A., Wellings, K., & Johnson, A. M. (2008). Prevalence of masturbation and associated factors in a British national probability survey. *Archives of Sexual Behavior, 37*:266–278.

29. Rubin, Z. (1973). *Liking and loving.* New York, NY: Holt, Rinehart, & Winston.

30. Fromm, E. (1956). *The art of loving.* New York, NY: Harper.

31. Lee, J. A. (1973). *The colours of love.* Ontario, Canada: New Press.

32. Sternberg, R. J. (1986). A triangular theory of love. *Psychological Review, 93*:119–135.

33. Sternberg, R. J. (1997). Construct validation of a triangular love scale. *European Journal of Social Psychology, 27*:313–335.

34. Sternberg, R. J. (1998). *Cupid's arrow: The course of love through time.* Cambridge, England: Cambridge University Press.

35. Rosen, R. C., & Bachmann, G. A. (2008). Sexual well-being, happiness, and satisfaction, in women: The case for a new conceptual paradigm. *Journal of Sex & Marital Therapy, 34*:291–297.

36. Sprecher, S. (2002). Sexual satisfaction in premarital relationships: Associations with satisfaction, love, commitment, and stability. *Journal of Sex Research, 39*(3):190–196.

37. National Marriage Project. (2009). *The state of our unions: Marriage in America 2009: Money & marriage.* Piscataway, NJ: Rutgers University. Retrieved on March 11, 2011, from http://www.virginia.edu/marriageproject/pdfs/Union_11_25_09.pdf

38. Popenoe, D. (2008). *Cohabitation, marriage and child wellbeing.* Piscataway, NJ: Rutgers University and The National Marriage Project. Retrieved on March 11, 2011, from http://www.virginia.edu/marriageproject/pdfs/NMP2008CohabitationReport.pdf

39. Centers for Disease Control and Prevention. (2010). Youth Risk Behavior Surveillance—United States, 2009. *Morbidity and Mortality Weekly Report, 59*(SS-5). Retrieved on March 14, 2011, from http://www.cdc.gov/mmwr/pdf/ss/ss5905.pdf

40. Centers for Disease Control and Prevention. (2010). Trends in the prevalence of sexual behaviors: National Youth Risk Behavior Survey, 1991–2009. Retrieved on March 14, 2011, from http://www.cdc.gov/HealthyYouth/yrbs/pdf/us_sexual_trend_yrbs.pdf

41. Elfenbein, D. S., & Felice, M. E. (2003). Adolescent pregnancy. *Pediatric Clinics of North America, 50*:781–800.

42. Schick, V., et al. (2010). Sexual behaviors, condom use, and sexual health of Americans over 50: Implications for sexual health promotion for older adults. *The Journal of Sexual Medicine, 7*(Suppl 5): 315–329.

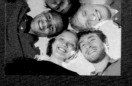

**Diversity in Health**
Khat

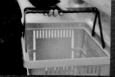

**Consumer Health**
Over-the-Counter
Medicines: Safety
and the FDA

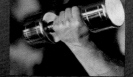

**Managing Your Health**
Falling Asleep Without
Prescriptions

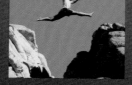

**Across the Life Span**
Drug Use and Abuse

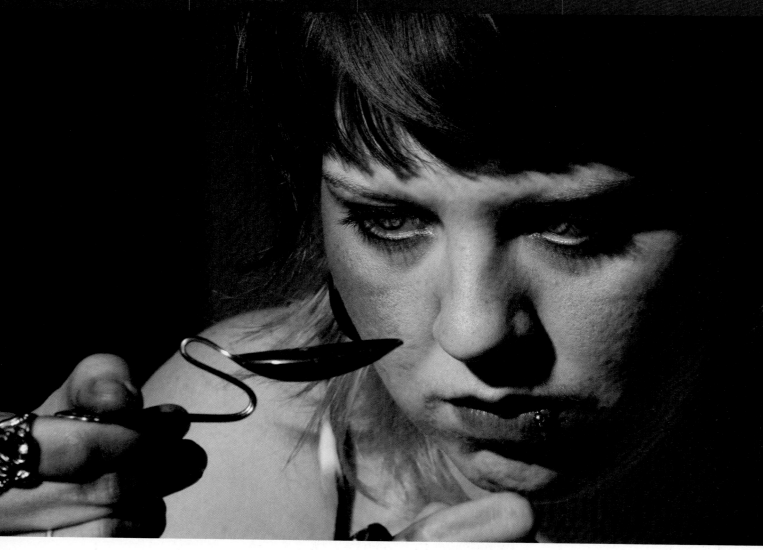

# Chapter Overview

Differences between drug use, misuse, and abuse

The effects of psychoactive drugs on the mind and body

Why people use psychoactive drugs

Patterns of drug use in the United States

How physiologic and psychological drug dependence
develops

The risk factors for drug dependence

The long-term effects of drug abuse

How the FDA regulates over-the-counter drugs

Goals and strategies for drug treatment and prevention

# Student Workbook

Self-Assessment: Are You Dependent on Drugs?

Changing Health Habits: Are You Using Drugs
Inappropriately?

# Do You Know?

How drugs can affect the brain?

If smoking marijuana is safer than smoking cigarettes?

Which dietary supplements contain drugs that may be
dangerous?

## CHAPTER 7

# Drug Use and Abuse

**D**rugs. For many people, this word produces thoughts of shadowy characters secretively injecting illegal and dangerous compounds into their veins. This word may also evoke images of boarded-up crack houses, young people cooking heroin to liquify it for injection, and women being assaulted while under the influence of date-rape drugs. To others, the word *drugs* brings positive thoughts, such as physicians prescribing medicines to relieve the signs and symptoms of illness. Other images might include your sitting comfortably in the dentist's chair while drugs block the pain of the drill, or a person with cancer being treated with powerful chemical therapies to eliminate deadly abnormal cells. What are drugs? Why do drugs elicit both negative and positive images?

**Drugs** are nonfood chemicals that alter the way a person thinks, feels, functions, or behaves. For thousands of years, people have taken naturally occurring drugs that produce medicinal benefits or **psychoactive** (mood-altering or mind-altering) effects. Nearly everyone uses drugs, for a variety of reasons. Most people have taken aspirin or other pain relievers to treat headaches, sipped cups of coffee or caffeinated soft drinks to stay awake, or

> "Drugs...can have serious negative effects on the health and well-being of individuals when used improperly."

**drugs** Nonfood chemicals that alter the way a person thinks, feels, functions, or behaves.

**psychoactive** Having mind-altering or mood-altering effects.

**drug misuse** The temporary and improper use of a legal drug.

drunk alcoholic beverages to celebrate special occasions or to complement meals. Each of these familiar products contains drugs that have beneficial uses, but they can have serious negative effects on the health and well-being of individuals when used improperly. Additionally, inappropriate drug use contributes to numerous social problems that plague our society, such as crime, unemployment, and family violence and dissolution.

This chapter examines the effects of certain drugs on the functioning of the brain, the general nature of drug use and abuse, and the various problems associated with the use of these chemicals. Summary **Table 7.7** at the end of this chapter lists the major types of drugs that affect brain functioning and provides examples of each. Because many Americans use alcoholic beverages and tobacco, Chapter 8 focuses on the effects of these products on health. Some people take steroid hormones to improve their appearance; see Chapter 11 for more information concerning the effects of steroids on health.

## Drug Use, Misuse, and Abuse

The typical American household has a supply of pain relievers, cold remedies, cough syrups, and other medications. Medications are drugs that have beneficial uses such as treating diseases or correcting physiologic abnormalities. Medicinal drugs are frequently misused. **Drug misuse** is the temporary and improper use of a legal drug. **Table 7.1** lists some typical misuses of drugs.

A prescription is necessary to legitimately purchase the most powerful and potentially hazardous medications. Most of the active compounds in prescription drugs have been tested scientifically for safety and effectiveness.

Nonetheless, mixing prescription drugs with other prescription or nonprescription drugs can be fatal. On January 22, 2008, actor Heath Ledger died from an accidental overdose of prescription drugs (**Figure 7.1**). The Academy Award nominee took a

### Table 7.1

### Typical Drug Misuse Behaviors

| Behavior | Example |
|---|---|
| Discontinuing the use of prescribed medications prematurely even though you have been instructed to take it for a longer period | Taking an antibiotic only until symptoms disappear |
| Mixing drugs | Taking barbiturates and drinking alcohol at a party (combining these depressant drugs can be fatal) |
| Taking more than the recommended dosage | Consuming ten multiple vitamin and mineral supplements instead of one daily |
| Saving and using medications past their expiration date | Taking a pain reliever that was prescribed 5 years ago |
| Sharing medicines | Giving your prescribed allergy medicine to a friend |

combination of painkillers, antianxiety drugs, and sleeping pills, and their combined effects led to his death. Together, these drugs can cause the brain and brainstem to stop sending messages to the heart and respiratory system. As happened with Ledger, the heartbeat and breathing stopped.

People can buy thousands of medicines without prescriptions, commonly called over-the-counter, or OTC, drugs. Many over-the-counter remedies contain chemicals that have not been evaluated scientifically. Although people often think that OTC drugs are completely safe, any substance that has druglike effects can be dangerous if used improperly. Aspirin and antihistamines, for example, are toxic (poisonous) when ingested in high doses. A later section of this chapter examines problems associated with the use of certain OTC drugs.

Foods are not considered drugs, but many foods contain substances such as caffeine that affect the body. Furthermore, when some vitamins and minerals are consumed in large doses, they have druglike activity in the body. For example, physicians occasionally prescribe large doses of niacin (a B vitamin)

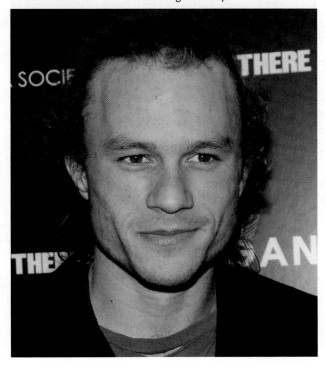

## Figure 7.1

**Mixing Prescription Drugs.** Academy Award nominee Heath Ledger died accidentally at the age of 28 from the abuse of prescription medications. The drugs Ledger took that resulted in his death included painkillers, tranquilizers, and antihistamines. Six prescription medications were found in Ledger's body.

**drug abuse** The intentional improper or nonmedical use of any drug.

to lower the blood cholesterol levels of certain patients. Many people, however, take massive doses of vitamins and minerals without consulting physicians because they think these nutrients are always safe to ingest. However, many vitamins and minerals are toxic when taken in such high doses. Chapters 9 and 16 discuss hazards associated with consuming large amounts of nutritional supplements.

In some instances, drug use becomes **drug abuse**, the intentional improper or nonmedical use of any drug. Drug abuse occurs whenever the use of a substance negatively affects the health and well-being of the user, his or her family, or society. People are more likely to abuse psychoactive drugs than other drugs because of their effects on the mind.

The government controls the use of most psychoactive drugs because of their potential for abuse. Title II of the Comprehensive Drug Abuse Prevention and Control Act of 1970, usually referred to as the Controlled Substances Act, is the legal foundation of narcotics enforcement in the United States. It classifies psychoactive substances into five drug sched-

ules according to their potential for abuse, medical usefulness, and safety (**Table 7.2**). Schedule I drugs have the most stringent control status. They are commonly abused, have little medicinal value (although the medicinal value of marijuana is hotly debated), and lack accepted safety for use. In the United States, it is illegal to use, possess, or sell Schedule I drugs. Schedule V drugs have the least stringent control status. They are infrequently abused, have important medicinal uses, and are considered safe when taken as directed. Schedule II, III, IV, and V drugs are available by prescription.

Officials with the Drug Enforcement Administration (DEA) evaluate medical and scientific information from the U.S. Department of Health and Human Services (HHS) before classifying a drug as a controlled substance. Although classified together, drugs in each schedule do not necessarily have the same potential for producing harmful effects. Heroin and marijuana are Schedule I drugs, for example, but the effects of abusing heroin are more serious than those of abusing marijuana. Additionally, drugs classified in a more stringently controlled schedule do not necessarily have a greater potential for producing harmful effects as drugs in a less stringently controlled schedule or drugs that are not scheduled. For instance, alcohol and nicotine are not scheduled drugs, yet the widespread abuse of these addictive substances is responsible for disabling and killing more people each year than the combined use of all controlled drugs.

People abuse illegal drugs such as cocaine, legally available psychoactive substances such as alcohol, some prescription drugs, and OTC remedies. Many individuals abuse a combination of legal and illegal drugs. Regardless of its legal status, no drug is completely safe. The risk that a drug will cause serious side effects largely depends on the type of drug, the amount taken over time, and the health of the person using the drug.

 **Healthy Living Practices**

☐ Because no drug is completely safe, consider the effects a drug can have on your health and well-being before using it.

## Table 7.2

### Drug Schedules

| Schedule | Examples of Drugs | Description |
|---|---|---|
| I | Heroin, LSD, mescaline, peyote, psilocybin, marijuana, GHB, China white | No current accepted medical use; high potential for abuse |
| II | Ritalin, PCP, Dilaudid, cocaine, methadone, Demerol, morphine, OxyContin, codeine, opium | Current accepted medical use; high potential for abuse |
| III | Paregoric, anabolic steroids, Tylenol with codeine, Vicodin, Marinol | Current accepted medical use; medium potential for abuse |
| IV | Rohypnol* ("roofies" or the "date-rape drug"), MDMA, Valium, Librium, Serax, Halcion, Darvon, Placidyl, phenobarbital, Xanax, khat | Current accepted medical use; low potential for abuse |
| V | Robitussin A–C, Lomotil, Motofen, Parepectolin | Current accepted medical use; lowest potential for abuse |

*Penalties for the possession, trafficking, or distribution of Rohypnol are the same as for Schedule I drugs.

Source: Data from U.S. Department of Justice, Drug Enforcement Administration.

# Psychoactive Drugs: Effects on the Mind and Body

## How Psychoactive Drugs Affect the Brain

Psychoactive drugs affect the nervous system—the "quick" communication network of the body—by changing the way the brain perceives and processes information received from the environment. Chapter 2 describes the nervous system, which includes the brain and spinal cord (central nervous system, or CNS) and the sensory and motor nerves that transmit messages to and from the central nervous system.

Psychoactive drugs interact with nerve cells in the brain, altering the activity of chemical transmitters that carry messages from one nerve to another. As a result, these drugs influence perceptions, thought processes, feelings, and behaviors. Many commonly abused drugs affect specific regions of the brain, referred to as reward centers because they have a positive influence on mood and alertness. As a result, when used initially, these drugs often produce **euphoria**, an intense feeling of well-being commonly called a "high." Although altering the normal internal chemical environment of the brain affects a person's mood and behavior, external conditions can modify these responses.

## What Happens to Drugs in the Body?

After being taken, psychoactive drugs enter the bloodstream and eventually reach the brain, where they produce their characteristic effects. As drugs circulate, the body may eliminate small amounts of these substances in urine, feces, or exhaled breath. In most cases, the remaining drugs undergo **detoxification**, the process of converting harmful substances into less dangerous compounds that can be excreted. Detoxification usually occurs in the liver. The body stores some drugs, primarily in fat, for days and possibly weeks after exposure, particularly when detoxification occurs slowly. Until the body completely eliminates a drug, small amounts of the substance may be detectable in blood or urine.

A state of **intoxication** occurs when the amount of a substance reaches poisonous levels in the body. This level varies among individuals, but genetic factors, body size, physical health, and prior drug exposure influence a person's ability to metabolize, or process, a drug. The signs and symptoms of intoxication include slurred speech, poor muscular coordination, and mental confusion.

An *overdose* occurs when an excessive amount of a drug circulates in the bloodstream and overwhelms the ability of the body to detoxify or eliminate the substance rapidly. Overdoses of OTC, prescription, and illegal drugs can damage or destroy tissues. In some instances, drug overdoses can be fatal. Table 7.7 (at the end of this chapter) describes some signs and symptoms of overdoses of various psychoactive drugs.

**Polyabuse**, abusing more than one drug at a time, is a common practice. For example, individuals often drink alcoholic beverages while they use heroin, barbiturates, cocaine, or other drugs. When people take different drugs that have similar actions, the effects of each drug may be greatly multiplied. This phenomenon, called **synergism**, can be deadly. Alcohol and barbiturates, for example, are depressant drugs that slow the functioning of the central nervous system. If a person drinks a few alcoholic beverages while taking barbiturates, the combined effects of these substances can depress respiration severely, producing coma or death. Polyabuse can cause drug interactions in addition to synergism that can have serious and even fatal outcomes. Many people are not aware

**euphoria (you-FOR-ee-a)** An intense feeling of well-being commonly called a "high."

**detoxification** The process of converting harmful substances into less dangerous compounds.

**intoxication** The state of being poisoned by a drug or other toxic substance.

**polyabuse** Abusing more than one drug at a time.

**synergism (SIH-ner-jism)** The multiplied effects produced by taking combinations of certain drugs.

that drinking alcohol while taking acetaminophen, a compound contained in popular over-the-counter pain relievers, can cause liver failure and death.

### Healthy Living Practices

☐ Do not combine drugs, including alcohol and OTC medicines, without consulting a physician or registered pharmacist. *Mixing drugs can kill you!*

### Figure 7.2

**Medical Marijuana.** As of early 2011, 17 states and the District of Columbia allowed the use of marijuana for medical purposes, and 12 states had legislation pending. In these states, registered outlets, such as the one in Denver, Colorado shown in this 2011 photo, sold marijuana to people with a license. A variety of medical marijuana strains are shown on the dispensary shelves.

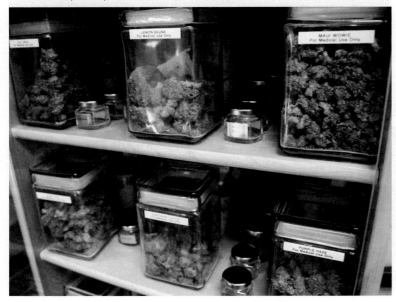

## Illicit Drug Use in the United States

### The Prevalence of Illicit Drug Use

*Illegal drugs*, such as heroin, lysergic acid diethylamide (LSD), and marijuana, are those having no currently accepted medical use in the United States, although some states allow medical marijuana use (**Figure 7.2**). Except for research purposes, it is illegal to buy, sell, possess, and use these drugs. They are listed as Schedule I drugs (see Table 7.2). Only registered, qualified researchers can obtain illegal drugs in this country.

Legal drugs are those whose sale, possession, and use as intended are not forbidden by law, but whose use may be restricted. Restricted drugs are called *controlled substances*, and they include narcotics, depressants, and stimulants. Controlled substances are available with a prescription. They are listed as Schedule

II to V drugs (see Table 7.2). The term *illicit drugs* is used by the Substance Abuse and Mental Health Services Administration to mean both illegal drugs and controlled substances held without a legal prescription.

Researchers conduct surveys and interviews to estimate the prevalence of illicit drug use in the United States. For example, the National Survey on Drug Use and Health samples tens of thousands of Americans 12 years of age or older annually. From the data they collected for 2009, researchers conclude that an estimated 21.8 million Americans (8.7% of the population aged 12 years and older) were current illicit drug users in that year, meaning they had used an illicit drug in the month prior to the interview (see Figure 7.9). The 2009 figure represents an increase of illicit drug users from 2008. In that year, 8% of the population currently used illicit drugs.[1] However, fewer Americans were using these substances than in the late 1970s. In 1979, researchers estimated that 25 million people in the United States used illicit drugs.

According to the 2009 National Survey on Drug Use and Health, more men than women take drugs currently, 10.8% and 6.6%, respectively, in that year, and certain segments of the American population use illicit drugs more than do other groups. Seventeen percent of unemployed adults were current users of illicit drugs in 2009; 8% of full-time employed adults took these substances. Among people aged 18 years and older in 2009, those who lacked high school diplomas had the highest rate of current illicit drug use (10.2%), and college graduates had the lowest rate of current use (6.1%).[1]

Rates of illicit drug use are especially high among teenagers and young adults. **Figure 7.3** shows that drug use peaks at ages 18 to 20 years, with more than one out of five persons in this age group reporting past-month illicit drug use in both 2008 and 2009. Current illicit drug use was reported by more than 10% of young people aged 16 to 29 years in 2008 and extended into the 30- to 34-year-old age group in 2009.

Since 1975, researchers at the University of Michigan's Institute for Social Research have conducted Monitoring the Future (MTF), an annual survey of American high school and college students, to ascertain their use of drugs. Data from the 2009 survey indicate that 36% of full-time college students aged 19 to 22 years took one or more illicit drugs during 2009, up from 30.6% in 1992. In 2009, 32.8% of college students used marijuana at least once during the year, up from 27.7% in 1992. Additionally, the use of LSD ("acid") rose in the mid-1990s from 1989, and has since begun to fall. In 2009, 2% of college students reported taking LSD during the previous 12 months. In 1994, this figure was about 5%; in 1989, it was 3.4%.[2]

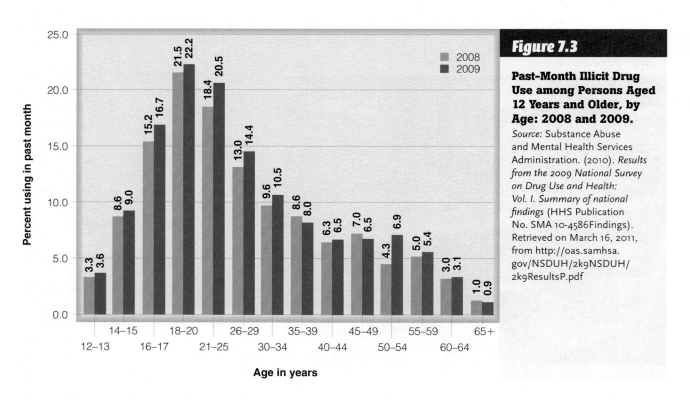

### Figure 7.3

**Past-Month Illicit Drug Use among Persons Aged 12 Years and Older, by Age: 2008 and 2009.**

*Source:* Substance Abuse and Mental Health Services Administration. (2010). *Results from the 2009 National Survey on Drug Use and Health: Vol. I. Summary of national findings* (HHS Publication No. SMA 10-4586Findings). Retrieved on March 16, 2011, from http://oas.samhsa.gov/NSDUH/2k9NSDUH/2k9ResultsP.pdf

## Why Do People Use Psychoactive Drugs?

Drug users often provide numerous reasons to explain why they began taking psychoactive substances. Most people begin taking mood-altering drugs for nonmedical purposes. Some individuals use alcohol or other drugs simply as a pleasurable experience. Others use drugs to cope with their psychological problems, reduce stress, or escape from unpleasant aspects of their lives. Curiosity often motivates many teenagers and young adults to experiment with drugs. Movies and advertisements may stimulate this curiosity by showing, for example, sophisticated and attractive people smoking cigarettes or cigars, or drinking alcoholic beverages while engaging in enjoyable activities (**Figure 7.4**). Additionally, teenagers may use drugs to experience new behaviors, relieve peer pressure, or enhance social interactions.

## Patterns of Psychoactive Drug Use

Drug experimentation and illicit use often occur during the teen years and peak between the ages of 18 and 20 years (see Figure 7.3). Most drug abusers in this age group begin by smoking cigarettes, and then they consume alcoholic beverages such as beer or wine. Some youth inhale chemicals such as those in aerosols and plastic cements to obtain their mind-altering effects. Alcohol, nicotine, marijuana, and inhalants are often referred to as "gateway" drugs because adolescents use these substances before moving on to other psychoactive drugs.[3]

Many adolescents stop experimenting with new drugs after using alcohol or nicotine. If they continue trying drugs, teenagers are likely to use marijuana next. Marijuana use increased among eighth, tenth, and twelfth graders in the United States in 2009 from 2008. Nearly 12% of eighth graders, nearly 27% of tenth graders, and nearly 33% of twelfth graders surveyed in the MTF study reported that they had tried marijuana in 2009.[2]

Any combination of stimulants, depressants, or hallucinogens may follow marijuana use. After trying these drugs, some young people move on to use opiates. However, not every youthful drug user follows this stepping-stone pattern of drug experimentation. For example, many teenagers who experiment with alcohol or marijuana do not try other psychoactive drugs.

The recreational use of illegal drugs generally declines with increasing age beyond age 20 years as traditional adult roles, including marriage, parenthood, and careers, are adopted. As they age, many individuals recognize that abusing illicit drugs can be self-destructive. Nevertheless, elderly persons who feel socially isolated and depressed, and those with a history of substance abuse, are at greater risk of abusing prescription drugs than are adolescents and young adults.[4]

## Drug Dependence

Most people who use psychoactive drugs such as alcohol or marijuana take them for pleasure, to relax, or to feel comfortable in social settings, which is termed *recreational drug use*. To assess your use of

### Figure 7.4

**Grammy-winning British singer Amy Winehouse at Balans café bar in Soho, London.** The media frequently portray sophisticated and attractive people smoking or binge drinking while engaging in enjoyable activities. As a result, some young people copy these unhealthy behaviors. Winehouse evidenced many other unhealthy behaviors. She died on July 23, 2011 at the age of 27, from accidental alcohol poisoning, drinking heavily after weeks of abstinence.

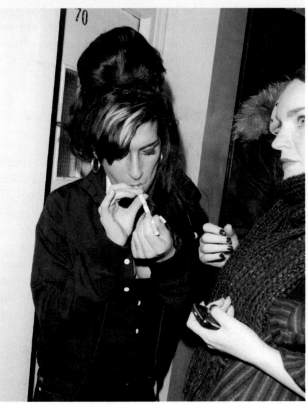

**drug dependence (addiction)** occurs when users develop a habitual pattern of taking drugs that produces a compulsive need, which is both physical and psychological.

**tolerance** An adaptation to drugs in which the usual dose no longer produces the anticipated degree of physical or psychological effects.

**withdrawal** A temporary physical and psychological state that occurs when certain drugs are discontinued.

drugs, complete the questionnaire in the exercise entitled "Are You Dependent on Drugs?" in the Student Workbook pages at the end of this book.

**Drug dependence** or **addiction** occurs when users develop a habitual pattern of taking drugs that produces a compulsive need, which is both physical and psychological. The terms *dependency* and *addiction* are often used interchangeably to describe any compulsive behavior that interferes with one's health, work, and relationships.

Dependent individuals are unable to avoid using drugs; most have a history of unsuccessful attempts to stop. Over time, these people escalate their intake of drugs even as they recognize that their actions are harmful to themselves and others. People who are dependent on drugs are so preoccupied with the need to obtain and use these substances that other aspects of their lives, such as handling the responsibilities of family and work, become less important.

## Physiologic and Psychological Dependence

When people take certain psychoactive drugs repeatedly over an extended period, their bodies make various physiologic adjustments to function as normally as possible. For example, dramatic chemical changes occur in the brains of chronic drug users that influence their thought processes and behaviors. As a result, these individuals display the characteristic signs and symptoms of *physical dependence* or *physical addiction*: drug tolerance and withdrawal.

After chronic exposure to certain drugs, the body develops **tolerance**, the ability to endure larger amounts of these substances while the adverse effects decrease. When this occurs, users discover that their usual dose of drugs no longer produces the desired degree of physical or psychological effects. To get the desired effects, people must take larger quantities, which results in increased tolerance. This upward

spiral is more difficult to break at each successive level, increasing the risk of overdose.

**Withdrawal** is a temporary physical and psychological state that occurs when certain drugs are discontinued. The signs and symptoms of withdrawal include trembling, anxiety, and pain. In cases of barbiturate addiction, withdrawal symptoms are so severe they can cause death. Table 7.7 at the end of this chapter indicates psychoactive drugs' potentials for producing tolerance, withdrawal, and addiction.

*Psychological dependence* is a person's need to use certain psychoactive drugs regularly to obtain their pleasurable effects and to relieve boredom, anxiety, or stress. Psychologically dependent people experience powerful cravings for these substances, which motivates drug-seeking behavior. However, it may be difficult to distinguish psychological dependence from physical dependence. As mentioned earlier, psychoactive drugs produce physiologic changes in the brain that influence behavior. Thus, these changes may affect a person's emotional responses, including feelings about the need to take psychoactive substances.

Not everyone who habitually uses or abuses psychoactive substances becomes dependent on their use. For example, individuals who drive after becoming drunk at bars or parties are abusing alcohol, but they are not necessarily alcoholics. It is difficult to determine when the habitual use of a psychoactive substance becomes a dependency. Scientists are interested in determining why some people seem to be more susceptible to drug dependency and addiction than others are.

## Risk Factors for Drug Dependency

Like many other health problems, there is no single risk factor for drug dependency. Substance addiction results from complex interactions among biological, personal, social, and environmental factors. Results of research conducted by the National Institute on Drug Abuse (NIDA) and reported in its most recent edition of *Preventing Drug Use Among Children and Adolescents: A Research-Based Guide* suggest that certain conditions in the home are probably the most crucial risk factors for children becoming drug abusers.[5] Such factors include home environments in which parents abuse drugs or suffer from mental illness; ineffective parenting, particularly with children who have difficult temperaments or conduct disorders; and a lack of mutual child–parent attachments

# Diversity in Health

## Khat

Which psychoactive drug is associated with weddings and weekends? If your answer is alcohol, you may be wrong with respect to certain cultures. In the East African countries of Somalia and Ethiopia, and on the nearby Arabian peninsula in Yemen, people chew khat, the leaf buds and leaves of the native bush *Catha edulis*, to celebrate weddings and other special events (see **Figure 7.A**). For centuries, people from these cultures have chewed or smoked khat or drunk tea brewed from its leaves as a socially acceptable and enjoyable pastime. Many homes in Somalia have a special room in which family members and their friends (primarily men) gather to munch khat and chat. Like alcohol and other psychoactive substances that are more familiar to Americans, khat contains chemicals that are known to produce both pleasurable and harmful side effects.

Khat contains cathionine, more potent and found in fresh leaves, and cathine, less potent and found in older leaves. These compounds are chemically similar to amphetamines and produce psychological and physiologic responses that resemble those produced by amphetamines and other stimulants. After using khat, people report feeling euphoric and alert; they have little desire to eat, sleep, or engage in sex. Additionally, khat users experience elevated blood pressures and heart rates. After the stimulating and mood-elevating effects of the drug subside, khat users feel anxious and irritable.

Khat impairs thought processes such as mental concentration and judgment; therefore, driving while under its influence can be hazardous. Men who use khat regularly may develop permanent impotence; women who use khat during pregnancy are at risk of giving birth to underweight newborns. Overdosing on khat can produce aggressive, paranoid, and psychotic behavior. Khat has also been found to be a significant risk factor for acute coronary syndrome, a range of life-threatening heart-related disorders.

In the early 1990s, thousands of Somalians and Ethiopians fled the civil unrest raging in their homelands and sought refuge in Western countries, including England and the United States. After settling in the West, many of these immigrants maintained their habit of using khat. To satisfy their demand, the immigrants purchase khat leaves that have been flown into North America or the United Kingdom from East Africa.

Concerned about the drug's effects on the central nervous system, officials at the U.S. Drug Enforcement Administration added cathine to its list of controlled substances in 1988 as a Schedule IV drug. In 1993, the Food and Drug Administration issued an import alert that recommended detention of khat by customs officials to prevent its entry into the United States. Currently, khat use does not pose a major drug enforcement problem.

*Sources:* Sources: Al-Hebshi, N. N., & Skaug, N. (2005). Khat (*Catha edulis*)— an updated review. *Addiction Biology, 10*:299–307; El-Wajeh, Y. A. & Thornhill, M. H. (2009). Qat and its health effects. *British Dental Journal, 206*:17–21; and Mwenda, J. M., Arimi, M. M., Kyama, M. C., & Langat, D. K. (2003). Effects of khat (*Catha edulis*) consumption on reproductive functions: A review. *East African Medical Journal, 80*:318–323.

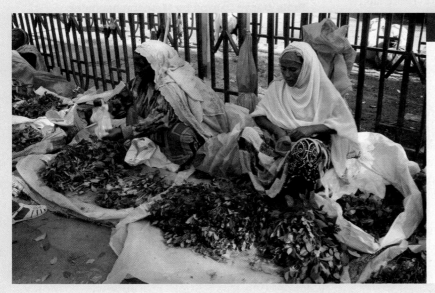

### Figure 7.A

**Women selling khat in Ethiopia.**

and parental nurturing. Risk factors for drug abuse that relate to a child's behavior outside of the home include inappropriately shy or aggressive behavior in the classroom; poor school performance; poor social skills; friendships with peers who use drugs; and a belief that parents, the school, peers, and the community approve of drug use. Conversely, *protective factors*, those associated with reduced potential for drug abuse, include strong family and school ties; parental monitoring of behavior with clear rules of conduct; involvement of parents in the lives of children; academic success in school; and the belief that parents, the school, peers, and the community do not approve of drug use.

 **Healthy Living Practices**

☐ To avoid the destructive effects of a drug dependency or addiction, do not use psychoactive substances unless you are under a physician's care.

 Stimulants

Throughout the world, people have used various stimulant drugs for thousands of years to relieve fatigue, suppress appetite, and improve mood. (See the Diversity in Health essay "Khat.") Stimulants enhance chemical activity in parts of the brain that influence emotions, sleep, attention, and learning. Within minutes after taking stimulants, users are more alert, excitable, and restless. Additionally, these drugs increase blood pressure levels and heart rates.

## Amphetamines and Methamphetamines

Synthetic stimulants are amphetamines, methamphetamines, and nonamphetamines (see Table 7.7). Amphetamines such as Dexedrine (dextroamphetamine) increase energy and alertness, lessen the need to sleep, produce euphoria, and suppress appetite. In the early 1980s, 21% to 22% of college students reported using amphetamines within the past year. Their use dropped significantly each year from 1983 to 1992, when only 3.6% of college students reported using this drug. From 1993 to 2001, their use rose again, ranging from 4.2% in 1993 to 7.2% in 2001. By 2009, 7.5% of full-time college students reported using amphetamines, but only 0.3% reported using

methamphetamines. Methamphetamine use in U.S. college students has declined since 1999.[2]

Methamphetamines ("speed") are powerful forms of amphetamines that have few medically approved uses. Methamphetamine is taken orally (usually as a pill), or the powder is snorted. It can also be injected or smoked. In small doses, methamphetamines produce euphoria, appetite loss, excessive perspiration, and pounding heartbeats. The effects of taking larger doses can be frightening: chest pains, irregular heartbeat, fever, hallucinations, and convulsions. People who drive while on methamphetamines exhibit erratic driving patterns and are often involved in high-speed collisions.

Methamphetamine use is associated with weakening of the heart muscle in young people (those aged 45 years or younger).[6] Overdoses of methamphetamines can be deadly by resulting in cardiovascular collapse or strokes. When taken by pregnant women, the drug can stunt fetal growth and negatively affect the development of the fetal brain.[7,8]

Brain damage is a hallmark of chronic methamphetamine abuse. **Figure 7.5** shows this damage in a user: The red areas are those with the greatest tissue loss. The limbic region, which is involved in drug craving, reward, mood, and emotion, lost 11% of its tissue in this user's brain. The hippocampus, which is involved in memory making, lost 8% of its tissue. The persons examined in the study were in their 30s and

### Figure 7.5

**Brain Decay Caused by Methamphetamine Use.** This magnetic resonance imaging (MRI) image of one hemisphere of the brain shows areas of brain-volume loss in a methamphetamine user.

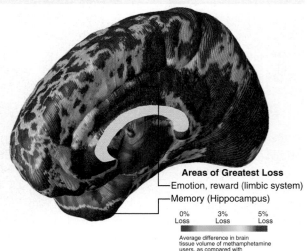

**Areas of Greatest Loss**
— Emotion, reward (limbic system)
— Memory (Hippocampus)

| 0% Loss | 3% Loss | 5% Loss |

Average difference in brain tissue volume of methamphetamine users, as compared with nonusers

## Figure 7.6

**Before and After Using Crystal Meth.** The mug shot on the left is of a woman who committed a felony prior to using crystal meth. The mug shot on the right is of the same woman after 2.5 years of using this drug.

*Source:* © Images from the Faces of Meth V 1, 2005 CD©, Multnomah County Sheriff's Office.

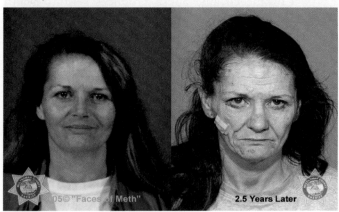

had used methamphetamine for 10 years, primarily by smoking it approximately every other day, using 4 g per week.[9] Withdrawal from methamphetamines often results in anxiety, fatigue, sleeplessness, paranoia, delusions, and severe depression.

In the 1980s, drug suppliers from Korea, Taiwan, and the Philippines introduced an illegal crystalline form of methamphetamine called *crystal meth* (also referred to as *meth, crank, ice,* and *glass*). An extremely potent and addictive drug, crystal meth can produce violent behavior and damage the liver, kidneys, and lungs as well as the physical appearance (**Figure 7.6**).

Both methamphetamine and crystal meth are synthetic drugs; that is, they are not made directly from plant material as are opium or cocaine but are made in laboratories from other chemicals, called precursor chemicals. Drug suppliers manufacture the drug using temporary homemade labs that they move from place to place to evade law enforcement.

The ingredients for making meth are lithium from batteries, acetone from paint thinner, lye, and ephedrine/pseudoephedrine, which are found in cold remedies and sinus medications. However, the Domestic Chemical Diversion Control Act of 1993 made it illegal to sell ephedrine over the counter (although it could still be sold in pills containing other active ingredients), and the Comprehensive Methamphetamine Control Act of 1996 placed additional controls on products containing ephedrine and pseudoephedrine. More recently, the Combat

Methamphetamine Epidemic Act enacted in 2006 placed restrictions on the amount of medications containing ephedrine and pseudoephedrine that could be sold in one day and over a 30-day period to an individual. To circumvent the law, methamphetamine "manufacturers" often use the drug ephedra (ma huang) as a substitute or have many individuals purchase the drugs up to the daily and monthly limit, a practice called "smurfing."

**Party Drugs** Amphetamines and methamphetamines are two drugs in a group called *party drugs* (*club drugs*). Party drugs also include alcohol, GHB, GBL, and Rohypnol (depressants); LSD (acid) and ketamine (special K) (both are hallucinogens); and MDMA (Ecstasy, a drug with mixed effects). Adolescents, teenagers, and young adults use these drugs at all-night parties and in other social situations to reduce anxiety, induce euphoria, or build energy to keep on dancing or partying. However, these drugs are not harmless "fun" drugs because they can have long-lasting negative effects on the brain. (We discuss these drugs in this chapter, with the exception of alcohol, which is discussed in Chapter 8.)

**Ritalin, Adderall, and Other Medically Useful Stimulants** Amphetamines and chemically related stimulants have a few medical uses, such as treatment of the sleep disorder narcolepsy, short-term weight loss, and attention control. One medicinally useful stimulant is Ritalin (methylphenidate), prescribed for people with attention disorders. Ritalin is abused, however, by persons who do not need the drug for its prescribed use but use it for its stimulant effect.

The annual prevalence of nonprescription Ritalin use for high school seniors from 1976 to 1993 was very low and ranged from 0.1% to 0.7%. In 1994, Ritalin use by high school seniors rose to 1% from 0.4% in 1993 and reached a peak of 3.9% in 2004. Since then, prevalence of use has fallen and was 1.3% in 2009.[10] In 2001, MTF researchers changed the way they asked the question about nonprescription Ritalin use, and the results yielded higher prevalence rates, from 5.1% in 2001, decreasing to 2.1% in 2009.[2] The results from asking both questions suggest an ongoing, gradual decline in Ritalin use in recent years.

The stimulant Adderall (amphetamine and dextroamphetamine) is more recently used for the treatment of attention-deficit hyperactivity disorder (ADHD), and the MTF researchers began asking questions of seniors regarding its use in 2007. In that year, 2.8% of high school seniors reported using the drug, and that figure rose to 3.3% by 2009.[10] Using a revised question as with Ritalin, the prevalence of Adderall use by seniors in 2009 was 5.4%.[2] MTF researchers suggest that the decrease in Ritalin use may be occurring because it is being replaced by Adderall use.

Among college students, the annual prevalence of Ritalin use is about the same as with high school seniors. MTF began asking the question of college students in 2002, using the revised format. Nonprescription prevalence of use for college students was 5.7% in 2002, but fell through 2009 to a rate of 1.7%. The annual prevalence of use for young adults aged 19 to 28 years not enrolled in college was lower than for college students from 2002 to 2008 but was the same in 2009 at 1.7%. Use of Adderall was high in college students in 2009 at 7.9% and was 4.9% for young adults not enrolled in college.[2]

# Cocaine

Cocaine is a white powdery substance extracted from the leaves of the coca bush, which is not the same plant as the cacao tree from which cocoa and chocolate are derived. Crack is a rock crystal form of cocaine that can be heated and its vapors smoked (inhaled); its name comes from the cracking sound that is heard during the heating process. The powdered form of cocaine can be snorted (inhaled through the nose) or dissolved in water and injected. Most people snort, rather than inject, cocaine.

This potent stimulant has some medical uses, particularly as an **anesthetic**, a substance that interferes with normal sensations. However, cocaine was the most widely used illegal stimulant in the United States during the late 1970s and early 1980s, a time during which the public was misinformed about the drug and its dangers. Additionally, many healthcare practitioners did not understand the dangers of cocaine use or its addictive nature, and, as a consequence, cocaine was viewed as glamorous and was used by many celebrities as well as millions of other Americans. The popularity of cocaine declined dramatically between 1985 and 1992, most likely from public understanding that accompanied increased knowledge about this drug and its dangerous effects.[3] The level of cocaine use has not changed significantly since 1992, but it has dropped somewhat in recent years. Experts estimate that approximately 1.6 million Americans were current cocaine users in 2009, down from 2.4 million in 2006 (see Figure 7.9).[1]

Cocaine is highly addictive. In laboratory studies of the drug's effects, animals prefer to self-administer cocaine rather than engage in reproductive behavior or obtain food. Many people who are dependent on cocaine demonstrate similar responses. Cocaine abusers often dissociate themselves from their families, friends, and associates.

Chronic cocaine abuse produces serious health problems (see Table 7.7). People who snort cocaine regularly often suffer from chronic irritation of their nasal passages. This irritation causes nosebleeds, and it can destroy the septum, the cartilaginous tissue that divides the area between the two nostrils (**Figure 7.7**). Additionally, snorting cocaine and smoking crack damage lung tissue and increase susceptibility to respiratory tract infections.

Long-term use of cocaine may interfere with normal sexual functioning. Men who use cocaine regularly often experience an inability to achieve erections and a reduced sexual drive. Women who are chronic users may experience infertility, menstrual problems, and difficulty achieving orgasms.

Cocaine use can have deadly consequences. People with hepatitis or AIDS can spread these diseases by sharing their used hypodermic needles with uninfected drug users. Additionally, cocaine use increases the risk of dying suddenly from life-threatening disorders of the circulatory system such as irregular and rapid heartbeat, high blood pressure, stroke, and heart attacks. Death is especially likely when people

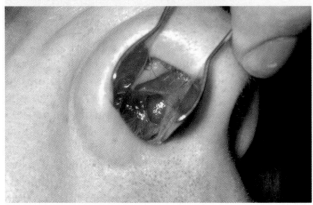

### Figure 7.7

**Perforated nasal septum.** The nostril is being held open with a nasal speculum, showing the nasal passage and mucosa. The septum divides the inner passageways. The perforation (hole) in the septum, a common result of snorting cocaine, may cause symptoms such as bleeding, crusting, whistling, and difficulty breathing.

take cocaine with other psychoactive substances such as alcohol and heroin. During the past two decades, several well-known individuals have died as a result of using cocaine, such as comedian/actor John Belushi, comic Chris Farley, and bassist John Entwistle of the rock band The Who.

While under the influence of cocaine, some individuals experience severe psychotic reactions, including paranoia, which may result in violent behavior. It is not uncommon for cocaine abusers to report having delusions such as the sensation that bugs are crawling beneath their skin. The psychological symptoms of cocaine intoxication also lead some users to attempt suicide, and a number of them succeed.

## Caffeine

Worldwide, caffeine is the most widely used psychoactive substance. Caffeine and its related chemical compounds occur naturally in several varieties of plants that we use to make foods and beverages, including coffee, tea, and cocoa. People may ingest caffeine when they consume caffeinated soft drinks or they take certain over-the-counter medications. **Table 7.3** lists the amounts of caffeine contained in certain beverages, foods, and over-the-counter products.

Caffeine has been generally recognized as a stimulant that causes limited dependence. The average American consumes about 200 mg of caffeine daily—the equivalent of about two cups of coffee or five cola beverages. Typical patterns of moderate caffeine consumption do not appear to be harmful to healthy persons.

The Center for Science in the Public Interest notes that—on the positive side—people who consume caffeine regularly have a lower risk of developing Parkinson's disease and gallstones. In addition, caffeine intake improves alertness and reaction time, lifts the mood, helps the body burn fat, blunts pain, and helps relieve headache pain. On the negative side, however, caffeine can disturb sleep and provoke migraine headaches in those prone to them. Consuming 200 mg or more per day may increase the risk of miscarriage.[11]

After abstaining from caffeine for about half a day, a person who is accustomed to taking the drug typically experiences withdrawal symptoms that include headache, tiredness, irritability, and depression. Individuals who consume more than 600 mg per day often experience psychological as well as physical problems known as *caffeinism*. The manifestations of caffeinism include nervousness, trembling, irritation of the stomach lining, insomnia, increased urine

## Table 7.3

### Caffeine Content of Popular Beverages, Foods, and Products

| Beverage, Food, or Product | Typical Amount/ Range (mg) |
| --- | --- |
| **Coffee** | |
| Cappuccino (2 oz) | 100 |
| Espresso (2 oz) | 100 |
| Brewed, drip method (5 oz) | 60–180 |
| Brewed, percolator (5 oz) | 40–170 |
| Instant (5 oz) | 30–120 |
| Decaffeinated, brewed (5 oz) | 2–5 |
| Decaffeinated, instant (5 oz) | 1–5 |
| **Tea** | |
| Brewed, U.S. brands (5 oz) | 20–90 |
| Brewed, imported brands (5 oz) | 25–110 |
| Instant (5 oz) | 25–50 |
| Iced (5 oz) | 28–32 |
| **Cocoa-Containing Products** | |
| Cocoa (5 oz) | 2–20 |
| Chocolate milk (5 oz) | 1–4 |
| Milk chocolate (1 oz) | 1–15 |
| Dark chocolate, semi-sweet (1 oz) | 5–35 |
| Chocolate-flavored syrup (1 oz) | 4 |
| **Soft Drinks (12 oz)** | |
| Dr. Pepper | 40 |
| Cola-type beverages | |
|     Regular | 30–46 |
|     Diet | 2–58 |
|     Caffeine-free | 0 |
|     Mountain Dew, Mello Yello | 52 |
|     Jolt | 75–100 |
| **Over-the-Counter Medications** | |
| Vivarin (1 pill) | 200 |
| Nōdōz (1 pill) | 100 |
| Anacin, Empirin, or Midol (2 pills) | 64 |

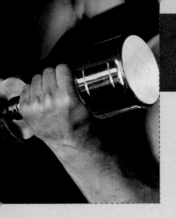

# Managing Your Health

## Falling Asleep Without Prescriptions

If you experience occasional sleepless nights, the following self-treatment tips for insomnia may be helpful:

1. Try to adhere to a regular sleeping and waking schedule, even on weekends, to foster natural sleep–wake timing.
2. Don't eat big meals or drink large amounts of fluids in the evening. Have a light snack before bedtime if you like, but avoid alcohol, caffeine, and OTC pain relievers that contain caffeine.
3. Reserve time for vigorous regular exercise earlier in the day and no closer than 2 hours before bedtime.
4. Practice a prebedtime relaxing routine, such as taking a warm bath or shower.
5. Keep your bedroom dark, cool, and as quiet as possible.
6. Practice progressive muscular relaxation while in bed (see Chapter 3 for details).
7. Don't stay in bed if you can't fall asleep; get out of bed and read a dull book. Avoid watching TV or any screen; the flickering light stimulates the brain. Return to bed when you begin to feel sleepy.
8. Take an over-the-counter (OTC) sleep aid only as a last resort. Recognize that most of these medications contain antihistamines that lose their effectiveness if used regularly.

---

production, diarrhea, sweating, and rapid heart rate. People who do not regularly consume caffeine or who are sensitive to it may develop caffeinism after taking as little as 250 mg of the drug daily.

 **Healthy Living Practices**

 If you have ill effects such as anxiety or sleep disturbances from consuming too much caffeine, gradually wean yourself from the drug to avoid its withdrawal symptoms, especially headaches.

## Depressants

Depressants produce **sedative** (calming) and **hypnotic** (trancelike) effects as well as drowsiness. These drugs slow the activity of the cerebral cortex, the part of the brain that is responsible for thought processes. Depressant drugs include alcohol, barbiturates such as phenobarbital (Luminal), and minor tranquilizers such as diazepam (Valium).

Dangerous side effects can result when people misuse depressants. All of these drugs slow the heart and respiratory rates, which increases the risk of dying from respiratory failure after taking an overdose. Combining depressants—for example, drinking alcohol while taking Valium—produces synergistic

(combined) effects. Such synergism of depressants can be life threatening.

Tolerance and dependency occur with regular use of depressants. Withdrawal from these drugs can cause *delirium* (mental confusion and disorientation) and *seizures* (abnormal brain activity that results in uncontrollable muscular movements). Some addicted people die while undergoing withdrawal from depressants.

## Sedatives and Tranquilizers

Physicians frequently prescribe sedatives and minor tranquilizers, especially for people suffering from insomnia or mild anxiety. In many instances, people can treat their mild anxiety or insomnia without powerful depressants. Anxious individuals can try to reduce their feelings of stress by practicing the relaxation techniques described in Chapter 3. The Managing Your Health feature "Falling Asleep Without Prescriptions" provides suggestions that may induce sleep without the use of depressants or other drugs. Prescription medications used to treat anxiety and sleep disorders are often abused. In 2007, 2 million people abused tranquilizers and 370,000 abused sedatives.[1]

## Rohypnol

*Rohypnol* (row-HIP-nole), commonly called *roofies* (along with a variety of other street names), is one of a few "date-rape drugs." (See the section titled "GHB and GBL" that follows.) While under the influence of Rohypnol, women are unable to resist rapists, and they cannot recall, for various lengths of time, what happened to them while under the influence. Because of concern about Rohypnol and other similarly abused sedative–hypnotics, Congress passed the Drug-Induced Rape Prevention and Punishment Act of 1996 to increase federal penalties for use of any controlled substance to aid in sexual assault. After 1996, Rohypnol use declined. It was used by only 1% of high school seniors in 2009 and less than 0.1% of college students, which appears on MTF tables as 0%.[2]

Although not approved for use in the United States, this drug is widely available in Mexico, Colombia, and Europe, where it is used for the treatment of insomnia. Like other depressants, its effects include sedation, muscle relaxation, and anxiety reduction. It also causes dizziness, loss of motor control, lack of coordination, slurred speech, confusion, and gastrointestinal disturbances, all of which can last 12 hours or more.

## GHB and GBL

Gamma hydroxybutyrate, better known as *GHB*, was formerly sold in health food stores as a dietary supplement to induce sleep and build muscle. Its over-the-counter sale was banned by the FDA in 1990. The longer periods of sleep it induced were supposed to allow release of human growth hormone, which has been linked with increased muscle mass. However, GHB users reported unpleasant side effects such as nausea and shaking. More dangerously, this drug has induced seizures and coma in some users and can also cause irregular heartbeat, slowed breathing, hypothermia, and vomiting.[12] With legislation passed in February 2000, GHB became a Schedule I drug.

In January 1999, the FDA warned consumers about a drug related to GHB: gamma butyrolactone, or *GBL*. After ingestion, the body converts GBL to GHB. Some products labeled as dietary supplements contain GBL and claim to build muscles, improve physical performance, enhance sex, reduce stress, and induce sleep. However, GBL-related products have been associated with reports of at least 55 adverse health effects, including seizures, vomiting, slowed breathing, slowed heartbeat rate, and coma. One death had been reported from GBL at the time of the FDA warning. The FDA considers GBL an unapproved drug. After the FDA warning, all but one manufacturer of GBL-related products agreed to recall these drugs and to stop their manufacture and distribution.

**sedatives** Drugs that produce calming effects.

**hypnotics** Drugs that produce trancelike effects.

**analgesics (an-al-GEEZ-iks)** Drugs that alleviate pain.

## Healthy Living Practices

- Do not accept drinks from casual acquaintances or strangers; they may contain dangerous drugs.
- Do not drive or operate machinery while under the influence of depressant drugs because these substances can impair your thought processes and muscular coordination.
- Do not drink alcohol while taking other depressants. The synergistic effect of combining these compounds can be deadly.

## Opiates

Opiates include *opium*, the dried sap extracted from seedpods of opium poppies shown in **Figure 7.8**, and drugs such as codeine, morphine, heroin, and Percodan (aspirin and oxycodone hydrochloride) that are derived from opium. Synthetic opiates include Darvon (propoxyphene) and Demerol (meperidine). These compounds have important medical uses as sedatives, analgesics, and narcotics. **Analgesics** alle-

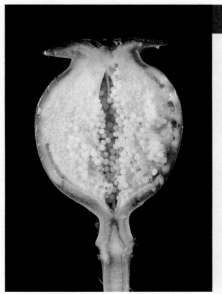

**Figure 7.8**

**Longitudinal Section Through a Seedpod of the Opium Poppy.** The dried sap extracted from opium poppy seedpods is used to make the narcotic opium. Some white sap can be seen on the cut edge of this seedpod.

viate pain; **narcotics** alter the perception of pain and induce euphoria and sleep. (Many people incorrectly use the term *narcotic* to describe any illegal drug.)

In addition to relieving pain, opiates slow the activity of the intestinal tract, so they are useful in treating severe diarrhea. In addition, physicians frequently prescribe codeine-containing syrups to subdue severe coughing. Despite their medicinal value, opiates are extremely dangerous when taken in an uncontrolled manner. These drugs are highly addictive; people who use opiates daily develop dependence and tolerance within a few weeks.

Using opiates, especially heroin, can cause a variety of serious health problems as well as death. Excessive doses of opiates depress the CNS, slowing respiration and reducing mental functioning. Such overdoses require immediate medical attention. Sharing needles that are used to inject heroin intravenously can cause life-threatening bacterial infections and viral diseases, such as AIDS and hepatitis.

## Opium and Heroin

After it enters this country, opium is chemically converted to heroin by drug dealers. They also add various materials, such as quinine or cornstarch, to dilute the drug's concentration. Substances that dilute the concentration of a drug are called *adulterants*. Because heroin abusers lack information concerning the potency of their drug purchases after chemical conversion by drug dealers, they risk taking overdoses or having allergic reactions to the adulterants.

Heroin is one of the most widely abused illegal drugs worldwide.[3] However, survey data indicate that it is not very popular with young people in the United States. Only 0.7% of American high school seniors and 0.4% of college students used heroin in 2009.[2] In the United States overall, only 0.2% of those aged 12 years and older used heroin in 2009 (see **Figure 7.9**).

## OxyContin and Vicodin

In 2001, news reports of abuse of the time-released opiate pain reliever OxyContin became common. OxyContin (oxycodone) is a medication prescribed primarily for patients with terminal cancer and other illnesses that cause moderate to severe chronic pain. By 2002, hundreds of people had died from OxyContin abuse, and researchers began collecting data on the use of OxyContin by high school students, college students, and adults. In 2009, the percentages of eighth, tenth, and twelfth graders, college students, and adults aged 19 to 28 years using OxyContin during the year prior to being surveyed (the annual prevalence) were 2.0%, 5.1%, 4.9%, 7.3%, and 6.0%, respectively. The annual prevalence of use of OxyContin has risen for all groups since 2002. The figures show that the highest use in 2009 was among college students.[2]

OxyContin is a time-release medication with the synthetic opiate oxycodone as its active ingredient.

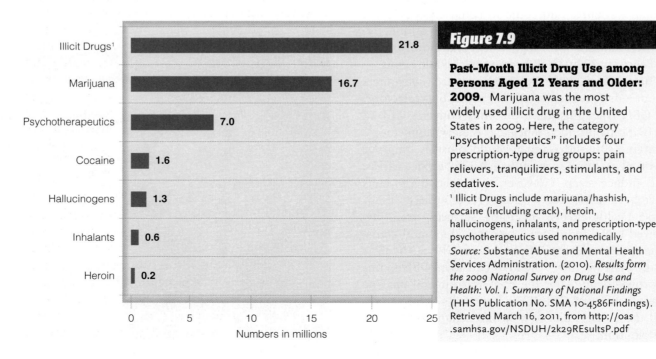

### Figure 7.9

**Past-Month Illicit Drug Use among Persons Aged 12 Years and Older: 2009.** Marijuana was the most widely used illicit drug in the United States in 2009. Here, the category "psychotherapeutics" includes four prescription-type drug groups: pain relievers, tranquilizers, stimulants, and sedatives.

[1] Illicit Drugs include marijuana/hashish, cocaine (including crack), heroin, hallucinogens, inhalants, and prescription-type psychotherapeutics used nonmedically.

*Source:* Substance Abuse and Mental Health Services Administration. (2010). *Results form the 2009 National Survey on Drug Use and Health: Vol. I. Summary of National Findings* (HHS Publication No. SMA 10-4586Findings). Retrieved March 16, 2011, from http://oas.samhsa.gov/NSDUH/2k29REsultsP.pdf

Persons who abuse this prescription medication chew, crush, or dissolve the pills, and then inject, inhale, or take them orally, which delivers the medication all at once rather than slowly over time. The result is a rapid and intense euphoria that does not occur when the drug is taken as prescribed, but such ingestion carries the dangers of opiates mentioned previously. Abusers also take OxyContin with other pills, marijuana, or alcohol, which can result in serious injury or death.

Vicodin (hydrocodone bitartrate and acetaminophen) is also a drug prescribed to reduce pain. Abuse of this drug is more prevalent than abuse of OxyContin. In 2009, the annual prevalence of abuse of Vicodin among eighth, tenth, and twelfth graders, college students, and adults aged 19 to 28 years was 2.5%, 8.1%, 9.7%, 8.4%, and 8.9%, respectively. The annual prevalence of use of Vicodin rose for all groups since 2002, but in 2009 the prevalence rate for eighth graders dropped to its 2002 level. In 2009, the annual prevalence of use was highest for twelfth graders.[2]

## Marijuana

*Marijuana* is the most widely used illicit drug in the United States. An estimated 16.7 million Americans aged 12 years and older were current users of marijuana in 2009 (Figure 7.9).

The marijuana plant (*Cannabis sativa*) contains the psychoactive compound delta-9-tetrahydrocannabinol, or THC. *Hashish* is a dried resin made from marijuana flowers, which contain a higher concentration of THC than the leaves of the plant. Also extracted from marijuana flowers, hashish oil contains a greater percentage of THC than hashish. A few drops of hashish oil added to a cigarette produce psychoactive effects that are the same as smoking a marijuana cigarette, or *joint*.

When people smoke marijuana or hashish, THC enters the brain rapidly. THC alters muscular coordination and normal thought processes such as mental concentration, problem solving, time perception, and short-term memory. Not only are these effects likely to decrease educational achievement, but also they can have serious consequences for drivers. Results of studies on the effects of marijuana on driving abilities reveal that marijuana impairs driving performance in a dose-related manner, just like alcohol does. In addition, recent use of marijuana appears to increase the risk of a driver's being involved in a car crash. Smoking marijuana and drinking alcohol together has significant additive effects on driving ability and sharply increases a driver's risk of a car crash, even at low doses.[13]

Marijuana and hashish smoke contain numerous irritants that can damage the bronchial tubes and lungs. Respiratory symptoms reported consistently by those who smoke these drugs on a regular basis include chronic bronchitis; shortness of breath; frequent coughing, wheezing, and phlegm production; and pneumonia. Long-term marijuana smokers have an increased risk for developing chronic obstructive pulmonary disease (COPD), which is a group of lung diseases that makes it hard to breathe. COPD can range from mild to life threatening. Physical and behavioral dependence occurs in about 7% to 10% of users and is more likely in those who begin using this drug at an early age.[13]

Although many users think that marijuana enhances their sexual responsiveness, results of some studies have found that the drug interferes with reproductive functioning. Men who use marijuana may experience a temporary reduction of their normal testosterone levels. Testosterone is a sex hormone that maintains sex drive and sperm production. This effect decreases the sperm count and increases the proportion of abnormal sperm, qualities that are associated with reduced fertility and an increased probability of fetal abnormalities. Babies born of women who smoked marijuana during their pregnancy face an increased risk of low birthweight and mild developmental abnormalities.[3,13]

Most Americans who smoke marijuana use the drug occasionally, particularly while they are in social settings. Although low-THC cannabis (the form generally available in the United States) rarely produces physical dependence when taken infrequently and in low doses, it can cause psychological dependence. Psychologically addicted persons mentally crave the euphoric effects of THC; experience a heightened sensitivity to and distortion of sight, smell, taste, and sound; have mood changes; and have a slowed reaction time.[3,13]

Among marijuana's medical uses is that it helps control seizures, reduces the fluid pressure in the eyes of people with glaucoma, eases the symptoms of wasting syndrome in AIDS patients, lessens muscle spasms in patients with muscle disorders such as multiple sclerosis, and reduces the pain of migraine headaches and peripheral neuropathy (a condition of the hands or feet that produces significant nerve pain). Patients usually smoke medical marijuana, eat it in baked goods, or drink it in tea. Marinol, a drug that contains synthetic THC, is an alternative to medical marijuana, but many patients become sick or significantly disoriented shortly after taking it.

As of February 2011, marijuana has been approved for medical use in the District of Columbia and 17 states: Alaska, Arizona, California, Colorado, Hawaii, Maine, Michigan, Montana, Nevada, Oregon, Washington, New Jersey, New Mexico, Oregon, Rhode Island, Vermont, and Washington. Laws in these states also remove state-level criminal penalties for cultivation, possession, and use of medical marijuana. As of mid-March 2011, the following 12 states had legislation pending to approve the use of medical marijuana: Connecticut, Delaware, Idaho, Illinois, Iowa, Kansas, Maryland, Massachusetts, New Hampshire, New York, Oklahoma, and West Virginia. Florida and Texas had legislation pending that was favorable to medical marijuana use but would not legalize it.

In June 2005, the U.S. Supreme Court ruled that federal authorities may prosecute patients whose physicians prescribe marijuana for their medical use, and that state laws do not protect users from the federal ban on the drug. Although against federal law, the sale, purchase, and use of medical marijuana by licensed individuals in accordance with state law was not prosecuted during the Obama administration (see Figure 7.2) until October 2011, when federal prosecutors in California targeted growers and dispensaries they believed were involved in drug trafficking. Many medical societies support legal protection for those using marijuana medically and support research into its usefulness as a medicinal treatment.

## Healthy Living Practices

☐ Smoking marijuana can impair your thought processes and ability to drive, damage your lungs, reduce your fertility, and lessen your motivation to work. To avoid these serious effects, abstain from using this drug unless prescribed for medical reasons.

 # Hallucinogens

When taken internally, hallucinogens produce *hallucinations*, abnormal and unreal sensations such as seeing distorted and vividly colored images. Many people report feeling pleasantly detached from their bodies or united with their environment while using hallucinogens. Hallucinogens, however, can produce frightening psychological responses such as anxiety, depression, and the feeling of losing control over your mind. The physical side effects of hallucinogens include elevated blood pressure, dilated pupils, and increased body temperature. Although chronic users of these drugs may develop psychological dependence and tolerance, physical addiction and withdrawal do not occur.

In the United States, the most potent and commonly abused hallucinogens are LSD, mescaline, psilocybin (SIGH-low-SIGH-bin), PCP, and ketamine. These drugs have no approved medical uses, and their recreational use is illegal. Native Americans, however, are permitted to use peyote, a cactus that contains mescaline, in certain religious rites.

## LSD

LSD (lysergic acid diethylamide) is a colorless, odorless, flavorless compound that is manufactured in pill, solution, and powder form. It is an extremely potent drug; taking very small amounts produces vivid hallucinations that can last up to 12 hours. While taking LSD, some people have severe psychotic reactions, such as paranoid delusions. Additionally, for weeks or months after taking LSD, some users may have "flashbacks" in which they experience mild hallucinations. Flashbacks usually subside over time and few long-term psychological problems seem to result from hallucinogen use. LSD can stimulate uterine contractions, so pregnant women should avoid it.

During the early 1980s, LSD use by college students declined dramatically, from 6.3% in 1982 to 2.2% in 1985. By 1992, however, LSD use among college students had climbed to 5.7% and peaked in 1995 at 6.9%. Use then steadily declined to 0.7% in 2005, with the exception of a spike in 1999 of 5.4%. After 2005, LSD use among college students began to climb again; in 2009, 2.0% of college students had used LSD in the past year.[2]

## Mescaline

A small, round, spineless cactus that grows in Mexico and Texas produces the hallucinogen mescaline, or peyote (**Figure 7.10**). After eating peyote, people have hallucinations that last 1 to 2 hours. These "trips" are milder and easier to control than LSD trips. Because pure mescaline is difficult to produce for illicit sale, most mescaline sold on the streets contains LSD as the psychoactive agent.

## Figure 7.10

**Peyote Cactus (*Lophophora williamsii*).** This small, round, spineless cactus grows in Mexico and Texas and produces the hallucinogen mescaline, or peyote.

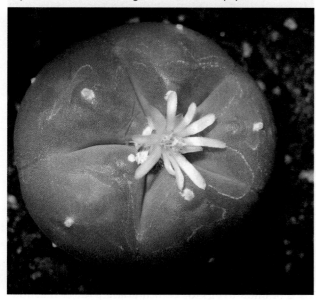

## Psilocybin

Many mushrooms, including several wild-growing varieties that are found throughout the United States, contain psilocybin. After eating these fungi, sometimes called *magic mushrooms*, people experience elevated blood pressure, body temperature, and pulse rate. Psilocybin produces euphoria and hallucinations, but these psychoactive effects are not as intense or long-lasting as those produced by LSD. Unpleasant responses to psilocybin ingestion include wide mood swings and uncontrollable movements of arms and legs. Although fatal overdoses from psilocybin have not been reported, users may die if they eat other wild mushrooms that are poisonous.

## PCP

PCP (commonly called *angel dust* or *rocket fuel*) is difficult to classify because the drug produces hallucinogenic, depressant, stimulant, or anesthetic effects depending on the dose in which it is taken. Within a few minutes after taking PCP, users begin to experience its psychoactive effects, which can last up to 6 hours.

Unlike other hallucinogenic drugs, high doses of PCP can cause severe toxic reactions. Taking 1 mg to 5 mg of PCP produces confusion and loss of muscular coordination; users also feel warm, sweaty, relaxed, and euphoric. As the level of intake increases to about 10 mg, users become confused, paranoid, and agitated; they act drunk, have hallucinations, and report numbness in their arms and legs. Taking 10 mg to 25 mg produces the signs and symptoms of PCP toxicity, including trancelike or psychotic behavior. Doses that exceed 25 mg to 50 mg can produce fever, convulsions, coma, elevated blood pressure, and death. People who survive the acute toxic effects of PCP often feel depressed and anxious. Additionally, they may show signs of brain damage such as confusion and disorientation that can take weeks to disappear.

## Ketamine

In the 1960s, drug researchers developed ketamine, a PCP analog that has fewer troublesome side effects than PCP. An **analog** is chemically similar to another drug and may or may not produce similar responses. Today, legally manufactured PCP analogs such as Ketalar (ketamine hydrochloride) have limited human and veterinary medical use as anesthetics.

Teens and young adults most commonly abuse ketamine by snorting the drug for its dreamlike or hallucinatory effects. In addition, the drug can be swallowed, smoked, drunk, or injected intramuscularly. Ketamine injection is highly risky because multiple injections typically occur during a single "session" in large groups, and the drug is drawn from shared bottles of liquid ketamine. These behaviors put ketamine injectors at risk of infectious diseases such as hepatitis C and HIV. At high doses, ketamine can cause delirium, amnesia, impaired motor function, high blood pressure, and potentially fatal respiratory problems. These effects are magnified when the drug is taken with sedatives or depressants, such as alcohol, which is a common practice.

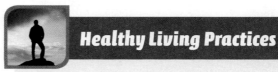

### Healthy Living Practices

☐ Do not eat wild mushrooms. Some are poisonous and can cause death.

# Inhalants

Inhalants are gases (fumes) that are breathed in and produce euphoria, dizziness, confusion, and drowsiness. Most inhalants are taken to induce mood changes, but nitrites are used as a sexual enhancer because they dilate (widen) blood vessels. **Table 7.4** lists the types of inhalants.

## Table 7.4

### Types of Toxic Inhalants and Common Examples

| Types of Toxic Inhalants | What Are They? | Examples |
| --- | --- | --- |
| volatile solvents  | Liquids that form gases at room temperature | Paint thinner, paint remover, dry-cleaning fluid, gasoline, glues, felt-tip marker fluids |
| aerosols | Sprays that contain propellants and solvents | Spray paint, spray deodorant, hairspray, fabric protector sprays |
| gases | Medical anesthetics and other gases used in everyday products | Examples of toxic gases: ether, chloroform, nitrous oxide (laughing gas) Examples of products containing toxic gases: whipped cream dispensers, butane lighters, propane tanks, refrigerants |
| nitrites | Chemicals that dilate blood vessels and relax muscles | Known as "poppers" or "snappers"; sold in small bottles labeled as video head cleaner, room odorizer, leather cleaner, or liquid aroma |

*Source:* Data from the National Institute on Drug Abuse.

Inhalants are taken into the body in a variety of ways. Fumes can be sniffed from a container, or aerosols can be sprayed directly into the nose or mouth. Alternatively, fumes or sprays can be sniffed directly or inhaled from a bag, a practice called "bagging." Another approach is "huffing," in which a rag is soaked with the inhalant and the rag is pressed to the mouth and nose. Nitrous oxide can be inhaled from balloons filled with the gas or from poppers, small bottles of the gas (see Table 7.4).

Inhalants irritate the mucous membranes lining the eyes, mouth, nose, throat, and lungs. Inhalant abusers often develop watery, reddened eyes and a persistent cough. Some users experience double vision, nausea, vomiting, fainting, and a ringing sensation in their ears. Many teenagers are unaware of the serious health effects of inhalant use: brain damage, irregular heartbeat, anemia, liver damage, kidney failure, coma, or death.

Inhalant use begins at young ages—sometimes in the fifth grade—and its use drops as students grow older. Inhalants are the second most widely used class of illicit drugs for eighth graders (after marijuana). In 2009, the annual prevalence for inhalant use for eighth graders was 8.1%; for tenth graders, 6.1%; and for twelfth graders, 3.4%. Lowest use was by college students and young adults at 1.2% and 0.9%, respectively.[2]

## Healthy Living Practices

☐ Use household products that release toxic fumes, such as paints, glues, and lighter fluids, in well-ventilated areas to avoid inhaling these chemicals.

# Designer Drugs: Drugs with Mixed Effects

People who have some knowledge of chemistry can alter the chemical structure of a controlled substance to make a new compound that is not classified as a controlled drug. The new compound, called a *designer drug,* usually produces psychoactive responses similar to the drug from which it was produced. Designer drugs are relatively easy and inexpensive to produce. Thus, people who make these drug analogs can reap considerable profits from selling them.

## Table 7.5

### Popular Designer Drugs

| Designer Drug | Original Drugs | Psychoactive Effects | Possible Health Risks |
|---|---|---|---|
| MPPP MPTP | Meperidine (Demerol) | Heroin-like euphoria (depressant) | Parkinsonian syndrome: drooling, uncontrollable skeletal muscle movements, muscle rigidity (permanent) |
| China white | Fentanyl (Sublimaze) | Euphoria, respiratory depression | Death from respiratory failure |
| Ecstasy, XTC, Adam, M & M, MDMA | Mescaline–methamphetamine | Euphoria, CNS stimulant, hallucinations | Panic, anxiety, paranoia, increased and irregular heart rate, fever, hypertension, brain damage, seizures, death |
| Love drug (MDA) | Mescaline–methamphetamine | Euphoria, talkativeness, increased need to make friends | Fever, rapid heart rate, hypertension, seizures, death |

After officials with the DEA determine that a designer drug has the potential to be abused, they can classify the compound as a controlled substance. However, underground chemists often avoid prosecution by continuing to modify the substance, producing new generations of the drug that the DEA does not control. **Table 7.5** lists some of the best-known designer drugs, their psychoactive effects, and potential health risks.

Designer drugs are often more toxic than the compounds from which they are derived. China white, for example, is 1,000 times more potent than its parent drug, fentanyl, a powerful synthetic opioid often used for general anesthesia or in the treatment of chronic pain. In 2008, the Centers for Disease Control and Prevention (CDC) reported that illicitly manufactured fentanyl and its analogs were responsible for more than 1,000 deaths in the United States from April 2005 to March 2007 alone.[14] This was the most recent report from the CDC on fentanyl deaths as of March 2011.

## Ecstasy

The illegal designer drug *Ecstasy*, or *MDMA* (3,4-methylenedioxymethamphetamine), became a controlled substance in 1985. Chemically similar to mescaline and methamphetamine, Ecstasy produces both hallucinogenic and stimulant effects. Ecstasy users report that the drug improves their self-esteem and increases their desire to have intimate contacts with other people. However, users may experience panic and anxiety, hallucinations, tremors, rapid heart rate, loss of coordination, and psychotic behavior. Some users report more serious side effects such as irregular heartbeat, hypertension, fever, memory loss, and seizures. Since the 1980s, several people have died after taking this drug.

The use of Ecstasy by high school students, college students, and young adults rose sharply between 1999 and 2001. Use declined since then in all three groups. In 2009, annual prevalence rates for eighth, tenth, and twelfth graders were 1.3%, 3.7%, and 4.3%, respectively. For college students and for young adults aged 19 to 28 years and not in college, the prevalence rate was 3.1%.[2]

## K2

K2 is a drug that is made in the laboratory and works in the brain much like the THC of marijuana. It is sprayed on herbal and spice plant products and smoked. First synthesized and used recreationally in the mid-1990s, K2 became popular again in 2006. Although nicknamed "fake weed," this drug is not marijuana and is much more potent and dangerous than marijuana. Some of K2's side effects are severe potentially life-threatening hallucinations; dangerously elevated blood pressure and heart rate; pale skin; vomiting; and seizures.

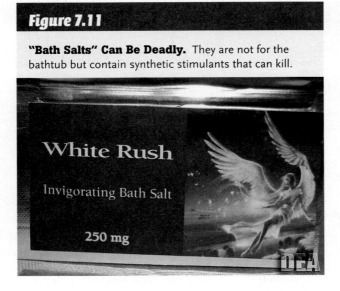

**Figure 7.11**

**"Bath Salts" Can Be Deadly.** They are not for the bathtub but contain synthetic stimulants that can kill.

White Rush

Invigorating Bath Salt

250 mg

## Bath Salts

Despite its name, this stimulant designer drug has nothing to do with the bath salts you put in your soaking tub. The name is only a disguise for a cocaine-like, life-threatening drug that raises the blood pressure and heart rate, increases the risk of heart attack and stroke, and can cause hallucinations, delusions, and paranoia—possibly long-term. Marketed under names like Zoom 2, Vanilla Sky, and Ocean Wave (**Figure 7.11**), reports of this drug began in 2010, and by 2011 legislation was under way to make "bath salts" a controlled substance.

## Over-the-Counter Drugs

The FDA regulates the production and marketing of prescription and nonprescription medications in the United States. To be sold in this country, an OTC medicine must be effective and safe when people follow the product information that comes with it (in packages or on labels). Although the FDA does not evaluate the safety or effectiveness of every OTC product that is marketed, the agency requires that active ingredients in products be evaluated for safety and usefulness. *Active* ingredients have an effect on the body; *inert* ingredients do not affect the body. Products that contain unsafe or ineffective ingredients or that have dishonest labeling cannot be sold. Herbal products that are sold as food supplements in health food stores are not regulated by the FDA. Some of these products contain substances that produce druglike effects and are toxic (see the Consumer

Health box in Chapter 1 and the one that follows in this chapter).

Individuals, physicians, and staff of healthcare facilities can report cases of harm that result from using medicinal and nutritional products. If you have any problem with a medication, medical device, or dietary supplement, report the problem to the FDA's MedWatch hotline by calling 1-800-332-1088 or go to www.fda.gov/MedWatch/report.htm.

Misuse and abuse of OTC medicines are common. As mentioned in the beginning of this chapter, the improper use of these medications can be harmful. Furthermore, some OTC products contain substances that can produce serious psychoactive effects, especially when they are taken in large doses.

An example of the potential dangers of abusing OTC medications is the tragic death of a 17-year-old track star in June 2007 from an overdose of methyl salicylate. This chemical compound is an active ingredient in a popular sports muscle pain cream and other OTC medications. The young woman used the sports cream liberally on her legs between runs while also using two other OTC medications containing methyl salicylate. This drug is an anticlotting agent, and at high doses it can cause internal bleeding, changes in heart rhythm, and liver damage. The death of the young woman emphasizes the need to use even seemingly harmless OTC medications according to directions and in moderation, and to remember that taking more than one medication simultaneously—even OTC preparations—may be risky.

## Look-Alike Drugs

The active ingredient in "stay-awake" pills is the stimulant caffeine. Some manufacturers produce caffeine-containing capsules or pills that look like prescription amphetamines or related prescribed stimulants. The production and sale of these look-alike drugs are difficult to regulate because they contain caffeine, an allowed substance. Frequently, people who sell street drugs misrepresent look-alike stimulants as amphetamines to unsuspecting users.

## Weight Loss Aids

Nearly anyone who has tried to lose weight knows that it is frustrating and that hunger seems to be constant. Many overweight people have taken various pills, powders, beverages, and foods for years to promote weight loss and prevent hunger. The Consumer Health box in Chapter 10 describes the potential harmful effects of these products and the drugs they contain.

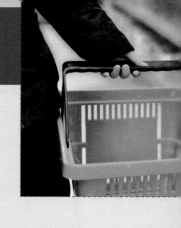

# Consumer Health

## Over-the-Counter Medicines: Safety and the FDA

To protect consumers, the Food and Drug Administration (FDA) regulates the testing, production, marketing, and labeling of medical devices and medications; the safety of foods and truthfulness of information on their labels; and the safety of cosmetics. A medical device or OTC medicine that is sold in the United States must be effective for its intended use and safe when its instructions are followed.

The FDA also requires that the active ingredients in OTC products be evaluated for safety and usefulness. Active ingredients have an impact on the body; inert ingredients do not affect the body. The FDA allows manufacturers of OTC products to use ingredients that are generally recognized as safe (GRAS), generally recognized as effective (GRAE), and generally recognized as honestly labeled (GRAHL). The FDA employs investigators who review information that appears on the labels of OTC products. Products that contain unsafe or ineffective ingredients, or that have labels displaying dishonest information, cannot be sold.

In 1998, the FDA proposed an easy-to-read and easy-to-understand labeling format for OTC drugs. **Figure 7.B** shows the information that must appear on the labels of an OTC medicinal product. Note that the label clearly displays warnings concerning the safe use of the product. Always follow instructions on the package or label concerning the use of any OTC medication.

Individuals, physicians, and staff of healthcare facilities can report cases of harm that result from using medicinal and nutritional products. If you have any problem with a medication, medical device, or dietary supplement, report the problem to the FDA's MedWatch hotline by calling 1-800-332-1088 or go to www.fda.gov/MedWatch/report.htm.

### Figure 7.B

**An OTC Label.** Certain information must appear on the labels of an OTC medicinal product. (a) Front of label, and (b) back of label.

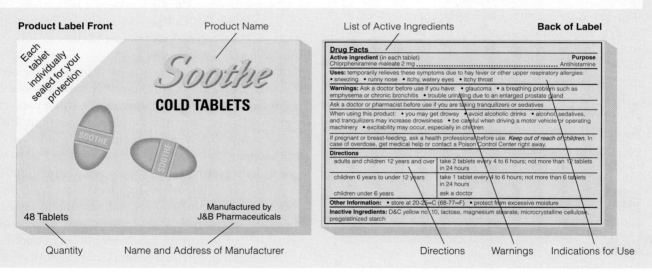

## Ephedrine/Ephedra

Ephedrine and pseudoephedrine are found in various OTC preparations such as weight loss aids and cold remedies, and they act as a stimulant, appetite suppressant, concentration aid, and decongestant. Because ephedrine and pseudoephedrine act as mild stimulants, some individuals misuse medicines that contain these compounds to pep themselves up.

However, ephedrine-containing drugs can produce high blood pressure, sleeplessness, irregular and rapid heart rate, and restlessness; taking high doses of either substance may evoke psychotic symptoms.

Ephedra, known in Chinese as ma huang, is a plant extract that is the source of ephedrine and pseudoephedrine. Many laws control the sale of ephedrine-, pseudoephedrine-, and ephedra-containing

## Figure 7.12

**Hazardous Herbs.** Numerous plants can be toxic. For example, when taken internally, comfrey (shown here) can cause hepatic veno-occlusive disease (VOD), in which some of the small veins of the liver are blocked. VOD can lead to liver failure and death.

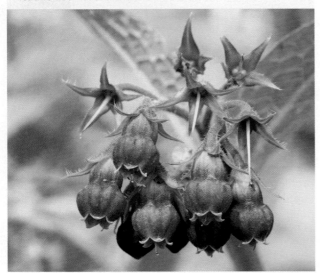

products. For example, in 2004 FDA officials banned the sale of ephedra-containing dietary supplements because of their dangerous side effects. The ban targeted supplements that had been advertised for weight loss, muscle building, and athletic performance. In 2003, ephedra was implicated in the death of 23-year-old Steve Bechler, a prospective pitcher for the Baltimore Orioles.

In addition to ephedra, numerous other herbs or plant extracts—such as lobelia, comfrey, yohimbine, *Ginkgo biloba*, or sassafras—contain substances that can produce harmful side effects when ingested as supplements or teas (**Figure 7.12**).

 **Healthy Living Practices**

☐ Ask your physician about the need to use over-the-counter medications. If it is necessary for you to take these drugs, follow the labels' instructions concerning their safe use. Your pharmacist is also a source of reliable information concerning the safe use of OTC drugs.

☐ Obtain reliable information concerning the safety and effectiveness of herbal products before you take them.

# Drug Treatment and Prevention

## Treating Drug Dependency

The goal of drug treatment is to stop the drug abuse and reduce the likelihood that abusers will return to their previous drug use behaviors. Currently, three major forms of long-term drug abuse treatment exist: methadone maintenance, outpatient drug-free programs, and residential therapeutic communities.

*Methadone maintenance* is used to treat addiction to opiates; methadone reduces the cravings for these drugs. This controversial treatment is often used after other attempts at treatment have failed. Methadone is taken orally, diluted in juice. When taken this way, the drug prevents opiate withdrawal symptoms and reduces cravings, but it does not produce euphoria or cloud the mind. In addition, it blocks the effects of heroin and other opiates, which reduces the desire of addicts to continue taking these drugs. Thus, methadone treatment helps people stop taking opiates while at the same time allowing them to go to work, go to school, and take care of themselves and their family. Some drug rehabilitation programs prescribe methadone during opiate detoxification and then taper off methadone use. However, other programs allow people to stay on methadone as long as they feel it is necessary.

Most abusers prefer *outpatient drug-free programs* that provide medical care and a wide variety of counseling and psychotherapy approaches while patients continue to live with their families and work in their communities. These programs do not include use of methadone.

Self-help groups are a popular and useful adjunct to professional outpatient drug treatment. Individuals recovering from drug dependency attend regular meetings to receive encouragement and social support from other former substance abusers. Alcoholics Anonymous (AA) is one of the oldest, most effective self-help programs and is described in Chapter 8. Many other community-based self-help programs that treat drug abuse, such as Narcotics Anonymous, are modeled after AA.

In severe cases, drug abusers may undergo detoxification and then live for several months in controlled environments called *residential therapeutic communities* or *group homes*. Living in these communities reduces the likelihood that patients will be exposed to drugs while they resocialize, or readjust to general society.

While in group homes, patients also receive medical care, social services, and psychological counseling. After they leave residential therapeutic communities, individuals usually attend community- or hospital-based counseling sessions to prevent *relapse,* the return to drug abuse. For people who lack health insurance, the high cost of medical care is a major barrier to obtaining treatment in a therapeutic community.

Most drug treatment programs that last fewer than 3 months have limited long-term effectiveness.[15] According to the Partnership for a Drug-Free America, results of studies show that length of time in drug treatment is the best single predictor of positive post-treatment outcomes. Many drug-dependent people need more than 3 months of outpatient care or living in controlled environments to change their substance-related behaviors and attitudes. Additionally, recovering addicts often need to acquire job skills while they are in therapy to improve their chances of becoming drug-free, productive members of society.

A considerable number of patients finish treatment but relapse within a few weeks or months of abstinence. Former addicts are more likely to relapse if they have severe mental illness or polyabuse, and if they return to communities where illicit drugs are available and are widely used. Recovering drug addicts are more likely to abstain from using drugs if they are married or in stable relationships, supported by their families, and employed. In 2009, 2.6 million Americans received treatment for their drug use, including alcohol use.[1]

# Antidrug Vaccines

Many drug treatment programs use medications to help individuals break their addictions. These medications help by suppressing drug withdrawal symptoms, reducing drug cravings, and helping reestablish proper brain function. One new type of drug that is being developed to help in drug treatment is the antidrug vaccine.

An antidrug vaccine works by stimulating the immune system to develop antibodies against a particular drug, such as an anticocaine vaccine or an antimorphine vaccine. These antibodies attach to the drug in the bloodstream, making the molecules of the drug too large to pass through the membranous blood–brain barrier. If the drug does not reach the brain, the vaccinated person will not feel the effects of the drug because the pleasure centers of the brain would not be stimulated. With no "reward" for taking the drug, the addicted person soon loses the craving sensations that are a part of drug addiction.

One problem is that drug vaccines do not always elicit a robust antibody response in an individual. If the antibody response is weak, only some of the drug would be bound by the vaccine and some would remain free and able to pass to the brain. In this situation, if the drug addict took a high-enough dose of the drug, he or she could likely attain their usual "high." Researchers are working to resolve problems such as this and also note that counseling and behavior therapy in conjunction with vaccines would likely produce the best results.[16]

# Preventing Drug Misuse and Abuse

The U.S. government devotes much of its drug prevention efforts to reducing the supply of illicit drugs. These efforts include destroying crops such as marijuana and coca plants; stopping the flow of illegal substances through U.S. borders; and prosecuting individuals who manufacture, sell, and purchase drugs illegally. Such measures, however, are not effectively reducing the demand for illicit drugs in this country. Many people think that social and economic programs to reduce poverty and unemployment would decrease the demand for illicit drugs. Additionally, educational programs that promote drug-free lifestyles, especially among children and young adults, may help reduce the prevalence of drug abuse.

The National Institute on Drug Abuse conducted research for 25 years to determine which drug prevention programs have the highest degree of long-term effectiveness. They found that successful prevention programs:

- Enhance protective factors and reverse or reduce known risk factors

- Use interactive methods such as peer discussion groups

- Target all forms of drug use

- Teach skills to resist drugs when offered

- Strengthen personal commitments against drug use

- Increase social skills and assertiveness

- Reinforce attitudes against drug use

Additionally, drug education programs that involve parents, media, and the community are more successful than programs that limit educational activities to classrooms.[17]

## Healthy Living Practices

☐ If you or someone you know is abusing drugs, obtain help from local substance abuse programs or from your healthcare practitioner.

## Across THE LIFE SPAN

### DRUG USE AND ABUSE

Pregnant drug users are at risk for miscarriage, *ectopic* ("tubal") pregnancy, and stillbirth (giving birth to a dead infant). Babies born to women who used cocaine, opiates, amphetamines, or marijuana regularly during pregnancy are more likely to be premature (born too soon) and smaller than infants who were not exposed to these drugs before birth. Compared to other infants, premature, underweight, and prenatally drug-exposed newborns are more likely to have serious health problems early in life. Drug-exposed newborns also tend to have smaller than normal head circumferences, a sign that brain growth has been negatively affected. Pregnant women should consult their physicians before taking any drug.

Adolescents who have certain risk factors are more likely to use alcohol and other drugs than adolescents without these characteristics. **Table 7.6** lists risk factors and protective factors in drug use prevention.

Despite living in situations that promote substance use and abuse, many young people abstain from taking psychoactive drugs. Teenagers who stay in high school, attend classes regularly, make good grades,

### Table 7.6

### Risk and Protective Factors for Drug Abuse Among Youth

| *Protective factors* |
| --- |
| Strong and positive family bonds |
| Parental monitoring of children's activities and peers |
| Clear rules of conduct that are consistently enforced within the family |
| Involvement of parents in the lives of their children |
| Success in school performance |
| Strong bonds with institutions, such as school and religious organizations |
| Adoption of conventional norms about drug use |
| *Risk factors* |
| Chaotic home environments, particularly in which parents abuse substances or suffer from mental illnesses |
| Ineffective parenting, especially with children with difficult temperaments or conduct disorders |
| Lack of parent–child attachments and nurturing |
| Inappropriately shy or aggressive behavior in the classroom |
| Failure in school performance |
| Poor social coping skills |
| Affiliations with peers displaying deviant behaviors |
| Perceptions of approval of drug-using behaviors in family, work, school, peer, and community environments |

*Source:* National Institute on Drug Abuse. (2002, February). Risk and protective factors in drug abuse prevention. *NIDA Notes, 16*(6). Retrieved on March 21, 2011, from http://archives.drugabuse.gov/nida_notes/nnvol16n6/Risk.html

The following ad promotes a book that describes how to eliminate addictive urges. Read the advertisement and evaluate it using the model for analyzing health-related information. The main points of the model are noted here; the model is fully explained in Chapter 1.

1. Which statements are verifiable facts, and which are unverified statements or value claims?
2. What are the credentials of the person who makes health-related claims? Does this person have the appropriate background and education in the topic area? What can you do to check the person's credentials?
3. What might be the motives and biases of the person making the claims?
4. What is the main point of the ad? Which information is relevant to the issue, main point, product, or service? Which information is irrelevant?
5. Is the source reliable? What evidence supports your conclusion that the source is reliable or unreliable? Does the source of information present the pros and cons of the topic or the benefits and risks of the product?
6. Does the source of information attack the credibility of conventional scientists or medical authorities?

Based on your analysis, do you think that this ad and the book are reliable sources of health-related information? Explain why you would or would not buy the book. Summarize your reasons for coming to this conclusion.

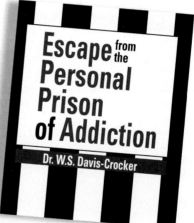

# Escape from the Personal Prison of Addiction

## Dr. W. S. Davis-Crocker

**Is your life being ruined by chemical addictions? Wouldn't it be wonderful to say "no" to drugs and to stick to it? Now you can learn a simple technique to take control of your destructive behaviors.**

After years of scientific research, Dr. W.S. Davis-Crocker has unlocked the neurobiochemical secrets of addiction. In her newest book, *Escape from the Personal Prison of Addiction,* Dr. Davis-Crocker, world-renowned author and founder of the Davis-Crocker Institute for the Study of Habituation, describes how to rid yourself of addictions painlessly.

Finally, there is hope for addicts. In just three days of practicing the advice in her book, your cravings for alcohol, cigarettes, heroin, and even chocolate will vanish! There is no need for you to use special medications or costly psychotherapy.

To order your copy of *Escape from the Personal Prison of Addiction,* call 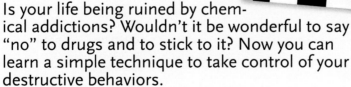. All major credit cards accepted.

Also register to attend Dr. Davis-Crocker's next seminar in your area. Enrollment is limited, so call the toll-free number now to reserve your seat, and we'll send you our informative pamphlet *Why Me?* at no charge.

## Table 7.7

## Summary of Psychoactive Drugs: Effects on the Body

| Drug Category | Trade or Other Names | Physical Dependence | Psychological Dependence | Tolerance | Possible Side Effects | Overdose Effects | Withdrawal Effects |
|---|---|---|---|---|---|---|---|
| Stimulants | Caffeine, cocaine (snow, big c), methamphetamine, crystal meth (crystals), Preludin, Ritalin, Dexadrine or "dex," black beauties, black hollies | Possible | High | Yes | Alertness, euphoria, increased pulse rate and blood pressure, sleeplessness, lack of appetite | Fever, hallucinations, convulsions, death | Prolonged sleep, irritability, depression, anxiety, moodiness, headaches |
| Depressants | Alcohol,* barbiturates (goofballs), Valium, Halcion, Quaalude, GHB, GBL, "roofies" (Rohypnol) | Varies | Varies | Yes | Slurred speech, drunken behavior | Depressed breathing, dilated pupils, coma, death | Depression, anxiety, sleeplessness, convulsions, death |
| Opiates | Heroin (China white), morphine, codeine-containing products, methadone, Demerol, OxyContin, Vicodin, Darvon, Percodan | Moderate to high | Moderate to high | Yes | Euphoria, sleepiness, depressed breathing, nausea | Slowed breathing, convulsions, coma, death | Teary eyes, watery nose, yawning, tremors, anxiety, abdominal cramps |
| Marijuana (cannabis) | Pot, hash, hashish oil, Acapulco gold, blunts, buds, Colombo, weed | Unknown | Moderate | Possible | Euphoria, relaxation, increased appetite, distorted time perception | Anxiety, paranoia | Anxiety, depression |
| Hallucinogens | LSD blotters, mescaline, STP, psilocybin, high doses of PCP, peyote, psychedelic mushrooms, ketamine | None (LSD and mescaline) Others: unknown | Unknown | Yes | Euphoria, hallucinations, poor time perception | Anxiety, psychotic behavior | None reported |
| Inhalants | Gasoline, paint thinners and removers, freon, aerosols, butyl nitrate | None | Possible | No | Euphoria, sleepiness, confusion, slurred speech | Brain, kidney, or liver damage; headaches; death | Anxiety |

## Table 7.7

### Summary of Psychoactive Drugs: Effects on the Body *(Continued)*

| Drug Category | Trade or Other Names | Physical Dependence | Psychological Dependence | Tolerance | Possible Side Effects | Overdose Effects | Withdrawal Effects |
|---|---|---|---|---|---|---|---|
| Drugs with mixed effects | Nicotine,* PCP, MDMA (Ecstasy) | Unknown | High (PCP) Unknown (MDMA) | Yes | Hallucinations and altered perceptions (PCP) | Psychosis, possible death (PCP) | Unknown |

*See Chapter 8.

*Sources: Drugs of abuse.* (2005). Washington, DC: U.S. Department of Justice, Drug Enforcement Administration; Goldberg, R. (2009). *Drugs across the spectrum.* Belmont, CA: Brooks/Cole; and Hanson, G. R., et al. (2011). *Drugs and society.* Sudbury, MA: Jones & Bartlett.

and get along well with their parents generally avoid using drugs. These children have personality traits that are collectively referred to as resiliency. Resilient children accept responsibility, adapt to change, manage stress, solve problems, and are achievement- and success-oriented. Resilient young people have the ability to remain psychologically, socially, and spiritually healthy even if their families are dysfunctional or not supportive.

The abuse of illicit drugs is not a widespread problem among older adults in the United States. However, many older adults take a variety of prescribed medications to treat problems such as insomnia, depression, hypertension, and heart disease. These aged individuals have a higher risk of becoming intoxicated from taking medications because their bodies do not detoxify and eliminate the substances as effectively as younger people do. More research is needed to determine medication levels that are safe and effective for elderly individuals.

The risk of serious drug interactions and drug synergism is high among aged people who take more than one prescribed drug. In many instances, elderly persons appear to have suffered a stroke, developed Alzheimer's disease, or become severely depressed when actually their confusion and weakness are the side effects of taking numerous prescribed medicines in bad combinations or the wrong amounts or schedules.

## Healthy Living Practices

☐ Do not use drugs of any kind during pregnancy without the approval of your physician.

# Summary

Drugs are nonfood chemicals that alter the way a person thinks, feels, functions, or behaves. Many drugs have beneficial uses as medicines, but these substances can have serious negative effects on the health and well-being of people who use them improperly. People often abuse psychoactive, or mood-altering, drugs. Drug abuse contributes to numerous social problems that plague our society, such as crime, unemployment, and family violence and dissolution.

By interacting with nerve cells in the brain, psychoactive drugs influence perceptions, thought processes, feelings, and behaviors. Additionally, environmental factors can affect how people act and feel while under the influence of psychoactive drugs.

In most instances, the liver converts drugs into less dangerous compounds that can be eliminated in urine, feces, or exhaled breath. When the body is unable to detoxify and eliminate excessive amounts of a drug rapidly, the characteristic signs and symptoms of intoxication occur. Drug overdoses and polyabuse may produce serious, even deadly, effects.

In 2009, an estimated 21.8 million Americans older than 12 years of age were current illicit drug users. Rates of illicit drug use are especially high among teenagers and young adults. Initially, these individuals typically use alcohol, nicotine, or inhalants; they then may move on to marijuana. Some persons experiment with or use other illicit drugs after marijuana. In general, illicit drug use declines after age 20 years.

Dependency and addiction describe any habitual behavior that interferes with a person's health, work, and relationships. Drug dependence or addiction occurs when users develop a pattern of taking drugs that usually produces a compulsive need to use these substances, a tolerance for them, and withdrawal when they are discontinued. The type of substance taken, the social environment of the person, his or her personality, and genetics influence an individual's chances of developing a drug dependency.

Depressants such as alcohol and barbiturates slow the activity of the cerebral cortex, producing sedative and hypnotic effects as well as drowsiness. Thus, people should not drive or operate machinery while under the influence of depressants. Misusing depressants can be deadly.

Stimulants enhance chemical activity in parts of the brain that influence emotions, sleep, attention, and learning. Caffeine is the most commonly consumed legal stimulant in this country. Stimulants such as Ritalin and cocaine have few medical uses. Cocaine is addictive and frequently abused. Methamphetamine use in U.S. college students has declined since 1999, from 3.3% in that year to 0.3% in 2009.

Opiates have important medical uses as sedatives, analgesics, and narcotics. When misused, opiates are highly addictive and extremely dangerous.

Marijuana, which contains THC as its major psychoactive compound, is the most widely used illicit drug in the United States. Although marijuana does not produce physiologic dependence, some people become compulsive users. Marijuana smoke contains numerous irritants that can damage the bronchial tubes and lungs.

Hallucinogens alter the brain's ability to perceive sensory information, producing abnormal and unreal sensations. In the United States, the most potent and commonly abused hallucinogens are mescaline, psilocybin, LSD, ketamine, and PCP. High doses of PCP and ketamine can be deadly.

Many common household products release toxic fumes that can produce psychoactive effects when inhaled. Teenagers may use inhalants before they move on to other psychoactive drugs. Inhalants can depress respiration, resulting in coma or death.

Designer drugs are made by altering the chemical structures of controlled substances. In some cases, these drug analogs are more toxic than the compounds from which they were derived.

The FDA regulates the production and marketing of all medications in the United States. Some health food and OTC products contain substances that are harmful or that produce psychoactive effects, especially when they are misused or abused.

The primary goal of drug treatment is to help abusers become drug-free. Drug treatment usually involves participation in outpatient treatment programs and self-help groups. Drug prevention programs that target school-age children typically provide information about drugs and teach drug resistance and refusal skills.

Drug use during pregnancy increases the risk of miscarriage, ectopic pregnancy, and stillbirth. Women who use cocaine, opiates, amphetamines, and marijuana regularly during pregnancy are more likely to give birth to premature and smaller infants than pregnant women who do not use these drugs.

The extent to which prenatal drug exposure influences the long-term mental and physical development of children is unclear.

Adolescents who are more likely to use drugs are those who have parents and friends who abuse drugs, are failing in school, have poor social coping skills, and have a lack of parent–child attachment.

Although drug abuse is rare among older adults, these individuals may experience harmful effects from taking prescribed medicines because they do not detoxify and eliminate drugs as effectively as younger individuals do or because they misuse or become confused by multiple prescriptions.

## Applying What You Have Learned

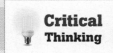

**Critical Thinking**

1. Why do people abuse certain drugs such as cocaine and not others such as aspirin? **Application**
2. Have you ever used a medication improperly? If your answer is yes, describe your misuse of the drug. **Analysis**
3. Plan an educational program for fifth-grade students that discourages illicit drug use. **Synthesis**

4. One of your friends thinks that marijuana is safe and that its use should be decriminalized. Evaluate this person's position by considering the health effects on the population if marijuana were legalized. **Evaluation**

| **Application** | **Analysis** | **Synthesis** | **Evaluation** |
|---|---|---|---|
| using information in a new situation. | breaking down information into component parts. | putting together information from different sources. | making informed decisions. |

**Key**

## Reflecting on Your Health

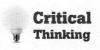

**Critical Thinking**

1. Do you use drugs responsibly? Explain why you do or do not.
2. Under what circumstances would you intervene to stop a friend from abusing drugs?
3. What are you currently doing or what would you do to encourage your children not to use illegal drugs?
4. What kinds of over-the-counter drugs do you use? Do you think that your use of these drugs is helpful or harmful to your health?
5. If you abuse drugs, do you think that your health or the health of others is adversely affected by your behavior? Why or why not? After reading this chapter and learning about the health effects of illegal drugs, are you motivated to stop your drug abuse? Why or why not?

## References

1. Substance Abuse and Mental Health Services Administration. (2010). *Results from the 2009 National Survey on Drug Use and Health: Vol. I. Summary of National Findings* (HHS Publication No. SMA 10-4586Findings). Retrieved on March 16, 2011, from http://oas.samhsa.gov/NSDUH/2k9NSDUH/2k9ResultsP.pdf

2. Johnston, L. D., et al. (2010). *Monitoring the future: National survey results on drug use, 1975–2009: Volume 2, college students and adults ages 19–45* (NIH Publication No. 10-7585). Bethesda, MD: National Institute on Drug Abuse. Retrieved on March 16, 2011, from http://www.monitoringthefuture.org/pubs/monographs/vol2_2009.pdf

3. Hanson, G., Fleckenstein, A. E., & Venturelli, P. J. (2012). *Drugs and society* (11th ed.). Sudbury, MA: Jones & Bartlett Learning.

4. Culberson, J. W., & Ziska, M. (2008). Prescription drug misuse/abuse in the elderly. *Geriatrics*, 63:22–31.

5. National Institute on Drug Abuse. (2003). *Preventing drug use among children and adolescents: A research-based guide* (2nd ed.). Washington, DC: U.S. Government Printing Office. Retrieved on March 16, 2011, from http://www.nida.nih.gov/pdf/prevention/RedBook.pdf

6. Yeo, K.-K., et al. (2007). The association of methamphetamine use and cardiomyopathy in young patients. *American Journal of Medicine*, 120:165–171.

7. Nguyen, D., et al. (2010). Intrauterine growth of infants exposed to prenatal methamphetamine: Results from the infant development, environment, and lifestyle study. *Journal of Pediatrics, 157*(2):337–339.

8. Roussotte, F., et al. (2010). Structural, metabolic, and functional brain abnormalities as a result of prenatal exposure to drugs of abuse: Evidence from neuroimaging. *Neuropsychology Review, 20*(4):376–397.

9. Thompson, P. M., Kayashi, K. M., Simon, S. L., Geaga, J. S., Hong, M. S., Sui, Y., et al. (2004). Structural abnormalities in the brains of human subjects who use methamphetamine. *Journal of Neuroscience, 24*:6028–6036.

10. Johnston, L. D., et al. (2010). *Monitoring the future: National survey results on drug use, 1975–2009: Volume 1, secondary school students* (NIH Publication No. 10-7584). Bethesda, MD: National Institute on Drug Abuse. Retrieved on March 17, 2011, from http://www.monitoringthefuture.org/pubs/monographs/vol1_2009.pdf

11. Schardt, D. (2008, March). Caffeine: The good, the bad, and the maybe. *Nutrition Action Health Letter,* Center for Science in the Public Interest. Retrieved on March 17, 2011, from http://www.cspinet.org/nah/02_08/caffeine.pdf

12. Drasbek, K. R., et al. (2006). Gamma-hydroxybutyrate—a drug of abuse. *Acta Neurologica Scandinavica, 114*:145–156.

13. Hall, W., & Degenhardt, L. (2009). Adverse health effects of nonmedical cannabis use. *Lancet, 374*(9698)1383–1391.

14. Centers for Disease Control and Prevention. (2008, July 25). Nonpharmaceutical fentanyl-related deaths—multiple states, April 2005 to March 2007. *Morbidity and Mortality Weekly Report, 57*:793–796.

15. National Institute on Drug Abuse. (2009). *Principles of drug addiction treatment: A research-based guide* (NIH Publication No. 09-4180). Washington, DC: National Institutes of Health, National Institute on Drug Abuse. Retrieved on March 21, 2011, from http://www.nida.nih.gov/PDF/PODAT/PODAT.pdf

16. Kinsey, B. M., et al. (2009). Anti-drug vaccines to treat substance abuse. *Immunology and Cell Biology*, *87*(4):309–314.

17. National Institute on Drug Abuse. (2004). Lessons from prevention research. *NIDA InfoFacts*. Retrieved from http://drugabuse.gov/pdf/infofacts/Prevention04.pdf

go.jblearning.com/alters6e

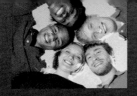
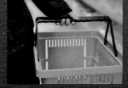
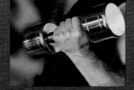
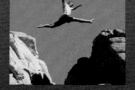
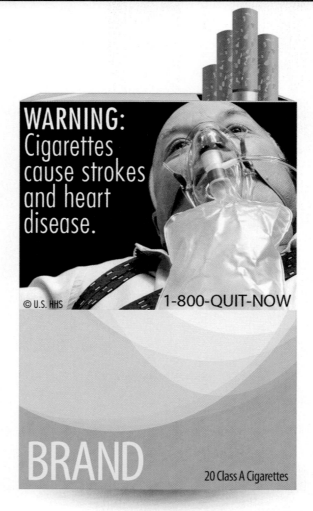

WARNING: Cigarettes cause strokes and heart disease.

© U.S. HHS

1-800-QUIT-NOW

BRAND

20 Class A Cigarettes

## Chapter Overview

Factors related to and consequences of alcohol abuse and dependence

Alcohol's effects on college students

How to control your alcohol consumption

How alcoholism is diagnosed and treated

Who uses tobacco products and why

The short- and long-term health effects of tobacco use

The benefits and process of quitting

## Student Workbook

Self-Assessment: Why Do You Smoke?

Changing Health Habits: Do You Want to Change a Smoking or Drinking Habit?

## Do You Know?

Whether clove cigarettes are safer than regular cigarettes?

The major reasons why college students drink?

How smoking can affect your sex life?

# CHAPTER 8

# Alcohol and Tobacco

The graphic and sobering warnings shown on the facing page are among those that were developed to appear on cigarette packs and advertisements by September 22, 2012. For 28 years—from 1984 to 2012—the health warning on cigarette packs in the United States is small and text-only. A major change occurred with the passage of the Tobacco Control Act, which was signed into law on June 22, 2009. With this law, the U.S. Food and Drug Administration (FDA) became empowered to regulate the manufacture, marketing, and distribution of tobacco products. The law also stipulates that the FDA develop color graphics—photos or drawings—to accompany nine new health warnings written to educate the American public about the dangers of smoking. The goal of the educational warnings is to reduce the rate of smoking in the United States to 12% by 2020. The new warnings were mandated to cover at least half of the front and back of each cigarette pack and at least one-fifth of the area of an advertisement. However, five tobacco companies filed a lawsuit against the federal government in August 2011. The companies contend that these huge graphics and accompanying statements advocate that people not buy cigarettes, rather than simply warning them of the risks of smoking.

Other countries also require graphic images and strong health warnings on their cigarette packages, including Australia, Brazil, Canada, Malaysia, Singapore, and Thailand. Do these warning labels work to deter people from smoking?

> *For 28 years—from 1984 to 2012—the health warnings on cigarette packs in the United States were small and text-only.*

To find out, researchers from the Centers for Disease Control and Prevention (CDC) asked smokers and nonsmokers aged 18 to 24 years to explain their reactions to large graphic and text cigarette warnings on packs of Canadian cigarettes compared to the much smaller text-only U.S. warnings.[1] The results from this investigation and other studies cited by the CDC revealed that the large graphic images along with specific information, such as those on the Canadian cigarette packs, were more likely to be noticed, read, and believed than the smaller, text-only, less-specific messages on U.S. cigarette packs. Percentages, facts, and corresponding graphic images had more effect on the thinking of young adults than did vague text-only messages such as "Quitting smoking now greatly reduces serious risks to your health." The CDC concluded that "stronger warnings on U.S. cigarette packages that include graphic images and factual messages may help consumers make more informed decisions about using tobacco products."

Smoking cigarettes and drinking alcohol are behaviors that begin in the preteen and teen years. Many in these age groups view smoking and drinking as acceptable because advertisements encourage such thinking, especially ads and products that target young people. Although tobacco companies are not allowed to advertise, market, and promote their products to those younger than 18 years as part of the 1998 Master Settlement Agreement (MSA) between the states and the tobacco industry, they still do. Results of a study conducted by researchers at the Cancer Prevention and Control Program at the University of California San Diego Cancer Center conclude that "recent RJ Reynolds advertising may be effectively targeting adolescent girls."[2] The researchers were referring to the Camel No. 9 advertising campaign, which associated the thin cigarettes with romance, glamour, and Chanel perfumes. One of the Camel No. 9 advertisements is shown in **Figure 8.1**.

Hanewinkel et al. studied cigarette ads versus non-cigarette ads and the effect of each on smoking initiation among adolescents and teens. The data revealed an association between cigarette ads and smoking initiation in youth aged 10 to 17 years but revealed no association between exposure to ads in general and smoking initiation in this age group. The researchers explain that cigarette ads are powerful mechanisms that draw young persons to smoking because they contain images to which this age group aspires—images of "masculinity (for boys), thinness (for girls), independence, extroversion, and sex appeal." The researchers note:

### Figure 8.1

**Camel No. 9 Cigarette Advertisement.** The magazine ads attracted adolescent and teen girls with flowery images and vintage fashion. The cigarette packs were a high-style glossy black with hot pink and teal blue borders. Promotional giveaways were hot pink as well and included cell phone jewelry and tiny purses.

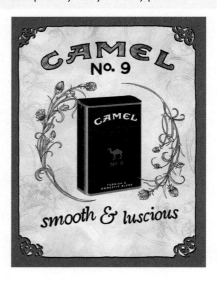

*Cigarette marketers have created brands with multiple aspirational images, each designed to fit the needs common among adolescents. Adolescents are in the process of identity formation, when they face emotional instability and social self-consciousness. Aspirational imagery used in cigarette advertising is especially appealing, because it associates the behavior, smoking, with characteristics adolescents are trying to assimilate.[3]*

Many medical researchers and healthcare professionals think that advertising alcohol and other drug-related products such as cigarettes encourages the use of all drugs. The practice of promoting alcohol and tobacco use is particularly dangerous because they are two primary "gateway" drugs. That is, most people who abuse drugs have followed a progression in drug use from alcohol and/or tobacco to marijuana and "hard" drugs.

Both tobacco and alcohol can have devastating effects on health. Before you read this chapter, consider taking the self-assessment for this chapter in the Student Workbook pages at the end of this text. The National Cancer Institute's quiz "Why Do You Smoke?" will help you understand the roots of your smoking behavior. If you do not smoke cigarettes or drink alcoholic beverages, you probably know family members, coworkers, or friends who may benefit from these self-assessments. Taking these tests could be their first steps to healthier lifestyles.

# Alcohol

## Alcohol Use, Abuse, and Dependence

Alcohol use is quite common in the United States. According to the 2009 National Survey on Drug Use and Health, 51.9% of Americans older than 12 years are current alcohol users, which means that they had at least one drink in the month before they took the survey.[4] This group includes binge alcohol users and heavy alcohol users. For the purposes of the survey, binge alcohol users had five or more drinks on the same occasion at least once in the month prior to the survey. Heavy alcohol users had five or more drinks on the same occasion on at least five days in the month prior to the survey. (All heavy alcohol users are also binge alcohol users.) **Table 8.1** lists the num-

**harmful use** Drinking alcoholic beverages while knowingly damaging one's physical and/or psychological health.

**alcohol abuse** Includes the symptoms of harmful use, but when drinking the abuser exhibits long-term social interaction problems and uses alcohol in physically dangerous situations.

**alcohol dependence (alcoholism)** A syndrome characterized by at least three of the following symptoms: a compulsion to drink, difficulty in controlling the amount of alcohol consumed, withdrawal symptoms when alcohol is not consumed, evidence of tolerance, progressive neglect of other interests because of drinking, and continuing to use alcohol despite its physical and psychological effects on the user.

ber of drinks consumed by light to heavier drinkers as measured in standard drinks.

Responsible drinkers do not allow drinking alcoholic beverages to threaten their physical or psychological health or interfere with their relationships or interactions with others. Additionally, their behavior while drinking does not threaten the health or well-being of others.

Alcohol use becomes **harmful use** when a person drinks alcoholic beverages while knowingly damaging his or her health. For example, a person who drinks heavily on a regular basis (see Table 8.1), gets injured often while drinking, or becomes depressed from drinking is engaging in harmful use.

**Alcohol abuse** includes the symptoms of harmful use but adds a social dimension. When drinking, the alcohol abuser has problems interacting with people in his or her family, in social settings, or at work. Typically, the abuser uses alcohol in physically dangerous situations, such as when driving a car. However, he or she does not develop tolerance to the drug, exhibit withdrawal symptoms when not drinking (see Chapter 7), or compulsively use alcohol. Both harmful use and alcohol abuse are patterns of behavior, not just one-time occurrences. Both are usually considered to be present if the behavior has occurred for at least 1 month or has occurred repeatedly over a longer period of time.

Alcohol abuse becomes **alcohol dependence**, or **alcoholism**, when certain other symptoms occur that are part of the *alcohol dependence syndrome*. **Table 8.2** lists the symptoms of this syndrome. A diagnosis of dependence is usually made if a person exhibits three or more of these symptoms over a year's time. According to the CDC, excessive alcohol use is the third leading cause of preventable death in the United States, accounting for approximately 79,000 deaths per year.[5]

| Table 8.1 | |
| --- | --- |
| **Drinking Levels as Shown in Standard Drinks*** | |
| **Drinking Level** | **Amount** |
| Abstainer | Fewer than 12 drinks in lifetime or no drinks in the past year |
| Light | Three or fewer drinks/week |
| Moderate | More than 3 drinks/week but no more than 7 drinks/week for women and no more than 14 drinks/week for men |
| Heavy or high-risk | Women: More than 3 drinks on any day or more than 7 drinks/week. Men: More than 4 drinks on any day or more than 14 drinks/week. |

*One standard drink is 0.5 oz absolute alcohol, 12 oz beer, 5 oz wine, or 1.5 oz 80-proof liquor. (Amounts for beer and wine vary depending on their alcohol content.)

Sources: U.S. Department of Agriculture and U.S. Department of Health and Human Services. (2010). *Dietary guidelines for Americans, 2010* (7th ed.). Washington, DC: U.S. Government Printing Office; and National Institute on Alcohol Abuse and Alcoholism.

## Table 8.2

## Alcohol Dependence Syndrome

Having three or more of the following symptoms over a year usually indicates alcohol dependence syndrome:

- A strong desire or compulsion to drink

- Difficulty in controlling the amount of alcohol consumed and when it is consumed

- Withdrawal symptoms when alcohol is not consumed, or consuming alcohol to avoid withdrawal symptoms

- Evidence of tolerance, that is, increased amounts of alcohol are needed to achieve the effects originally produced by lower amounts

- Progressive neglect of other interests because of drinking, while spending an increased amount of time obtaining and drinking alcohol, and recovering from its effects

- Continued use of alcohol despite clear evidence of its physical and/or psychological effects on the user

# Factors Related to Alcohol Abuse and Dependence

About 100 years ago, alcoholics were thought simply to have a "weak character" or to suffer from "moral weakness." Since that time, especially within the past 50 years or so, scientists have gathered evidence showing that alcoholism has a variety of origins, many of them biological. In addition, research results show the importance of the interactions among heredity, brain effects, and psychological, social, and developmental factors in the development of alcoholism. Researchers are increasingly studying the roles of the interaction between genes and the environment in alcohol use and dependence.[6] A cause of alcoholism is unknown.

**Heredity** For centuries, people have observed that alcoholism runs in families. Researchers have explored environmental and hereditary (genetic) factors of alcoholics to determine which are significant in the development of alcoholism.

By studying the family history of alcoholics, scientists determined that people who have a first-degree relative (parent, brother, or sister) with alcoholism have a higher risk of developing alcoholism than do people in the general population. Scientists estimate this risk to be from four to seven times higher. Sons of alcoholic fathers are at greatest risk. Additionally, data from adoption, twin, and animal studies indicate that there is a genetic component to alcoholism.

Scientists also study the reactions of people at risk for developing alcoholism (those who have a first-degree alcoholic relative) compared to those not at risk for alcoholism. In general, those at risk do not react to the consumption of alcohol with the same intensity as those not at risk. Some scientists think that persons at risk for alcoholism may not perceive that they are becoming intoxicated until they have had far more to drink than those not at risk for alcoholism.

Two other genetically linked factors are thought to influence the development of alcoholism: behavior and temperament. *Behavior* is the way people act—what they do. *Temperament* means disposition—the characteristic way in which people emotionally respond to the things and people around them. Behavior and temperament are thought to be inherited traits that are modified by interactions with the environment. Certain characteristics of behavior and temperament appear to be associated with enhanced risk for alcoholism: hyperactivity, impulsivity, aggression, short attention span, quickly changing emotions, slowed ability to calm oneself following stress, thrill-seeking behavior, and inability to delay gratification.

**Brain Effects** When a person drinks alcoholic beverages, various behavioral changes occur that are commonly called **intoxication**, impairment of the functioning of the central nervous system (the brain and spinal cord). *Table 8.3* lists the changes that characteristically take place as a person consumes more and more alcohol. In this table, alcohol consumption and blood alcohol concentrations (BACs) are listed as ranges because the number of drinks as related to the body weight determines the concentration of alcohol in the blood. That is, in general, the larger the person, the greater the amount of alcohol that must be consumed for a specific blood alcohol concentration. Blood alcohol concentrations also rise more quickly in women than in men. One of the reasons for this occurrence is that women have proportionately more fat and less water in their bodies than do men. Alcohol is more soluble in water than in fat; therefore, if a woman drinks the same amount as a man, her generally smaller size and lower water content result in a higher concentration of alcohol in watery body tissues such as the blood. Additionally, the stomach enzyme that breaks down alcohol before it reaches the bloodstream is less active in women than it is in men.

Why do certain changes take place in the body when a person consumes alcoholic beverages? The answer has to do with how alcohol affects interactions among nerve cells in the brain. As discussed in Chapter 7, psychoactive drugs (including alcohol) act at communication points among nerve cells. Psychoactive drugs interfere with the normal activity of the chemicals that carry nerve impulses from one nerve cell to another. The manner of this interference varies among drugs.

Alcohol acts on parts of the brain that are responsible for drives and emotions, as well as the part of the brain that coordinates skeletal muscle movements. It also affects the "thinking" part and reward centers in the brain.

Many people drink alcohol to "get drunk," but other factors often contribute to excessive alcohol consumption. Anxious people, for example, may use alcohol to relieve their anxieties. Researchers think that persons with a family history of alcoholism are more likely to be motivated to drink alcohol to get "high," while persons with no family history of alcoholism are more likely to be motivated by anxiety.

At high doses, alcohol also has effects that are aversive; that is, they are sufficiently unpleasant (such as nausea and vomiting) that people often lose their desire to drink. Severe aversive effects, such as unconsciousness, result in a person's inability to continue drinking. Therefore, aversive effects help curb excessive alcohol consumption.

Chronic drug users develop **tolerance** to the drug; that is, increased amounts of alcohol are required

**intoxication** Impairment of the functioning of the central nervous system as a result of ingesting toxic substances such as alcohol.

**tolerance** A physiologic response in chronic users of drugs in which increased amounts of the drug are required to achieve effects previously produced by lower amounts.

to achieve effects previously produced by lower amounts. Tolerance develops because the chronic use of the drug stimulates liver enzymes to break down the drug with increasing swiftness. Also, brain cells become less responsive to the drug over time. Tolerance develops for both the pleasant and unpleasant effects of alcohol consumption, so chronic drinkers do not experience the aversive effects as quickly as do occasional drinkers. Therefore, their alcohol consumption is not curbed as quickly.

**Psychological, Social, and Developmental Factors** People drink for reasons other than to experience the "brain effects" of feeling good or reducing anxiety. Similarly, people curb their drinking or abstain from drinking for reasons other than aversive brain effects that may stimulate nausea and vomiting. Many of these reasons are *psychological*, having to do with thoughts, feelings, attitudes, and expectations about alcohol. Some of the reasons are *social*, relating to interactions with friends, relatives, and coworkers. Still other reasons are *developmental*, relating to the psychological, social, and biological changes in individuals over time and as they mature.

## Table 8.3

### Effects of Various Levels of Alcohol Consumption on Inexperienced Drinkers

| Number of Standard Drinks | Blood Alcohol Concentration (BAC)* | Effects |
|---|---|---|
| 1–2 | 0.02 to 0.06% | Euphoria; reduction in anxiety |
| 3–5 | 0.08 to 0.15% | Impairment of judgment, motor coordination, and emotional control; involuntary rapid eye movements; double vision; speech disorders; may be accompanied by aggressive behavior as alcohol level rises |
| 7–8 | 0.20 to 0.25% | Sedation; impairment of ability to learn and remember information |
| 12–18 | 0.40 to 0.50% | Loss of adequate respiration; dangerously low blood pressure; dangerously low internal body temperature; coma or death may result |

*Blood alcohol concentration is expressed in percentages: A BAC of 0.05% means an alcohol concentration of 5 milliliters (ml) for every 10,000 ml of blood.

People often consume alcoholic beverages because they expect positive psychological effects from their drinking, such as enhancing social interactions, feeling pleasurable effects, or producing sedation. People develop their expectations concerning alcohol from experience, observation, and what they are told. In fact, a person's beliefs about alcohol can be predictive of their future drinking habits: Heavy drinkers tend to view the positive effects of alcohol as arousing, while light drinkers tend to view the positive effects as sedating.

Individuals often consume alcohol to ease their social interactions or because it's the thing to do in a particular social setting. With adolescents and young adults, peers may pressure one another to drink alcohol. The section titled "Alcohol and College Students," which follows, explores the role of peer pressure in the drinking patterns of college students. Cultural factors are additional important social reasons for drinking alcohol. In many cultures, people consume alcohol with meals or as a part of other traditional social activities.

Abusive and alcohol-dependent drinking patterns often begin in adolescence. A wide variety of factors affects children as they mature and influences the development of patterns of drinking alcoholic beverages. The biggest early risk factor for alcohol abuse and dependence is having a parent who is an alcoholic or who abuses alcohol. Children of alcoholics are 4 to 10 times more likely to become alcoholics than are children of nonalcoholics. Additionally, a child reared in an alcoholic family has a greater risk of developing alcoholism than a child who is not reared in such an environment.[7]

Another way in which parents influence their children is by their parenting practices. Teenagers who report receiving high levels of nurturing and support from their parents also report fewer alcohol-related problems than teenagers who report little parental nurturing and support. Teenagers who report feeling close to their parents drink alcoholic beverages less frequently than teenagers who report that they do not feel close to their parents. Children are more likely to use alcohol if their parents are not involved in their activities, there is a lack of, or inconsistent, discipline, and the parents have low educational aspirations for the children. Positive family relationships, involvement, and attachment appear to discourage youths' initiation into alcohol use.

Psychological, social, and developmental factors all interact with genetic factors to result in a certain kind of behavior. These interactions explain why not all alcoholics have a family history of alcoholism, and why not all persons with a family history of alcoholism become alcoholics. These dynamic interactions occur throughout life, with varying contributions from genes and environment at different times.

## Alcohol and College Students

Alcohol abuse is a serious problem that often appears to begin or accelerate during the college years. In fact, the most abused drug among college students is alcohol. Most studies of alcohol use by college students examine psychological and social issues; those issues are discussed here. However, there are also economic, political, and ecological factors of college alcohol use, such as the alcohol environment on college campuses and their surrounding communities.

Studies show that college students drink alcohol for a variety of reasons. **Table 8.4** lists the primary reasons that students give to explain why they drink. However, there are differences between moderate and heavy drinkers with regard to their reasons for drinking.

Moderate drinkers who do not abuse alcohol do not cite many reasons for their drinking. They drink to feel more comfortable in social situations or to relieve stress. They do not drink with any goal in mind such as getting drunk.

Heavy drinkers who abuse alcohol, however, often state many reasons for their drinking, including the reasons listed in Table 8.4, but their drinking tends to be escapist and goal-oriented. They often drink to get drunk. Results of studies show that college students who drink heavily believe that drinking is part of the college experience and that it is something they are entitled to do as undergraduates. College men are more likely to think this way than women. In addition, college students who are heavy drinkers tend to have been drinkers in high school and have friends who drink.[8]

Additional student characteristics correlate with alcohol abuse as well. Although any student may abuse alcohol, abusers are more likely to be younger students with low self-esteem, high levels of anxiety, a mildly assertive personality, and at least one alcoholic parent. The freshman and sophomore years are the most likely times for students to exhibit alcohol abuse. Additionally, students who are fraternity/sorority members and who are athletes are more likely than nonfraternity/sorority members or nonathletes to abuse alcohol.[8,9]

## Table 8.4

### College Students: Major Reasons for Drinking

| Reason | Category |
| --- | --- |
| It makes them feel good | Enhancement |
| They want to get drunk | Enhancement |
| It helps them feel more comfortable in social situations | Social |
| It helps them relax | Coping |
| It puts them in a better mood | Coping |
| It helps relieve tension and stress | Coping |
| It helps them feel more accepted by their peers | Conformity |

*Sources:* Patrick, M. E., et al. (2011). Drinking motives, protective behavioral strategies, and experienced consequences: Identifying students at risk. *Addictive Behaviors, 36*:270–273; LaBrie, J. W., et al. (2007). Reasons for drinking in the college student context: The differential role and risk of the social motivator. *Journal of Studies on Alcohol and Drugs, 68*:393–398; Ham, L. S., & Hope, D. A. (2003). College students and problematic drinking: A review of the literature. *Clinical Psychology Review, 23*:719–759.

Drinking alcohol during the college years poses many risks for students, including driving after drinking, getting behind in schoolwork, and getting into trouble with campus or local police. In fact, many students who abstain from alcohol do so because they want to avoid such risks. Alcohol can also be a vehicle for date-rape drugs. The Managing Your Health box "Drinking and Date-Rape Drugs: Safety Tips for Women" provides guidelines to help women avoid ingesting these dangerous substances in alcoholic beverages. **Table 8.5** lists the primary reasons some students abstain from drinking alcohol.

**Binge Drinking and Drinking Games** College men who belong to fraternities, especially those who live in fraternity houses, make up a large proportion of students who drink heavily. Drinking in fraternities, as in other campus social groups including many sororities, is perceived as promoting a feeling of unity and cohesiveness among their members. A Harvard School of Public Health survey found that about 75% of college students who lived in fraternities and sororities binge drank versus about 55% of students who lived in off-campus housing alone or with a roommate, 45% who lived in residence halls, 30% who lived off-campus with parents, and 27% who lived off-campus with a spouse.[10]

**Table 8.6** shows binge drinking prevalence, frequency, and intensity by sex and age group in 2009. Those aged 18–24 years, including those attending and those not attending college, had the highest

## Table 8.5

### College Students: Major Reasons for Not Drinking

College students report that they abstain from drinking alcohol because of:

- Disapproval/Lack of interest (against religious/moral convictions)

- Risks and negative effects (hangovers/alcoholism/medication interactions)

- Social responsibility (might interfere with job/family/school/relationships)

- Loss of control (negatively affects mood/effects unpleasant)

- Lack of availability (expense/hard to obtain)

- Health concerns (in training/fattening/bad for health)

*Source:* Adapted from Johnson, T. J., & Chen, E. A. (2004). College students' reasons for not drinking and not playing drinking games. *Substance Use & Misuse, 39*:1139–1162.

overall prevalence of binge drinking at 25.6%. That is, one out of every four people in this age group who responded to the binge drinking telephone survey reported at least one binge drinking episode during the preceding month. The table shows that the preva-

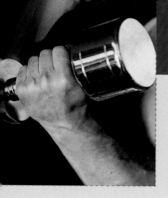

# Managing Your Health

## Drinking and Date-Rape Drugs: Safety Tips for Women

- When you can, drink from tamper-proof bottles or cans and open them yourself.
- If at a bar or club, accept drinks only from the bartender or server. Try to watch your drink being prepared.
- Always keep your drink with you, even in the restroom.
- If you leave your drink or lose sight of it for any reason, discard it and get a fresh drink.
- Don't trust someone to watch your drink. Even a friend can get distracted.

- Don't share or exchange drinks.
- Don't take a drink from a punch bowl or container that is passed around.
- Don't drink anything that has an unusual taste or appearance, although a date-rape drug dissolved in alcohol may not change the taste of your drink.
- If your drink changes color, suddenly becomes "fizzy," or appears to have something floating in it, discard it. Someone likely tried to drug you.
- Don't mix drugs with alcohol.
- Limit your drinking to one to two drinks to remain aware and able to follow safety procedures.
- If you feel ill or lightheaded while drinking away from home, tell a friend, call a cab, and return home. If you feel extremely ill, go to an emergency room.

## Table 8.6

### Binge Drinking Prevalence, Frequency, and Intensity, by Sex and Age Group—United States, 2009*

| Sex/Age Group | Prevalence | | Frequency[†] | | Intensity[§] | |
|---|---|---|---|---|---|---|
| | No. | % | No. | No. of Episodes | No. | No. of Drinks |
| **Sex** | | | | | | |
| Men | 154,834 | 20.8 | 25,212 | 4.6 | 23,409 | 8.5 |
| Women | 254,011 | 10.0 | 18,703 | 3.1 | 17,687 | 5.7 |
| **Age group (yrs)** | | | | | | |
| 18–24 | 12,312 | 25.6 | 2,950 | 4.1 | 2,713 | 9.1 |
| 25–34 | 35,441 | 22.5 | 7,415 | 3.9 | 6,983 | 8.0 |
| 35–44 | 57,057 | 17.8 | 9,891 | 3.9 | 9,375 | 7.3 |
| 45–64 | 173,869 | 12.1 | 19,464 | 4.2 | 18,233 | 6.5 |
| ≥65 | 130,166 | 3.8 | 4,195 | 5.4 | 3,792 | 5.5 |
| Total | 408,845 | 15.2 | 43,915 | 4.1 | 41,096 | 7.5 |

\* Respondents were from all 50 states and the District of Columbia.

[†] Average number of binge drinking episodes during the preceding 30 days.

[§] Average largest number of drinks consumed by binge drinkers on any occasion during the preceding 30 days.

Source: Kanny D., et al. (January 14, 2011). Binge drinking—United States, 2009. *Morbidity and Mortality Weekly Report*, 60:101–104.

lence of binge drinking decreases as age increases. Although those aged 18–24 years did not have the highest number of binge drinking episodes during the preceding month (frequency), they did have the highest average number of drinks consumed by binge drinkers on any occasion during the preceding month (intensity).

Binge drinking is often accompanied by drinking games. There is a high prevalence of drinking games on college campuses, with approximately two-thirds of college students engaging in these activities.[11] **Table 8.7** lists specific motives for playing drinking games. Compare this table with Table 8.4 and you will see some similarities. Although some motives for playing drinking games seem specific to the games (e.g., competition), current research has not conclusively established that the motives for playing drinking games are separate from the general motives for drinking.

In drinking games, participants follow rules that specify when and how much they must drink and that mandate certain verbal, physical, or memory skills. When players make mistakes or are cued by game rules, they are required to drink. The more game players drink, the more they make mistakes, and the amount of alcohol they consume increases. The danger of unconsciousness, coma, and death increases as alcohol consumption increases.

---

### Table 8.7

### College Students: Major Reasons for Playing Drinking Games

- Competition and thrills
- Conformity (to fit in)
- Novelty (to try something different)
- Fun and celebration
- Social lubrication
- Sexual manipulation (in order to have sex with someone or get a date)
- Boredom
- Coping (to forget about problems)

*Source:* Adapted from Johnson, T. J., & Sheets, V. L. (2004). Measuring college students' motives for playing drinking games. *Psychology of Addictive Behaviors, 18*(2):91–99.

---

What can you do to help an intoxicated person avoid serious medical consequences or death? A person who has slurred speech, a staggering walk, double vision, and is not alert (but is able to be aroused by voice) should be stopped from drinking and taken away from the source of the alcohol. A person with signs of more severe intoxication, such as not making sense, urinating on himself or herself, breathing irregularly, vomiting repeatedly, and not being able to be aroused with a strong stimulus like a slap, should be taken to an emergency room immediately.

**Alcohol-Related Injury Deaths in College Students** One sobering statistic is that more than 5,000 alcohol-related deaths occur each year among those aged 18 to 24 years (including college and noncollege individuals), which is more than the number of U.S. soldiers killed in the Iraq war. Ralph Hingson and colleagues of the National Institute on Alcohol Abuse and Alcoholism made this comparison. The researchers also determined that among college students aged 18 to 24 years, approximately 1,600 are killed each year as a result of alcohol-related injuries. About three-fourths of these deaths are from alcohol-related car crashes and one-fourth from other alcohol-related causes, such as drownings, falls, gunshots, and alcohol/drug poisonings.[12]

## How the Body Processes Alcohol

When an alcoholic beverage is consumed, the alcohol in the drink is absorbed into the bloodstream from the stomach and intestinal tract. The blood transports alcohol to the "detoxification center" of the body—the liver. The liver breaks down harmful substances such as drugs, changing them into compounds that are safer or easier to excrete.

The liver can break down only a certain amount of alcohol per hour, no matter how much has been consumed. That rate depends, in part, on the concentration of enzymes that break down alcohol in the liver, and this concentration varies among individuals. Nevertheless, alcohol is absorbed into the bloodstream more quickly than it can be broken down by the liver, and the excess alcohol stays in the blood. Therefore, the intake of alcohol needs to be controlled to prevent its accumulation in the blood, resulting in an increase in the blood alcohol level.

The stomach also breaks down some alcohol. Eating food while drinking alcoholic beverages results

The following news release appeared on the website of the National Institute on Alcohol Abuse and Alcoholism. It was posted on November 12, 2010. Read the news release and explain why you think it is a reliable or an unreliable source of information. Use the model for analyzing health information to guide your thinking; the main points of the model are noted here. A full explanation of the model can be found in Chapter 1.

1. Which statements are verifiable facts, and which are unverified statements or value claims?
2. What are the credentials of the person (in this case press office) who makes health-related claims? Does this press office have the appropriate background and education in the topic area? What can you do to check the credentials of this press office?
3. What might be the motives and biases of the press office making the claims?
4. What is the main point of the article? Which information is relevant to the issue, main point, product, or service? Which information is irrelevant?
5. Is the source reliable? What evidence supports your conclusion that the source is reliable or unreliable? Does the source of information present the pros and cons of the topic or the benefits and risks of the product?
6. Does the source of information attack the credibility of conventional scientists or medical authorities?

Based on your analysis, do you think that this article is a reliable source of health-related information? Summarize your reasons for coming to this conclusion.

## NIH-Supported Study Finds Strategies to Reduce College Drinking

by NIAAA Press Office

Highly visible cooperative projects, in which colleges and their surrounding communities target off-campus drinking settings, can reduce harmful alcohol use among college students, according to a report by researchers supported by the National Institute on Alcohol Abuse and Alcoholism (NIAAA), part of the National Institutes of Health.

"This innovative, important study is a valuable contribution to the search for solutions to the alcohol problems that beset colleges and universities throughout the country," says NIAAA Acting Director Kenneth R. Warren, PhD.

As reported online in the *American Journal of Preventive Medicine*, researchers led by Robert Saltz, PhD, conducted the Safer California Universities study of college and community alcohol prevention strategies at 14 large public universities in California.

"Other investigators have noted the need for studies of multi-strategy cooperative prevention approaches to reduce harmful college drinking," notes Dr. Saltz, a senior research scientist at the Prevention Research Center in Berkeley, Calif. "Our study addresses that need." Beginning in 2003, Dr. Saltz and his colleagues conducted random surveys of students from each of the participating schools. The survey documented that heavy drinking at off-campus parties was a common problem. Policy and enforcement interventions were implemented in 2005 and 2006 at half of the universities, with the other half also monitored for comparison. Interventions included nuisance party enforcement operations, surveillance to prevent alcohol sales to minors, drunken driving checkpoints, social host ordinances, and use of campus and local media to increase the visibility of the interventions.

To assess the effectiveness of the interventions, the researchers measured the proportion of drinking occasions in which students got drunk in various settings. They found significantly greater reductions in the incidence and likelihood of intoxication at off-campus parties and at bars and restaurants for students at the intervention universities. Students at intervention universities also reported a lower likelihood of drinking to intoxication the last time they attended an off-campus party, a bar or restaurant, or other drinking settings. The greatest reductions were found at universities with the highest intensity of intervention implementation, achieved through heavy publicity and highly visible enforcement activities.

"Nearly as significant was that we saw no concurrent increase in drinking at non-targeted settings such as parks, beaches, or residence halls," Dr. Saltz says. "Some fear that more rigorous alcohol control measures will merely drive college student drinking to other, presumably more dangerous, settings, but that was not the case here."

"These findings should give college administrators and surrounding communities some degree of optimism that student drinking is amenable to a combination of well-chosen, evidence-based universal prevention strategies," says Dr. Saltz. "Here, one set of alcohol control strategies was found to be effective, but other combinations may work as well, or even better."

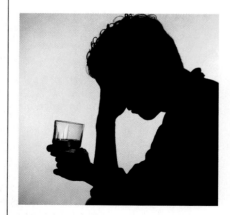

*Source:* Retrieved April 1, 2011, from http://www.nih.gov/news/health/nov2010/niaaa-12.htm.

in the alcohol being held in the stomach for a longer time with the food. Therefore, more of it gets broken down in the stomach, and less alcohol enters the bloodstream. A person who drinks while eating will have a slower rise in the blood alcohol level than will a person who drinks on an empty stomach. Conversely, aspirin and cimetidine (an ulcer drug) inhibit the breakdown of alcohol in the stomach. A person who takes either of these drugs along with alcohol will have a quicker rise in the blood alcohol level than will a person who does not take these drugs when drinking alcohol.

# Consequences of Alcohol Abuse and Dependence

**Diseases and Conditions** The harmful use and abuse of alcohol result in multiple effects on the body that are serious threats to health. Alcohol consumption does not affect all individuals in the same way; various effects result from differences among abusers' genetic makeup, general health, and drinking patterns. Despite these differences, however, excessive alcohol consumption exerts its most serious effects on the liver, cardiovascular system, immune system, reproductive system, and brain. It also affects how vitamins are used by the body and can result in vitamin deficiencies. In pregnant women, it has devastating effects on the fetus.

*Diseases of the Liver*  Because the liver is the major detoxification site for alcohol, it is particularly prone to harm by chronic alcohol consumption. Years of drinking can result in three types of liver disease: fatty liver, alcoholic hepatitis, and cirrhosis of the liver. The symptoms of each may overlap, and a person can have more than one of these conditions simultaneously. Women tend to develop these conditions at lower levels of alcohol intake than men do (see "Factors Related to Alcohol Abuse and Dependence" in this chapter).

Nearly 90% of heavy drinkers develop a *fatty liver* because alcohol stimulates the buildup of fat in liver cells. This process begins immediately upon drinking: Fat accumulation has been found in the livers of young men after only one night of heavy drinking. Most liver cells are not specialized for fat storage, and their ability to perform their normal functions declines when they store fat. These liver cells eventually die; the scar tissue that remains produces cirrhosis.

Approximately 15% to 30% of alcoholics develop liver cirrhosis (**Figure 8.2**). This disease develops as alcohol begins to kill liver cells. Liver cells have the

**Figure 8.2**

**A Healthy and an Unhealthy Liver (with Cirrhosis).** (a) Healthy liver tissue is smooth and dark red/brown. (b) The liver with cirrhosis develops scar tissue and nodules (bumps) as it works to repair damage.

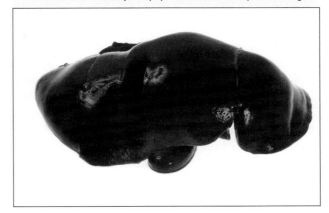

(a)

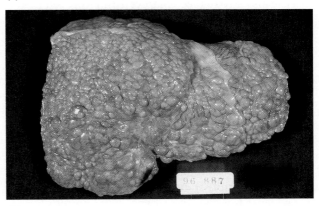

(b)

ability to regenerate, much like skin heals from a small cut. However, if cell damage is extensive, the liver cannot produce new cells quickly enough to replace destroyed ones. Connective tissue cells fill the spaces left by the dead cells, similar to the way scar tissue may fill the gap of tissue caused by a severe cut. However, connective tissue is not functional liver tissue, and the liver's ability to perform its many important functions declines. Eventually the person must have a liver transplant or he or she will die.

Approximately 40% of chronic abusers develop *alcoholic hepatitis*. Hepatitis is an inflammation of the liver, which can be caused by hepatitis viruses or by toxic chemicals such as alcohol. A severe case of hepatitis can result in death.

The majority of individuals who develop cirrhosis of the liver have been drinking heavily for 10 to 20 years. Women, however, are more at risk than men for liver disease. Because women detoxify alcohol less efficiently than men do, the concentration of alcohol in their blood rises more quickly than in men when both consume the same number of drinks. Therefore, serious forms of alcoholic liver disease occur more frequently in women than in men. Additionally, women are more likely than men to develop these conditions at lower levels of alcohol consumption and after shorter periods of alcohol dependence. Hereditary factors and body weight, as well as sex, appear to play a role in susceptibility to liver disease. Obese alcoholics have a higher risk of having alcoholic liver disease than nonobese alcoholics, and heavy alcohol consumption increases the severity of liver disease associated with obesity.[13]

**Cardiovascular Disease and Cancer** There is considerable evidence that limiting alcohol consumption to 1 oz or less of ethanol per day (two drinks or less) decreases the risk of death from coronary artery disease and stroke (see Chapter 12). However, heavier drinking is associated with cardiovascular diseases such as cardiomyopathy (heart muscle disease), hypertension (high blood pressure), arrhythmias (disturbances in heart rhythm), and stroke.[14]

Alcohol abuse is a risk factor for certain cancers. The heavy consumption of alcohol can cause cancers of the esophagus and liver. It is also associated with the development of stomach cancer and increases the likelihood of larynx and mouth cancer. People who smoke cigarettes and drink alcohol, even in moderate amounts, multiply their risk of cancer of the esophagus because together these drugs have a multiplier effect. That is, when people take both drugs routinely, their risk of cancer is much higher than if the risk of each was added.[15]

Even when not abused, alcohol can raise the risk of cancer. Consuming three-quarters to one drink per day raises a woman's risk of developing breast cancer by 9%. The risk increases as consumption increases. Consuming two to three drinks per day raises breast cancer risk by 43%. Additionally, data suggest that women who drink alcohol while taking estrogen in postmenopausal estrogen replacement therapy may increase their breast cancer risk more than if they used either one alone.[16,17]

**Immune System Suppression** The immune system (see Chapter 14), which protects the body from invasion by pathogens, also suffers as a result of chronic alcohol abuse. This behavior impairs the functioning of the immune system, predisposing the drinker to infectious diseases such as colds, pneumonia, and tuberculosis. Chronic alcohol abuse even suppresses the activity of certain immune system cells that defend the body against the spread of cancer.

*Detrimental Effects on the Reproductive System* Alcohol affects the reproductive systems of both men and women. It affects the functioning of the testes, decreasing the amount of the sex hormone, testosterone, these organs produce. Alcoholic men often experience shrinking of the testicles, impotence, and loss of libido, or sex drive. In women, alcohol affects the functioning of the ovaries. The menstrual periods of alcoholic women are often irregular or cease altogether. As a result, alcoholic women often have difficulty becoming pregnant. Alcoholic women also have a higher rate of early menopause than nonalcoholic women. During pregnancy, alcohol consumption can have devastating effects on the fetus. This topic is discussed in the Across the Life Span section of this chapter.

*Detrimental Effects on the Brain* Alcohol consumption has multiple effects on the brain. Chronic alcoholics may experience brain disorders. One of the most serious is the Wernicke-Korsakoff syndrome. This syndrome includes mental confusion, abnormal eye movements, and an inability to coordinate skeletal muscles, which results in abnormal posture and a staggering walk. Scientists have discovered that this syndrome may be to the result of the alcoholic's inability to use the B vitamin thiamin properly. Some alcoholics are deficient in this vitamin (and many other nutrients) because their diets consist primarily of alcohol rather than food. In either case, if given thiamin, the alcoholic can be cured of the abnormal eye movements, posture, and gait if he or she stops drinking. However, the person is left with anterograde amnesia—the inability to remember new information for more than a few seconds.

Another effect of alcohol on the brain is intoxication, the impairment of the central nervous system (see Table 8.3). *Withdrawal* is also a brain effect of alcohol, but only in alcohol-dependent individuals who stop drinking or reduce their alcohol intake. Withdrawal symptoms usually occur about 24 to 36 hours after an alcoholic stops drinking. Typically, the alcoholic experiences mild agitation, shaking, anxiety, loss of appetite, restlessness, and insomnia. Five percent to 15% of alcoholics experience grand mal seizures (convulsions) during withdrawal. Additionally, a small percentage of alcoholics have severe withdrawal symptoms that include hyperactivity, hallucinations, disorientation, and confusion. This severe withdrawal syndrome is called *delirium tremens*, or *DTs*.

Some researchers suggest that a *hangover* is a mild form of withdrawal that can occur in anyone who consumes alcoholic beverages heavily during a session of drinking. The signs of a hangover can include headache, mental slowness, dry mouth, fatigue, diarrhea, anxiety, stomach pains, and tremors. If the "mild withdrawal" explanation is true, it explains why consuming additional alcohol temporarily relieves hangover effects.

In addition to alcohol causing hangovers, other substances in alcoholic beverages may cause hangovers too. Alcoholic beverages contain certain acidic compounds that have toxic effects on the body. These compounds differ among types of alcoholic beverages and affect whether someone will experience a hangover. Another compound called formaldehyde (a preservative of dead animals) is produced by the body when it cannot keep up with the breakdown of alcohol being consumed. The buildup of formaldehyde contributes to a hangover. Additionally, alcohol causes the body to lose water. This dehydration occurs in brain cells as well as other body cells. Pain accompanies their rehydration.

Whatever the causes of a hangover, home remedies such as taking vitamins, getting in a cold shower, or drinking coffee will not cure the "morning-after" pain of drinking too much. Time alone will cure a hangover.

### Effects on Behavior and Safety

*Serious and Fatal Injuries* Statistics show that alcohol use and abuse are related to serious and even fatal injuries. Alcohol frequently contributes to water-related accidents, motor vehicle accidents, general aviation crashes, domestic and nondomestic violence including sexual assault and rape, suicides, and homicides.

Data show that 32% of all fatal motor vehicle crashes in 2009 were alcohol-related.[18] Other types of injury fatalities are also more likely for current drinkers as compared to abstainers and prior drinkers, including unintentional falls, fires, drownings, and poisonings. Current drinkers are also more likely to commit suicide or to be intentionally killed by another person.

*Automobile Accidents* Drinking and driving are potentially deadly because alcohol impairs the perceptual, intellectual, and motor skills needed to operate motor vehicles safely. Traffic accidents are the leading cause of death among people aged 5 to 24 years, the second leading cause of death after other unintentional injuries in children aged 1 to 4 years, and the fifth leading cause of death after cancer, heart

disease, other unintentional injuries, and suicide in adults aged 25 to 44 years.[19] In all states, the District of Columbia, and Puerto Rico, the legal blood alcohol concentration (BAC) limit for operating an automobile is 0.08%. It is a criminal offense to operate a motor vehicle at or above that limit. All states have a lower unlawful BAC threshold for youth younger than 21 years, and in some cases, younger than 18 years. **Figure 8.3** shows approximate BAC by body weight and the time from the first drink. Note the number of drinks a person can have over a period of time before he or she is considered legally drunk. Also realize that some impairment occurs after a person consumes only one drink.

Alcohol-related fatal automobile accidents occur more frequently at certain times of the day and during certain days of the week than others. For example, in 2009 on weekend nights, 52% of drivers and motorcycle riders younger than 21 years and 72% of those 21 years and older who were killed in single-vehicle crashes had a BAC of 0.08% or higher. In contrast, the percentage of weekend daytime accident deaths resulting from alcohol impairment was much lower: 21% of those younger than 21 years and 31% of those 21 years and older. In addition, far fewer alcohol-related fatalities occurred during weekdays than on weekends. The National Highway Transportation Safety Administration (NHTSA) notes that a BAC of 0.08 g/dL or higher indicates alcohol-impaired driving.[20]

**Figure 8.4** shows that the percentage of traffic fatalities resulting from alcohol-related crashes peaks between midnight and 3 A.M. A comparatively low percentage of traffic fatalities are alcohol-related between 6 A.M. and 3 P.M., but the percentage rises throughout the late afternoon and evening until the midnight-to-3 A.M. peak. A significant percentage occurs from 3 A.M. to 6 A.M. as well. The statistics in the previous paragraph, together with these, show that a person driving at night and in the early morning hours, especially on weekends, is more likely to be involved in a fatal alcohol-related motor vehicle accident than when driving during the day and during the week. Using the subway system in safe areas, walking in safe areas away from the street, or staying at home during these peak alcohol-related traffic fatality times are strategies to consider to help lower your risk of being involved in an alcohol-related car crash.

Alcohol-impaired driving fatalities dropped from 48% of total traffic fatalities in 1982 to 32% in 2009. The drivers with the highest percentage of intoxi-

## Figure 8.3

**Blood Alcohol Concentration (BAC) by Weight and Gender.** These graphs show the approximate BACs of men and women in various weight ranges. All states have set 0.08% as the legal BAC limit while driving for those 21 years and older. All states have lower thresholds for those younger than 21 years of age. However, you may be convicted of driving under the influence (DUI) of alcohol if evidence exists that your driving is impaired. Commercial drivers may be convicted of a DUI at a BAC of 0.04%.

*Source:* "Female Alcohol Impairment Chart" and "Male Alcohol Impairment Chart" from "Blood Alcohol Concentration by Weight and Gender" formulation and computation by the Pennsylvania Liquor Control Board, Bureau of Alcohol Education. Used by permission.

Alcohol Impairment Chart: Female

| Approximate Blood Alcohol Percentage | | | | | | | | | |
|---|---|---|---|---|---|---|---|---|---|
| Drinks | Body Weight in Pounds | | | | | | | | |
| | 90 | 100 | 120 | 140 | 160 | 180 | 200 | 220 | 240 | |
| 0 | .00 | .00 | .00 | .00 | .00 | .00 | .00 | .00 | .00 | Only safe driving limit |
| 1 | .05 | .05 | .04 | .03 | .03 | .03 | .02 | .02 | .02 | Impairment begins |
| 2 | .10 | .09 | .08 | .07 | .06 | .05 | .05 | .04 | .04 | Driving skills affected |
| 3 | .15 | .14 | .11 | .10 | .09 | .08 | .07 | .06 | .06 | Possible criminal penalties |
| 4 | .20 | .18 | .15 | .13 | .11 | .10 | .09 | .08 | .08 | |
| 5 | .25 | .23 | .19 | .16 | .14 | .13 | .11 | .10 | .09 | |
| 6 | .30 | .27 | .23 | .19 | .17 | .15 | .14 | .12 | .11 | Legally intoxicated |
| 7 | .35 | .32 | .27 | .23 | .20 | .18 | .16 | .14 | .13 | Criminal penalties |
| 8 | .40 | .36 | .30 | .26 | .23 | .20 | .18 | .17 | .15 | |
| 9 | .45 | .41 | .34 | .29 | .26 | .23 | .20 | .19 | .17 | |
| 10 | .51 | .45 | .38 | .32 | .28 | .25 | .23 | .21 | .19 | |

Your body can get rid of one drink per hour
Each 1 1/2 oz. of 80 proof liquor, 12 oz. of beer or 5 oz. of table wine = 1 drink.

Alcohol Impairment Chart: Male

| Approximate Blood Alcohol Percentage | | | | | | | | |
|---|---|---|---|---|---|---|---|---|
| Drinks | Body Weight in Pounds | | | | | | | |
| | 100 | 120 | 140 | 160 | 180 | 200 | 220 | 240 | |
| 0 | .00 | .00 | .00 | .00 | .00 | .00 | .00 | .00 | Only safe driving limit |
| 1 | .04 | .03 | .03 | .02 | .02 | .02 | .02 | .02 | Impairment begins |
| 2 | .08 | .06 | .05 | .05 | .04 | .04 | .03 | .03 | |
| 3 | .11 | .09 | .08 | .07 | .06 | .06 | .05 | .05 | Driving skills affected |
| 4 | .15 | .12 | .11 | .09 | .08 | .08 | .07 | .06 | Possible criminal penalties |
| 5 | .19 | .16 | .13 | .12 | .11 | .09 | .09 | .08 | |
| 6 | .23 | .19 | .16 | .14 | .13 | .11 | .10 | .09 | |
| 7 | .26 | .22 | .19 | .16 | .15 | .13 | .12 | .11 | Legally intoxicated |
| 8 | .30 | .25 | .21 | .19 | .17 | .15 | .14 | .13 | Criminal penalties |
| 9 | .34 | .28 | .24 | .21 | .19 | .17 | .15 | .14 | |
| 10 | .38 | .31 | .27 | .23 | .21 | .19 | .17 | .16 | |

Your body can get rid of one drink per hour
Each 1 1/2 oz. of 80 proof liquor, 12 oz. of beer or 5 oz. of table wine = 1 drink.

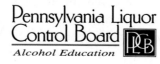

Pennsylvania Liquor
Control Board
*Alcohol Education*

cation in fatal crashes (0.08% BAC or higher) were young adults aged 21 to 24 years (35% of this group), followed closely by those aged 25 to 34 years (32%) and 35 to 44 years (26%).[20]

For safety, women who drink and drive must remember that their BACs rise more quickly than the BACs of males who consume the same number of drinks. Both sexes must also remember that the risk of fatal crashes rises rapidly with increasing BAC. As **Figure 8.5** shows, compared to persons with no alcohol in their blood, drivers with BACs between 0.050% and 0.079% have a 5-fold increased risk of having a fatal car crash, while males aged 16–20 years have a 10-fold increased risk at this same BAC level. Male and female drivers aged 21–34 years with BAC levels between 0.80% and 0.99% (legally drunk) have a 13-fold increased risk, and those aged 35 years and older have a 6-fold risk. However, while driving at this BAC level, young men aged 16–20 years have a 24-fold risk of being killed in a car crash, and that increases to an 83-fold risk at a BAC level of 0.100% to 0.149%. At the same BAC level, others have about an 11- to 13-fold increased risk of killing themselves in a car crash. Not shown in Figure 8.5 is the fact that young men aged 16–20 years have more than a 2,000-fold increase of being killed while driving with a BAC level of 0.150% and over. Others have an 84- to 88-fold increased risk.

*Airplane Accidents* Alcohol also impairs the ability of pilots to fly aircraft. Alcohol has not been directly implicated in U.S. commercial airline crashes; however, it appears to play a more prominent role in general aviation crashes. Alcohol has been shown to impair flight performance in pilots when they drink and up to 8 hours after drinking.[21] Chaturvedi and colleagues from the Federal Aviation Administration Aerospace Medical Institute found that 101 pilots (6%) out of the 1,587 pilots killed in the aviation accidents they studied had alcohol in their blood at the time of the crash.[22]

*Water-Related Accidents* Alcohol is also a significant factor in water-related accidents. Researchers estimate that alcohol consumption is associated with between 30% and 70% of adult drownings.[23] The highest percentages are associated with males older than 25 years. Most alcohol-related drownings are associated with motor vehicle accidents, but alcohol is also present in the blood of more than half the drowning victims who were swimming, boating, or rafting when they died. Alcohol also contributes to diving accidents that leave victims with serious spinal cord injuries.

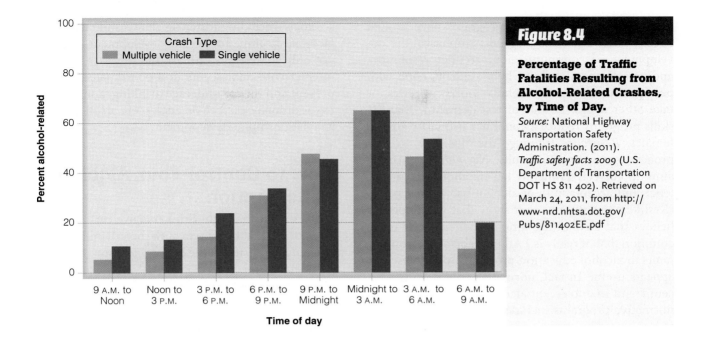

**Figure 8.4**

**Percentage of Traffic Fatalities Resulting from Alcohol-Related Crashes, by Time of Day.**
*Source:* National Highway Transportation Safety Administration. (2011).
*Traffic safety facts 2009* (U.S. Department of Transportation DOT HS 811 402). Retrieved on March 24, 2011, from http://www-nrd.nhtsa.dot.gov/Pubs/811402EE.pdf

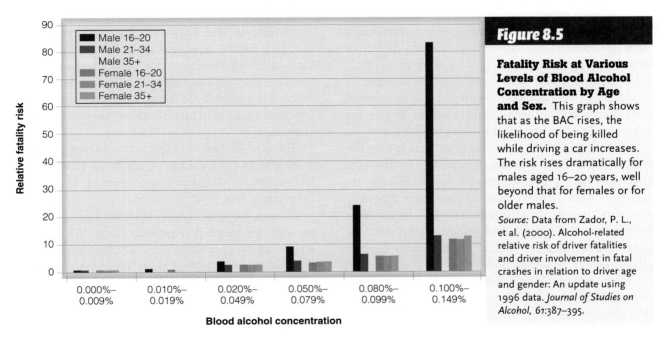

**Figure 8.5**

**Fatality Risk at Various Levels of Blood Alcohol Concentration by Age and Sex.** This graph shows that as the BAC rises, the likelihood of being killed while driving a car increases. The risk rises dramatically for males aged 16–20 years, well beyond that for females or for older males.
*Source:* Data from Zador, P. L., et al. (2000). Alcohol-related relative risk of driver fatalities and driver involvement in fatal crashes in relation to driver age and gender: An update using 1996 data. *Journal of Studies on Alcohol,* 61:387–395.

# Prevention

Because many people begin drinking alcoholic beverages during adolescence, prevention programs often target younger children to educate them about alcohol before they reach their teenage years. Prevention efforts include school-based programs for children in grades 5 through 10, but most target fifth and sixth graders. Because this time is developmentally critical as students move from elementary school to middle school or junior high, those who have experimented with alcohol may begin to misuse it at this time.

There is a variety of school-based programs. *Affective education* seeks to influence students' feelings about themselves and alcohol by helping them develop self-esteem as well as problem-solving and decision-making abilities. In addition, these programs promote an understanding of how alcohol use can interfere with personal values and goals. Results of research show that such programs have limited effectiveness. *Life skills programs* emphasize the development of communication, conflict resolution, and assertiveness skills to help students cope with peer pressure to drink alcohol, smoke cigarettes, or take other drugs. Results of research show that life skills programs reduce alcohol use primarily among females. *Resistance training*—the "Just say no" approach—shows mixed results. *Normative education* aims to correct erroneous beliefs about the prevalence and acceptability of alcohol use among peers. (Results of survey research show that young people believe that alcohol use among their peers is more common than it really is.) Adding normative components to alcohol education programs for adolescents appears useful. In fact, normative education is a recent trend in adolescent alcohol education. Current normative programs include teaching students how to resist peer influence and often incorporate activities and events outside of the classroom.

Prevention efforts that focus on the entire population of drinkers are called *environmental approaches*. Such approaches are important because 51.9% of Americans aged 12 years or older were current alcohol users in 2009,[4] and many drinkers experience moderate to severe alcohol-induced impairment at least occasionally. These drinkers are all at risk for alcohol-related injuries and health problems.

Beginning in 1989, one prevention strategy for the general population was the requirement by the U.S. government to place warnings on alcoholic beverage containers. However, survey data show that only about one-fourth of adults realize that the labels exist. Researchers have not found evidence that warning labels reduce alcohol consumption and its health-related effects. Another prevention strategy was the establishment of 21 as the minimum age for purchase and consumption of alcohol. Evidence shows that this strategy significantly reduced youth drinking and related problems such as alcohol-related traffic accidents in those younger than age 21 years.[24]

In 2007, in response to the finding that alcohol was the number one abused substance by America's youth, the acting Surgeon General of the United States, Kenneth P. Moritsugu, issued *The Surgeon General's Call to Action to Prevent and Reduce Underage Drinking*.[25] This report notes that parents of adolescents do not recognize how widespread alcohol use is in this population and how the brains of adolescents are particularly susceptible to the negative effects of alcohol use. Noting that alcohol use by America's youth is influenced by many factors, the report develops six goals, including fostering changes in society that facilitate healthy adolescent development, engaging not only adolescents but also the social systems that interact with adolescents in a coordinated effort to prevent and reduce underage drinking, and conducting additional research on adolescent alcohol use and its relationship to development.

## How to Control Your Alcohol Consumption

Studies show that light drinkers have certain behavior patterns that help them curb their drinking. These attributes are listed in the Managing Your Health box "Guidelines for Safer Drinking" and are effective rules for controlling alcohol consumption.

## Diagnosis and Treatment of Alcoholism and Alcohol Abuse

According to the 2009 National Survey on Drug Use and Health, approximately 1.5 million Americans received treatment for alcohol abuse during the year prior to the survey.[4] Various types of treatments are available for those who need help. Screening techniques help identify those persons who need treatment.

The CAGE screening test is considered one of the most effective screening devices for alcohol abuse or alcoholism. A variety of other screening instruments is available also.

Healthcare professionals who determine that their patients are alcohol dependent refer them to substance abuse specialists for evaluation and possible treatment. Patients that show nondependent problem drinking are often encouraged to participate in brief intervention programs.

In the past, physicians and substance abuse practitioners thought that an alcoholic could not be helped until he or she "hit bottom" and then asked for help. A person who did not ask for help was considered to be denying his or her alcoholism and lacking motivation to change. Current thinking regards motivation as a process of behavioral change rather than a trait that people have or do not have.

Before treatment, the role of clinical intervention is to help the patient understand the serious dangers inherent in his or her abusive or dependent drinking behavior. Once the alcoholic realizes the need to change his or her behavior, he or she tries to decide what course of action to take. The clinician helps the

# Managing Your Health

## Guidelines for Safer Drinking

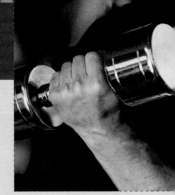

1. If you choose to drink, plan ways to drink that promote safety behind the wheel and safety for health. Considering some of the following points should help.
2. Eat before you drink and while you are drinking.
3. Drink alcoholic beverages slowly. Consider watering down your drinks or alternating alcoholic drinks with nonalcoholic drinks.
4. For safety behind the wheel, set a limit on the amount of alcohol you can drink per hour. Use the chart in Figure 8.3 to determine how many drinks you can have per hour and still maintain a BAC of 0.05% or below. If you are a 120-pound woman, for example, you can have only one drink per hour to stay below a BAC of 0.05%. Count drinks to stay within your limit.
5. For health safety, men should consume no more than 2 drinks per day/14 drinks per week, and women should consume no more than 1 drink per day/7 drinks per week.
6. Refuse drinks you do not want and that do not fit within your plan.
7. Cultivate alternatives to drinking to help you relax, such as meditating.
8. Learn to socialize without drinking. For example, use fun venues or fun foods as a social lubricant instead of alcohol.

patient select a course of action or treatment program that best suits his or her needs.

Both inpatient and outpatient programs exist. *Inpatient treatment*, in which the alcoholic resides at a treatment facility, is sometimes used for the early phases of treatment, particularly acute detoxification. During this time, the patient abstains from alcohol and experiences withdrawal symptoms (see "Detrimental Effects on the Brain" in this chapter). Approximately 10% to 13% of patients need medication during this time to help them reduce potentially life-threatening effects of withdrawal. During the detoxification period, patients participate in group therapy and alcohol education sessions for several hours daily. Recovering alcoholics usually live with patients to help them through the process. Such programs usually last 28 days. Near the end of this process the alcoholic's family is usually asked to participate in treatment.

Because of rising medical costs, acute detoxification, as well as further treatment, may take place in outpatient programs. Such programs, developed over the past 25 years, have been extremely successful. Approximately 90% of patients are now treated in outpatient facilities. In these programs, the patient spends a specific amount of time at the treatment facility but lives at home.

After a person has sought treatment for alcohol abuse or dependence, the next stage in behavior change is *maintenance*. For long-term maintenance treatment, recovering alcoholics take part in group meetings and attend individual counseling sessions once or twice a week at outpatient facilities, participate in self-help group meetings, and sometimes participate in family therapy. The maintenance period usually lasts 1 year.

Sometimes *relapse* occurs. During a relapse, a recovering alcoholic returns to his or her drinking habits. Relapse can be triggered by a variety of factors such as stress, depression, alcohol craving, negative life events, and interpersonal tensions. To recover once again, the patient goes through the stages of behavior change. Treatment to prevent an initial or repeated relapse often involves self-help groups.

Alcoholics Anonymous (AA) is the best known and most widely available of the self-help groups. Governed by its members, the organization's philosophy is that alcoholism is a physical, emotional, and spiritual disease for which there is no cure. Recovery is a lifelong process that involves attention to AA's Twelve Steps, which are listed in **Table 8.8**. AA also has related support groups for family members and friends of alcoholics, such as Alateen and Al-Anon.

Although not as well known, other self-help groups exist. The Secular Organization for Sobriety (SOS) is a group similar to AA, except its program does not include spiritual aspects. The Rational Recovery (RR) program is also a secular organization and emphasizes the importance of alcoholics becom-

## Table 8.8

### The Twelve Steps of Alcoholics Anonymous

1. We admitted we were powerless over alcohol—that our lives had become unmanageable.

2. Came to believe that a Power greater than ourselves could restore us to sanity.

3. Made a decision to turn our will and our lives over to the care of God as we understood Him.

4. Made a searching and fearless moral inventory of ourselves.

5. Admitted to God, to ourselves, and to another human being the exact nature of our wrongs.

6. Were entirely ready to have God remove all these defects of character.

7. Humbly asked Him to remove our shortcomings.

8. Made a list of all persons we had harmed, and became willing to make amends to them all.

9. Made direct amends to such people wherever possible, except when to do so would injure them or others.

10. Continued to take personal inventory and when we were wrong promptly admitted it.

11. Sought through prayer and meditation to improve our conscious contact with God, as we understood Him, praying only for knowledge of His will for us and the power to carry that out.

12. Having had a spiritual awakening as the result of these Steps, we tried to carry this message to alcoholics, and to practice these principles in all our affairs.

*Source:* "The Twelve Steps" are reprinted with permission of Alcoholics Anonymous World Services, Inc. (AAWS). Permission to reprint the Twelve Steps does not mean that AAWS has reviewed or approved the contents of this publication, or that AAWS necessarily agrees with the views expressed herein. AA is a program of recovery from alcoholism only—use of the Twelve Steps in connection with programs and activities which are patterned after AA, but which address other problems, or in any other non-AA context, does not imply otherwise.

ing aware of their irrational beliefs, self-perceptions, and expectancies to be successful in changing their behavior. These groups suggest abstinence as a preferred drinking goal but emphasize personal choice. One self-help approach for women is Women for Sobriety. This group emphasizes women's issues such as assertiveness, self-confidence, and autonomy as part of the change process.

## Healthy Living Practices

☐ To be a responsible drinker, do not allow your drinking to threaten your health, endanger the safety of others, or interfere with business or personal relationships.

☐ If drinking alcohol is damaging your physical and/or psychological health, you should seek medical help.

☐ If you use alcohol in physically dangerous situations, have developed a tolerance to alcohol, exhibit withdrawal symptoms when you are not drinking, and compulsively use alcohol, you are probably alcohol dependent and should seek medical help.

☐ Be sure to eat while drinking alcoholic beverages so that less alcohol will enter the bloodstream.

☐ If you consume alcohol and are male, drink only 1 oz of ethanol per day (2 drinks) or less to decrease the risk of coronary artery disease and stroke. The safest alcohol consumption level for women is 0.5 oz of ethanol per day (1 drink). Heavier alcohol consumption is associated with a variety of conditions and diseases.

☐ Do not drive after consuming alcoholic beverages. Alcohol impairs many of the skills needed to operate motor vehicles safely. As your blood alcohol concentration increases, your risk of having a car crash increases significantly.

# Tobacco

## Types of Tobacco Products

Cigarettes are the most prevalent tobacco product in the United States. In 2009, an estimated 58.7 million Americans smoked cigarettes, representing 23.3% of the population age 12 years and older.[4]

Smoking rates increase with age to the early 20s, and then generally decline with age. In 2009, 8.9% of youths aged 12 to 17 years were current cigarette smokers, 33.1% of young adults aged 18 to 20 years

**Figure 8.6**

**Past Month Cigarette Use Among Persons Aged 12 Years or Older, by Age: 2009.** This graph shows that persons aged 21–25 years had the highest prevalence of current smoking in 2009. In general, smoking prevalence declined as age decreased and increased from that peak. There was a slight increase in smoking prevalence in those aged 45 to 54 years from those aged 40 to 44 years, however.
*Source:* Substance Abuse and Mental Health Services Administration. (2010). Results from the 2009 National Survey on drug use and health: Vol. I. Summary of national findings (HHS Publication No. SMA 10-4586Findings). Retrieved on March 16, 2011, from http://oas.samhsa.gov/NSDUH/2k9NSDUH/2k9ResultsP.pdf

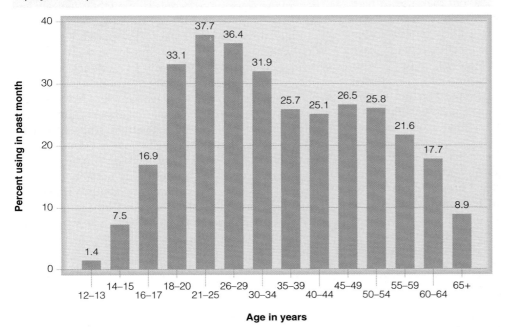

were current smokers, and 37.7% of those aged 21 to 25 were current smokers. Use then declined with age: 36.4% of those aged 26 to 29 years were current smokers, as were 34% of those aged 26 to 34 years. By age 35 years and older, the percentage of those who were current smokers dropped to 20.4%.[4] **Figure 8.6** shows the proportion of current smokers in each age group, with the younger and older groups broken down in more detail.

The prevalence of smoking is high in college students. In 1991, 35.6% of college students smoked at least once during the past year. This percentage rose throughout the 1990s to a peak of 44.5% in 1999. The percentage has fallen since then to 29.9% in 2009, which is below 1991 levels.[26]

The prevalence of smoking in high school students is lower than in college students. However, the Consumer Health box "Kreteks and Bidis: Unwrapping the Facts" describes types of cigarettes that were becoming popular particularly with high school students,

so much so that University of Michigan Monitoring the Future researchers, who track drug, alcohol, and tobacco use among the nation's youth, added a question about these products in 2001. The popularity of kreteks (clove cigarettes) and bidis (small, strong, flavored cigarettes) declined between 2001 and 2009. Nonetheless, in 2009 5.5% of high school seniors smoked kreteks and 1.5% smoked bidis.[26]

Smoking cigars and pipes is not as popular in the American population as is smoking cigarettes. Most cigar and pipe smokers are male. In 2009, 8.7% of males were current cigar smokers versus 2.0% of females, and 1.4% of males were current pipe smokers versus 0.2% of females.[4]

*Smokeless tobacco,* which includes *snuff* and *chewing tobacco,* is not very popular in the American population either. Snuff, the most popular form of smokeless tobacco, is powdered or finely cut tobacco. It may be used loose or wrapped in a paper pouch. Although snuff can be inhaled, most users in the United

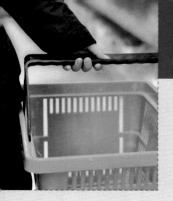

# Consumer Health

## Kreteks and Bidis: Unwrapping the Facts

Kreteks (clove cigarettes) and bidi cigarettes (small, strong-smelling brown cigarettes) appeared to be popular with American youth in the late 1990s, but their use by high school seniors declined from 10.1% in 2001 to 5.5% in 2009. Clove cigarettes, developed in Indonesia in the early 1900s and presently manufactured there, have been imported into the United States since 1968. Bidis, manufactured primarily in India and other Southeast Asian countries, were not widely used in the United States until the mid-1990s. In 2000, 9.2% of high school seniors smoked bidis, but by 2009 that figure had fallen to 1.5%.

Clove cigarettes look much like tobacco cigarettes and are made with or without filter tips. Most are wrapped with white paper, but some have brown or black coverings. Clove cigarettes contain approximately 40% ground cloves and 60% tobacco, although the specific amount varies among manufacturers and brands. Clove oil is added as well, often discoloring the cigarette paper. As these cigarettes burn, the cloves make a crackling sound. (Kretek means "crackle.")

Many users of clove cigarettes think that they are less dangerous to smoke than regular cigarettes because 40% of their content is cloves rather than tobacco. However, they are making an incorrect assumption. Clove cigarettes are rolled tighter than regular cigarettes, resulting in a denser product. Put simply, there is less air in clove cigarettes than in regular cigarettes, so the tobacco content of kreteks is similar to that of regular cigarettes. Additionally, tests show that clove cigarettes deliver, on average, twice as much tar, nicotine, and carbon monoxide as do moderate tar-containing American cigarettes.

Clove cigarettes also contain an anesthetic called eugenol (a natural component of the cloves), which can cause allergic reactions in some. This anesthetic numbs the backs of smokers' throats and windpipes. Researchers think that this numbing effect is the reason that smokers inhale kretek smoke more deeply and retain it in their lungs longer than when smoking regular cigarettes. They also suspect that this numbing effect may encourage smoking by people who might otherwise find smoking cigarettes harsh and distasteful.

Bidis are wrapped in leaves (much like cigars) and tied with a string. They are smaller and thinner than regular cigarettes and come in flavors such as cherry, mango, chocolate, and strawberry. Young people smoke bidis because they like the flavor and find bidis cheaper and easier to buy than regular cigarettes. Additionally, they perceive bidis to be safer than smoking regular cigarettes. As with clove cigarettes, however, this assumption is false. Tests show that bidis produce approximately three times the amount of carbon monoxide and nicotine as American cigarettes and about five times the amount of tar. Additionally, smokers inhale more often and more deeply when smoking bidis than when smoking regular cigarettes because the leaf wrapper does not burn well.

Are smoking kreteks and bidis safe alternatives to smoking regular cigarettes? The answer is an emphatic no! In fact, the data show that these alternative smoking products pose even greater health risks than regular cigarettes do.

*Source:* Johnston, L. D., et al. (2010). *Monitoring the Future national survey results on drug use, 1975–2009: Volume 1, secondary school students* (NIH Publication No. 10-7584). Bethesda, MD: National Institute on Drug Abuse. Retrieved March 17, 2011, from http://www.monitoringthefuture.org/pubs/monographs/vol1_2009.pdf

# Diversity in Health

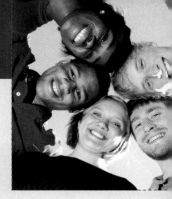

## Tobacco Drinking?

To North Americans, the phrase "using tobacco" usually means smoking cigarettes, cigars, or pipes. Occasionally, we might envision a person using chewing tobacco or placing a pinch of snuff between the gums and cheek. But various cultures use tobacco in other ways—including some ways that may be new to you.

Drinking liquid tobacco is one of the oldest methods of tobacco use. The members of certain tribal populations in South America, particularly those living in Guiana, the upper Amazon, and the mountainous regions of Ecuador and Peru, drink tobacco juice. The drinking of tobacco has also been reported in other South American regions, including northwestern coastal Venezuela, northwestern Colombia, and a few scattered places in Bolivia and Brazil.

The various groups of people who drink tobacco juice prepare it in different ways. The leaves may be first pounded, chewed, or shredded. Sometimes they are left untreated. Then, the tobacco leaves are placed in water; sometimes other ingredients are added such as salt, pepper, or plant materials such as tree bark. The mixture is boiled and then strained to obtain the liquid. Usually it is then set aside to allow much of the water to evaporate. The remaining material has the consistency of a paste, syrup, or jelly. The syrups and jellies are usually liquid enough to drink by mouth or pour in the nose. People from some areas squirt the juice from one person's mouth to another.

Various tribes of the northernmost extension of the Andes in Colombia and Venezuela and in parts of the northwest Amazon make a thick extract of tobacco called ambil that they rub across their teeth, gums, or tongue. This thick, black gelatin is made by boiling tobacco leaves for hours or days and then thickening the extract with starch. Recipes vary; some tribes add pepper, avocado seeds, sugar, or tapioca. Ambil is sometimes ingested with other tobacco products or hallucinogenic drugs.

Using chewing tobacco is practiced by about 2% to 3% of the population in the United States. It is more widely practiced in South America and the West Indies. A person who uses tobacco in this way usually sucks or sometimes chews tobacco quids, which are simply pieces of tobacco made for this purpose. However, the South American and West Indian practices of preparing quids may seem unusual to North Americans. South American and West Indian recipes may include soil, ashes, salt, or honey with the finely crushed tobacco leaves. (North American quids are also flavored in various ways.) South American Indians generally swallow the juices from the tobacco, rather than spit them out.

Another practice among South American Indians that may seem unusual to North Americans is the use of to-

bacco as an enema or suppository. Generally, these native people use tobacco in this manner to treat constipation or worm infestations. Various tribes of Indians who reside in the mountains of Peru also use tobacco in this way during certain rituals.

People in different cultures often adopt different health-related behaviors. What seems unusual to persons in one culture may not seem unusual to individuals from another. In fact, tobacco drinking may be entering the American culture in trendy restaurants. An increasing number are including tobacco items on the menu or in the bar because the law does not allow their customers to light up their favorite cigarettes or cigars. Therefore, restaurateurs have developed alternatives to smoking. In some eateries, tobacco leaves are used as overnight wraps for fish before the fish are smoked. Tobacco juice is being used as an ingredient in sauces and desserts. And an alcoholic beverage has been developed called a nicotini (**Figure 8.A**), which includes "tea" brewed from tobacco leaves.

Tobacco drinking? It may be happening at the table next to yours, and its health effects are still to be determined.

*Sources:* Donovan, L. (2008, March 12). With nicotini, no need to light up. *Chicago Sun Times*, p. S1; Pino, D. (2010, November 17). Now on the menu: Tobacco. *SF Weekly* (California); U.S. Department of Health and Human Services. (1992). *Smoking and health in the Americas: A 1992 report of the Surgeon General, in collaboration with the Pan American Health Organization* (DHHS Publication No. CDC 92-8419). Atlanta, GA: Author, pp. 19–31.

### Figure 8.A

**The Nicotini.** Nicknamed the liquid cigarette, the nicotini is made by soaking tobacco leaves overnight in vodka or other spirits. Nicotine is a powerful, toxic drug, and the amount served in nicotinis is not regulated. Drinking a nicotini may result in unpleasant and harmful side effects.

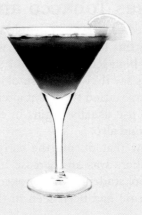

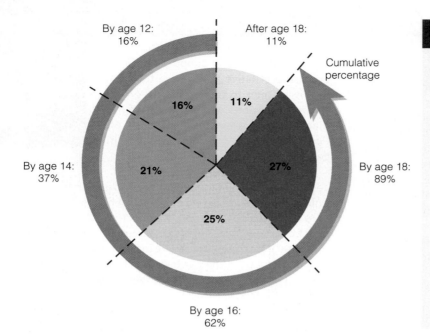

By age 12:
16%

After age 18:
11%

Cumulative percentage

16%

11%

By age 14:
37%

21%

27%

By age 18:
89%

25%

By age 16:
62%

**Figure 8.7**

**Age at Which Adults Say They Started Smoking.** Most smokers started this habit when they were in their teens or preteens. *Sources:* Substance Abuse and Mental Health Services Administration; Office on Smoking and Health, Centers for Disease Control and Prevention

States today place snuff between the cheek and gum. This practice is called *dipping*.

*Chewing tobacco* is loose leaf tobacco or a plug of compressed tobacco, which is sometimes called a *quid*. It is placed in the cheek. It can be chewed, as its name suggests, or, more often, it is sucked. During the time that snuff or chewing tobacco remains in the mouth, it forms a liquid that smokeless tobacco users usually spit out. For this reason smokeless tobacco is often called spitting tobacco. In 2009, 6.7% of males currently used smokeless tobacco versus 0.3% of females.[4]

Worldwide, a variety of other tobacco products exists besides those mentioned here. Additionally, methods of tobacco use vary among cultures. The Diversity in Health essay "Tobacco Drinking?" describes a few tobacco-related practices of various South American cultures.

## Who Uses Tobacco and Why?

As mentioned earlier, most people who smoke cigarettes began this habit when they were adolescents, primarily in high school. **Figure 8.7** shows the ages at which adults say they started smoking. Only 11% of adult smokers started this habit after age 18. Smokeless tobacco use usually begins in early adolescence or in childhood also.

Data show that during the early 1990s through 1996/1997 there was an increase in the percentage of high school students who smoked cigarettes daily, after a decrease had been seen in the prevalence of

smoking by high school seniors from 1976 through 1992. However, those percentages have declined steadily through 2009 (**Figure 8.8**). Nevertheless, 19.5% of high school students responded that they were current cigarette smokers on the national Youth Risk Behavior Survey in 2009,[27] despite all that is known today about the health consequences of cigarette smoking.

**Psychosocial Reasons for Using Tobacco Products** Adolescents initially try tobacco products for a variety of reasons. Adolescents who have family members or friends who smoke cigarettes or use smokeless tobacco are more likely to begin these habits than teenagers who do not observe these behaviors in people close to them. Many adolescents try smoking, chewing, or dipping simply to experiment. Others use tobacco as a way to feel older and more independent, as a response to advertising, or as a response to social pressure. The influence of peers is the most important factor in determining when and how adolescents first try cigarettes.

Certain characteristics of adolescents make them more likely to use tobacco: low self-esteem, susceptibility to peer pressure, a sensation-seeking nature, a rebellious personality, depression or anxiety, low academic achievement, and a low level of knowledge about the immediate health risks of smoking. Additionally, adolescents who think that their parents do not care about them or adolescents who are alone much of the time are more likely to try smoking. Girls are significantly less likely to begin smoking if they are involved in an organized sport. However, participation in sports does not affect boys' initiation into smoking.

**Nicotine Addiction** Why do teenagers and adults continue smoking and using smokeless tobacco? Most people continue because they are addicted to **nicotine**. Nicotine is a psychoactive drug that acts at communication points among nerve cells in the brain, as do other psychoactive drugs. It becomes addicting during the first few years of use.

The many reasons that people say they continue to smoke (other than craving or being addicted to cigarettes) include the following:

- It is arousing and gives them energy.
- It helps concentration.
- It lifts the mood.
- It reduces anger, tension, depression, and stress.
- It is a habit.
- It is a pleasurable activity.

However, some of the pleasure of smoking (as well as using smokeless tobacco) is really the relief of the symptoms of nicotine withdrawal. During the day, as a person smokes, he or she builds up tolerance

to nicotine. Nicotine withdrawal symptoms become more pronounced between each successive cigarette. To relieve these symptoms (**Table 8.9**), most cigarette addicts smoke more as the day goes on. Overnight, the level of nicotine in the blood drops and tolerance decreases; thus, the smoker is resensitized to the effects of nicotine. The first cigarette of the day is usually quite satisfying to the smoker as the cycle of tolerance and then resensitization begins once again.

## The Health Effects of Tobacco Use

In 1964, U.S. Surgeon General Luther Terry issued a landmark report that linked cigarette smoking with the development of lung cancer and other diseases. Since that famous report, scientists have learned a great deal about the health consequences of smoking and smokeless tobacco use, and the Surgeon General's Office has issued 30 more tobacco-related reports. In these reports, cigarette smoking is recognized as the leading source of preventable illness and death in

### Figure 8.8

**Cigarettes: Trends in Daily Use by Eighth, Tenth, and Twelfth Graders.**

*Source:* Johnston, L. D., et al. (2010). *Monitoring the future:oN national survey results on drug use, 1975–2009: Volume 1, secondary school students* (NIH Publication No. 10-7584). Bethesda, MD: National Institute on Drug Abuse. Retrieved on March 17, 2011, from http://www.monitoringthefuture.org/pubs/monographs/vol1_2009.pdf

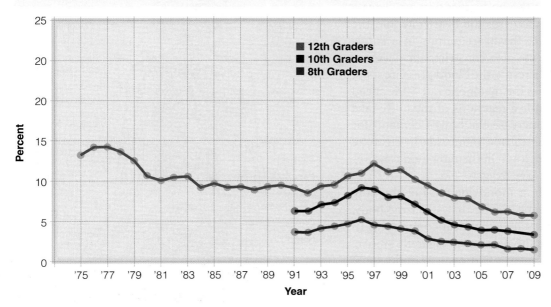

**Table 8.9**

## Typical Symptoms of Nicotine Withdrawal

| | |
|---|---|
| Anxiety/tension | Heart palpitations |
| Cough/dry mouth/nasal drip | Impatience |
| Craving cigarettes | Insomnia |
| Depression | Irritability |
| Difficulty concentrating | Loss of energy/fatigue |
| Disorientation | Restlessness |
| Dizziness | Stomach or bowel problems/nausea |
| Excessive hunger | Sweating |
| Frustration | Tightness in chest |
| Headaches | Tremors |

*Sources*: Adapted from Shiffman, S., West, R., & Gilbert, D. (2004). Recommendation for the assessment of tobacco craving and withdrawal in smoking cessation trials. *Nicotine and Tobacco Research, 6*:599–614; Gritz, E. R., Carr, C. R., & Marcus, A. C. (1991). The tobacco withdrawal syndrome in unaided quitters. *British Journal of Addiction, 86*(1):57–69.

the United States. Every year, approximately 443,000 people die in the United States as a result of using tobacco products.[28] **Figure 8.9** shows the cancers and chronic diseases to which smoking has a causal link.

**Immediate Effects of Nicotine and Carbon Monoxide** After entering the body, nicotine produces a variety of effects. It increases the heart rate and the amount of blood that the heart pumps in a single beat. However, nicotine also constricts, or narrows, the blood vessels. As a result, the blood pressure rises. Nicotine also increases the metabolic rate—the speed at which all the chemical reactions of the body take place. These effects increase the body's demand for oxygen. However, the carbon monoxide in cigarette smoke binds to hemoglobin in the red blood cells, reducing its ability to carry oxygen.

Nicotine and carbon monoxide are not the only components of cigarette smoke that affect the body. There are more than 4,000 chemical compounds in the gases and particles that make up cigarette smoke. Some are poisonous, such as hydrogen cyanide; some are irritating to the lungs and mucous membranes, such as particulate matter; and some cause cancer,

such as the tars—sticky substances similar to road tar. The rest of this section describes specific health effects of smoking tobacco and using smokeless tobacco products.

**Respiratory Illnesses** The windpipe and its major subdivisions are lined with microscopic hairlike structures called *cilia*, which are embedded in a layer of sticky mucus. This mucus traps inhaled particles and microbes. As the cilia beat, the mucus moves upward, sweeping this debris up and out of the air passageways.

Inhaled cigarette smoke paralyzes the cilia. With continued smoking, the cilia are damaged. Cigarette smoke also irritates the airways and tar builds up on the cilia, causing excess mucus to be produced. The chronic cough of smokers, usually called *smoker's cough*, is a result of the body's attempt to remove this excess, stationary mucus.

**Acute bronchitis** is an inflammation of the mucous membranes of the bronchi, which is usually

**Figure 8.9**

**Smoking Cigarettes Can Cause These Cancers and Chronic Diseases.**

*Source:* U.S. Department of Health and Human Services. (2010). *How tobacco smoke causes disease: The biology and behavioral basis for smoking-attributable disease: A report of the Surgeon General.* Atlanta, GA: Author. Retrieved on April 3, 2011, from http://www.surgeongeneral.gov/library/tobaccosmoke/report/full_report.pdf

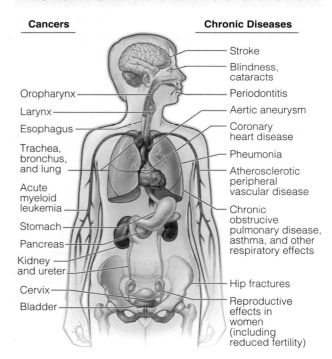

| Cancers | Chronic Diseases |
|---|---|
| Oropharynx | Stroke |
| Larynx | Blindness, cataracts |
| Esophagus | Periodontitis |
| Trachea, bronchus, and lung | Aertic aneurysm |
| Acute myeloid leukemia | Coronary heart disease |
| Stomach | Pheumonia |
| Pancreas | Atherosclerotic peripheral vascular disease |
| Kidney and ureter | Chronic obstrucive pulmonary disease, asthma, and other respiratory effects |
| Cervix | Hip fractures |
| Bladder | Reproductive effects in women (including reduced fertility) |

caused by a viral infection. However, smokers are more susceptible than nonsmokers to acute bronchitis because of their impaired and irritated bronchi. The signs and symptoms of this disease are soreness or tightness in the chest, slight fever, cough, chills, and a vague feeling of weakness or discomfort. Bronchitis with accompanying high fever, breathlessness, and yellow, gray, green, or bloody sputum is serious and the person should seek medical attention immediately.

**Chronic bronchitis** is usually caused by cigarette smoking, but cigar and pipe smoking may also be causes. Chronic bronchitis is a persistent inflammation and thickening of the lining of the bronchi caused by the constant irritation of smoke. As the lining of these airways thickens, breathing becomes more difficult and coughing increases. The cells lining the bronchi produce additional mucus, causing congestion in the lungs and further hampering breathing. The signs and symptoms of chronic bronchitis are shortness of breath and a chronic cough that produces considerable amounts of mucus. Chronic bronchitis is a serious disease that can result in death. In addition to bronchitis, smoking is also a risk factor for *pneumonia*, an inflammation of the lungs that is caused by a variety of bacteria and viruses.

Smoking is also the main cause of **emphysema** (**Figure 8.10**), a condition in which the air sacs of the lungs lose their normal elasticity. Some air sacs become overstretched and eventually rupture, resulting in larger air sacs with less surface area over which gas exchange can take place. Under these conditions, the lungs can no longer accommodate normal amounts of air. Also, without the normal elasticity of the lungs, a person can no longer inhale and exhale normally. Breathing becomes a continual effort.

The lung damage of emphysema can never be repaired. As the disease progresses, the heart becomes increasingly overworked. Because the blood it is pumping is oxygen poor, the body sends signals to the heart to pump more blood more quickly. Eventually the person with extensive lung damage dies, usually from heart failure. However, if emphysema is detected early (especially before symptoms develop), its destructive effects can be halted by stopping smoking.

People with chronic bronchitis and emphysema are said to have **chronic obstructive pulmonary disease (COPD)**. Cigarette smoking is the major cause of COPD; it would probably be a minor health problem if people did not smoke. Smoking is thought to be responsible for approximately 108,000 deaths

**acute bronchitis** A temporary inflammation of the mucous membranes of the bronchi.

**chronic bronchitis** A persistent inflammation and thickening of the lining of the bronchi.

**emphysema (EM-fih-SEE-mah)** A chronic condition in which the air sacs of the lungs lose their normal elasticity, impairing respiration.

**chronic obstructive pulmonary disease (COPD)** A syndrome that includes chronic bronchitis, asthma, and emphysema and that is characterized by extreme difficulty in breathing.

## Figure 8.10

**A Healthy Lung and Lung from a Person with Emphysema.** (a) The healthy lung is smooth, a deep pink, and relatively uniform in color. (b) Because of emphysema, some of the alveoli have ruptured, creating tiny craters within the lung, which are difficult to see in this picture. Note the blackened tissue as a result of years of smoking.

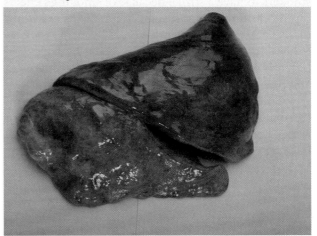

(a)

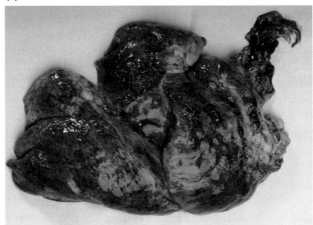

(b)

**cardiovascular disease (CVD)** Disorders of the heart and blood vessels.

**periodontal (PER-ee-oh-DON-tal) disease** A disorder of the tissues that support the teeth.

from COPD per year, or 85% to 90% of all COPD deaths.[29]

**Cardiovascular Disease** Thirty-one percent of people who die from smoking-related causes die from **cardiovascular disease (CVD)**, or dysfunction of the heart and blood vessels.[30] There is a variety of cardiovascular diseases, including *coronary artery disease (CAD)*, *hypertension* (chronic high blood pressure), and stroke (blood vessel disease of the brain). *Atherosclerosis*, the buildup of fatty deposits in the arteries, is an important cardiovascular disease process that is an underlying cause in CAD and stroke. These diseases are discussed in detail in Chapter 12.

According to the National Stroke Association, cigarette smokers are more than twice as likely as nonsmokers to have a stroke because of smoking's effects on the cardiovascular system. As many as one-third of CVD deaths in the United States each year are attributable to cigarette smoking.[30] Using smokeless tobacco is a significant CVD risk factor also, but cigar and pipe smoking are less significant.

Women who take oral contraceptives (birth control pills) and who smoke cigarettes increase their risk of heart attack several times. Oral contraceptives increase the risk of developing blood clots, which can block already narrowed arteries in persons with atherosclerosis, a disease that smokers have an increased risk of developing. For these reasons, smoking while taking oral contraceptives also increases the risk of peripheral vascular disease and stroke.

Smokers often think that smoking low-yield ("light") cigarettes poses fewer health risks than smoking regular-strength cigarettes. Light cigarettes, which began to be marketed in the 1960s in response to health concerns, are lower in tar and nicotine. However, research data show that smokers generally puff on these cigarettes longer and inhale more deeply than when smoking regular cigarettes. Also, they often smoke more light cigarettes than they would regular cigarettes, so they may take in as much tar, nicotine, and other noxious and cancer-causing compounds than if they smoked regular cigarettes. Scientists have found no evidence that smoking low-tar and low-nicotine cigarettes reduces the risk of coronary heart disease.[28]

When a smoker quits, his or her risk of heart disease begins dropping immediately. The time it takes for a former smoker's risk of death from heart attack to reach that of a nonsmoker's varies from 3 to 9 years. The recovery time depends on the number of years a person smoked and how many cigarettes he or she smoked per day. However, if a smoker has already developed heart disease before quitting, the risk of heart attack will not return to that of a nonsmoker, although it will be lower than if he or she had continued smoking.

**Cancer** Cancer is a group of diseases in which certain cells exhibit abnormal growth. Cancers can arise in various locations in the body and then spread to others. The most prevalent forms of cancer in the United States are discussed in Chapter 13, which also describes lifestyle changes you can make in addition to quitting smoking that will reduce your chances of developing these cancers. Guidelines for early detection are listed in Chapter 13.

Cancer is the second biggest killer of Americans, and tobacco use is responsible for about 30% of cancer deaths and 87% of lung cancer deaths annually in the United States.[31] Tobacco use causes or is related to cancers of the lungs, larynx, oral cavity, esophagus, kidneys, bladder, pancreas, stomach, and cervix (see Figure 8.9). Lung cancer is the most prevalent form of cancer caused by tobacco use.

**Periodontal Disease** Smoking tobacco and using smokeless tobacco can have serious effects on the oral cavity. These effects can range from embarrassing problems such as bad breath and stained teeth to life-threatening conditions such as oral cancer (**Figure 8.11**).

People who use tobacco products regularly, often develop **periodontal disease**, commonly known as gum disease. Periodontal disease is actually more than just disease of the gums. It is a disease of all the supporting tissues around the teeth, which include the gums, the bone in which the teeth are embedded, and the ligaments that hold the teeth to the bone.

People can develop periodontal disease for a variety of reasons, such as poor dental hygiene, overzealous brushing that damages the gums, and clenching and grinding of the teeth. Using tobacco products is especially destructive to the gums and often is a cause of severe periodontal disease. Nicotine narrows the blood vessels in the gums, reducing the amount of oxygen that reaches these tissues. As a result, the gum tissue becomes less resistant to infection. Additionally, good oral hygiene and proper periodontal

## Figure 8.11

**Gruen Von Behrens, After Using Smokeless Tobacco.** Gruen began using smokeless (spit) tobacco at age 13, and by age 17 he had oral cancer and a 25% chance of survival. Formerly a star baseball player, Gruen can no longer play sports, and after 40 operations he is still missing his lower teeth and jawbone. His body rejected a bone transplant that would have created a new jaw. Gruen is now a spokesperson for Oral Health America's National Spit Tobacco Education Program (NSTEP), warning audiences of the dangers of using smokeless tobacco.

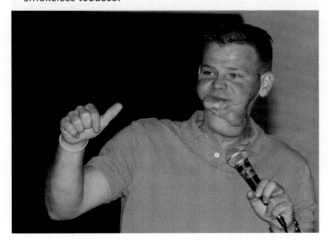

## Figure 8.12

**Advanced Leukoplakia.** This precancerous condition often develops on the mucous membranes of the mouths of those who use smokeless tobacco products.

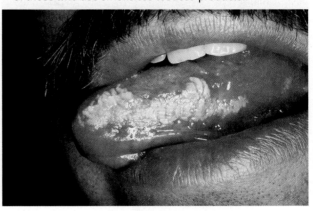

treatment are often ineffective when a person with periodontal disease continues to use tobacco.

Young people who use smokeless tobacco products often develop periodontal disease. Gum recession most often occurs at places where smokeless tobacco is held in the mouth. Additionally, *leukoplakia*, a disease characterized by precancerous white patches that develop on the mucous membranes of the mouth (**Figure 8.12**), is common in adolescents who use these products. Approximately 5% of these lesions become cancerous within 5 years. However, if a smokeless tobacco user discontinues use, the leukoplakia regresses and may disappear.

**Osteoporosis** Smoking cigarettes can lead to lower bone density, or osteoporosis, which occurs most frequently in postmenopausal white women. This disease is serious because it places women at risk for bone fractures, back pain, and other accompanying problems. Hip fractures are particularly serious; the death rate for people who sustain hip fractures is 20% to 24% higher in the year following the fracture than for people of the same age who did not sustain this injury.[32] (Osteoporosis is discussed in more detail in Chapter 9.)

## Environmental Tobacco Smoke

In the past three decades, nonsmokers have become increasingly aware that smoke in their indoor environments could pose a health risk. This smoke, termed **environmental tobacco smoke (ETS)** or *secondhand smoke*, is made up of the sidestream smoke emitted from a lit cigarette, cigar, or pipe and the smoke exhaled by smokers.

In 1986, the National Research Council (NRC) and the United States Surgeon General's Office compiled research data to assess the health effects of exposure to ETS.[33,34] Both landmark reports conclude that ETS can cause lung cancer in adult nonsmokers. In 2006, the Surgeon General's Office released another report on secondhand smoke: *The Health Consequences of Involuntary Exposure to Tobacco Smoke.*[35] At the press release of the report, Surgeon General Richard H. Carmona stated, "The debate is over. The science is clear: secondhand smoke is not a mere annoyance, but a serious health hazard that causes premature death and disease in children and nonsmoking adults."

Conclusions from these reports prompted the designation of governmental and other public buildings, many workplaces, and restaurants in many states as smoke-free environments to reduce the effects of ETS

## Figure 8.13

### The Health Consequences of Repeated Exposure to Secondhand Smoke.

*Source:* U.S. Department of Health and Human Services. (2010). *How tobacco smoke causes disease: The biology and behavioral basis for smoking-attributable disease: A report of the surgeon general.* Atlanta, GA: Author. Retrieved on April 3, 2011, from http://www.surgeongeneral.gov/library/tobaccosmoke/report/full_report.pdf

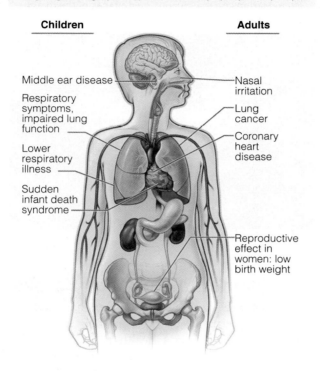

on the public. By 1993, nearly 82% of indoor workers were restricted from smoking in their workplaces.[36] By 2006, almost all workplaces, governmental buildings, and public places in the United States were smoke free.[35] However, if a "smoke-free" area is adjacent to a smoking area it will contain unacceptable levels of airborne pollutants unless the two areas have separate ventilation systems.

**Figure 8.13** shows the health consequences of repeated exposure to secondhand smoke for both children and adults. Avoiding secondhand smoke will help you stay healthier. The Managing Your Health box includes tips on how to say no to secondhand smoke.

## Quitting

Most smokers want to quit. In a 2010 Gallup poll, 75% of smokers told Gallup interviewers that they would like to give up cigarettes. Eighty-six percent of smokers said that they think second-hand smoke is very or somewhat harmful to health. And 96% of smokers reported that they think smoking is very or somewhat harmful to health.[37]

**Benefits of Quitting**  At any age, there are many reasons to stop smoking cigarettes. Some of those reasons are to lower your risk of various diseases and conditions including certain cancers, heart attack, stroke, and chronic lung disease; in pregnant women, to reduce the risk of having a low-birth-weight baby; to stop exposing your family and other people around you to second-hand smoke; to rid yourself of a stale cigarette odor on your body and breath; and to rid yourself of an expensive addiction to nicotine.

On quitting, an addicted smoker experiences some or all of the nicotine withdrawal symptoms listed in Table 8.9. These unpleasant psychological and physiologic conditions peak 1 to 2 days following quitting but subside during the following weeks. The two withdrawal symptoms that last the longest are the urge to smoke and an increased appetite. However, using a nicotine replacement therapy product, such as the nicotine patch, nicotine gum, or nicotine inhaler; buproprion (an antidepressant used to treat nicotine dependence); or varenicline (Chantix) during the early cessation period may help reduce these symptoms and make quitting easier. Varenicline eases withdrawal symptoms by providing some nicotine effects to the brain while simultaneously blocking the effects of nicotine from cigarettes. Of these therapies, varenicline appears to be the most effective.[38]

*Electronic cigarettes*, or *e-cigarettes*, which are marketed as an alternative cigarette and as a quitting aid, have been cited by the FDA for "unsubstantiated claims and poor manufacturing practices."[39] For example, the FDA found nicotine in e-cigarettes labeled as having no nicotine and similarly labeled e-cigarettes as delivering differing amounts of nicotine.[40] Most e-cigarettes are manufactured to look like cigarettes and contain a stainless steel shell encasing a heating element, a chemical-containing cartridge, and an atomizer that vaporizes the chemicals when heated (**Figure 8.14**). The vapor is inhaled.

A promising quitting aid is the nicotine addiction vaccine, which was in late-stage clinical trials in early 2011. The vaccine, called NicVAX, works by stimulating the body to produce antibodies against nicotine so that the drug cannot get to the brain, stimulate pleasure centers, and reinforce the craving for nicotine.

During the quitting process as withdrawal symptoms subside, former smokers report that favorable

# Managing Your Health

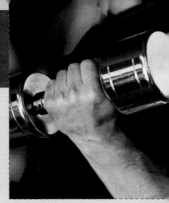

## How to Say No to Secondhand Smoke

If you live with a smoker:

- Ask him or her not to smoke in your home. Discuss how his or her habit puts you and others living there at risk.
- If he or she is unwilling to go outside, suggest ways to limit the exposure to smoke for you and others. Maybe a room could be set aside for smoking—one that is seldom used by other members of the household. Some smokers protect others at home by smoking near an open window or when no one is around.
- Keep rooms well ventilated. Open windows.
- Support smokers who decide to quit.

When visitors come:

- Ask all smokers who visit not to smoke in your house or apartment, but to please smoke outside.
- Do not keep ashtrays around.

In others' homes or in vehicles:

- Tell friends and relatives politely that you would appreciate their not smoking while you are there.
- Let people know when their smoke is causing immediate problems. If it is making your allergies worse, making you cough or wheeze, or making your eyes sting, say so. Some smokers put their cigarettes away when they see the discomfort it causes.

If you have children:

- Insist that babysitters, grandparents, and other caregivers not smoke around your children.
- Help children avoid secondhand smoke if smokers do use tobacco around them. Have them leave the room or play outside while an adult is smoking. Air rooms out after smoking occurs.
- Keep smokers away from places in which children sleep.

When smoking is allowed at the workplace:

- Talk to your employer about the company's smoking policy. Give your employer copies of the Environmental Protection Agency (EPA) report on the harmful effects of environmental tobacco smoke. Call 1-800-438-4318 to obtain this report.
- Ask to work near other nonsmokers and as far away from smokers as possible.
- Ask smokers if they would not smoke around you.
- Use a fan and open windows (if possible) to keep air moving.
- Hang a Thank You for Not Smoking sign in your work area.
- Volunteer to help develop a fair company policy that protects nonsmokers.
- Contact the local Lung Association, the American Cancer Society, or the National Cancer Institute (1-800-4-CANCER) for information concerning smoking cessation programs that can be conducted at your workplace.

When you are in public places:

- Always take the nonsmoking options that are available in rental cars, hotels, and restaurants.
- If a restaurant puts you at a table near smokers (even if you are in a nonsmoking section), ask to move.
- Keep children out of smoking areas.

*Source:* Adapted from National Cancer Institute. (n.d.). I mind very much if you smoke. Retrieved April 3, 2011, from http://dccps.nci.nih.gov/tcrb/i_mind_if_you_smoke/mindsmo.html

---

psychological changes occur over time, such as enhanced self-esteem and an increased sense of self-control. Because smoking cigarettes has negative effects on the respiratory system, a person who quits notices that it is easier to breathe. Smoking cessation reduces the rate at which symptoms such as cough, mucus production, and wheezing occur after an initial period of clearing mucus from the lungs subsides. It also reduces the incidence of respiratory infections such as bronchitis and pneumonia. (Pneumonia can be deadly for people who have chronic diseases.) Also, after sustained abstinence from smoking cigarettes, persons with COPD have less chance of dying from this disease than they did before they quit.

Quitting also has positive effects on the cardiovascular system. Data show that the smoker who quits cuts his or her elevated risk of coronary heart disease in half only 1 year after quitting. The degree of risk

## Figure 8.14

**The Anatomy of an E-cigarette.** An electronic cigarette has a stainless steel casing that is often manufactured to look like a filter-tipped cigarette but that may look like a pen or a thumb drive for those who wish to conceal their use of the product. Internally, the e-cigarette contains a heating element, a chemical-containing cartridge, and a vaporizing unit.

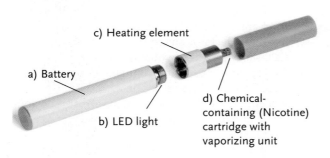

c) Heating element

a) Battery

b) LED light

d) Chemical-containing (Nicotine) cartridge with vaporizing unit

that remains then declines gradually. At 15 years, a former smoker reaches the risk level of a nonsmoker for coronary heart disease and death.[41] The more cigarettes a person smoked and the earlier a person started to smoke, the longer the recovery time. Because the risk of cardiovascular disease increases as the number of cigarettes smoked increases, smoking fewer cigarettes can be a way to lower CVD risk if an individual has little success quitting. However, smoking low-yield (low tar and nicotine) cigarettes does not appear to reduce risk. Among persons diagnosed with cardiovascular disease, smoking cessation markedly reduces the risk of additional heart attacks and cardiovascular death. The benefits of quitting exist for people of all ages. Older individuals should not think that it is "too late" to quit.

Quitting reduces cancer risk. In 5 years after quitting, the excess risk has been cut in half of developing mouth, throat, esophagus, and bladder cancers, and the excess risk of cervical cancer has been eliminated. In 10 years after quitting, the excess risk of dying from lung cancer is cut in half and the risk of cancer of the larynx and pancreas decreases.[41] **Figure 8.15** is a visual summary of the health benefits of quitting smoking.

**The Process of Quitting** Cigarette smoking is an addiction, and an addicted smoker who is quitting goes through the same process of behavioral change as does anyone addicted to any drug. For a smoker to

contemplate quitting, he or she must understand and accept that cigarette smoking is dangerous or must have other reasons for quitting that are important to him or her. Then, the smoker begins to see the potential benefits and negative effects associated with quitting. For example, the smoker may realize that nicotine is a drug and that he or she is addicted to this drug. Quitting will stop the addiction. However, along with this positive behavior (stopping the addiction) comes negative consequences: withdrawal symptoms. To be prepared to quit, the smoker should analyze both the negative and positive aspects of change and prepare to deal with the negative aspects. Often, discussion with a medical practitioner is helpful. Also, if a smoker analyzes the reasons he or she smokes (see "Why Do You Smoke?" in the Student Workbook pages at the end of this text), the smoker will be better equipped to handle the consequences of quitting (see the Managing Your Health box "Tips for Quitters").

Once the smoker realizes the need to quit, he or she should decide what course of action to take. Should it be quitting "cold turkey" or cutting down at first? (If a person is addicted to nicotine, stopping "cold turkey" may be best. The assessment activity "Why Do You Smoke?" can help identify addiction.) Will the smoker join a smoking cessation program or stop without group support? Again, the advice of a medical practitioner may be helpful at this stage. A smoker can also call the American Lung Association, the American Heart Association, the American Cancer Society, or the National Cancer Institute for free literature on quitting and information on smoking cessation programs. Many programs are available, and the smoker needs to select the program that suits his or her needs best. Medication may also be helpful at this stage, such as a nicotine replacement product, buproprion, or varenicline to lessen the withdrawal symptoms from nicotine. Also, the smoker may enlist the support of family and friends through the quitting process.

After the first 6 months, which is considered the *quitting period*, the former smoker enters the period of *maintenance*, which lasts 6 months also. Some quitters who join smoking cessation programs continue to attend group meetings for support. Others get continued support from friends, family members, or other former smokers.

As with other addictions, sometimes *relapse* occurs. During a relapse, a former smoker returns to smoking habits. Relapse can be triggered by a vari-

**Figure 8.15**

**The Health Benefits of Quitting Smoking.** The risks of developing many diseases and conditions drop dramatically, in varied lengths of time, after a person quits smoking.

*Source:* Centers for Disease Control and Prevention. (2004). The benefits of quitting. Retrieved on April 4, 2011, from http://www.cdc.gov/tobacco/data_statistics/sgr/2004/posters/benefits/index.htm

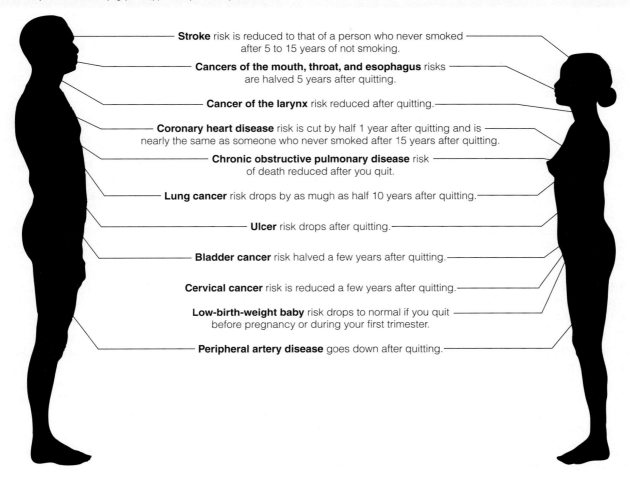

**Stroke** risk is reduced to that of a person who never smoked after 5 to 15 years of not smoking.

**Cancers of the mouth, throat, and esophagus** risks are halved 5 years after quitting.

**Cancer of the larynx** risk reduced after quitting.

**Coronary heart disease** risk is cut by half 1 year after quitting and is nearly the same as someone who never smoked after 15 years after quitting.

**Chronic obstructive pulmonary disease** risk of death reduced after you quit.

**Lung cancer** risk drops by as mugh as half 10 years after quitting.

**Ulcer** risk drops after quitting.

**Bladder cancer** risk halved a few years after quitting.

**Cervical cancer** risk is reduced a few years after quitting.

**Low-birth-weight baby** risk drops to normal if you quit before pregnancy or during your first trimester.

**Peripheral artery disease** goes down after quitting.

ety of factors such as stress, depression, a craving for cigarettes, negative life events, and interpersonal tensions. To quit, the relapsed smoker goes through the stages of behavior change once again.

One barrier to quitting is the smoker's fear of gaining weight. In fact, about 25% of smokers cite this possibility as the reason for not quitting. Likewise, about 25% of people who quit relapse because they begin to gain weight and are afraid of gaining more. This fear is not unfounded—80% of persons who quit smoking gain weight. Data show, however, that the average weight gain is only 6 to 9 pounds and the risk of large weight gain is extremely low. Individuals who smoked heavily gain the most weight after quitting.

People gain weight when they stop smoking for two reasons: They eat more (often to put something other than a cigarette into their mouths) and their metabolism slows slightly. To combat this effect, as part of your smoking cessation plan be sure to include an exercise program to maintain your metabolic rate. Also, keep lots of fat-free, low-calorie snacks handy, such as slices of vegetables with low-fat dip, fruits, pretzels, and sugar-free gelatin.

## Prevention

Prevention programs developed in the 1980s reflect an understanding that smoking begins in early adolescence and that young people go through stages in

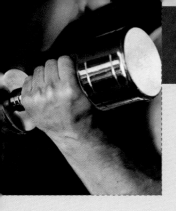

# Managing Your Health

## Tips for Quitters

If you smoke and have not responded to the questions in the assessment activity in the Student Workbook pages at the end of this text titled "Why Do You Smoke?" do so now. Then, read the suggestions for quitting that specifically address each reason you smoke. If you tailor your plan to quit smoking to match the reasons that you smoke, the cessation process will be easier.

### Reason: "Smoking gives me energy."

- Get enough rest to feel refreshed and alert.
- Exercise regularly to raise your overall energy level.
- Take a brisk walk instead of smoking if you start feeling sluggish.
- Eat regular, nutritious meals for energy.
- Drink lots of cold water to refresh you.
- Avoid getting bored, which can make you feel tired.

### Reason: "I like to touch and handle cigarettes."

- Pick up a pen or pencil when you want to reach for a cigarette.
- Play with a coin or handle nearby objects.
- Put a plastic cigarette in your hand or mouth.
- Hold a real cigarette if the touch is all you miss.
- Eat regular meals to avoid confusing the desire to eat with the desire to put a cigarette in your mouth.
- Take up a hobby such as knitting or carpentry that keeps your hands busy.
- Eat low-fat, low-sugar snacks such as carrot sticks or bread sticks.
- Suck on sugar-free hard candy.

### Reason: "Smoking gives me pleasure."

- Enjoy the pleasures of being tobacco free, such as how good foods taste; how much easier it is to walk, run, and climb stairs; and how good it feels to be in control of the urge to smoke.
- Spend the money you save on cigarettes on another kind of pleasure, such as a shopping spree or a night out.
- Remind yourself of the health benefits of quitting. Giving up cigarettes can help you enjoy life's other pleasures for many years to come.

### Reason: "Smoking helps me relax when I'm tense or upset."

- Use relaxation techniques to calm down when you are angry or upset. Deep breathing exercises, muscle relaxation, and imagining yourself in a peaceful setting can make you feel less stressed.
- Exercise regularly to relieve tension and improve your mood.
- Take action to alleviate situations that cause stress.
- Avoid stressful situations.
- Get enough rest and take time to relax each day.
- Enjoy relaxation. Take a long, hot bath. Have a massage. Lie in a garden hammock. Listen to soothing music.

### Reason: "I crave cigarettes and am addicted to nicotine."

- Ask your medical practitioner about using a nicotine patch or nicotine gum to help you avoid withdrawal symptoms.
- Go "cold turkey." Tapering off probably won't work for you because the moment you put out one cigarette you begin to crave the next.
- Keep away from cigarettes completely. Get rid of ashtrays. Destroy any cigarettes you have. Try to avoid people who smoke and smoke-filled places like bars.
- Tell family and friends you've quit smoking.
- Remember that physical withdrawal symptoms last about 2 weeks. Hang on!

### Reason: "Smoking is a habit."

- Cut down gradually. Smoke fewer cigarettes each day or only smoke them halfway down. Inhale less often and less deeply. After several months it should be easier to stop completely.
- Change your smoking routines. Keep your cigarettes in a different place. Smoke with your opposite hand. Do not do anything else while smoking. Limit smoking to certain places, such as outside or in one room at home.
- When you want a cigarette, wait 1 minute. Do something else instead of smoking.
- Be aware of every cigarette you smoke. Ask yourself, "Do I really want this cigarette?" You may be surprised at how many you can easily pass up.
- Set a date for giving up smoking altogether and stick to it.

*Source:* Adapted from National Cancer Institute. (1993). *Learning why you smoke can teach you how to quit.* Washington, DC: U.S. Department of Health and Human Services.

## Healthy Living Practices

- ☐ If you are a smoker, make a plan for quitting and follow through on your plan. Expect quitting to be difficult at times. Consider using an organized program, medication, or both to help you quit. To combat weight gain when quitting, exercise and keep lots of fat-free, low-calorie snacks handy.

- ☐ If you have or plan to have children, consider discussing the health effects of smoking with them when they are very young to discourage them from starting the habit.

- ☐ Do not allow your children to be near someone who is smoking. Children are particularly susceptible to the damaging effects of tobacco smoke.

- ☐ If you have bronchitis with accompanying high fever, breathlessness, and yellow, gray, green, or bloody sputum, seek medical attention immediately.

- ☐ If you have a smoker's cough that produces considerable amounts of mucus and shortness of breath, seek medical attention immediately because you may have chronic bronchitis, a serious disease.

- ☐ See your healthcare provider regularly for an evaluation of your respiratory system.

- ☐ If you are a nonsmoker, avoid areas where cigarette smoke is present. Breathing in this smoke increases your risk of developing heart disease, lung cancer, and various respiratory diseases and conditions.

- ☐ If you use tobacco products, you can reduce your risk of developing various cancers, cardiovascular disease, and periodontal disease by quitting.

- ☐ If you are female and smoke cigarettes, you have a higher risk of developing osteoporosis than nonsmoking women. To reduce this risk, stop smoking.

the development of smoking behavior (see the section titled "Psychosocial Reasons for Using Tobacco Products" earlier in this chapter). Today's programs also recognize that a child's social environment is the most important determinant of whether he or she will smoke. Therefore, prevention programs now target seventh and eighth graders, reaching children before most start smoking. Their focus is on help-

**fetal alcohol spectrum disorders (FASDs)** A variety of incurable conditions and birth defects caused by alcohol exposure during prenatal development.

**fetal alcohol syndrome (FAS)** The most severe FASD. Children born with FAS may suffer mental retardation and have characteristic facial anomalies, growth deficiency, and central nervous system abnormalities.

ing young people develop skills to identify and resist social influences to smoke, such as advertising and peer pressure. Additionally, they educate adolescents about the short-term negative effects of tobacco use. Understanding short-term consequences positively affects adolescent behavior more than knowledge of long-term effects. Data show that several types of prevention programs delay or reduce youth tobacco use for periods of 1 to 5 years and more. Effective prevention programs engage the school, parents, and media.

Other programs have been developed that focus on smokeless tobacco use. The goal of these programs is to counter the perception that smokeless tobacco is a safe alternative to smoking cigarettes.

Reducing the availability of cigarettes to adolescents is another prevention measure. Unfortunately, adolescents can get cigarettes quite easily even though the sale of tobacco products to minors is illegal in all states and the District of Columbia. One of the goals of *Healthy People 2020* is to enforce laws that prohibit sales to minors to reduce the percentage of minors who successfully purchase cigarettes to 5%.

## Across THE LIFE SPAN

### THE EFFECTS OF ALCOHOL AND TOBACCO USE

Fetuses and infants are significantly affected by the alcohol and tobacco use of their mothers. Babies of women who consume alcohol while pregnant may be born with certain incurable birth defects caused by alcohol exposure during prenatal development. These disorders range in their severity and effects; the phrase **fetal alcohol spectrum disorders (FASDs)** refers to the entire group of disorders. The various effects seen in FASDs include growth deficiencies, brain dysfunctions, distinctive facial features, and structural birth defects. One of the most severe of these disorders is **fetal alcohol syndrome (FAS)**.

**Figure 8.16**

**Garrison Lee, a Victim of Fetal Alcohol Syndrome, Who Has Lived on the Streets of Gallup, N.M., for 11 Years.** Garrison exhibits features characteristic of FAS: small eye openings, a broad, thin upper lip, and a flattened nose bridge and mid-face.

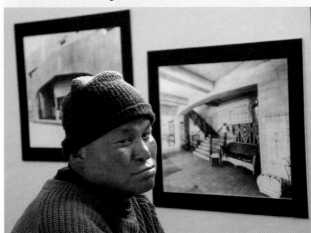

The predominant feature of FAS is brain effects and may include mental retardation. This syndrome is also characterized by slowed growth both before and after birth; other central nervous system defects, such as behavioral problems, and skull or brain malformations; and characteristic facial features that include small eye openings, a broad thin upper lip, and a flattened nose bridge and midface (**Figure 8.16**).

Researchers have not determined an exact relationship between the amount and timing of drinking during pregnancy and the effects on the fetus. Thus, *there is no safe level of alcohol consumption during pregnancy.* Women who are pregnant, who are trying to get pregnant, or who are of childbearing age, sexually active, and not using contraception consistently and well should refrain from drinking to avoid exposing their fetus to alcohol in the womb. In 2009, the prevalence of current alcohol consumption in pregnant women aged 15 to 44 years was 10.0%, and the prevalence of binge drinking was 4.4%. Heavy alcohol use was rare (0.8%).[4]

Maternal smoking during pregnancy can harm not only the fetus, but the pregnant woman as well. Abruptio placentae occurs when the placenta separates from the uterus, resulting in hemorrhage (life-threatening bleeding). (The placenta is an organ shared with the mother through which the fetus obtains nutrients and oxygen, and excretes wastes.) Maternal smoking is associated not only with abruptio placentae but also with placenta previa, in which the placenta implants abnormally and covers the opening of the cervical canal. As this opening dilates at the beginning of the birth process, bleeding and severe hemorrhage can occur.

Smoking during pregnancy also reduces the flow of blood in the placenta, limits the nutrients that reach the fetus, and causes an average reduction in birth weight.[42] Additionally, the fetuses or infants of women who smoke during pregnancy are 25% to 30% more likely to die between 28 weeks of gestation and 4 weeks after birth than those of women who do not smoke. Babies born of mothers who smoke also have a higher than average incidence of death from *sudden infant death syndrome (SIDS)* and from respiratory diseases. The sudden, unexpected death of an apparently healthy infant, SIDS occurs while the baby is sleeping. It is the most common cause of death of children between the ages of 2 weeks and 1 year.

During 2008–2009, the percentage of women who smoked during pregnancy was 15.3%. Pregnant young women 18 to 25 years old had the highest rate of smoking among pregnant women—22.0%.[4]

Another age group of persons strongly affected by alcohol and tobacco use is the elderly. Because older adults are more physically vulnerable to the effects of alcohol, they may develop alcohol problems even though their formerly unproblematic patterns of drinking have not changed. Alcohol also reacts adversely with many medications. Elderly persons taking medications for various conditions may appear to be reacting adversely to their medications rather than experiencing an alcohol problem. Additionally, if alcohol worsens their health, their healthcare providers may prescribe additional or different medications. A vicious cycle of drug interactions and health complications may continue until the healthcare practitioner recognizes that the patient has an alcohol problem.

Older adults face special harm from smoking because most people older than 65 years of age who smoke have been doing so for 30, 40, or 50 years. As a result, a disproportionate number of elderly persons develop life-threatening diseases such as cancer and emphysema because these diseases usually take decades to develop.

Among those older than 65 years, the death rate of current smokers is twice that of people who never smoked. Smoking is associated with a variety of other ailments that are often seen in older adults, such as cataracts (a loss of transparency of the lens of the eye), delayed healing of broken bones, periodontal problems, ulcers, high blood pressure, brain hemorrhages, and skin wrinkles. Additionally, heavy smoking in middle age more than doubles the risk of Alzheimer's disease and other dementias later in life.[43]

From prenatal development to the elderly years, no one who uses alcohol or tobacco products, or breathes in smoke from others' use, can escape their health effects. Except in pregnant women, one drink per day for women and two drinks per day for men may confer health advantages, however.

## Healthy Living Practices

- [ ] Do not consume alcoholic beverages when pregnant because alcohol exposure can result in incurable lifelong disabilities in the fetus.
- [ ] Smoking during pregnancy is associated with serious, and possibly deadly, health effects in both the mother and the fetus.

# Summary

Drinking alcohol and smoking cigarettes are behaviors that often begin in adolescence. Alcohol use is quite prevalent in the United States; 51.9% of Americans use alcohol. Some people use alcohol responsibly, not allowing their drinking to threaten their health or interfere with their relationships. In contrast, the harmful user drinks alcoholic beverages while knowingly damaging his or her health. The alcohol-dependent person, or alcoholic, additionally develops tolerance to the drug, exhibits withdrawal symptoms when not drinking, compulsively uses alcohol, and may exhibit other behaviors that are a part of the alcohol dependence syndrome.

The cause of alcoholism is unknown. However, alcoholism has a genetic (hereditary) component. People abuse alcoholic beverages and become alcohol dependent for psychological, social, and developmental reasons as well.

When a person drinks alcoholic beverages, various behavioral changes that are commonly called intoxication result from impairment of the central nervous system. The harmful use and abuse of alcohol results in multiple effects on the body that are significant threats to health. Excessive alcohol consumption exerts its most dangerous effects on the liver, cardiovascular system, immune system, reproductive system, and brain. Alcohol use and abuse are also related to serious and even fatal injuries.

Approximately 1.5 million Americans were treated for alcohol abuse and dependence in 2009. Alcohol abuse and dependence are often detected by the use of screening tests. Healthcare professionals who determine that their patients are alcohol dependent refer them to substance abuse specialists for evaluation and possibly treatment. Patients who show nondependent problem drinking are often encouraged to participate in brief intervention programs. Self-help groups support the alcoholic on a long-term basis to help prevent relapse into abusive or dependent behaviors.

Cigarettes are the most prevalent type of tobacco product used in the United States today. Approximately 23% of Americans smoked cigarettes regularly in 2009. Most people who smoke cigarettes and use smokeless tobacco began this habit when they were adolescents. Adolescents initially try tobacco products for a variety of reasons: to do what parents or peers do, to experiment, to feel older and more independent, or to join certain social groups. Adolescents most likely to use tobacco have particular characteristics such as low self-esteem, high susceptibility to peer pressure, and a sensation-seeking nature.

Most teenagers and adults continue to smoke and use smokeless tobacco because they are addicted to the psychoactive drug nicotine. Nicotine, like all psychoactive drugs, acts on certain communication points among nerve cells in the brain.

Cigarette smoking is the leading source of preventable illness and death in the United States because many of the 4,000 chemical compounds in cigarette smoke affect the body adversely. Every year, approximately 443,000 people die in the United States as a result of using tobacco products.

Inhaled cigarette smoke affects the airways by damaging the cilia that sweep debris from this region, by causing the airways to secrete excess mucus, and by irritating and inflaming the airways. As a result, smokers suffer chronic cough and are at high risk for a variety of respiratory infections, such as acute and chronic bronchitis and pneumonia. Smoking is also the main cause of emphysema, a condition in which the air sacs of the lungs have lost their usual elasticity so that a person cannot inhale and exhale normally.

Thirty-one percent of people who die from smoking-related causes die from cardiovascular disease. Scientists have found no evidence that smoking low-tar and low-nicotine cigarettes reduces the risk of coronary heart disease.

Cancer is the second-biggest killer of Americans, and tobacco use is responsible for about 30% of cancer deaths annually in the United States. Lung cancer is the most prevalent form of cancer caused by tobacco use. Smokeless tobacco use does not cause lung cancer, but it does cause cancers of the larynx, oral cavity, and esophagus. These cancers are also caused by smoking cigarettes, cigars, and pipes.

People who use tobacco products regularly often develop periodontal disease, which is a disease of the supporting structures of the teeth. Eventually, if periodontal disease is not treated and controlled, the teeth become loose and fall out.

Smoking cigarettes causes a loss of bone density in women. This condition is serious because it places women at risk for bone fractures, back pain, and other accompanying problems.

Environmental tobacco smoke (ETS), the side-stream smoke emitted from a lit cigarette, cigar, or pipe and the smoke exhaled by smokers, can cause lung cancer in adult nonsmokers. Chronic ETS exposure is also a risk factor for cardiovascular disease and heart attack. Additionally, children of parents who smoke have an increased frequency of respiratory symptoms such as coughing and wheezing, and lower respiratory tract infections such as bronchitis and pneumonia.

Seventy-five percent of smokers say they would like to quit smoking. Quitting has major and immediate health benefits for people of all ages.

Cigarette smoking is an addiction, and an addicted smoker who is trying to quit goes through the same process of behavioral change as does anyone addicted to any drug. Quitting is easier if the smoker analyzes why he or she smokes and develops or chooses a method of quitting that addresses these reasons.

Successful smoking-prevention programs reflect an understanding that smoking begins in early adolescence and that a child's social environment is the most important determinant of whether he or she will smoke. Prevention programs help young people develop the skills to identify and resist social influences to smoke.

Fetuses and infants are significantly affected by the alcohol and tobacco use of their mothers. The syndrome of fetal effects from alcohol consumption during pregnancy is called fetal alcohol spectrum disorders (FASDs). One of the most severe of these disorders is fetal alcohol syndrome. Children born with FAS may suffer mental retardation and have characteristic facial anomalies, growth deficiency, and central nervous system abnormalities. Maternal smoking during pregnancy can harm the pregnant woman and her fetus, placing both at risk for developing several serious conditions.

Another age group of persons strongly affected by alcohol and tobacco use is the elderly. Older adults are more physically vulnerable to the effects of alcohol and are more likely to be taking a variety of medications that may interact negatively with alcohol.

Smoking is associated with a variety of ailments in older adults. Among those older than 65 years, the death rate of current smokers is twice that of people who have never smoked.

## Applying What You Have Learned

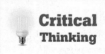
**Critical Thinking**

1. Using the information in this chapter, write a paragraph that would describe what you might say to a friend to discourage him or her from abusing alcohol. **Application**

2. Analyze your reasons for smoking or those of a smoking friend or relative by using the assessment "Why Do You Smoke?" located in the Student Workbook section. Then, list the essential elements of a smoking cessation program for yourself or for that individual. **Synthesis**

3. For the past two decades or so, researchers have viewed alcoholism from a "biomedical" point of view. Many researchers thought that it was only a matter of time before a gene for alcoholism would be found. Recently, many researchers have agreed that biology plays a role in addiction but suggest that biology is only one factor in the development of alcoholism. What other factors are involved? Does Alcoholics Anonymous appear to address this variety of factors in its 12 steps

go.jblearning.com/alters6e

to recovery? State the reasons for your answers. **Evaluation**

4. List all the places where you are regularly exposed to environmental tobacco smoke. Decide

whether you should change any of your activities to reduce your exposure to ETS. State the reasons for your answer. **Evaluation**

**Key**

**Application**
using information in a new situation.

**Synthesis**
putting together information from different sources.

**Evaluation**
making informed decisions.

# Reflecting on Your Health

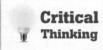

**Critical Thinking**

1. Describe your attitudes toward alcoholics before reading this chapter. Have your attitudes changed after reading this chapter? Why or why not?

2. If you drink alcohol, what motivates your use of this drug? Are you comfortable with your patterns of drinking and reasons for doing so? Why or why not? If you are uncomfortable with your drinking patterns, what can you do to change them?

3. If you were out with friends who were drinking, would you attempt to stop someone from driving who was clearly unfit to get behind the wheel? If not, why not? If so, what strategy might be suc-

cessful? Why do you think this strategy would work?

4. If you are a smoker, what do you do to avoid having others breathe your secondhand smoke? If nothing, what might you do in the future? If you are a nonsmoker, what do you do to avoid breathing others' secondhand smoke? If nothing, what might you do in the future?

5. Do you smoke bidis or clove cigarettes? If so, why did you start smoking these products? After reading the Consumer Health feature in this chapter, do you think you will continue this practice? Why or why not?

# References

1. O'Hegarty, M., et al. (2007, April). Young adults' perceptions of cigarette warning labels in the United States and Canada. *Preventing Chronic Disease, 4*(2):A27. Retrieved on March 22, 2011, from http://www.cdc.gov/pcd/issues/2007/apr/06_0024.htm

2. Pierce, J. P., et al. (2010). Camel No 9 cigarette-marketing campaign targeted young teenage girls. *Pediatrics, 125*(4):619–626.

3. Hanewinkel, R., et al. (2011). Cigarette advertising and teen smoking initiation. *Pediatrics, 127*(2):e271–e278.

4. Substance Abuse and Mental Health Services Administration. (2010). *Results from the 2009 National Survey on Drug Use and Health: Vol. I. Summary of National Findings* (HHS Publication No. SMA 10-4586Findings). Retrieved on March 16, 2011, from http://oas.samhsa.gov/NSDUH/2k9NSDUH/2k9ResultsP.pdf

5. Centers for Disease Control and Prevention. (2010, October 5). Vital signs: Binge drinking among high school students and adults—United States, 2009. *Morbidity and Mortality Weekly Report, 59*:1–6.

6. van der Zwaluw, C. S., & Engels, R. C. M. E. (2009). Gene–environ-

ment interactions and alcohol use and dependence: Current status and future challenges. *Addiction, 104*:907–914.

7. Enoch, M. A. (2006). Genetic and environmental influences on the development of alcoholism: Resilience vs. risk. *Annals of the New York Academy of Sciences, 1094*:193–201.

8. Wechsler, H., & Nelson, T. F. (2008). What we have learned from the Harvard School of Public Health College Alcohol Study: Focusing attention on college student alcohol consumption and the environmental conditions that promote it. *Journal of Studies on Alcohol and Drugs, 69*:481–490.

9. Turrisi, R., et al. (2006). Heavy drinking in college students: Who is at risk and what is being done about it? *Journal of General Psychology, 133*:401–420.

10. Wechsler, H., et al. (2002). Trends in college binge drinking during a period of increased prevention efforts: Findings from 4 Harvard School of Public Health college alcohol study surveys: 1993–2001. *Journal of American College Health, 50*:203–217.

11. Ahern, N. R., & Sole, M. L. (2010). Drinking games and college students part 1: Problem description. *Journal of Psychosocial Nursing, 48*(2):17–20.

12. Hingson, R. W., et al. (2009, July). Magnitude of and trend in alcohol-related mortality and morbidity among U.S. college students ages 18–24, 1998–2005. *Journal of Studies on Alcohol and Drugs* (Suppl 16):12–20.

13. Addolorato, G., et al. (2006). Understanding and treating patients with alcoholic cirrhosis: An update. *Alcoholism: Clinical and Experimental Research, 33*(7):1136–1144.

14. Klatsy, A. L. (2010). Alcohol and cardiovascular health. *Physiology and Behavior, 100*(1):76–81.

15. Khan, N., et al. (2010). Lifestyle as risk factor for cancer: Evidence from human studies. *Cancer Letters, 293*(2):133–143.

16. Zhang, S. M., et al. (2007). Alcohol consumption and breast cancer risk in the Women's Health Study. *American Journal of Epidemiology, 165*:667–676.

17. Li, Y., et al. (2009). Wine, liquor, beer and risk of breast cancer in a large population. *European Journal of Cancer, 45*(5):843–850.

18. National Highway Transportation Safety Administration. (2010). *Traffic safety facts: Alcohol-impaired driving, 2009 Data* (U.S. Department of Transportation, DOT HS 811 385). Retrieved on March 24, 2011, from http://www-nrd.nhtsa.dot.gov/Pubs/811385.pdf

19. Kochanek, K. D., et al. (2011). Deaths: Preliminary data for 2009. *National Vital Statistics Reports, 59*(4):1–68. Retrieved on March 24, 2011, from http://www.cdc.gov/nchs/data/nvsr/nvsr59/nvsr59_04.pdf

20. National Highway Transportation Safety Administration. (2011). *Traffic safety facts 2009* (U.S. Department of Transportation DOT HS 811 402). Retrieved on March 24, 2011, from http://www-nrd.nhtsa.dot.gov/Pubs/811402EE.pdf

21. Mumenthaler, M. S., et al. (2003). Psychoactive drugs and pilot performance: A comparison of nicotine, donepezil, and alcohol effects. *Neuropsychopharmacology, 28*:1366–1373.

22. Chaturvedi, A. K., et al. (2005). Toxicological findings from 1587 civil aviation accident pilot fatalities, 1999–2003. *Aviation, Space, and Environmental Medicine, 76*(12):1145–1150.

23. Driscoll, T. R., et al. (2004). Review of the role of alcohol in drowning associated with recreational aquatic activity. *Injury Prevention, 10*(2):107–113.

24. Wagenaar, A. C., & Toomey, T. L. (2010). The effects of minimum legal drinking age 21 laws on alcohol-related driving in the United States. *Journal of Safety Research, 41*(2):173–181.

25. U.S. Department of Health and Human Services. (2007). *The Surgeon General's call to action to prevent and reduce underage drinking.* Atlanta, GA: Author.

26. Johnston, L. D., et al. (2010). *Monitoring the future: National survey results on drug use, 1975–2009: Volume 1, secondary school students* (NIH Publication No. 10-7584). Bethesda, MD: National Institute on Drug Abuse. Retrieved on March 17, 2011, from http://www.monitoringthefuture.org/pubs/monographs/vol1_2009.pdf

27. Centers for Disease Control and Prevention. (2010). Youth risk behavior surveillance—United States, 2009. *Morbidity and Mortality Weekly Report, 59*(SS-5). Retrieved April 3, 2011, from http://www.cdc.gov/mmwr/pdf/ss/ss5905.pdf

28. U.S. Department of Health and Human Services. (2010). *How tobacco smoke causes disease: The biology and behavioral basis for smoking-attributable disease: A report of the Surgeon General.* Atlanta, GA: Author. Retrieved on April 3, 2011, from http://www.surgeongeneral.gov/library/tobaccosmoke/report/full_report.pdf

29. American Lung Association. (2011). *Chronic obstructive pulmonary disease (COPD) fact sheet.* Retrieved on April 3, 2011, from http://www.lungusa.org/lung-disease/copd/resources/facts-figures/COPD-Fact-Sheet.html

30. American Heart Association. (2011). *Smoking and cardiovascular disease.* Retrieved on April 3, 2011, from http://www.heart.org/HEARTORG/GettingHealthy/QuitSmoking/QuittingResources/Smoking-Cardiovascular-Disease_UCM_305187_Article.jsp

31. American Cancer Society. (2010). *Cancer facts and figures 2010.* Atlanta, GA: Author. Retrieved on April 3, 2011, from http://www.cancer.org/acs/groups/content/@epidemiologysurveilance/documents/document/acspc-026238.pdf

32. International Osteoporosis Foundation. (2010). Facts and statistics about osteoporosis and its impact. Retrieved on April 3, 2011, from http://www.iofbonehealth.org/facts-and-statistics.html#factsheet-category-16

33. Centers for Disease Control and Prevention. (1986). *The health consequences of involuntary smoking—a report of the Surgeon General* (DHHS Publication No. [CDC] 87–8398). Rockville, MD: U.S. Department of Health and Human Services, Public Health Service.

34. National Research Council. (1986). *Environmental tobacco smoke: Measuring exposure and assessing health effects.* Washington, DC: National Academy Press.

35. U.S. Department of Health and Human Services. (2006). *The health consequences of involuntary exposure to tobacco smoke: A report of the Surgeon General.* Atlanta, GA: Author.

36. Farrelly, M. C., Evans, W. N., & Sfekas, A. E. (1999). Impact of workplace smoking bans: Results from a national survey. *Tobacco Control, 8*:272–277.

37. Gallup Organization. (2010). Tobacco and smoking. Retrieved on April 3, 2009, from http://www.gallup.com/poll/1717/Tobacco-Smoking.aspx

38. McNeil, J. J., et al. (2010). Smoking cessation—recent advances. *Cardiovascular Drugs and Therapy, 24*(4): 359–367.

39. U.S. Food and Drug Administration. (2010, September 9). FDA acts against 5 electronic cigarette distributors. Retrieved on April 4, 2011, from http://www.fda.gov/NewsEvents/Newsroom/PressAnnouncements/2010/ucm225224.htm

40. U.S. Food and Drug Administration. (2010, September 9). E-Cigarettes: Questions and answers. Retrieved on April 4, 2011, from http://www.fda.gov/ForConsumers/ConsumerUpdates/ucm225210.htm

41. American Cancer Society. (2011). When smokers quit—what are the benefits over time? Retrieved on April 4, 2011, from http://www.cancer.org/healthy/stayawayfromtobacco/guidetoquittingsmoking/guide-to-quitting-smoking-benefits

42. Andersen, M. R., et al. (2009). Smoking cessation early in pregnancy and birth weight, length, head circumference, and endothelial nitric oxide synthase activity in umbilical and chorionic vessels: An observational study of healthy singleton pregnancies. *Circulation, 119*:857–864.

43. Rusanen, M., et al. (2011). Heavy smoking in midlife and long-term risk of Alzheimer disease and vascular dementia. *Archives of Internal Medicine, 171*(4):333–339.

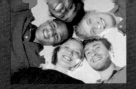
**Diversity in Health**
Asian American Food

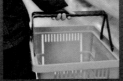
**Consumer Health**
Dietary Supplements

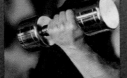
**Managing Your Health**
Trimming Unhealthy Fats
from Your Diet

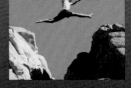
**Across the Life Span**
Nutrition

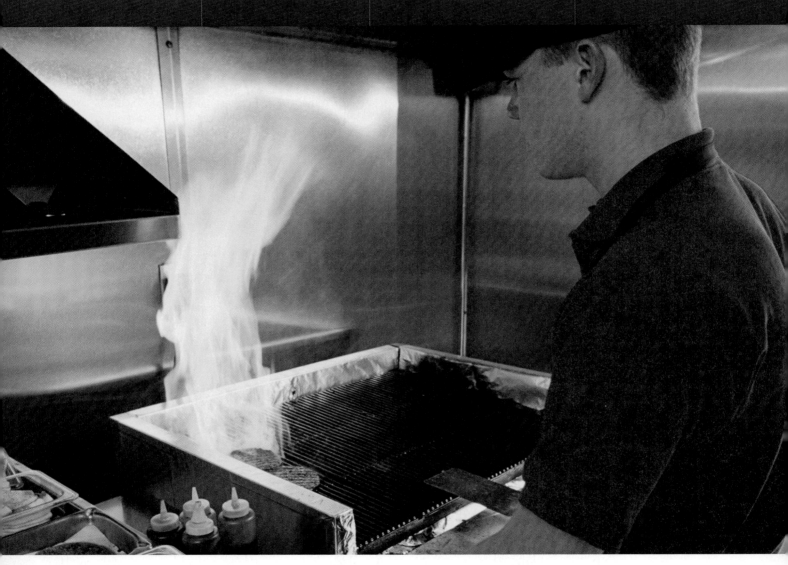

# Chapter Overview

The basic principles of nutrition

How your body digests and uses the food you eat

The functions and sources of nutrients

How to plan a nutritious diet

How malnutrition affects health

# Student Workbook

Self-Assessment: Assessing the Nutritional Quality of Your
Diet | Diabetes Risk Test | Using MyPlate

Changing Health Habits: Are You Ready to Improve Your
Diet?

# Do You Know?

Which foods might help prevent cancer?

How to judge the nutritional adequacy of your diet?

If any vitamins are poisonous?

## CHAPTER 9

# Nutrition

**H**amburger, cola, french fries, pizza, potato chips, tofu, yogurt, olive oil, nonfat milk, mango, and wheat germ—which of these foods do you eat regularly? Have you eaten chutney, trifle, black beans, calamari, sushi, or hummus? How often do you buy soft drinks and snacks from vending machines? During the past week, how many times did you eat at fast-food restaurants? Why do you eat certain foods and not others? Before deciding what to eat, do you consider the nutritional value of food? When asked if they care about what they eat, three students who were enrolled in a college health class responded as follows:

*Do I care about what I eat? Well, it depends on how hungry I am. If I am hungry enough, I'll eat anything, except some processed meats. I don't care about the amount of fat, calories, or nutritional value in foods. All I care about is how much the food costs and how much it takes to fill me up. I'm young and healthy and have hardly any body fat—I've been eating greasy, cheap, fast foods for years.*

*I care about what I eat, but my diet doesn't show it. When I wake up, I don't have time to eat. After class I eat burritos or pizza rolls before going to work. After work, I usually stop at a fast-food place. ... I eat lots of french*

> ## "Which of these foods do you eat regularly?"

**diet** One's usual pattern of food choices.

*fries. I do want to eat better, but it's hard when you're always on the go.*

*I'm not concerned about what I eat. People call me the "fast-food queen" because that's all I eat. I know fast food is not always healthy, but I'm going to school full-time and working. It's hard finding time to buy food and cook it.*

If you are like these students, taste, cost, and convenience are the most important factors that influence your food choices. You may not be aware, however, that many other factors, including food advertising and moods, can also influence your diet. Although people usually associate **diet** with losing weight, the term actually refers to one's usual pattern of food choices. A healthful diet provides substances that are necessary for life, but most people do not eat simply to satisfy their nutritional needs.

Your diet reflects not only your food likes and dislikes but also your lifestyle, financial status, and educational, cultural, religious, and ethnic backgrounds. Additionally, certain foods have social significance. When you watch a major sports event at a friend's apartment with a group of people, do you help share the cost of pizzas that are delivered?

Some foods have personal emotional meanings. People often use such foods, especially sweets, to lift their mood when they are feeling sad or distressed.

Do you head for the kitchen not because you are hungry, but because you are bored or lonely? At other times, do you reward yourself for achieving a desired goal by eating a favorite food? Eating food to feel better, substitute for social activity, or reward yourself can result in a nutritionally inadequate diet and unwanted weight gain.

For many young adults, selecting a nutritionally inadequate diet has a major effect on their current and future health. Poor diet can reduce the effectiveness of the *immune system*, the body's defense against many acute illnesses, including the common cold and other infectious diseases. Poor food choices can result in *anemia*, a group of conditions characterized by an insufficient number of properly formed red blood cells. People who have anemia lack the energy to carry out their normal activities and exercise without tiring easily. For women, unhealthy diets can increase the risk of having a baby born too early or with birth defects. Poor diet is also a major risk factor for serious chronic diseases that are the major killers of Americans: cardiovascular disease (*CVD*), which includes heart disease and stroke; diabetes; obesity; Alzheimer's disease; kidney disease; and possibly, certain cancers (**Figure 9.1**). Sensible lifelong eating and physical activity habits play important roles in maintaining good health and preventing these chronic diseases. By making specific dietary changes, people can improve their chances of enjoying good health now and later in life.

This chapter highlights the nutrients, their major food sources and roles in the body, and the benefits

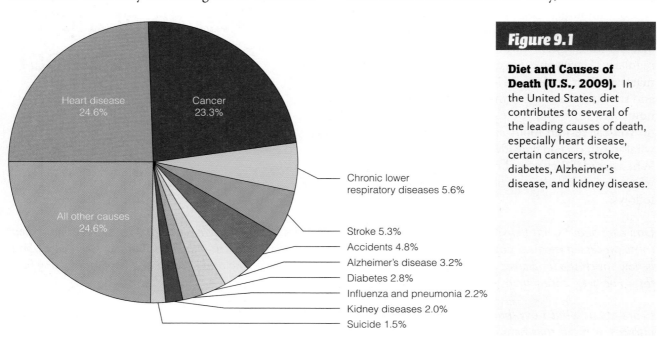

Chronic lower
respiratory diseases 5.6%

Stroke 5.3%

Accidents 4.8%

Alzheimer's disease 3.2%

Diabetes 2.8%

Influenza and pneumonia 2.2%

Kidney diseases 2.0%

Suicide 1.5%

### Figure 9.1

**Diet and Causes of Death (U.S., 2009).** In the United States, diet contributes to several of the leading causes of death, especially heart disease, certain cancers, stroke, diabetes, Alzheimer's disease, and kidney disease.

of choosing a nutritious diet. The information in this chapter will help you evaluate the nutritional adequacy of your diet and plan nutritious menus.

## Basic Nutrition Principles

### What Are Nutrients?

Nutrition is the study of the way the body processes and uses **nutrients**, substances in food that are needed for growth, repair, and maintenance of cells. In addition to these functions, some nutrients regulate cellular activity or supply energy. **Table 9.1** lists the six classes of nutrients, describes some of their roles in the body, and identifies their major food sources. In general, carbohydrates and fats supply energy; vitamins and minerals participate in chemical reactions that regulate body processes; and proteins provide the material for tissue (cellular) growth,

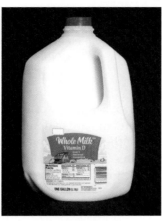

Vitamin-D fortified milk.

repair, and maintenance. Water transports materials in the body and also participates in numerous chemical reactions.

The human body can *synthesize* (produce) certain nutrients. For example, exposing skin to sunlight enables the body to make vitamin D. Other nutrients are essential; that is, the diet must supply nutrients that the body does not make or does not make in the amounts needed for good health. Nutritional deficiency diseases can develop when diets contain inadequate amounts of essential nutrients. These diseases are uncommon in the United States because we have a wide variety of foods available to eat. Additionally, many commonly eaten foods and certain beverages are *enriched* or *fortified* with vitamins and minerals. Enriched bread, for example, has iron and certain B vitamins added to it. Milk is usually forti-

## Table 9.1

### The Six Classes of Nutrients

| Nutrient Class | Major Roles in the Body | Rich Food Sources |
|---|---|---|
| Carbohydrates | Energy | Grain products, beans, vegetables, fruits, honey, sugar-sweetened soft drinks, and candy |
| Lipids | Triglycerides: energy<br><br>Cholesterol: most steroid hormones, bile production, skin maintenance, vitamin D synthesis, and nerve function | Vegetable oils, nuts, margarines, fatty meats, cheeses, cream, butter, and fried foods |
| Proteins | Growth, repair, and maintenance of all cells; production of enzymes, antibodies, and certain hormones | Dried beans, peas, nuts, soy products, meats, shellfish, fish, poultry, eggs, and dairy products (except cream and butter) |
| Vitamins | Metabolism, reproduction, development, and growth | Widespread in foods: nuts, beans, peas, fruits and vegetables, whole grains, meats, enriched breads and cereals, fortified milk |
| Minerals | Metabolism, development, and growth | Widespread in foods: nuts and whole grains; meats, fish, and poultry; dairy products; vegetables and fruits; enriched breads and cereals |
| Water | Essential for life: many chemical reactions require water; it helps maintain normal body temperature, and dissolves and transports nutrients | Water, nonalcoholic and caffeine-free beverages, fruits, vegetables, and milk (nearly every food contributes water to the diet) |

**phytochemicals** A group of nonnutrients that are produced by plants and may have beneficial effects on the body.

**antioxidants** Compounds that protect cells from free-radical damage.

**probiotics** Microorganisms that may provide healthful benefits when consumed

**digestion** The process of breaking down large food molecules into smaller molecules that the intestinal tract can absorb.

fied with vitamins A and D, and you can purchase orange juiced that has been fortified with calcium.

## What Are Nonnutrients?

Some foods contain substances that you can live without. Many of these *nonnutrients* are naturally found in plants and have beneficial effects on the body. Other nonnutrient substances, such as pesticide residues or lead, enter food unintentionally and can be hazardous to health.

Plants produce **phytochemicals**, a large group of nonnutrients that may provide health benefits. Many phytochemicals, including betacarotene, lutein, and anthocyanin, are antioxidants. **Antioxidants** prevent or reduce the formation of *free radicals*, unstable and highly reactive atoms or compounds that can cause cellular damage. Such damage may contribute to heart disease, certain cancers, and the aging process. There is no scientific evidence, however, that people benefit from taking pills that contain phytochemicals.

Therefore, nutrition experts recommend that people eat a variety of fruits, vegetables, and whole grains daily to obtain a natural array of these substances. Dark green, yellow, orange, red, and purple fruits and vegetables tend to have the most antioxidant phytochemicals, so let color be your key to selecting the richest food sources of antioxidants (**Figure 9.2**). **Table 9.2** lists some phytochemicals as well as their food sources and possible effects on the body.

## Natural, Health, Organic, and Functional Foods

Food manufacturers can label their products as *natural* if they are minimally processed and contain no artificial additives such as synthetic colors or flavors. So-called natural foods are not necessarily more nutritious than foods that do not carry this description. Many consumers think natural foods such as honey, herbal teas, and cider vinegar are *health foods* because they have medicinal benefits. Although these foods provide nutrients, there is little or no scientific evidence to support claims that they prevent or treat various health conditions. Regardless of whether it is natural or manufactured, a "healthy" food contributes to your nutrient needs and is safe to eat. Herbs, for example, may contain beneficial phytochemicals, but some are natural sources of toxic substances and should be avoided.

Food producers can label their fruits, vegetables, and meat and poultry products as *organic* if they meet certain standards. Fruits and vegetables, for example, must be grown without the use of synthetic pesticides and fertilizers. Advertisers sometimes refer to their products as organic to imply that these items are superior. Although organically grown foods may contain less pesticide residue, they are not more nutritious than similar foods that have been grown using conventional farming methods. Chemists classify compounds as organic if they contain carbon. Carbohydrates, fats, proteins, and vitamins contain carbon; therefore, they are organic compounds. Because most foods naturally consist of these nutrients, all foods are organic.

Functional foods, sometimes called *nutraceuticals*, are manufactured with ingredients that have scientifically established medicinal benefits. A person must eat a certain amount of these foods

**Figure 9.2**

**Color Palette for Good Health.** Add colorful fruits and vegetables to your meals and snacks to boost your intake of antioxidant phytochemicals.

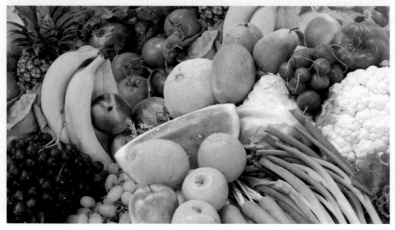

## Table 9.2

### Phytochemicals

| Phytochemicals | Major Plant Sources | Possible Disease-Fighting Properties |
|---|---|---|
| Allium | Garlic, onions, leeks | Enhances immune function; may reduce risk of certain cancers |
| Indoles, isothiocyanates (includes sulforaphane) | Broccoli, cabbage, watercress, kale, cauliflower, bok choy, collard and mustard greens, brussels sprouts | May inhibit cancer tumor growth |
| Ellargic acid | Nuts (especially walnuts), grapes, apples, berries | Has antioxidant activity; may inhibit tumor growth |
| Flavonoids (includes anthocyanin) | Soy products, apples, artichokes, red grapes and wines, tea, onions, berries, red cabbage | Have antioxidant activity; may reduce risk of heart disease and certain cancers |
| Polyphenols | Black and green tea, red wine | Inhibit tumor growth; may reduce risk of heart disease |
| Monoterpenes | Citrus peel oils, citrus fruits, cherries | Anticancer agents |
| Carotenoids (includes beta-carotene, lutein, and lycopene) | Dark orange, yellow, and green fruits and vegetables; tomatoes | May reduce risk of cancer, but more research is needed |
| Phytic acid | Whole wheat (bran and germ) | May reduce risk of certain cancers and heart disease |

*Sources:* Dietary flavonoids and risk of coronary heart disease. (1994). *Nutrition Reviews, 52*(2):59–68; Marwick, C. (1995). Learning how phytochemicals help fight disease. *Journal of the American Medical Association, 274*:1328–1330; A garden of phytochemicals. (1995). *University of California of Berkeley Wellness Letter, 12*(1):6–7.

regularly to obtain the desired effects. For example, a phytochemical that can lower blood cholesterol levels has been added to certain margarines and salad dressings. In the future, a variety of other specially formulated foods with health benefits will be available in supermarkets, including those that reduce the appetite or risk of heart disease.

**Probiotics** are live bacteria that may benefit health. Many different kinds of bacteria naturally reside in the large intestine. If certain bacteria overpopulate this region, diarrhea and serious infections can result.

Eating foods that contain certain kinds of microbes (*probiotics*) regularly may help maintain or regain the normal balance of bacteria in the large intestine. Some brands of yogurt contain probiotics. *Prebiotics* are substances in certain foods that support probiotics.

## What Happens to the Food You Eat?

Humans eat a wide variety of plants, animals, and animal products to obtain nutrients and other beneficial substances. In their natural state, many nutrients are in complex forms that the body cannot use. During the process of **digestion**, the gastrointestinal tract (diges-

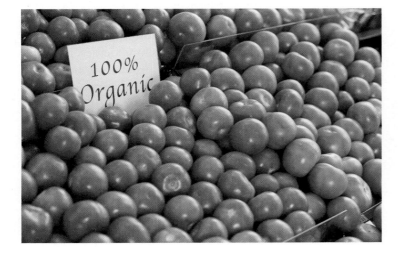

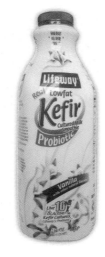

tive system) breaks down complex food substances into nutrients (**Figure 9.3**). Various *enzymes*, compounds that speed up chemical changes, participate in the process of digestion.

**Absorption** is the passage of nutrients through the walls of the intestinal tract and eventually into the blood. After nutrients enter the bloodstream, many are transported to the liver, where they are processed or stored.

By the time any remaining food material enters the colon (the major segment of the large intestine), most of its nutrients have been absorbed. This residue, which makes up some of the *feces* or *stool*, remains in the rectum until the individual has a bowel movement to eliminate the waste. The entire process

of digesting the food, absorbing its nutrients, and eliminating fecal residue generally takes about 1 to 3 days.

The kidneys play an important role in maintaining the body's normal nutrient levels by filtering excess *water-soluble* nutrients from the blood so that they can be eliminated in the urine. A water-soluble nutrient dissolves in water. Many nutrients, such as proteins, B vitamins, and vitamin C, are water-soluble. *Fat-soluble* nutrients such as cholesterol and vitamin A do not dissolve in water, and the kidneys cannot eliminate them easily. Fat-soluble nutrients generally circulate until the liver or fat cells remove them for storage.

Nutrient toxicities occur when the body cannot use or store excess nutrients, especially minerals and fat-soluble vitamins. For example, signs of vitamin A toxicity include nausea, vomiting, headaches, bone pain, hair loss, liver damage, birth defects, and, even, death (see Table 9.7 later in this chapter). People rarely eat enough food to obtain excessive amounts of nutrients. Nutrient toxicities, however, are more likely to occur from taking too many pills (*dietary supplements*) that contain the substances.

**Energy from Foods Metabolism** refers to all of the chemical reactions that take place in the body. These reactions are necessary to power muscular movements, synthesize and repair tissues, release and use energy, and produce enzymes and hormones. To carry out metabolic activities, cells need the energy stored in fat, certain

## Figure 9.3

**The Digestive System.** The stomach and small intestine break down large compounds in foods into smaller molecules that can be absorbed through the intestinal walls.

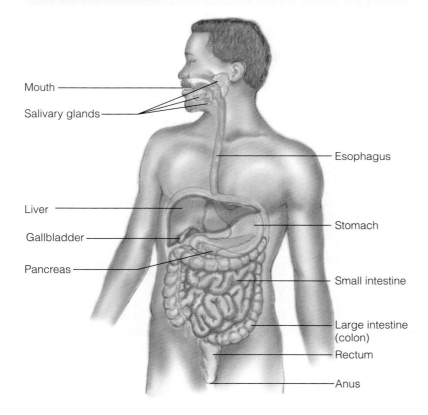

Mouth

Salivary glands

Esophagus

Liver

Gallbladder

Pancreas

Stomach

Small intestine

Large intestine (colon)

Rectum

Anus

carbohydrates, and to a small extent, protein. Oxygen, which enters the body from the lungs, is needed to release the stored energy. This energy powers cell activities and helps maintain body temperature.

The amount of energy in foods is expressed as a number of *kilocalories*, commonly referred to as "calories." A **calorie** is a unit of energy. Foods containing carbohydrates, fats, proteins, and the nonnutrient alcohol provide calories. Proteins and most carbohydrates supply 4 calories per gram, alcohol provides 7 calories per gram, and fat provides 9 calories per gram. The body cannot extract energy from water, vitamins, and minerals; therefore, these nutrients do not provide calories. The following sections provide some basic information about the six major classes of nutrients.

# Energy-Supplying Nutrients

## Carbohydrates

**Carbohydrates** include sugars and starches. The simplest carbohydrates are sugars called *monosaccharides* and *disaccharides*. *Glucose*, *fructose* (fruit sugar), *sucrose* (table sugar), and *lactose* (milk sugar) are the major simple sugars in our diets. Fruits, vegetables, milk, and honey are naturally rich sources of simple sugars.

*Starches* are complex carbohydrates that contain hundreds of glucose molecules. Grains, beans, and certain vegetables such as potatoes are rich sources of starch. Plant foods supply most of the carbohydrates in the diet. Except for honey and milk, most animal foods do not contain carbohydrates.

During digestion, the large starch molecules are broken down to release glucose molecules, and sucrose molecules are broken down to release glucose and fructose molecules. The small intestine absorbs these monosaccharides, and the liver converts much of the fructose to glucose. Eventually, the glucose molecules enter the bloodstream and can be used by cells.

**Glucose**, commonly referred to as "blood sugar," is the most important monosaccharide in the human body. All cells, especially nerves, metabolize glucose for energy. A healthy body carefully maintains a normal blood glucose level.

Plants make lignin and certain carbohydrates that the human small intestine cannot digest. This material is called **dietary fiber**, or simply fiber. Soluble forms of fiber swell or dissolve in water; insoluble forms remain relatively unchanged in water. Apples, bananas, citrus fruits, carrots, kidney beans, psyllium seeds, and oats are rich sources of *soluble fiber*. Brown rice, wheat bran, and whole-grain wheat products are rich sources of *insoluble fiber*. Plants usually contain mixtures of these forms of fiber. *Table 9.3* lists fiber-rich foods; note that none are from animal sources.

In the United States, carbohydrates constitute about 44% to 47% of the typical person's caloric intake. Many nutrition experts think Americans should increase their total carbohydrate intake to 65% of calories, primarily from starchy high-fiber foods. Recommendations for simple carbohydrate intake range from 10% to 25% of calories. Foods that contain high amounts of the simple carbohydrates sucrose and an-

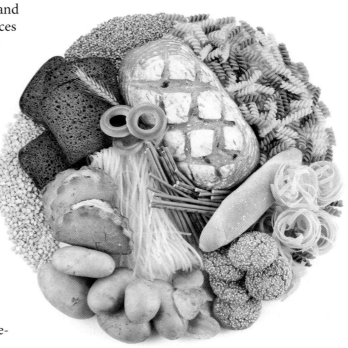

## Table 9.3

### Fiber-Rich Foods

| | |
|---|---|
| Whole-grain products | Whole-wheat flour, high-fiber wheat bran cereals, psyllium,* oat bran,* oatmeal,* brown rice, whole-grain crackers, buckwheat groats, barley,* wheat germ |
| Dried beans and peas | Lentils, pinto beans, lima beans, kidney beans,*navy beans, split peas |
| Fruits | Bananas,* berries, oranges,* figs, grapefruits,* fruits with edible peels (e.g., apples,* peaches, pears) |
| Vegetables | Vegetables with edible peels (e.g., potatoes), brussels sprouts, broccoli, okra, cabbage, peas, turnips, spinach, sweet potatoes, carrots* |

*Rich source of soluble fiber.

## Table 9.4

### Other Names for Sugars

| |
|---|
| Sucrose |
| Table sugar, raw sugar, turbinado sugar |
| Granulated cane juice or evaporated cane juice |
| Confectioner's or powdered sugar |
| Brown sugar |
| Invert sugar |
| Maple syrup |
| Molasses or blackstrap molasses |
| Honey |
| Date sugar |
| Corn syrup, cultured corn syrup, or high-fructose corn syrup |
| Fruit sugar |
| Levulose |
| Fruit juice concentrate |
| Concentrated fruit juice sweetener |
| Glucose or dextrose |
| Polydextrose |
| Maltose |
| Maltodextrin |

other form of sugar called high fructose corn syrup (HFCS) are often poor sources of vitamins and minerals. Thus, eating a lot of sugary foods can displace more nutritious foods from a person's diet. It can be difficult to identify sugars in foods by the ingredients listed on the label. **Table 9.4** lists names for various sugars.

Most nutrition experts recommend that Americans reduce their intake of sucrose and high fructose corn syrup by consuming fewer regular soft drinks, candies, and bakery items. Sugar substitutes such as rebaudiana (a form of stevia), aspartame (Nutrasweet), sucralose, and saccharin are available in packets for consumers to use. Food manufacturers may also use sugar substitutes to sweeten sugar-free gums, candies, and diet soft drinks. When consumed in normal amounts by healthy people, these sweeteners are safe and contribute few or no calories to diets.[1]

**Carbohydrates and Health** According to the U.S. Department of Agriculture (USDA), each American consumed about 64 pounds of sucrose and other caloric sweeteners in 2009.[2] High fructose corn syrup (HFCS) and sucrose are the primary caloric sweeteners in soft drinks, candies, desserts, and many processed foods. These simple carbohydrates are blamed for numerous health problems, including diabetes, hyperactivity, mental illness, and criminal behavior. Does scientific evidence support these claims?

Despite popular beliefs, there is no scientific evidence that sucrose or other sugars cause or contribute to hyperactivity, mental illness, or criminal behavior. Sucrose cannot be absorbed by the intestinal tract. During digestion, the sugar is broken down into glucose and fructose, which are sources of energy for the body.

The only disorder clearly associated with carbohydrate consumption is tooth decay. Carbohydrates can stick to teeth, providing food for bacteria in the mouth. As the bacteria metabolize carbohydrates, they produce acids that destroy the enamel of teeth, and decay results. Good oral hygiene practices, including brushing and flossing after meals and snacks, can reduce the risk of dental decay.

Some people avoid eating table sugar, which is made from sugar beets or sugar cane, but will use honey as a sweetener because they think it is more "natural" and nutritious than sugar. Although honey contains very small amounts of phytochemicals,

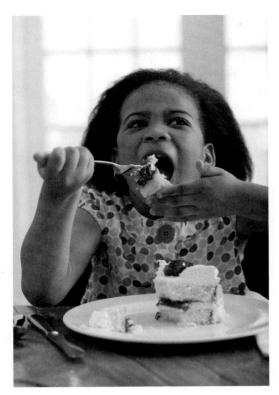

Contrary to popular myth, eating sugar does not make children hyperactive.

it has essentially the same nutritional value as other sugars.

Honey should not be added to baby foods because it may contain spores of *Clostridium botulinum*, a bacterium that produces a dangerous toxin. This toxin affects nerves, causing loss of muscle functioning, which can be life threatening when it impairs breathing. Infants who eat contaminated honey are at risk of developing infantile botulism because their stomachs do not produce enough acid to kill the bacterial spores. Children older than 1 year and adults produce sufficient amounts of stomach acid, so they can eat honey safely.

*Diabetes Mellitus* **Diabetes mellitus**, often simply called diabetes, is a group of chronic diseases characterized by an inability to metabolize carbohydrates properly. This abnormality also affects metabolism of proteins and fats. A person with diabetes produces no insulin or insufficient amounts of insulin or has cells that do not respond normally to insulin. *Insulin*, a hormone that is produced in the pancreas (see Figure 9.3), helps glucose enter cells. Without the normal action of insulin, the cells cannot carry out their metabolic activities properly, and glucose builds up in the blood. High blood glucose levels can lead to

serious chronic health disorders, including hypertension, loss of vision, and nerve damage. In the United States, poorly controlled diabetes is a major cause of kidney failure, blindness, and lower limb amputations. Furthermore, having diabetes greatly increases one's risk of heart disease and stroke. Each year, thousands of people die as a result of diabetes. In 2009, diabetes was the seventh leading cause of death in the United States.[3]

In 2010, nearly 26 million Americans had diabetes; 7 million of these people were unaware that they had the disease.[4] The two most prevalent forms of diabetes are *type 1 diabetes* and *type 2 diabetes*. Most people with diabetes have type 2. **Table 9.5** lists the common signs and symptoms of each type.

Type 1 diabetes is caused by an inappropriate immune system response to an infection (autoimmune disease) that damages the cells of the pancreas that make insulin. People with this condition require daily injections of insulin because the pancreas does not produce the hormone. Some people with type 1

### Table 9.5

### Common Signs and Symptoms of Diabetes Mellitus

**Type 1 Diabetes**

(Generally develops in childhood and young adulthood)

- Lack of energy
- Listlessness
- Frequent urination
- Excessive thirst
- "Fruity" odor in breath
- Increased appetite with weight loss
- Vision problems

**Type 2 Diabetes**

Usually few symptoms, but when they exist:

- Excessive thirst
- Frequent urination
- Vision problems
- In women, recurrent vaginal infections
- Skin sores that do not heal

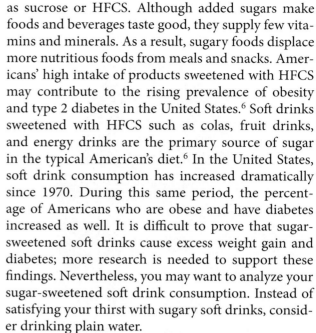

diabetes wear a small device that pumps insulin into their bodies. Although type 1 diabetes is often called juvenile diabetes, the label is misleading because type 1 can strike at any age. The majority of cases, however, are diagnosed in childhood.

People with type 2 diabetes are usually older than 40 years and have excess body fat (*obesity*) and a family history of diabetes. Since 1997, the prevalence of type 2 diabetes has increased dramatically in the United States, particularly among black and Hispanic Americans.[5] Moreover, this form of the disease is becoming more common among children and adolescents, as rates of obesity increase among younger members of the population.

Obesity contributes to type 2 diabetes, especially when one has a family history of the disorder. In many instances, people with type 2 diabetes can improve their blood glucose levels by losing their excess body fat. Regular physical activity can also reduce high blood glucose levels, and adopting a physically active lifestyle helps people achieve and maintain healthy body weights.

Poor diet also contributes to the development of type 2 diabetes. When too much glucose enters the bloodstream after a high-carbohydrate snack or meal, the pancreas may respond by releasing an excess of insulin. High blood insulin levels may increase the risk of heart disease, obesity, and type 2 diabetes. Scientists have measured the intestinal absorption rates of many commonly eaten carbohydrate-rich foods and assigned *glycemic index* (*GI*) values to them. Foods with high GIs (over 70), such as white, short-grained rice, increase blood glucose levels more than foods with low GIs (under 55), such as kidney beans. People may reduce their risk of type 2 diabetes by eating diets that contain more low-GI than high-GI foods. Among nutrition experts, however, the contribution of a high-GI diet to the development of type 2 diabetes is controversial.

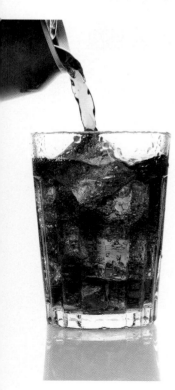

Poor diets often contain high amounts of *added sugars*, such as sucrose or HFCS. Although added sugars make foods and beverages taste good, they supply few vitamins and minerals. As a result, sugary foods displace more nutritious foods from meals and snacks. Americans' high intake of products sweetened with HFCS may contribute to the rising prevalence of obesity and type 2 diabetes in the United States.[6] Soft drinks sweetened with HFCS such as colas, fruit drinks, and energy drinks are the primary source of sugar in the typical American's diet.[6] In the United States, soft drink consumption has increased dramatically since 1970. During this same period, the percentage of Americans who are obese and have diabetes increased as well. It is difficult to prove that sugar-sweetened soft drinks cause excess weight gain and diabetes; more research is needed to support these findings. Nevertheless, you may want to analyze your sugar-sweetened soft drink consumption. Instead of satisfying your thirst with sugary soft drinks, consider drinking plain water.

Type 2 diabetes can often be controlled by dietary modifications and regular exercise. Many affected persons, however, need to take medications, some of which increase the production of insulin by the pancreas. Some people with type 2 diabetes need daily insulin injections. By carefully controlling their blood sugar levels through diet, exercise, and, if necessary, medication, people with diabetes can often lessen the long-term damaging effects of the disease.

You may be able to reduce your risk of type 2 diabetes by losing excess weight and increasing physical activity.[7] It is also important to have routine health checkups that include diabetes testing because many people with type 2 diabetes are not aware that they have the disorder. You may want to take the diabetes quiz in the Student Workbook at the end of this text to assess your risk of developing this disease.

*Metabolic Syndrome* About one-fourth of American adults have *metabolic syndrome*, a condition that increases the risk of CVD and type 2 diabetes.[8] People with metabolic syndrome have excess abdominal fat and at least two of the following health problems: hypertension (chronically elevated blood pressure), high blood glucose, high blood triglycerides (fat), and low HDL ("good") cholesterol levels. People who have large waistline measurements generally have excess *visceral* fat, deposits of **adipose cells** that are located deep within the abdomen. Adipose cells store fat, but the tissue also secretes substances that have important immune functions. Storing too much fat disrupts the normal functioning of visceral fat cells. As a result, these cells secrete *C-reactive pro-*

*tein* and other factors that are thought to contribute to systemic inflammation—inflammation that occurs throughout the body. Systemic inflammation may be partially responsible for heart disease, hypertension, and type 2 diabetes. Losing excess body fat can reduce levels of inflammatory substances and lower the risk of these chronic conditions.

Poor dietary habits such as eating a diet that lacks fruits, vegetables, and other fiber-rich foods contribute to metabolic syndrome. By exercising regularly, maintaining a healthy body weight, and eating plenty of fiber-rich foods, people may be able to avoid this common condition.

***Lactose Intolerance*** *Lactose* (milk sugar) is composed of two monosaccharides. During digestion, lactose is broken down, releasing its component simple sugars. Many older children and adults, however, cannot digest lactose. Such lactose-intolerant people may experience intestinal bloating, cramps, and diarrhea if they consume milk or other products that contain the sugar. Lactose intolerance affects millions of Americans. Members of certain minority groups, especially people with Asian or African ancestry, are more likely to be affected than Caucasians.[9]

Because milk is an excellent source of the mineral nutrient calcium, it is important that lactose-intolerant people consume alternative calcium-rich foods, such as cheese, yogurt, broccoli, turnip and mustard greens, and some types of tofu. People with this condition can add a special enzyme to milk and other foods that contain lactose before consuming them. The enzyme breaks down lactose, reducing the risk of unpleasant side effects. Also, supermarkets often sell fresh milk that has been treated with the enzyme. Affected individuals, however, can often consume small amounts of lactose-containing foods without experiencing discomfort.

***Fiber and Health*** Fiber provides some important health benefits. By eating more high-fiber cereals, people may reduce their risk of developing metabolic syndrome, a condition that often precedes type 2 diabetes. Table 9.3 lists some foods that contain fiber and indicates which are rich sources of *soluble* and *insoluble* fiber. Soluble fiber slows the absorption of glucose from the digestive tract, which is beneficial for people who already have diabetes. Furthermore, eating a high-fiber diet, particularly one with plenty of soluble fiber, can reduce the risk of heart disease (see Chapter 13). Soluble fiber lowers blood cholesterol levels by reducing cholesterol absorption in the small intestine. Elevated blood cholesterol levels are associated with increased risk of CVD.

Many Americans are concerned with their bowel habits; they spend millions of dollars a year on laxatives that promise "regularity." Eating fiber-rich foods can prevent **constipation**, a condition characterized by having fewer than three bowel movements per week.[10] *Insoluble fiber* contributes to the formation of softer, larger stools that stimulate the muscles of the colon, producing the urge to have bowel movements more frequently.

Constipation results when stools are too small and hard to stimulate the colon regularly. A constipated individual often has to strain while having bowel movements, increasing the pressure on veins in the rectum. This pressure can result in **hemorrhoids**, which are painfully swollen veins in the rectal and anal areas. Straining during bowel movements causes **diverticulosis**, a chronic condition in which the lining of the colon forms small pouches called *diverticula* (**Figure 9.4**). Fecal material that becomes lodged in some of these little pouches can cause serious bleeding and inflammation (diverticulitis). Diverticulitis can be life threatening if an inflamed pouch ruptures and spills fecal material into the abdominal cavity. Diverticulosis commonly occurs in Americans older than 50 years, but the condition often produces no serious symptoms.

In addition to eating more fiber-rich foods, you may prevent constipation by consuming adequate amounts of water. Regular exercise may also improve bowel functioning.[10] If constipation persists, or if you have intestinal pain, blood in your stools, or rectal bleeding, check with a physician to rule out serious health problems.

Can eating a high-fiber diet reduce your chances of developing certain cancers of the intestinal tract? Over the past few years, several population studies have provided conflicting findings concerning fiber intake and the risk of colon and rectal cancer. Some medical researchers have found no association between

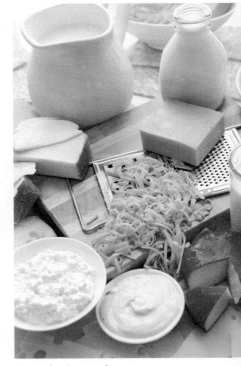

Dairy foods are often sources of lactose.

high-fiber diets and risk of these cancers, but others have determined that eating such diets lowers the risk. More research is needed to clarify the role of dietary fiber in gastrointestinal health. Chapter 13 discusses colon and rectal cancer, including risk factors.

The typical American consumes less than 20 g of fiber a day. Medical experts think individuals should consume at least 25 g of fiber by eating more fruits, vegetables, beans, and whole-grain cereal products each day. During processing, grains often lose their vitamin, mineral, and fiber-rich parts. White flour, for example, is a refined grain product made from wheat kernels. Compared to whole-wheat flour, white flour contains very little fiber. Replacing refined flour products, such as white bread, with whole-grain foods is an easy way to increase the fiber content of your diet. Some "100% wheat" breads contain little fiber; use the nutrient label to compare the fiber content of breads.

## Lipids

Dietary **lipids** include cholesterol and triglycerides. About 95% of the lipid content in foods are **triglycerides**, commonly called *fats* and *oils*. Because each cell contains triglycerides, it is not surprising that a small amount of fat is necessary for health. Compared to carbohydrates, fat is a more concentrated source of calories. The body stores energy in its fat deposits, which insulate the body from cold temperatures, give the body shape, and protect internal organs from jarring movements.

Each triglyceride has three fatty acids. Scientists classify fatty acids into three types—*saturated*, *monounsaturated*, and *polyunsaturated*—according to their chemical structures. Although the triglycerides found in foods contain mixtures of these three types of fatty acids, one type usually predominates. **Figure 9.5** indicates the amounts of lipid as well as the percentages of saturated, monounsaturated, and polyunsaturated fatty acids in a tablespoon of various fats and oils.

Animal foods generally contain more saturated fat than do plant foods. Olive, peanut, and canola oils are rich sources of monounsaturated fat; corn, safflower, cottonseed, and walnut oils are high in polyunsaturated fat. Oils from palm kernels or coconuts, commonly called tropical oils, are unusual in that they are from plants but contain large amounts of saturated fat.

Animal foods also contain **cholesterol**, a compound that is structurally different from a triglyceride. Despite its reputation for being a troublemaker, cholesterol has several very important functions in the body. Cell membranes contain cholesterol, and the body uses this lipid to produce steroid hormones, vitamin D, and bile, a substance needed for proper fat digestion. Even if you could avoid eating foods that contain cholesterol, your liver and small intestine would make this essential compound.

Only animals produce cholesterol; therefore, the compound is found in animal and not plant foods. Meats, whole-milk products, and egg yolks supply most of the cholesterol in the typical American diet. **Table 9.6** lists cholesterol-rich foods and the amount of cholesterol in each serving.

### Figure 9.4

**Diverticula.** Diverticula are small pockets of the large intestine's inner lining that protrude through the outer wall of the large intestine. Diverticula can become infected and rupture.

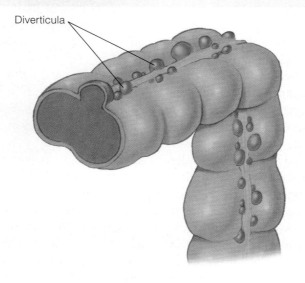

Diverticula

## Figure 9.5

**Fatty Acid Content of Common Fats and Oils*.**

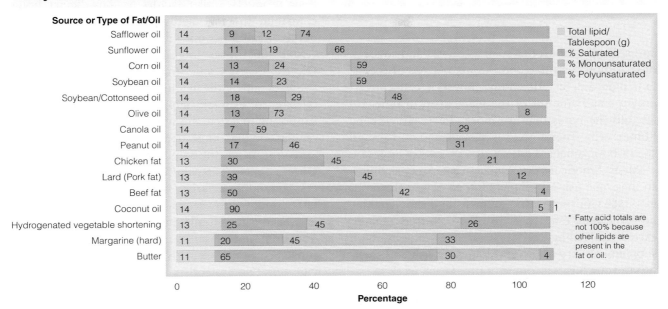

Source or Type of Fat/Oil

| Source | Total lipid/Tablespoon (g) | % Saturated | % Monounsaturated | % Polyunsaturated |
|---|---|---|---|---|
| Safflower oil | 14 | 9 | 12 | 74 |
| Sunflower oil | 14 | 11 | 19 | 66 |
| Corn oil | 14 | 13 | 24 | 59 |
| Soybean oil | 14 | 14 | 23 | 59 |
| Soybean/Cottonseed oil | 14 | 18 | 29 | 48 |
| Olive oil | 14 | 13 | 73 | 8 |
| Canola oil | 14 | 7 | 59 | 29 |
| Peanut oil | 14 | 17 | 46 | 31 |
| Chicken fat | 13 | 30 | 45 | 21 |
| Lard (Pork fat) | 13 | 39 | 45 | 12 |
| Beef fat | 13 | 50 | 42 | 4 |
| Coconut oil | 14 | 90 | 5 | 1 |
| Hydrogenated vegetable shortening | 13 | 25 | 45 | 26 |
| Margarine (hard) | 11 | 20 | 45 | 33 |
| Butter | 11 | 65 | 30 | 4 |

Percentage: 0, 20, 40, 60, 80, 100, 120

* Fatty acid totals are not 100% because other lipids are present in the fat or oil.

## Table 9.6

### Cholesterol in Foods

| Food | Serving Size | Cholesterol (mg) |
|---|---|---|
| Beef liver | 4 oz | 545 |
| Egg | 1 large | 212 |
| Yolk | | 212 |
| White | | 0 |
| Shrimp | 3 oz | 167 |
| Turkey, ground cooked | 4 oz | 116 |
| Beefsteak | 4 oz | 94 |
| Ice cream (rich = 16% fat) | 1 cup | 90 |
| Sherbet (2% fat) | 1 cup | 10 |
| Yogurt, plain low-fat | 1 cup | 14 |
| Whole milk | 1 cup | 33 |
| Reduced-fat (2%) milk | 1 cup | 18 |
| Nonfat milk | 1 cup | 4 |
| Butter | 1 tablespoon | 31 |
| Swiss cheese | 1 oz | 26 |
| Cream cheese | 1 oz | 10 |
| Bacon | 3 slices | 16 |

**Lipids and Health** If you used to drink whole or reduced-fat (2%) milk, how did you react when you first tasted nonfat milk? Did you think the milk was watery or "thin"? The fat contained in or added to foods makes them taste rich and flavorful. Fat in food also increases the absorption of vitamins A, D, E, and K and many phytochemicals. Nutrition experts recommend that adults should obtain about 20% to 35% of their total calories from fat.[11]

Diets that supply too much saturated fat are associated with an increased risk of heart disease. High intakes of saturated fat can increase blood cholesterol levels. Although eating foods that contain cholesterol may also raise blood levels of this lipid, saturated fat tends to increase blood cholesterol levels to a much greater extent.

Diets that contain high amounts of certain unsaturated fatty acids, the *omega-3 fatty acids*, may reduce inflammation in the body, which may lower the risk of heart decrease.[12] Rich food sources of omega-3 fatty acids include fatty fish and shellfish from cold water, such as wild salmon, herring, tuna, mackerel, and shrimp. Plant foods such as canola and soybean oils, walnuts, and flax and pumpkin seeds also contain omega-3 fat. The body, however, can convert only a small amount of the plant form of omega-3 fat into the types that are more effectively used by human cells. Therefore, it is best to rely on fish and shellfish for omega-3 fats.

Many Americans do not like to eat fish or shellfish, so they take fish oil supplements to obtain the omega-3 fats. Consuming too many fish oil supplements, however, may interfere with blood clotting, making excessive bleeding likely. Instead of relying on fish oil supplements, try to include coldwater fish and shellfish in your meals a couple of times each week.

Unlike the typical American (Western) diet that contains large amounts of red meat and few fruits and vegetables, traditional food choices of Mediterranean populations supply smaller amounts of meat, fried foods, and sweets and larger amounts of plant foods, fish, and olive oil (see the inside back cover). The risk of heart disease is lower for individuals who consume the traditional Mediterranean diet.[13] The Diversity in Health essay discusses the traditional Asian diet, which also contains less animal protein and saturated fat than Western diets do.

*Trans Fats* Not all foods made with vegetable oil have healthful properties. *Hydrogenation* is a food processing technique that partially hardens the oil so that it can be made into shortening and sticks of margarine. This process alters the natural chemical structure of some unsaturated fatty acids in vegetable oils, forming *trans fatty acids*. In the body, trans fatty acids behave like saturated fats, raising unhealthy forms of cholesterol in blood.[12] To reduce your intake of trans fatty acids, use soft or liquid margarines, eat less commercial cake frostings, and avoid baked goods and fried foods, which are

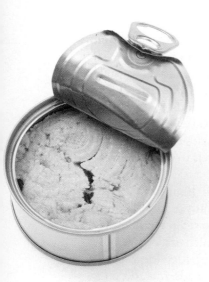

Tuna is an excellent source of omega-3 fat.

often made with hydrogenated fats. In response to consumer concerns, many restaurant chains and food manufacturers have eliminated trans fats from their products. Other factors besides dietary lipids contribute to heart disease; Chapter 12 discusses in depth this number one killer of Americans.

**Fat Substitutes** Engineered compounds such as Olestra, Oatrim, and Simplesse are used to replace some or all of the fat in certain processed foods. Olestra, for example, supplies no calories because it cannot be digested and absorbed. A 1-oz serving of regular tortilla chips supplies 130 calories and contains 6 g of fat; the same amount of chips fried in Olestra contains 76 calories and no fat. For consumers demanding a variety of fat-free snack foods that taste good, Olestra seems to be a good fat substitute. However, eating foods made with Olestra may produce some unpleasant side effects. Additionally, the substance interferes with the absorption of certain vitamins. Food scientists are currently developing fat replacers that taste good, do not cause side effects, and are chemically stable when heated.

**Setting Limits** The typical American diet contains too much fat, especially the unhealthy kinds of fat (saturated and trans fats) from dairy products, meats, baked goods, and processed snack foods. College students and other busy people often consume more fat than is necessary by eating greasy snacks and fast foods regularly. Popular fast foods, such as cheeseburgers, pizza, fried chicken and fish, french fries, and milk shakes, contain large amounts of saturated fat. Many fast-food restaurants, however, offer less fatty items such as roast chicken, low-fat yogurt, bean burritos, and meatless salads. The Managing Your Health feature "Trimming the Unhealthy Fats from Your Diet" provides some practical ways to reduce your intake of saturated and trans fats.

Most food labels provide nutrition information concerning the amounts of total fat, saturated fat, trans fat, and cholesterol in food products. A later section of this chapter describes how to use this information to control the amount and type of fat in your diet.

## Proteins

Your body needs **proteins** to build, maintain, and repair cells; to form structural components such as hair and nails; and to make enzymes, antibodies, and numerous hormones. Although carbohydrates and fats are its primary fuels, the body derives a small amount of energy from protein. Proteins consist of **amino acids**. During digestion, proteins in plant or

# Diversity in Health

## Asian American Food

Asian populations consume large quantities of rice, wheat noodles, and vegetables combined with eggs or a small amount of meat (usually seafood, poultry, fish, or pork). The traditional Asian diet is high in starch and fiber and usually low in fat, especially saturated fat. Stir-frying vegetables and meats in a lightly oiled wok and steaming foods are popular Asian cooking methods that add fewer calories than deep-fat frying and preserve more vitamins and minerals than boiling. To season their foods, most Asian cooks use low-fat items such as garlic, ginger, and sauces made from mustard and soybeans.

Not all features of the traditional Asian diet are healthful. Asian meals contain little or no dairy products; therefore, the amount of calcium in these diets is usually low. Among the residents of northern Japan, the consumption of soy sauce as well as fermented and pickled foods adds excessive amounts of sodium to diets and may contribute to the relatively high incidence of certain cancers and hypertension. After immigrating to the United States, many Asians adopt Western food preferences and preparation practices. For example, American-style Chinese meals often include larger portions of meat and breaded, deep-fat fried foods.

Some people experience an adverse reaction when they eat Asian or other foods to which the flavor enhancer *monosodium glutamate* (MSG) has been added. After eating food that contains MSG, persons who are sensitive to the compound may report a "tight" sensation in the face and chest, headache, and pain and reddening of skin, especially on the face. Results of clinical studies, however, fail to show consistently that MSG causes adverse reactions in most people.[14]

When you eat at Chinese, Japanese, Thai, and other Asian American restaurants, select menu items carefully. Choose plenty of steamed vegetables and rice or noodles to accompany the entrée. Avoid dishes containing foods that have been dipped in batter and fried, avoid or limit your intake of fried wontons and egg rolls, and do not add soy sauce to your food. If you react adversely to MSG, many cooks, upon request, will prepare your food without it.

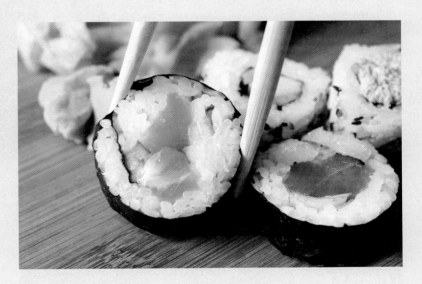

animal foods are broken down, releasing amino acids for absorption. Human cells use about 20 different amino acids to synthesize the thousands of proteins in the body. The cells can make 11 of these amino acids; the other 9 amino acids are essential and must be supplied by the diet. If the diet lacks the essential amino acids, the body is unable to grow properly or carry out vital functions.

Most foods, even plant foods, contain some protein. Animal foods generally contain adequate amounts of each essential amino acid; these foods are *complete* or high-quality protein sources. Most plants are sources of *incomplete* or low-quality protein because they either contain insufficient amounts or lack one or more of the essential amino acids. The best plant sources of essential amino acids are soybeans, quinoa, whole grains, seeds, nuts, peas, and lentils (**Figure 9.6**). Fruits do not contain appreciable amounts of essential amino acids.

**Proteins and Health** Animal products, especially meat, fish, poultry, eggs, milk, and milk products, contribute almost two-thirds of the protein in the typical American's diet.[15] Although eating large amounts of protein does not harm most healthy individuals, generous portions of animal foods contribute excessive amounts of saturated fat to the diet. Diets

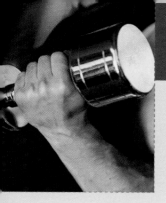

# Managing Your Health

## Trimming Unhealthy Fats from Your Diet

Americans can reduce the amount of unhealthy fats in their diets by changing the ways they select and prepare their food. The following tips can help you trim unwanted fat from your diet.

- Avoid breaded and fried vegetables, chicken, fish, and meats.
- Eat less red meat and more poultry and fish.
- Avoid sausage, bacon, and fatty luncheon meats.
- Eat boiled or baked instead of fried potatoes.
- Trim all visible fat from meats before cooking them.
- Chill cooked chili, stews, soups, sauces, and gravies. Then, skim off the fat before reheating and serving these foods.
- Substitute fat-free ("skim") milk for whole or reduced-fat (2%) milk.
- Substitute reconstituted, nonfat dry milk in recipes that use milk or cream.
- Eat low-fat or fat-free frozen yogurt and ice milk.

- Replace hard cheeses with part-skim or low-fat cheeses.
- Substitute fat-reduced cream cheese for regular cream cheese.
- Substitute plain low-fat or fat-free yogurt for sour cream in recipes.
- Skim frostings from cakes; commercial frostings are often made with hydrogenated shortening, which is 100% fat and contains trans fats.
- When eating two-crust pies, eat the filling and only one crust; discard the remaining crust.
- Replace shortening in recipes with oil or margarine.

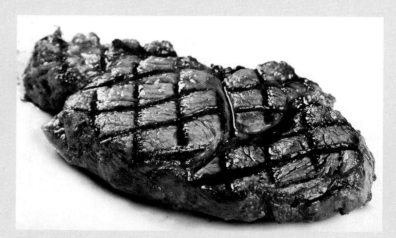

---

**Figure 9.6**

**Soybean Products.** Tofu and other processed soybean products are excellent plant sources of protein.

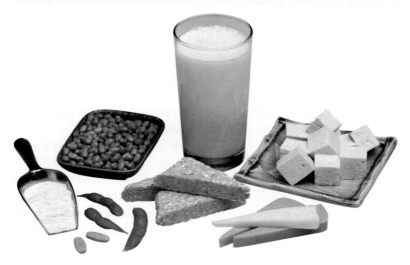

that contain high amounts of saturated fat are associated with increased risk of heart disease, the number one killer of Americans.

Many athletes and bodybuilders think it is necessary to consume large quantities of animal foods and protein supplements to increase their muscle mass. This practice does not build bigger muscles; instead, the body must metabolize the extra amino acids for energy or convert them into body fat. Additionally, the kidneys need more water to eliminate the excess amino acid by-products. The most effective way to enhance muscle mass is to combine a nutritionally adequate diet with a program of muscle-strengthening exercises.

Animal foods are among the most expensive items on the typical American's grocery list. You can reduce your food costs and decrease your saturated fat intake by substituting certain plant foods for meat and other animal protein sources. The following section discusses vegetarianism, a way to reduce your animal protein intake without sacrificing the nutritional adequacy of your diet.

*Vegetarianism* A growing number of Americans are consuming plant-based, or *vegetarian*, diets that contain little or no animal foods. Many people associate meat with protein, but processed soybean foods, such as tofu, soymilk, and soy nut butter; quinoa; various beans, peas, and lentils; nuts; seeds; and foods made from cereal grains (for example, wheat and oats) are among the best sources of protein from plants.

There are several types of vegetarian diets. The vegan, or total vegetarian, diet consists of plant foods only. Other vegetarian diets include some animal foods. For example, the *lacto-vegetarian* diet contains dairy products, and the *lacto-ovo-vegetarian diet* includes eggs as well as dairy products. Some people who eat fish or poultry still call themselves vegetarians because they do not eat *red* meats. There are so many different plant-based diets, it is difficult to estimate the number of Americans practicing some form of vegetarianism.

Are vegetarian diets nutritious? Plant-based diets may promote good health because they contain more fiber, antioxidants, and phytochemicals and less saturated fat and cholesterol than the traditional meat-rich Western diet. Generally, the nutritional adequacy of a vegetarian diet varies according to the degree of its dietary restrictions. Animal foods are rich sources of essential amino acids as well as certain minerals and vitamins. Plant foods, on the other hand, generally lack one or more essential amino acids.

In the past, nutrition experts advised vegans to consume mixtures of plant foods that supplied all the essential amino acids in one meal because it was believed the body did not save essential amino acids and was unable to make proteins unless all of them were available at one time. Now it is known that the body can conserve essential amino acids after a meal or snack and use them for protein production later in the day. Although it is not necessary to combine plant foods to obtain the proper mix of amino acids, combinations such as peanut butter on toast or red beans and rice make vegetarian meals nutritious, inexpensive, and easy to prepare. Most vegetarians can obtain adequate amounts of essential amino acids and other nutrients by eating a variety of plant foods, consuming dairy products, and taking a multiple vitamin/mineral supplement.

Thus, with careful planning, most plant-based diets can be nutritionally adequate.[16] If you are interested in learning specific details about vegetarian cookery and menu planning, you can obtain this information from registered dietitians (RDs) or University Outreach Extension nutritionists in your area.

*Food Allergies* A 3-year-old child develops hives—small, itchy, swollen, reddened areas on her skin—soon after she eats eggs. Her older brother must avoid peanuts and foods that may contain peanuts because he can experience *shock*, a drop in blood pressure and loss of consciousness that can be deadly if not treated immediately. These reactions are the result of food allergies, the immune system's inappropriate response to harmless proteins (*allergens*) in certain foods. In the United States, 6% to 8% of children and about 4% of adults are allergic to one or more foods.[17] Proteins in cows' milk, eggs, peanuts, tree nuts (such as cashews and walnuts), wheat, soybeans, fish, and shellfish are most likely to cause allergic reactions in susceptible people. Food manufacturers must identify ingredients that are common food allergens on labels (**Figure 9.7**).

Hives are the most common sign of food allergy; other signs include *eczema*, a scaly skin rash; asthma symptoms, such as wheezing and difficulty breathing; and vomiting and diarrhea. Shock (anaphylaxis) occurs when the entire body reacts to the allergen. As mentioned earlier, shock can be fatal.

If you think you or someone you know has a food allergy, consult an allergist/immunologist, a physician who specializes in the diagnosis and treatment

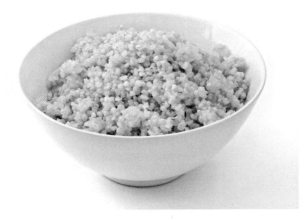

Quinoa (keen'-wah) is a vegetable that is often prepared like cooked cereal.

**celiac disease** A condition characterized by hypersensitivity to gluten.

of allergies. Special skin and blood tests are used to identify food allergies (**Figure 9.8**). Alternative medical procedures to diagnose allergies, such as food specific IgG tests, leukocyte cytotoxic tests, sublingual and intradermal provocation tests, electrodermal (VEGA) testing, and applied kinesiology, are inappropriate and unproven.[18]

In the case of a true food allergy, the best treatment is to avoid the offending food. Additionally, the allergic person should be prepared to treat shock by taking antihistamines or administering injectable *epinephrine*, a naturally produced substance that raises blood pressure. Parents of children with food allergies must read labels carefully to check ingredients for allergens. They should inform their children's adult caregivers, teachers, and the parents of their

children's friends about the allergy and the importance of not offering foods that may contain allergens to their children. Although most children outgrow milk, egg, and wheat allergies, they are likely to remain allergic to peanuts, tree nuts, fish, and shellfish throughout their lives.

*Celiac Disease* People with **celiac disease** are hypersensitive to *gluten*, a protein in wheat, rye, and barley. When a person with the disease consumes gluten, his or her immune system responds by causing an inflammation of the lining of the small intestine. The inflammation damages the lining, and the body cannot absorb nutrients from food as a result.

Signs and symptoms of celiac disease include malnutrition; fatigue; arthritis; skin rash; abdominal bloating and pain; chronic diarrhea; vomiting; pale, foul-smelling stools; and weight loss. Children with the disease are irritable and fail to grow properly.

Celiac disease is an *autoimmune disorder* (see Chapter 3). People with this chronic condition are also likely to have other autoimmune diseases, such as type 1 diabetes, rheumatoid arthritis, and Sjögren's syndrome.[19] Celiac disease has a genetic basis, so people who have family members with the condition are more likely to develop the disease.

The only cure for celiac disease is the complete avoidance of gluten-containing foods and products, such as lipstick, that may contain gluten. Many supermarkets have sections devoted to gluten-free foods, and in major urban areas, some restaurants have chefs that prepare meals in gluten-free kitchens for their customers with celiac disease. For people

### Figure 9.7

**Labeling Food Allergens.** The Food Allergen Labeling and Consumer Protection Act requires food manufacturers to identify common food allergens that may be in packaged foods on their products' labels.

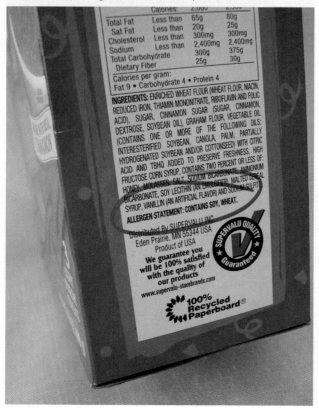

### Figure 9.8

**Skin Testing for Food Allergy.** Skin testing that is performed by a physician is an effective method of diagnosing food allergies.

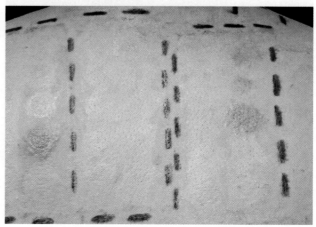

with celiac disease, a gluten-free diet is critical for maintaining good health. Gluten-free foods are not necessarily "low-calorie" or useful for people who do not have the condition but want to lose weight. For more information about celiac disease, visit the website of the American Celiac Disease Alliance at http://www.americanceliac.org.

## Healthy Living Practices

▢ To reduce your risk of obesity, heart disease, type 2 diabetes, and certain digestive tract disorders, exercise regularly and consume at least 25 g of fiber each day by eating more fruits, vegetables, beans, and whole-grain cereal products.

▢ To lower your risk of diabetes and heart disease, reduce your fat intake to 20% to 35% of your daily calories, limit your intake of saturated fat, avoid trans fat, and reduce your cholesterol intake to 300 or fewer milligrams per day.

▢ You can reduce the amount of cholesterol and saturated and trans fat in your diet by consuming low-fat yogurt and nonfat milk and by eating less cheese, fatty meat, fried food, and fat-laden bakery goods and snack foods.

▢ Many fast foods are high in saturated fat. If you eat at fast-food restaurants regularly, reduce your intake of meat and fried foods by selecting salads or grilled chicken or fish items.

▢ If you eat large amounts of red meat and other animal foods, consider eating less and consuming more fatty, cold-water fish; beans; nuts; and whole-grain cereals instead.

# Non-Energy-Supplying Nutrients

## Vitamins

**Vitamins** are organic compounds that have numerous functions in the body. Vitamins help regulate growth; release energy from carbohydrates, fats, and proteins; and maintain tissues. Although many vitamins participate in the chemical reactions that release energy, they do not provide calories.

**vitamins** A class of organic nutrients that help regulate growth; release energy from carbohydrates, fats, and proteins; and maintain tissues.

Scientists classify vitamins according to their ability to dissolve in water or fat. Vitamin C and the eight B vitamins are water-soluble; vitamins A, D, E, and K are fat-soluble. The body does not store most water-soluble vitamins to any appreciable extent, whereas fat-soluble vitamins are stored in the liver and body fat and can accumulate to toxic levels. *Table 9.7* lists most of the vitamins as well as their major roles in the body and rich food sources.

Compared to the energy-supplying nutrients and water, the body requires very small amounts of vitamins. Diets that include a wide variety of foods can meet the vitamin needs of healthy individuals. Some persons, however, take nutrient supplements that provide several times the recommended levels of vitamins to treat or prevent illness. Taking more of a nutrient than the body needs is not necessarily better. Cells use limited amounts of each vitamin daily. In many instances, excessive amounts of these nutrients accumulate in the body and cause harmful side effects. Vitamins A, B6, and niacin are very toxic when taken in large doses. Table 9.7 provides information concerning the signs and symptoms of vitamin toxicity disorders.

**Antioxidants** The chemical structures of certain compounds, particularly polyunsaturated fatty acids, make them vulnerable to damage by free radicals. Free radical formation produces chemical changes in cells that may contribute to the development of cardiovascular disease (diseases of the heart and blood vessels), certain cancers, degenerative changes in the eye, and other chronic health conditions.

Many foods contain antioxidants that can protect cells by preventing or reducing the formation of free radicals. These antioxidants include vitamins E and C and a variety of phytochemicals such as beta-carotene, a yellow-orange pigment in plants that the body converts to vitamin A. Table 9.2 lists some phytochemicals that have antioxidant activity and their major food sources; *Table 9.8* lists foods commonly consumed in the United States that have high antioxidant activity per serving.

Since the 1980s, scientists have been investigating the possible risks and benefits of eating diets rich in antioxidants or taking antioxidant supplements. No strong scientific data support the popular belief that vitamin C prevents the common cold, but taking the

**Table 9.7**

## Major Vitamins

| Vitamin | Major Functions | Rich Food Sources | Deficiency Signs/ Symptoms | Toxicity Signs/ Symptoms |
|---|---|---|---|---|
| A and provitamin A (beta-carotene) | Vision in dim light, growth, reproduction, maintains immune system and skin, antioxidant | Liver, milk, dark green and leafy vegetables; carrot, sweet potato, mango, oatmeal, broccoli, apricot, peach, and romaine lettuce | Poor vision in dim light, dry skin, blindness, poor growth, respiratory infections | Intestinal upset, liver damage, hair loss, headache, birth defects, death (beta-carotene has low toxicity) |
| D | Bone and tooth development and growth; immune system functioning | Few good food sources other than eggs, fortified milk, and orange juice | Weak, deformed bones (rickets) | Growth failure, loss of appetite, weight loss, death |
| E | Antioxidant: protects cell membranes | Vegetable oils, whole grains, wheat germ, sunflower seeds, almonds | Anemia (rarely occurs) | Intestinal upsets, bleeding problems |
| C | Scar formation and maintenance, immune system functioning, antioxidant | Citrus fruits, berries, potatoes, broccoli, peppers, cabbage, tomatoes, fortified fruit drinks | Frequent infections, bleeding gums, bruises, poor wound healing, depression (scurvy) | Diarrhea, nosebleeds, headache, weakness, kidney stones, excess iron absorption and storage |
| Thiamin | Energy metabolism | Pork, liver, nuts, dried beans and peas, whole-grain and enriched breads and cereals | Heart failure, mental confusion, depression, paralysis (beriberi) | No toxicity has been reported |
| Riboflavin | Energy metabolism | Milk and yogurt, eggs and poultry, meat, liver, whole-grain and enriched breads and cereals | Enlarged, purple tongue; fatigue; oily skin; cracks in the corners of the mouth | No toxicity has been reported |
| Niacin | Energy metabolism | Protein-rich foods, peanut butter, whole-grain and enriched breads and cereals | Skin rash, diarrhea, weakness, dementia, death (pellagra) | Painful skin flushing, intestinal upsets, liver damage |
| Vitamin $B_6$ | Protein and fat metabolism | Liver, oatmeal, bananas, meat, fish, poultry, whole grains, fortified cereals | Anemia, skin rash, irritability, elevated homocysteine levels | Weakness, depression, permanent nerve damage |
| Folate (folic acid) | DNA production | Leafy vegetables, oranges, nuts, liver, enriched breads and cereals | Anemia, depression, spina bifida in developing embryo, elevated homocysteine levels | Hides signs of $B_{12}$ deficiency; may cause allergic response |
| $B_{12}$ | DNA production | Animal products | Pernicious anemia, fatigue, paralysis, elevated homocysteine levels | No toxicity has been reported |

vitamin may shorten the duration of the infection.[20] Vitamin C may also reduce the risk of developing heart disease, but its usefulness in preventing diabetes, cancer, and Alzheimer's disease is not supported by scientific evidence.[20]

Should you take large doses of vitamins, especially antioxidant vitamins, to prevent disease? Nutrition experts are divided over the issue of antioxidant vitamin supplementation. The cells in your body make antioxidants. Some scientists think modern humans are exposed to much higher levels of environmental hazards, such as air pollution and pesticide residues, than their ancestors. These conditions may increase the body's need for antioxidants beyond the amounts that are made or can be obtained from food, making supplementation necessary. Other scientists think plant foods are the best source of antioxidants. Unlike nutrient supplements, plant foods contain mixtures of vitamins and phytochemicals that collectively may provide healthful benefits. Taking large doses of antioxidant vitamins may have harmful side effects, including promoting the growth of cancer cells.

In 1999–2000, 35% of adult Americans reported taking multiple vitamin supplements that contain three or more vitamins.[21] Unless medically necessary, taking these supplements is an economically wasteful and risky practice. By eating a variety of whole-grain products, fruits, and vegetables daily, you are less likely to encounter toxicity problems because these foods naturally supply vitamins in smaller quantities.

## Minerals

**Minerals** are a group of elements such as calcium, iron, and sodium. Several minerals are nutrients that have a wide variety of roles in the body. For example,

> **minerals** A class of inorganic nutrients that includes several elements, such as iron, calcium, and zinc.

the mineral nutrient magnesium regulates chemical reactions; other mineral nutrients are structural components of certain organic molecules, like the iron in red blood cells and calcium in bones. The body needs very small amounts of minerals, compared to the energy-supplying nutrients and water. Excesses of any mineral can create imbalances with other minerals or can be toxic.

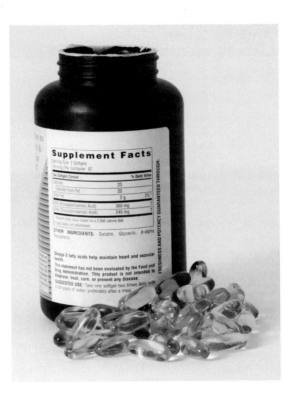

## Table 9.8

### Antioxidant-Rich Foods

| | | | | |
|---|---|---|---|---|
| Blackberries | Cranberries | Blueberries | Cranberry juice | Pineapple juice |
| Walnuts | Coffee | Cloves, ground | Cherries, sour | Guava nectar (beverage) |
| Strawberries | Raspberries | Grape juice | Wine, red | |
| Artichokes (cooked) | Pecans | Chocolate, baking, unsweetened | Power bar, chocolate | |

*Source:* Halvorsen, B. L., et al. (2006). Content of redox-active compounds (i.e., antioxidants) in foods consumed in the United States. *American Journal of Clinical Nutrition, 84*(1):95–135.

Table 9.9 lists some essential minerals, describes their major roles, and identifies common foods that contain high amounts of these substances. The following section provides information about calcium and iron, two minerals that have considerable health importance for Americans.

**Calcium** Calcium is the most plentiful mineral in the body. You may be aware that calcium is necessary for the development of strong bones and teeth, but this mineral has other important roles as well, such as regulating blood pressure and participating in muscular movements. The body carefully maintains the level of calcium in the blood within a specific range. When the level is too high, the bones can remove and store the excess. If the amount of calcium in the blood begins to drop below normal levels, the bones release some of the mineral from storage, returning the level to normal.

## Table 9.9

## Some Essential Minerals

| Mineral | Roles | Rich Food Sources | Deficiency Signs/Symptoms | Toxicity Signs/Symptoms |
|---------|-------|-------------------|---------------------------|-------------------------|
| Calcium | Builds and maintains bones and teeth, regulates muscle and nerve function, regulates blood pressure and blood clotting | Milk products; fortified orange juice, tofu, and soy milk; fish with edible small bones such as sardines and salmon; broccoli; hard water | Poor bone growth, weak bones, muscle spasms, convulsions | Kidney stones, calcium deposits in organs, mineral imbalances |
| Potassium | Maintains fluid balance, necessary for nerve function | Whole grains, fruits, and vegetables, yogurt, milk | Muscular weakness, confusion, death | Heart failure |
| Sodium | Maintains fluid balance, necessary for nerve function | Salt, soy sauce, luncheon meats, processed cheeses, pickled foods, snack foods, canned and dried soups | Muscle cramping, headache, confusion, coma | Hypertension |
| Magnesium | Regulation of enzyme activity, necessary for nerve function | Green leafy vegetables, nuts, whole grains, peanut butter | Loss of appetite, muscular weakness, convulsions, confusion, death | Rare |
| Zinc | Component of many enzymes and the hormone insulin, maintains immune function, necessary for sexual maturation and reproduction | Meats, fish, poultry, whole grains, vegetables | Poor growth, failure to mature sexually, improper healing of wounds | Mineral imbalances, gastrointestinal upsets, anemia, heart disease |
| Selenium | Component of a group of antioxidant enzymes, immune system function | Seafood, liver, and vegetables and grains grown in selenium-rich soil | May increase risk of heart disease and certain cancers | Hair and nail loss |
| Iron | Oxygen transport involved in the release of energy | Clams, oysters, liver, red meats, and enriched breads and cereals | Fatigue, weakness, iron-deficiency anemia | Iron poisoning, nausea, vomiting, diarrhea, death |

As it adjusts to the demands of bearing the body's weight, bone tissue undergoes a continual process of being built, torn down, and rebuilt. After about 40 years of age, the bones of most people begin to break down at a faster rate than they rebuild. As bones gradually lose mineral density, they become weak and brittle. Fragile bones break easily, and sometimes shatter because they cannot support the body. Although any bone can be affected, bones in the hip, spine, and wrist are most likely to break. This condition, **osteoporosis**, threatens the health of millions of aging Americans, especially older adult women. In the United States, 40 million Americans either have osteoporosis or are at risk of the disorder; most of these persons are older women.[22] Men usually have denser bones than women, which may explain why most aging men are not affected by osteoporosis to the same extent as aging women are.

Fractures are associated with an increased risk of permanent disability or death, particularly if the fracture immobilizes the person; immobility increases the likelihood that fatal blood clots or pneumonia will develop. A painful and disabling condition known as "dowager's hump" can occur when bones in the upper spine are so weak that they experience small compression fractures over time while trying to support the weight of the skull. As these bones heal into wedge shapes, the upper spine assumes an abnormal curvature (**Figure 9.9**). As a result, people with osteoporosis often "shrink"—they lose some of their height.

As one ages, a calcium-rich diet and weight-bearing physical activity help build and maintain strong bones. After *menopause*, however, such practices may not be enough to prevent osteoporosis or slow its progress. Within the first 5 to 10 years after menopause, even healthy women are susceptible to losing a large percentage of their bone mass. Why?

The hormone *estrogen* stimulates bones to maintain their mass and retain calcium. A sign of normal estrogen production is regular menstrual cycles. A woman has reached menopause when her estrogen levels drop dramatically and her menstrual cycles have ceased. As women approach this time of life, those who have a history of regular menstrual cycles are more likely to maintain their bone mass than those who had irregular or absent menstrual cycles.

Besides being a postmenopausal woman, other characteristics increase one's risk of osteoporosis. The condition may be inherited, and members of certain racial groups are more susceptible to osteoporosis than others. African Americans tend to have larger bone masses that afford some protection against osteoporosis. On the other hand, slender, small-boned people of European and Asian ancestry are more likely than people with large bones to develop osteoporosis.

Certain lifestyle choices can increase a person's risk of osteoporosis. Young people with low-calcium diets are likely to have less-dense bones that are susceptible to osteoporosis as they grow older. Cigarette smoking and alcohol consumption can accelerate bone loss. Furthermore, young women who exercise excessively may disrupt their body's normal estrogen production and menstrual cycles. This reduction in estrogen levels can lead to premature bone loss.

Special x-rays are used to diagnose bone loss clinically.

### Figure 9.9

**Dowager's Hump.** In people with osteoporosis, the bones in the upper spine develop small compression fractures. These bones heal into wedge shapes, and the upper spine assumes a deformed, curved shape known as "dowager's hump."

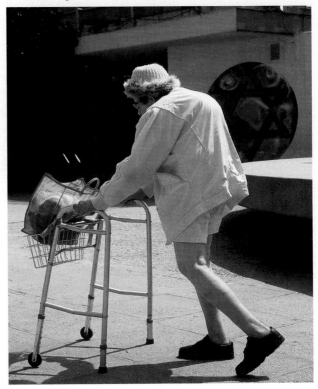

To treat menopausal women who are at risk of osteoporosis, physicians often prescribe hormone replacement therapy, that is, synthetic hormones that contain estrogen or a combination of estrogen and progesterone. Nonhormonal treatments are available also. Women who are approaching menopause should consult their physicians about their risks of developing osteoporosis and their treatment options.

Most medical experts recommend that young men and women adopt behaviors that maximize their bone mass. If you are concerned about your risk of developing osteoporosis, consume foods that supply calcium such as those shown in **Figure 9.10**.

If you do not consume dairy products or foods fortified with calcium, ask your physician about alternative ways to obtain this mineral, such as calcium-containing supplements or antacids. In addition to calcium, vitamin D and the mineral magnesium are important for bone health. Adopting healthful lifestyles, such as refraining from smoking, reducing alcohol consumption, and engaging in physical activities that place stress on your bones, such as walking, weight lifting, or jogging, can help maintain your skeleton's structural integrity.

Osteoporosis can occur at any age. If you think your risk of developing this condition is high, ask your doctor to perform a bone density test. By treating osteoporosis in its early stages, substantial bone loss can be prevented.

**Iron** Most of the body's iron is found in the hemoglobin molecules within the red blood cells. Hemoglobin combines with oxygen in the lungs and transports it to cells throughout the body. Oxygen is necessary to release the energy stored in glucose.

*Anemia* results when the body produces abnormal red blood cells. In cases of iron-deficiency anemia, the bone marrow forms red blood cells that are smaller and contain less hemoglobin than normal cells. Without sufficient hemoglobin, the red blood cells carry less oxygen than usual as they circulate. Anemic individuals often report feeling tired because their cells are unable to obtain adequate amounts of energy.

Iron deficiency is one of the most prevalent nutritional disorders in the United States. Many individuals, especially premenopausal women, are at risk of becoming iron deficient because they do not consume enough iron-rich food to replace the iron lost each month in menstrual blood. Individuals undergoing rapid growth, such as infants, children, teenagers, and pregnant women, have high needs for iron and are at risk of iron deficiency. If untreated, severe iron deficiency can cause iron-deficiency anemia. This type of anemia often occurs in people who lose a lot of blood.

To ensure adequate iron intake, you can eat the iron-rich foods listed in Table 9.9. Normally, the small intestine does not absorb much of the iron in

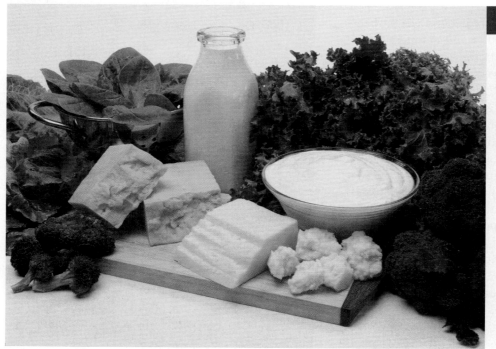

**Figure 9.10**

**Calcium-Rich Foods.** Some of the richest food sources of calcium are low-fat milk and yogurt, and greens. Although most cheeses are high in saturated fat, they are good sources of calcium.

foods, especially the iron in plants. You can enhance the absorption of plant sources of iron by eating them with meat or vitamin C–rich foods. In addition to eating more foods that contain iron, people with iron-deficiency anemia may need to take iron supplements.

Annually, thousands of young children unintentionally poison themselves, a few of them fatally, after ingesting toxic amounts of iron-containing supplements. Many of these cases involve unsupervised young children who take overdoses of flavored vitamin/mineral supplements, thinking they are candy. To prevent such tragedies, store nutrient and other dietary supplements like other medications, making them inaccessible to children.

*Hemochromatosis* An estimated 5 in 1,000 white Americans have *hemochromatosis*, a genetic condition that increases the intestinal absorption of dietary iron.[23] The iron accumulates in their organs and reaches toxic levels by the time they are middle-aged. These people are often unaware that they have the potentially fatal condition until it causes serious conditions such as diabetes, liver damage, and heart disease. A simple blood test can detect this treatable disorder. People with hemochromatosis should not take supplements that contain iron and should limit their intake of iron-rich foods.

## Water

Water is essential for life on earth. You can survive weeks, months, and even years without one of the other nutrients, but you cannot survive for more than a few days without water. Water has many functions in the body: dissolving and transporting materials, eliminating wastes, lubricating joints, and participating in numerous chemical reactions.

About 60% of an adult's body is water. To function properly, the body maintains its fluid levels within specific limits, generally by increasing or decreasing urine production. Although it carefully conserves water, the body loses water when one perspires, urinates, exhales, and defecates. Drinking plain water and fluids such as milk, juices, and soft drinks replenishes the body's water. Most foods, especially fruits and vegetables, also supply water.

Advertisements often promote beer as a thirst quencher; however, drinking alcoholic beverages does not replace body water. Alcohol acts as a diuretic, a compound that increases urinary losses of water. Caffeine is also a diuretic, but its effects are less than alcohol's.

According to a report issued by an expert panel of the National Institute of Medicine, the daily recommended amounts of water from food and beverages are about 16 cups for men and 11 cups for women.[24] In general, Americans' water intake is adequate. Dehydration occurs when the normal level of body water declines, and the affected individual does not consume replenishing fluids. The symptoms of dehydration include weakness, confusion, and irritability. During prolonged fevers or bouts of diarrhea or vomiting, the body can lose substantial amounts of water, causing dehydration. These conditions cause the loss of minerals such as sodium and potassium as well. If untreated, severe dehydration is usually fatal. Chapter 11 provides more information about dehydration and heat-related illnesses.

Healthy people can become dehydrated while working or exercising in hot conditions. Is it helpful to consume sports drinks under these situations? In addition to water and glucose, sports drinks contain small amounts of the minerals sodium and potassium; therefore, these beverages may be beneficial for individuals engaging in prolonged, strenuous physical activities in which considerable sweating occurs. Most people, however, can maintain their fluid and mineral balance by eating a variety of foods and by drinking water before and during the activity.

### Healthy Living Practices

- ☐ To obtain all of the vitamins and minerals you need, eat a wide variety of foods each day; include whole grains, dairy products, fruits, and vegetables.
- ☐ Store dietary supplements like other medications, making them inaccessible to children.
- ☐ If you are hot or exercising heavily, to prevent dehydration, drink plenty of water and other beverages that do not contain caffeine or alcohol.
- ☐ To increase the likelihood that you will maintain your bone mass as you age, consume adequate amounts of calcium-rich foods, drink less alcohol, do not smoke, and engage in weight-bearing exercise regularly.

# The Basics of a Healthful Diet

When you eat a milk-chocolate candy bar or some french-fried potatoes, you probably know that these foods contain carbohydrate and fat, but you may be surprised to learn that they also supply some protein, water, and even vitamins and minerals. Most foods are mixtures of nutrients that contain relatively large quantities of water, carbohydrate, fat, or protein, with much smaller quantities of vitamins and minerals. Candy bars and french fries are commonly called "junk" foods because they contain considerable calories from fat and sugar. Dietitians, however, generally refer to such foods as "empty-calorie" rather than junk foods.

A nutritious diet has two key features: *nutrient adequacy* and *nutrient balance*. The foods in a nutritionally adequate and balanced diet contain all essential nutrients in the proper proportions. By selecting a wide variety of foods, you can usually obtain all essential nutrients. Many people upset the nutritional balance of their diets by consuming more food than they need, by making poor food choices, or by taking massive doses of nutrient supplements. Eating too much food can make one overweight; eating too much salty food may raise one's blood pressure; ingesting too many supplements can cause nutrient toxicity disorders. "Everything in moderation" is the best approach to planning nutritionally adequate and well-balanced diets.

How much of each nutrient do you need for optimal health? How can you be certain that your diet is nutritionally adequate? The following information provides answers to these questions.

## Nutrient Requirements and Recommendations

A **nutrient requirement** can be defined as the minimum amount that prevents an average person from developing the nutrient's deficiency disease. A re-
quired level of a nutrient, however, is not necessarily an optimal amount. By obtaining only the required levels of most vitamins, for example, the body does not have amounts to store in various tissues. The body relies on its nutrient reserves if nutritious food becomes unavailable. Thus, nutrition experts recommend that people consume more than just the required amounts of many nutrients.

To determine whether a diet supplies amounts of certain nutrients that can prevent deficiency diseases, nutritionists now use a complex set of standards called the **Dietary Reference Intakes (DRIs)**. The DRIs are composed of four different recommendations for nutrient and energy intake levels, including the *Recommended Dietary Allowances* (*RDAs*), which at one time were the only standards for planning nutritious diets and analyzing the nutritional adequacy of diets. To establish the RDA for a nutrient, scientists take the required level and add a certain amount to provide a margin of safety. For example, the current RDA for vitamin C is 90 mg/day for men and 75 mg/day for women (nonsmokers). The average person, however, requires only about 8 to 10 mg of vitamin C each day to prevent scurvy, the vitamin's deficiency disease. Therefore, most people will not develop scurvy even if their intake does not meet 100% of the RDA.

The DRIs include a set of values called the "Tolerable Upper Intake Level" or simply "UL." The UL is the maximum average daily intake amount for a nutrient that is unlikely to be harmful. Therefore, regularly consuming amounts of a nutrient that exceed its UL is likely to cause toxicity signs and symptoms. The adult UL for vitamin C, for example, is 2,000 milligrams per day. Tables 9.7 and 9.9 indicate toxicity signs and symptoms for certain vitamins and minerals, respectively.

You can evaluate the nutritional adequacy of your diet by using the RDAs or other DRI values. A brief version of the DRI tables is shown in Appendix C. Complete the activity "Assessing the Nutritional Quality of Your Diet" in the Student Workbook section at the end of this text. If your usual intake of a nutrient is between 75% and 100% of the recommended amount, you probably are not at risk of developing that nutrient's deficiency disease. If you need to boost your intake of one or more nutrients, you can identify foods that are rich sources of the nutrient by using food composition tables, such as those on this text's accompanying website, and eat more of these foods.

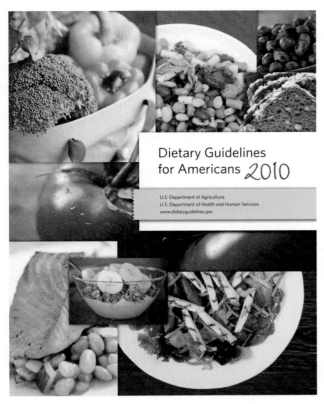

© U.S. Department of Agriculture and U.S. Department of Health and Human Services. *Dietary Guidelines for Americans, 2010.* 7th Edition, Washington, DC: U.S. Government Printing Office, December 2010.

## The Dietary Guidelines

Every 5 years, the U.S. Department of Agriculture (USDA) and the Department of Health and Human Services issue the *Dietary Guidelines for Americans*, a publication that provides general recommendations for a healthful diet. The *Guidelines* focus attention on the association between diet and chronic diseases, such as type 2 diabetes and cardiovascular disease. These guidelines provide basic advice concerning lifestyle behaviors that relate to nutritional health, such as choosing nutrient-dense foods, being more physically active, and following food safety practices. The key recommendations of the 2010 *Dietary Guidelines* are described here.

*Balance calories with physical activity to achieve and maintain healthy weight.*

1.  Prevent and/or reduce excess body fat by improving dietary practices and increasing physical activity.
    - Focus on the total number of calories consumed.

- Monitor food intake by recording what you eat.
- Consume smaller sized portions or low-calorie options.
- Eat a nutrient-dense breakfast.
- Limit the amount of time spent sitting.

2.  Control total calorie intake to manage body weight. For people who are overweight or obese, consume fewer calories.
    - Increase intake of plant foods, such as whole grains, vegetables, and fruits.
    - Reduce intake of sugar-sweetened beverages, such as regular soft drinks, fruit drinks, and energy drinks.
    - Monitor the 100% fruit juice intake of children, especially those who are overweight or obese.
    - Avoid excess intake of alcoholic beverages.

3.  Increase physical activity and reduce time spent being inactive (sedentary).
    - Balance calorie intake with calorie needs throughout the life span.

*Foods and food components to reduce.*

1.  Limit sodium intake to less than 2,300 mg/day. People older than 50 years of age or who are African American or have hypertension, diabetes, or chronic kidney disease should limit their sodium intake to 1,500 mg/day.
2.  Consume less than 10% of calories from unhealthy saturated fats by replacing them with foods that are rich sources of healthy mono-unsaturated and polyunsaturated fats.
3.  Consume less than 300 mg of cholesterol daily.

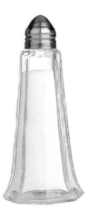

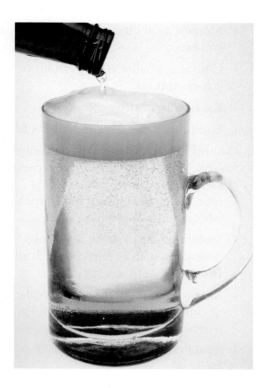

4. Avoid foods that contain trans fatty acids, such as solid fats and foods that are made with partially hydrogenated oils.
5. Reduce intake of calories from foods that contain solid fats and added sugars, such as cakes, cookies, and pastries.
6. Limit consumption of refined grains, especially those with added solid fat, sugar, and sodium.
7. If alcohol is consumed, limit intake to up to one drink per day (women) and two drinks per day (men). Only adults of legal age should consume alcohol.

*Foods and nutrients to increase.*

1. Increase vegetable and fruit intake.
2. Eat a variety of colorful vegetables, especially dark green, red, and orange vegetables, and beans and peas.
3. Consume at least half of all grain products as whole grains. Replace foods made with refined grains with those made from whole grains.
4. Increase intake of fat-free or low-fat milk and milk products or substitutes, such as yogurt, cheese, or fortified soy beverages.
5. Choose protein foods from a variety of sources, including seafood, lean meat and poultry, eggs, beans and peas, soy products, and unsalted nuts and seeds.

6. Increase the amount and variety of fish and shellfish in your diet by replacing some meat and poultry with such foods.
7. Replace solid fats with vegetable oils.
8. Choose foods that provide more potassium, dietary fiber, calcium, vitamin D. These foods include vegetables, dried beans and peas, fruit, whole grains, and milk and milk products.

*Build healthy eating patterns.*

1. Select an eating pattern that meets nutrient and energy needs over time.
2. Account for all foods and beverages consumed and evaluate the nutritional quality of your eating pattern.
3. Prepare, eat, and store foods by following food safety recommendations to reduce risk of foodborne illnesses.

## MyPlate

In spring 2011, the USDA introduced **MyPlate**, a practical guide for planning healthful diets that incorporates recommendations from the 2010 *Dietary Guidelines*. MyPlate has five primary food groups: grains, vegetables, fruits, dairy, and protein foods (**Figure 9.11**).

MyPlate provides "Daily Food Plans," amounts of foods to include in meals and snacks from the food groups that meet recommended nutrient intakes at 12 different calorie levels, ranging from 1,000 to 3,200 calories/day. Thus, a person can use MyPlate to

### Figure 9.11

**MyPlate.** The USDA's MyPlate interactive tool at www.choosemyplate.gov can be used to plan nutritious menus and evaluate the nutritional quality of a person's diet.

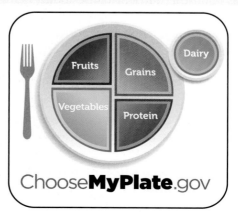

plan menus that meet his or her energy and nutrient needs. For example, a very physically active 22-year-old male may need 3,000 calories/day, whereas his physically inactive 20-year-old female friend might only need 1,600 calories/day. Appendix D provides the 12 food intake patterns as well as sample menus for a 2,000-calorie/day food pattern.

To obtain more information about MyPlate, access the USDA's interactive website (www.choosemyplate.gov/index.html). By clicking on the glass or section of the plate that represents one of the five major food groups, you will learn more about the foods in that particular group.

**Oils and Empty Calories** The MyPlate website includes information about oils and *empty calories.* Some fatty foods, such as olives, nuts, and seafood, naturally contain healthful oils. Depending on a person's total daily caloric intake, MyPlate indicates an amount of oils to consume each day. Empty calories are sugars and fats added to foods. Fats and sugars can make foods very tasty, but in many instances, such foods are not as nutritious as foods without these ingredients. Alcohol is also an empty-calorie food. MyPlate sets a limit for the number of empty calories to consume each day. The dietary plan has no recommendation for alcohol intake.

Diets that contain too many empty-calorie foods may contribute to excess body fat, heart disease, diabetes, and alcoholism. Additionally, these items can displace more nutrient-dense foods from your diet. Consuming a reasonable amount of empty-calorie foods may be acceptable if your diet is nutritionally adequate and you are physically active and need the extra calories to fuel physical activity. The Student Workbook section at the end of this text includes an activity that enables you to use MyPlate to evaluate the nutritional adequacy of your daily food choices.

## Using Nutritional Labeling

The FDA requires nearly every packaged food to have nutritional labeling. Consumers can use food labeling to determine and compare the nutritional value of most packaged foods. **Figure 9.12** illustrates the Nutrition Facts label and provides tips for using this information. A new format may be introduced in 2012.

Many consumers want to know how many grams of fat and calories are in a serving of packaged food. This information appears at the top of the Nutrition Facts label (see Figure 9.12). People can also monitor the amounts of cholesterol, sodium, and fiber in packaged foods. The Nutrition Facts label indicates these amounts by weight and as percentages of es-

tablished nutrient labeling standards called the *Daily Values* (*DVs*).

Health officials at the FDA used various sources of nutritional information to determine the DVs for many nutrients and for fiber. As you can see in Figure 9.11, the lower part of the Nutrition Facts label shows two sets of DVs. One set of DVs is for people who consume 2,000 calories each day; the other set is for those who consume 2,500 calories daily. The DVs for total fat, saturated fat, cholesterol, and sodium are maximum amounts. Most Americans should keep their daily intake of these nutrients below these amounts.

Specific information concerning the nutritional content per serving of the food product appears on the upper half of the label. In addition to showing amounts of fat, saturated fat, cholesterol, sodium, total carbohydrate, fiber, sugar, and protein by weight, the Nutrition Facts label displays most of this information as percentages of the DVs for a 2,000-calorie diet. Percentages of the DVs for key vitamins and minerals are shown below the second bold line.

According to the information near the top of the Nutrition Facts label shown in Figure 9.12, a serving of the product supplies 250 calories, 110 of which are from fat. To determine the percentage of calories from fat, divide the calories from fat (110) by the number of calories in the serving (250), and multiply the figure by 100. Forty-four percent of the calories in this food are from fat. Because most health experts recommend that healthy Americans eat no more than 35% of their total calories from fat, you might decide to purchase other food products that contain lower percentages of calories from fat.

Another approach to controlling your fat intake is to eat foods with a variety of fat contents, but your intake should not exceed 65 g of fat per day, the DV for a 2,000-calorie diet. For example, you might eat a 1-oz. serving of corn chips that contains 6 g of fat and supplies 40% of its calories from fat. The other foods eaten on this day should provide no more than 59 grams of fat (65 − 6 = 59).

Not everyone thinks that the Nutrition Facts label is easy to use or helpful. Because the percentage of total calories from fat is not listed, people cannot easily compare the fat content of packaged food products. Additionally, many adult Americans need to consume lower amounts of calories and fat than the DVs. Furthermore, most people eat a variety of foods,

**Figure 9.12**

**Nutrition Facts.** Most packaged foods have nutrient facts on their labels. People can use this information to evaluate the nutritional quality of their food. In 2012, the government may introduce a new nutrient label format.

1. **Serving Size** This section shows how many servings are in the package. *Remember*: all nutrition information on the label is based on one serving.

2. **Amount of Calories** The calories listed are for one serving. "Calories from fat" are also for one serving.

3. **Consume Adequate Amounts of These Nutrients** Get the most nutrition for your calories—compare the calories to the nutrients to make a healthier food choice.

4. **Limit These Nutrients** Too much total fat (especially saturated fat and trans fat), cholesterol, and sodium may increase your risk of certain chronic diseases.

5. **Choose "Healthy" Carbohydrates** Fiber and sugars are types of carbohydrates. Healthy sources like fruits, vegetables, beans, and whole grains can reduce the risk of heart disease and improve digestive functioning. Limit foods with added sugars (sucrose, glucose, fructose, corn or maple syrup) which add calories but not other nutrients such as vitamins and minerals.

6. **The Daily Value is a Key to a Balanced Diet** The % DV is a general guide to help you link nutrients in a serving of food to their contribution to your total daily diet. It can help you determine if a food is high or low in a nutrient—5% or less is low, 20% or more is high. The % DV is based on a 2,000-calorie diet.

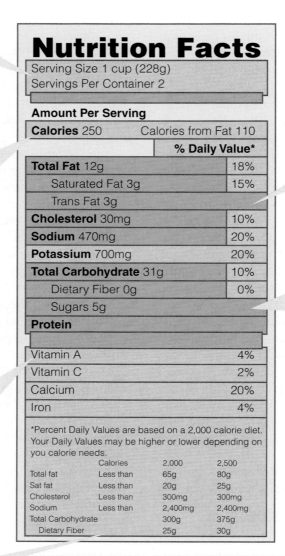

# Nutrition Facts

Serving Size 1 cup (228g)
Servings Per Container 2

**Amount Per Serving**

| Calories 250 | Calories from Fat 110 |
| --- | --- |

| | **% Daily Value\*** |
| --- | --- |
| **Total Fat** 12g | 18% |
| Saturated Fat 3g | 15% |
| Trans Fat 3g | |
| **Cholesterol** 30mg | 10% |
| **Sodium** 470mg | 20% |
| **Potassium** 700mg | 20% |
| **Total Carbohydrate** 31g | 10% |
| Dietary Fiber 0g | 0% |
| Sugars 5g | |
| **Protein** | |

| Vitamin A | 4% |
| --- | --- |
| Vitamin C | 2% |
| Calcium | 20% |
| Iron | 4% |

\*Percent Daily Values are based on a 2,000 calorie diet. Your Daily Values may be higher or lower depending on you calorie needs.

| | | Calories | 2,000 | 2,500 |
| --- | --- | --- | --- | --- |
| Total fat | Less than | | 65g | 80g |
| Sat fat | Less than | | 20g | 25g |
| Cholesterol | Less than | | 300mg | 300mg |
| Sodium | Less than | | 2,400mg | 2,400mg |
| Total Carbohydrate | | | 300g | 375g |
| Dietary Fiber | | | 25g | 30g |

some of which is fresh or prepared in restaurants. As a result, these people will probably underestimate the amounts of calories and nutrients in their diet if they rely only on the information provided by food labels.

You can learn more about the calories and nutrients in your foods and beverages by using the "What's in the Food You Eat" search tool at www.ars.usda.gov/Services/docs.htm?docid=17032.

## What About Foods Sold in Restaurants?

In 2010, the U.S. federal government passed legislation that required restaurants and food vendors with more than 20 locations to inform consumers about caloric and nutrient contents of products sold at these outlets. The goal of the legislation was to provide accurate and easy-to-understand information about the nutritional value of prepared foods. By considering this information, consumers would be able to make more educated decisions concerning their food choices when purchasing meals and snacks. At the time of this writing, the specific details of the guidelines had not been established.

## Do You Need Vitamin or Mineral Supplements?

Do you buy dietary supplements such as the ones listed in **Table 9.10**? If your answer is yes, why do you take them? Millions of Americans purchase dietary

---

### Table 9.10

#### Nutritional Dietary Supplements

| Supplement | Major Claims | Health Risks/Benefits |
|---|---|---|
| Apple cider vinegar | Cures arthritis, promotes weight loss, reduces blood cholesterol level | No scientific evidence to support claims. |
| Beta-carotene | Reduces risk of cancer and heart disease; antioxidant | Acts as antioxidant, but supplements may stimulate cancer cell growth. |
| Choline | Improves memory | No scientific evidence to support claim. |
| Chondroitin sulfate | Treats arthritis (often combined with glucosamine) | No scientific evidence to support claims. |
| Coenzyme Q-10 | Reverses signs of aging and disease; antioxidant | Helps cells generate energy and may have medicinal benefits, but more research is needed. |
| DHEA | Slows aging process, increases muscular strength, and cures numerous ailments | Does not slow rate of aging or cure ailments; long-term effects of taking this naturally occurring hormone are unknown. |
| Fish oil | Prevents heart disease and stroke, cures rheumatoid arthritis, reduces risk of Alzheimer's disease | Reduces inflammation by suppressing the body's immune response and lowers elevated triglyceride levels. May interfere with blood clotting, increasing the risk of hemorrhagic stroke. Cod liver oil contains vitamins A and D, which are toxic when taken in large doses. |
| Garlic | Lowers blood cholesterol levels | Does not lower cholesterol consistently, and can cause allergic reaction and unpleasant body odor and interfere with prescription blood thinners. |
| Glucosamine sulfate | Treats arthritis | May slow the destruction of cartilage in knee joint. |
| Lysine | Prevents herpes simplex viral outbreaks from recurring | No scientific evidence to support claim. |
| Melatonin | Treats insomnia and jet lag | Scientific evidence suggests this hormone can treat certain sleep disorders, but information about its long-term safety is lacking. |
| SAM-e | Relieves pain and depression | More research is needed to support claims and determine health risks; may increase risk of heart disease. |
| Yogurt (containing live bacterial cultures) | Slows aging process, prevents and cures vaginal yeast infections | No scientific evidence to support these claims, but it may improve intestinal health |

---

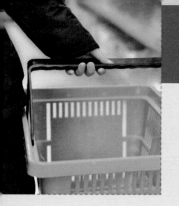

# Consumer Health

## Dietary Supplements

Provisions of the 1994 Supplement and Health Education Act allow manufacturers to classify vitamin and mineral pills, protein or amino acid preparations, and certain hormones as "dietary supplements." As mentioned in Chapter 1, the FDA does not regulate dietary supplements as extensively as it regulates medicinal drugs. For example, a pharmaceutical company that is developing a new drug to treat diabetes must submit the medication to thorough testing and provide scientific evidence of its safety and effectiveness as a treatment before the drug can be introduced into the marketplace. Thus, the process of approving a new medication generally takes several years. When the medication finally becomes available, purchasing it is likely to require a physician's prescription.

Dietary supplement manufacturers do not need to provide the FDA with scientific evidence that a supplement is safe for humans or provides measurable health benefits before they can market the product. As a result, many supplements contain ingredients that have not been scientifically tested for safety or effectiveness. Even if an ingredient in a dietary supplement is known to cause serious side effects, the product can still be sold through Internet outlets or in health food stores, pharmacies, and supermarkets without a prescription. If the FDA collects enough convincing evidence that a dietary supplement is dangerous, then the agency can ask manufacturers to remove the product from the marketplace voluntarily or require them to stop distributing it. Table 9.10 lists popular nutritional dietary supplements and their claimed health benefits and notes their potential risks.

The FDA requires manufacturers to provide certain information on dietary supplement labels. The label must show the product's name, state that it is a supplement, provide a list of ingredients, and indicate the net weight of the product's contents. The label also needs to display the name and address of the product's packer, distributor, or manufacturer. Additionally, supplements must have a Supplement Facts label that lists the product's ingredients and includes other information, such as the suggested daily dose.

The FDA allows manufacturers to make certain claims about a dietary supplement's nutrient content, health benefits, and structure/function usefulness. If manufacturers indicate that a dietary supplement treats a specific nutritional deficiency, supports health in some manner, or reduces the risk of a health condition, such claims must be followed by the disclaimer "This statement has not been evaluated by the Food and Drug Administration. This product is not intended to diagnose, treat, cure, or prevent any disease." To learn which kinds of health-related claims have been approved by the FDA, visit www.fda.gov/Food/LabelingNutrition/LabelClaims/ucm111447.htm.

According to the FDA, many consumers of dietary supplements want to know if health claims for these products on labels or in advertisements and printed material are truthful. Such claims do not require FDA approval before they can be used, but manufacturers are supposed to provide evidence to support the claims if the agency asks them to do so. The FDA, however, lacks sufficient funding and personnel to investigate all questionable or misleading claims.

supplements, especially multivitamin/multimineral products that contain mixtures of vitamins and minerals. Approximately 40% of adult Americans take at least one multivitamin/multimineral supplement.[25] In 2010, sales of dietary supplements, which include vitamin and mineral pills, herbal products, and certain hormones, were estimated to be almost $29 *billion* in the United States.[26]

Many people take vitamin and mineral supplements to reduce the risk of heart disease, osteoporosis, and other serious chronic diseases. By carefully selecting a variety of foods and eating recommended amounts from the major food groups, healthy adults should be able to obtain enough nutrients without supplementation. Some people, however, need to supplement their diets with certain nutrients. Pregnant and breastfeeding women need more iron, calcium, and folic acid than what is available in foods. Some vegetarians need more calcium, iron, zinc, and vitamins B12 and D. Elderly persons may benefit from extra vitamins D and B12.

Nutrient supplements do not contain all of the substances found in food that benefit health; therefore, they are not substitutes for nutrient-dense foods. If your diet is nutritious and you still want to take a multiple vitamin and mineral supplement as an "insurance policy," choose a reasonably priced product that contains no more than 100% of the DV for each of the vitamins and minerals listed on the label. The supplement should meet United States Pharmacopeia (USP) standards for strength, purity, and ability to dissolve. Vague advertising statements or labeling declarations, such as "meets laboratory standards for quality," do not guarantee product quality. Vitamin and mineral pills are dietary supplements. The Consumer Health feature "Dietary Supplements" provides information about claims made for dietary supplements.

## Healthy Living Practices

- To plan well-balanced, nutritious daily menus, you can follow the recommendations of the latest dietary guidelines and MyPlate.

- Use the Nutrition Facts on food labels to compare the nutritional content of packaged foods and plan nutritious meals and snacks.

- If you want to take a multiple vitamin and mineral supplement, choose a product that meets United States Pharmacopeia (USP) standards and supplies no more than 100% of each nutrient's DV.

## Malnutrition: Undernutrition and Overnutrition

**Malnutrition** results when a person's usual food intake supplies inadequate or excessive amounts of nutrients. *Under*nutrition occurs when a diet does not contain enough nutrients; *over*nutrition results from consuming excessive amounts of nutrients. Undernutrition can be especially devastating for children. Undernourished youngsters often develop nutritional deficiency diseases; as a result, they may not grow properly or perform physical and mental tasks optimally. In parts of the world where many babies are not vaccinated against common childhood diseases, undernourished children often die from infections such as measles.

Undernutrition also occurs in the United States. During 2009, the people living in about 15% of U.S.

**malnutrition** Overnutrition or undernutrition that results when diets supply improper amounts of nutrients.

households were uncertain about having or unable to obtain enough food for all members because of lack of resources.[27] Even some people with adequate incomes are marginally nourished because they choose diets that supply barely enough vitamins and minerals. Such individuals may experience more frequent infections and take longer to recover from illnesses than those who are well nourished. Alcoholics, people with anorexia nervosa, and individuals with chronic digestive system diseases are also at risk for undernutrition.

People living in countries with high standards of living are more likely to suffer from the ill effects of *over*nutrition rather than undernutrition. Individuals who eat too much sugar and fat may develop obesity, which increases their risk of diabetes, hypertension, and heart disease. The following chapter discusses obesity and weight management.

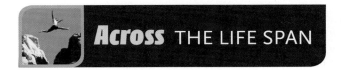

## Across THE LIFE SPAN

### NUTRITION

From conception until birth, the developing embryo/fetus depends on its mother to supply the nutrients it needs for development and growth. Women often become more health-conscious during pregnancy, and as a result, they may select more nutritious diets. A woman's nutritional status prior to conception, however, has a significant impact on the health of her baby. By consuming a nutritious diet before becoming pregnant, a woman can build optimal nutrient reserves that prepare her body for the nutritional demands of pregnancy. During pregnancy, malnourished women have a higher risk than well-nourished mothers-to-be of miscarrying, having premature or underweight infants, and delivering babies with birth defects.

Consuming diets that supply adequate folate (a B vitamin) is critical, especially during the first 4 weeks of pregnancy when the *neural tube*, the embryonic region that forms the brain and spinal cord, develops. Occasionally, the neural tube fails to develop properly, resulting in *spina bifida* and related defects. Spina bifida occurs when a section of the spine does not fuse to form the channel that encases and protects the spinal cord. In severe cases, the spinal cord protrudes from the infant's back, seriously impairing the child's ability to control the lower part of its body.

Many pregnant women are not even aware of their pregnancy when the neural tube is forming. To maximize the amount of folate in their tissues, women should eat plenty of folate-rich foods, especially enriched breads and cereals, lentils, fruits, and green leafy vegetables (see Table 9.7), *before* pregnancy. During pregnancy, women should eat nutritious diets, obtain medical care, and take their prescribed doses of prenatal vitamin and mineral supplements. Before taking other supplemental nutrients, pregnant women should always check with their physicians. Consuming excessive amounts of nutrient supplements during pregnancy increases the risk of certain birth defects.

Current infant feeding recommendations include the following: provide breastmilk and a supplement that contains vitamin D and iron for at least the first 12 months of life. Iron-fortified infant formulas are acceptable alternatives, but every healthy pregnant woman should consider the benefits of breastfeeding her baby. Breastmilk is the most suitable food for infants. Caregivers should not feed fresh whole or reduced-fat cows' milk to babies before their first birthday. Furthermore, babies should not be fed solid foods before they are 4 months of age.

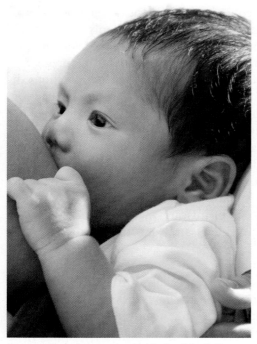
Breastmilk is the most suitable food for infants.

Breastmilk offers many health benefits to infants and their mothers. Babies who consume breastmilk have reduced risks for sudden infant death syndrome, childhood leukemia, ear infections, asthma, childhood obesity, and diabetes.[28] The proteins in human milk will not cause allergies like those in formulas do. Women who breastfeed can also obtain important health benefits—they have lower risks of type 2 diabetes, breast cancer, and ovarian cancer than do women who do not breastfeed.

Breastfeeding is economical and convenient; mothers can breastfeed anywhere they feel comfortable doing so. Individuals who are interested in breastfeeding can obtain educational materials and advice from members of the *La Leche League*, an organization with groups in many U.S. communities.

Many women do not breastfeed because they want to return to a job, they lack the support of family and friends, or they are uncomfortable with this practice. These women should follow their pediatrician's advice concerning the use of commercially prepared infant formulas.

Parents often describe their preschool-aged children as picky eaters because they do not seem to be as hungry or interested in eating as when they were infants. However, most children eat enough calories to maintain their normal growth pattern. During this period, children often establish their food preferences and eating habits; well-informed, responsible adults can serve as role models, teaching youngsters how to choose nutrient-dense foods.

Eating a nutritious breakfast is an important habit to develop early in life. The child who routinely skips breakfast and eats too many sugary snacks can develop borderline or overt nutritional deficiencies. This child often lacks energy, has difficulty concentrating on school work, and experiences behavioral problems. In severe cases, a malnourished child fails to grow properly.

Adolescents experience rapid growth during puberty, and their appetites increase accordingly. Teenagers often become overly concerned with their body size and shape. As a result, boys may experiment with dietary supplements to increase muscle mass. To lose weight, girls may skip meals or choose diets that limit nutritious foods, such as calcium-rich dairy products. Growing adolescents require plenty of calcium to maximize bone mass. An obsession with body size can foster poor eating practices and eating disorders that last into adulthood.

Older adults who consumed a nutritious diet and have exercised regularly since their youth are more

# Analyzing Health-Related Information

The following advertisement promotes a dietary supplement, garlic oil tablets, to relieve fatigue. Read the ad and evaluate it using the model for analyzing health-related information. The main points of the model are noted here; the model is fully explained in Chapter 1.

1. Which statements are verifiable facts, and which are unverified statements or value claims?
2. What are the credentials of the person who makes the health-related claims? Does this person have the appropriate background and education in the topic area? What can you do to check the person's credentials?
3. What might be the motives and biases of the person making the claims?
4. What is the main point of the ad? Which information is relevant to the product? Which information is irrelevant?
5. Is the source reliable? What evidence supports your conclusion that the source is reliable or unreliable? Does the source of information present the pros and cons of the topic or the benefits and risks of the product?
6. Does the source of information attack the credibility of conventional scientists or medical authorities?

Based on your analysis, do you think that this ad is a reliable source of health-related information? Summarize your reasons for coming to this conclusion.

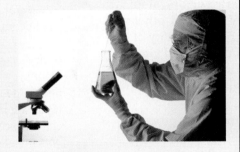

## RUSSIAN SCIENTISTS DISCOVER NEW TREATMENT FOR FATIGUE!

**Kiev, Russia**—Russian researchers working under the direction of famed doctor Igor X. Ivanamiraculsky of Minsk have discovered that Russian garlic oil is a safe and effective treatment for chronic fatigue. In hundreds of double-blind studies performed at the Minsk Institute of Food Research, college students, athletes, and even elderly persons who took the garlic oil capsules reported having 25% more energy than those persons taking placebos. These results are nothing short of amazing!

Now, you can benefit from Dr. Ivanamiraculsky's discovery. For the first time, the doctor's energy-boosting garlic oil pills are available in the United States. No prescription is needed for this 100% completely natural energizer. Just ask for odor-free GARGOIL at your local pharmacy or health-food store. Satisfaction guaranteed! If you are not completely satisfied after taking GARGOIL, return the unused portion to the place of purchase for a refund. Remember to be careful and follow the label's instructions; some people report feeling too energized after taking GARGOIL! Accept no garlic oil substitutes—ask for GARGOIL.

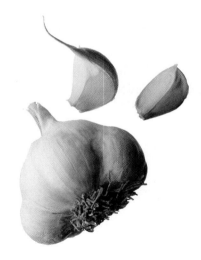

## Figure 9.13

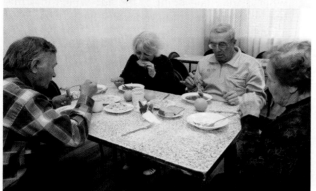

**Nutrition for Older Adults.** Many older adult Americans participate in congregate meal programs within their community.

likely to enjoy good health than those who ate poor diets and were inactive. However, physical, psychological, social, and economic factors often influence the quality and quantity of the elderly person's food intake. As one ages, production of acid and other stomach secretions decreases, reducing the ability of the small intestine to absorb calcium, iron, and vitamins D and B12. Therefore, older adults should ask their physicians about the need to take certain nutrient supplements.

Many elderly persons are unable to shop for groceries or prepare foods because of arthritis and strokes. Older individuals who are psychologically depressed, socially isolated, or financially impoverished often lack the interest or the resources to prepare nutritious meals. These people are at risk of becoming malnourished. Many communities offer federally subsidized nutrition programs such as Meals-on-Wheels and congregate meals for those who are at least 60 years old. The Meals-on-Wheels program relies on community volunteers to deliver a hot meal, milk, and fresh fruit to homebound people as often as five days a week. More mobile aged individuals can participate in congregate meal programs in which they visit community centers where hot meals are served five days a week (**Figure 9.13**). Besides providing a nourishing meal, these sites enable elderly participants to interact socially. Frequent contact with other people can reduce an elderly person's risk of depression, a health problem that often affects isolated aged people.

## Healthy Living Practices

- To increase your chances of having a healthy baby, improve the quality of your diet *before* you become pregnant.
- Excesses of certain nutrients can produce birth defects, so ask your physician for advice before you take nutrient supplements during pregnancy.
- If you are a woman who plans to have children, consider the benefits of breastfeeding, especially during their first 12 months of life.

# CHAPTER REVIEW

## Summary

Nutrients are substances in foods that supply energy; regulate body processes; and provide material for growth, maintenance, and repair of tissues. The six classes of nutrients are carbohydrates, lipids, proteins, vitamins, minerals, and water. Many foods also contain nonnutrients, substances that are not essential but may have healthful benefits. Phytochemicals may prevent various chronic diseases, including certain cancers.

During digestion, food is broken down into nutrients that can be absorbed. Cells metabolize carbohydrates, fats, and proteins for energy. The amount of energy stored in food is measured in calories. Cells cannot release energy from water, vitamins, and minerals.

Carbohydrates, the sugars and starches, are a major source of energy for the body. The only disorder that is clearly associated with excessive carbohydrate consumption is tooth decay. Plant foods supply dietary fiber and phytochemicals. Diets rich in fiber may reduce the risks of diverticulosis, hemorrhoids, constipation, and heart disease.

Many medical experts think Americans eat too much fat, especially saturated fat and trans fat. Eating excessive amounts of these lipids is associated with an increased risk of obesity, heart disease, and certain cancers.

Protein is essential for tissue growth, repair, and maintenance and for producing enzymes, antibodies, and certain hormones. The average American consumes more than twice the amount of protein needed, particularly from animal foods. One way to reduce the amount of animal foods in the diet is to eat more protein from plants. Vegetarian diets are associated with lower risks of chronic conditions such as heart disease.

Vitamins and minerals regulate body processes; some minerals are structural components of tissues. Overdoses of many vitamins and most minerals can cause nutritional imbalances and be toxic; therefore, unless medically indicated, people should avoid taking high doses of nutrient supplements.

A lifetime of inadequate calcium intake coupled with low estrogen levels after menopause increases a woman's risk of osteoporosis. Iron deficiency is a common nutritional problem, especially among women of childbearing age. Dehydration is a serious condition that results when water intake is inadequate or water losses are excessive.

The key features of a nutritious diet are nutrient adequacy and nutrient balance. By selecting a variety of foods and by avoiding the indiscriminate use of nutrient supplements, one's diet can be nutritionally adequate and balanced.

A requirement for a nutrient is the smallest amount that prevents a deficiency disease. Dietary Reference Intakes (DRIs) are standards for planning nutritious diets and determining the nutritional adequacy of diets. MyPlate and the *Dietary Guidelines* are practical daily menu-planning guides. Nutrient labeling can help consumers select nutritious foods. Malnutrition occurs when diets supply too little or too many nutrients.

The quality of a woman's diet before and during pregnancy has an impact on the health of her developing child. During the first year of life, human milk is the best food for infants; solid foods should not be fed to babies until they are 4 months old. Without proper supervision, children and teenagers may skip meals or select inadequate diets. Physical, psychological, economic, and social factors contribute to the risk of malnutrition among older adults.

# Applying What You Have Learned

**Critical Thinking**

1. Explain how you would use nutrient labeling information to choose food products that are low in fat. **Application**
2. Keep a food record for one day. Analyze this day's food choices by using the "Tracker" at the MyPlate web site (http://www.mypyramidtracker.gov/). **Analysis**
3. Consider the results of your food record. Which foods can you eat to improve your food intake? **Evaluation**
4. Plan a menu for a day (meals, snacks, and beverages) that meets MyPlate's recommended amounts of foods for a person of your age, sex, weight, height, and physical activity level. You'll need to visit www.choosemyplate.gov to do this activity. **Synthesis**

**Key**

| **Application** | **Analysis** | **Synthesis** | **Evaluation** |
|---|---|---|---|
| using information in a new situation. | breaking down information into component parts. | putting together information from different sources. | making informed decisions. |

# Reflecting on Your Health

**Critical Thinking**

1. After reading this chapter, what changes can you make to improve your diet? How is your present diet different from what you ate as a child or while in high school? Why do you think your present diet is better or worse than your past diet?
2. What factors influence your food choices? How willing are you to try new foods? What new foods have you eaten in the past year?
3. Do you use nutrition labels? If you do, which information do you think is most important? How does nutritional labeling help you be a better consumer? If you do not use nutrition labels, why not?
4. Do you take dietary supplements? If you do, which supplements do you take? Why do you take them?
5. Females: Would you or did you breastfeed your children? Explain why you would or did breastfeed your children. Males: Would you want or did the mother of your children breastfeed them? Why or why not?

# References

1. American Dietetic Association. (2004). Position of the American Dietetic Association: Use of nutritive and nonnutritive sweeteners. *Journal of the American Dietetic Association, 104*(2):255–275.

2. Haley, S., & McConnell, M. (2010). Sugar and sweeteners outlook. *USDA Outlook* (SSS-M-261). Retrieved on March 15, 2011, from http://www.ers.usda.gov/Publications/SSS/2010/May/SSSM261.pdf

3. Kochanek, K. D., et al. (2011). Deaths: Preliminary data for 2009.

4. *National Vital Statistics Reports, 59*(4):1–69.

5. U.S. National Institute of Diabetes, Digestive and Kidney Diseases, National Diabetes Information Clearinghouse. (2011, February). *National diabetes statistics, 2011* (NIH Publication No. 11-3892). Retrieved on February 28, 2011, from http://www.diabetes.niddk.nih.gov/dm/pubs/statistics/#fast

6. Centers for Disease Control and Prevention, National Center for Chronic Disease Prevention and Health Promotion. (2011, January). Age-adjusted incidence of diagnosed diabetes per 1,000 population aged 18–79 years, by race/ethnicity, United States, 1997–2009. Data and trends, National Diabetes Surveillance System. Retrieved on April 25, 2011, from http://www.cdc.gov/diabetes/statistics/incidence/fig6.htm

7. Malik, V. S., et al. (2010). Sugar-sweetened beverages and risk of metabolic syndrome and type 2 diabetes. *Diabetes Care, 33*(11):2477–2483.

8. U.S. Centers for Disease Control and Prevention. (2011, April). Diabetes Public Health Resource: Prevent diabetes. Retrieved on April 26, 2011, from http://www.cdc.gov/diabetes/consumer/prevent.htm

9. U.S. National Institutes of Health, National Heart Lung and Blood Institute. (2010, January). What is metabolic syndrome? Retrieved on April 25, 2011, from http://www.nhlbi.nih.gov/health/dci/Diseases/ms/ms_whatis.html

10. National Institutes of Health, National Digestive Diseases Information Clearinghouse. (2009). Lactose intolerance. Retrieved on April 25, 2011, from http://digestive.niddk.nih.gov/ddiseases/pubs/lactoseintolerance/

11. American Gastroenterological Association. (2008). Patient center: Understanding constipation. Retrieved on April 25, 2011, from http://www.gastro.org/patient-center/digestive-conditions/constipation

12. Otten, J. J., et al. (2006). *Dietary Reference Intakes: The essential guide to nutrient requirements*. Institute of Medicine of the National Academies. Washington, DC: National Academies Press.

13. Position of the American Dietetic Association and Dietitians of Canada. (2007). Dietary fatty acids. *Journal of the American Dietetic Association, 107*(9):1599–1611.

14. Buckland, G., et al. (2009). Adherence to the Mediterranean diet and risk of coronary heart disease in the Spanish EPIC Cohort Study. *American Journal of Epidemiology, 170*(12):1518–1529.

15. Williams, A. N., & Woessner, K. M. (2009). Monosodium glutamate "allergy": Menace or myth? *Clinical and Experimental Allergy, 39*(5):640–646.

16. U.S. Department of Agriculture, Economic Research Service (2011). U.S. Food Supply: Nutrients contributed from major food groups, 1970 and 2004. Retrieved on April 28, 2011, from http://www.ers.usda.gov/Data/FoodConsumption/NutrientAvailIndex.htm

17. American Dietetic Association. (2009). Position of the American Dietetic Association: Vegetarian diets. *Journal of the American Dietetic Association, 109*(7):1266–1282.

18. National Institutes of Health, National Institute of Allergy and Infectious Diseases. (2010). Food allergy: Quick facts. Retrieved on April 28, 2011, from http://www.niaid.nih.gov/topics/foodallergy/understanding/pages/quickfacts.aspx

19. Gerez, I. F. A., et al. (2010). Diagnostic tests for food allergy. *Singapore Medical Journal, 51*(1):4–9.

20. National Institutes of Health, National Digestive Diseases Information Clearinghouse. (2008). *Celiac disease* (NIH Publication No. 08-4269). Retrieved on April 28, 2011, from http://digestive.niddk.nih.gov/ddiseases/pubs/celiac/index.htm

21. U.S. National Institutes of Health. (2011, April 18). Vitamin C (ascorbic acid). *Medline Plus*. Retrieved on April 29, 2011, from http://www.nlm.nih.gov/medlineplus/druginfo/natural/1001.html

22. Rock, C. L. (2007). Multivitamin-multi-mineral supplements: Who uses them? *American Journal of Clinical Nutrition, 85*(Suppl):277S–279S.

23. National Institutes of Health, National Institute of Arthritis and Musculoskeletal and Skin Diseases. (2011, January). What is osteoporosis? Retrieved on April 29, 2011, from http://www.niams.nih.gov/Health_Info/Bone/Osteoporosis/osteoporosis_ff.asp

24. National Institutes of Health, National Digestive Diseases Information Clearinghouse. (2007). Hemochromatosis. Retrieved on April 30, 2011, from http://digestive.niddk.nih.gov/ddiseases/pubs/hemochromatosis/index.htm

25. Food and Nutrition Board, National Institute of Medicine. (2004). *Dietary reference intakes for water, potassium, sodium, chloride, and sulfate*. Washington, DC: National Academy Press.

26. Gahche, J., et al. (2011, April). Dietary supplement use among U.S. adults has increased since NHANES III (1988–1994). *NCHS Data Brief* No. 61. Retrieved on April 30, 2011, from http://www.cdc.gov/nchs/data/databriefs/db61.htm

27. Mast, C. (2011, January 7). Supplement sales continue strong growth trajectory in 2010. *Nutrition Business Journal*. Retrieved on April 30, 2011, from http://newhope360.com/supplements/supplement-sales-continue-strong-growth-trajectory-2010

28. Nord, M., et al. (2010). *Household food security in the United States, 2009* (Economic Research Report No. ERR-108). Retrieved on April 30, 2011, http://www.ers.usda.gov/publications/err108/

29. U.S. Department of Health and Human Services. (2010, November). *The health benefits of breastfeeding*. Retrieved on April 30, 2011, from http://www.healthcare.gov/news/factsheets/breastfeeding.html

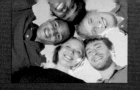
**Diversity in Health**
The Plight of the Pima

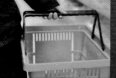
**Consumer Health**
Dietary Supplements:
Weight Loss Aids

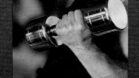
**Managing Your Health**
General Features of Reliable
Weight Reduction Plans

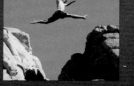
**Across the Life Span**
Weight Management

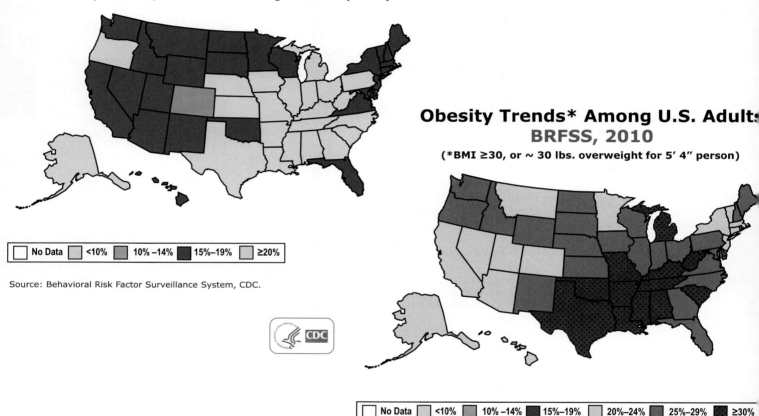

## Obesity Trends* Among U.S. Adults
### BRFSS, 2000
(*BMI ≥30, or ~ 30 lbs. overweight for 5′ 4″ person)

| No Data | <10% | 10%–14% | 15%–19% | ≥20% |

Source: Behavioral Risk Factor Surveillance System, CDC.

## Obesity Trends* Among U.S. Adults
### BRFSS, 2010
(*BMI ≥30, or ~ 30 lbs. overweight for 5′ 4″ person)

| No Data | <10% | 10%–14% | 15%–19% | 20%–24% | 25%–29% | ≥30% |

Source: Behavioral Risk Factor Surveillance System, CDC.

## Chapter Overview

The definitions of overweight and obesity

How your body uses the energy from foods

How to determine your percentage of body fat

The causes of obesity

How to manage your weight

## Student Workbook

Self-Assessment: How Much Energy Do You Use Daily?

Changing Health Habits: Altering Caloric Intake and
  Physical Activity

## Do You Know?

How to shed fat and gain muscle?

What causes "middle-age spread"?

How to lose weight and keep it off?

## CHAPTER 10

# Body Weight and Its Management

I n 2009, about 63% of American adults were overweight or obese.[1] A person who is **overweight** has more fat, muscle, bone, and/or body water than a person whose weight is normal. Being overweight is not necessarily un-healthy, but overweight people who have too much body fat are at risk of becoming *obese*. In this chapter, we use the term overweight to refer to *overfat*. **Obesity** is a condition characterized by excessive and unhealthy amounts of body fat. As these maps indicate, the prevalence of obesity in the United States rose rapidly between 2000 and 2010. In 2000, 20% or more of the adult population in 22 states was obese. Ten years later, 20% or more of adults in every state was obese. What is the prevalence of obesity in your state?

Overweight and obesity are the most common nutritional disorders in the United States.[2] These conditions often result from a combination of two behavioral risk factors—poor diet and physical inactivity. In this country, an increasing number of people are dying of causes related to these risk factors.[3]

People who do not have "weight problems" often think overweight and obese individuals lack the willpower to control their eating and weight. It is true that a person gains body fat by eating more food energy (calories) than

> "In 2009, about 63% of American adults were overweight or obese."

**overweight** A condition in which the body has more fat, muscle, bone, and/or body water than a person whose weight is normal. Overweight people have BMIs of between 25 and 30.

**obesity** A condition in which the body has an excessive and unhealthy amount of fat. Obese people have BMIs of 30 or more.

**adipose cells** Specialized cells that store extra food energy as fat.

**body mass index (BMI)** A standard that correlates body weight with the risk of developing chronic health conditions associated with obesity.

lograms) by height (meters squared), or kg/m$^2$. BMI correlates body weight with the risk of developing chronic health conditions associated with excess body fat.

To estimate your BMI, multiply your weight in pounds by 705. Then, divide that number by your height in inches squared. For example, if you weigh 150 lb and your height is 6'7", multiplying your weight times 705 equals 105,750 and squaring your height equals 4,489. Dividing 105,750 by 4,489 produces approximately 23.56. Thus, your BMI is 23.56. You can also determine your BMI by using the interactive BMI calculator at the National Heart Lung and Blood Institute's website (www.nhlbisupport.com/bmi/).

**Table 10.1** indicates weight classifications according to BMIs. Adults with BMIs below 18.5 are classi-

needed and that losing the excess weight involves a considerable amount of motivation and commitment. However, overweight and obesity result from a complex combination of biological, psychological, environmental, cultural, and socioeconomic influences. Thus, shedding excess fat to achieve a healthy body weight is not an easy task. According to most medical experts, obesity is a chronic metabolic disease that is extremely difficult to treat.

This chapter examines factors that contribute to the development of excess body fat, identifies health problems associated with this condition, and discusses various weight loss methods. Some individuals are underweight and want to increase their muscle mass; therefore, this chapter also provides information concerning healthy ways to gain weight.

## Overweight and Obesity

A healthy body is not fat free; a small amount of fat is essential for the normal functioning of all cells. Additionally, the body has specialized cells called **adipose cells** that store the extra energy from food as triglyceride (fat). If a person eats more food energy than is needed, his or her fat cells continue storing fat and increasing in size. Under certain conditions, additional fat cells can develop, further enlarging the fat mass, and this person soon notices that his belts are too small or her slacks are too tight as a result.

### Body Mass Index

How much extra fat must a person have to be considered overweight? At what point does an overweight person become obese? Most health experts use the **body mass index (BMI)** instead of height/weight tables to determine whether an individual weighs too much. BMI is calculated by dividing weight (ki-

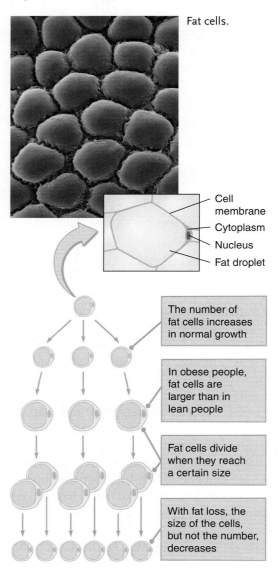

Fat cells.

Cell membrane
Cytoplasm
Nucleus
Fat droplet

The number of fat cells increases in normal growth

In obese people, fat cells are larger than in lean people

Fat cells divide when they reach a certain size

With fat loss, the size of the cells, but not the number, decreases

Adipose (fat) cells.

## Table 10.1

### Weight Classifications

| BMI | Weight Classification |
|---|---|
| Below 18.5 | Underweight |
| 18.5–24.9 | Healthy |
| 25.0–29.9 | Overweight |
| 30–39.0 | Obese |
| 40.0 and higher | Morbidly or extremely obese |

## Table 10.2

### Classifying Body Weight Based on BMI

| Height (in.) | Overweight (BMI 25.0 to 29.9) Lower Limit (lb) | Obese (BMI 30 or more) Lower Limit (lb) |
|---|---|---|
| 58 | 119 | 143 |
| 59 | 124 | 148 |
| 60 | 128 | 153 |
| 61 | 132 | 158 |
| 62 | 136 | 164 |
| 63 | 141 | 169 |
| 64 | 145 | 174 |
| 65 | 150 | 180 |
| 66 | 155 | 186 |
| 67 | 159 | 191 |
| 68 | 164 | 197 |
| 69 | 169 | 203 |
| 70 | 174 | 207 |
| 71 | 179 | 215 |
| 72 | 184 | 221 |
| 73 | 189 | 227 |

*Source:* National Institutes of Health, National Heart, Lung, and Blood Institute. (1998). *Clinical guidelines on the identification, evaluation, and treatment of overweight and obesity in adults.* Bethesda, MD: Author.

fied as *underweight*. Healthy BMIs are between 18.5 and 24.9. Adults with BMIs between 25.0 and 29.9 are *overweight*; those with BMIs of between 30.0 and 39.9 are *obese*. People who have BMIs of 40 or more are often referred to as morbidly, extremely, or super obese.

By using your BMI as a guide, you can determine whether your weight is in the overweight or obese range for your height (**Table 10.2**).

You can also use the graph shown in **Figure 10.1** to determine if your weight is within the healthy BMI range. Find your height, without shoes, on the left-hand side of the graph and place your left index finger on that point. Then, find your weight, without clothing, on the bottom line of the graph, and place your right index finger on that point. Move your left finger to the right and your right finger up until they meet. Note which range that point is in. Is your weight in the healthy BMI range?

Defining overweight and obese as certain BMIs can produce inaccurate conclusions, especially for very muscular people. For example, athletic individuals may have a BMI of 26 and be overweight according to Figure 10.1. Because muscle is denser than fat, an athletic muscular person can be heavier but healthier than a physically inactive (sedentary) individual who is the same height.

## The Prevalence of Obesity

The prevalence of obesity has reached epidemic proportions in the United States. Since 1980, obesity rates have doubled for American adults. In 2005–2006, 34% of Americans 20 years of age or older were obese.[1] American children are growing fatter too. Since 1980, the prevalence of obesity among children and adolescents who are 2–19 years of age has almost tripled. In 2009, approximately 17% of American children and adolescents were obese.[4] American infants and preschool children are also fatter than in the past.[5]

An objective of *Healthy People 2010* was to reduce the prevalence of excess body fat to 40% of the adult American population.[6] However, Americans did not meet this objective by 2010. A later section of this chapter discusses factors that contribute to the rising prevalence of overweight in the United States.

The United States is not the only country experiencing a rapid increase in the prevalence of obese people. The World Health Organization (WHO) recognizes obesity as a global health problem. The worldwide prevalence of obesity (*globesity*) is rising rapidly, especially in nations with developed market

**Figure 10.1**

**BMI Graph.** Find your BMI by following the instructions provided in the text.

*Source:* National Heart Lung and Blood Institute. (n.d.). Body mass index table 1. Retrieved on September 17, 2011, from http://www.nhlbi.nih.gov/guidelines/obesity/bmi_tbl.htm

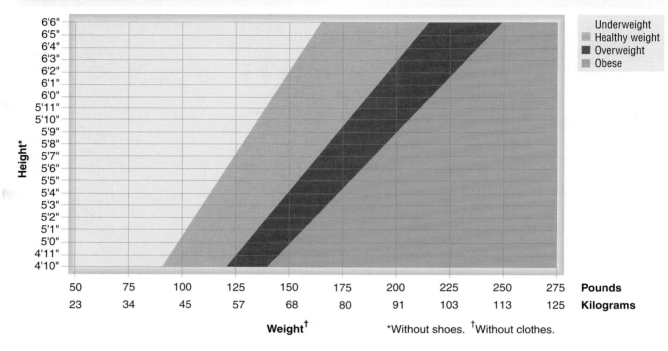

## How Does Excess Body Fat Affect Health?

Excess body fat, particularly obesity, contributes to many serious and disabling health problems. Obese people have greater risks than lean people of developing *gout*, a condition that affect joints; *carpal tunnel syndrome*, a painful nerve disorder involving the wrist and hand; and *sleep apnea*, a condition in which one stops breathing periodically while sleeping. Obese people are also more likely to suffer from metabolic syndrome, gallbladder disease, hypertension, diabetes, and heart disease. Obesity significantly increases the risk of cancers of the large intestine (colon), breast (postmenopausal women), uterus, kidney, and esophagus.[8] Compared to people who have healthy body weights, obese individuals are more likely to die prematurely.[9] In the United States, excess body fat contributes to more than 90,000 cancer deaths each year.[10]

economies such as those in western Europe. Globally, an estimated 500 million people, or more than 1 in 10 adults, were obese in 2008; remarkably, undernourished people can be living in the same families as obese persons.[7]

Surgery is riskier for obese people because physicians have more difficulty estimating the amount of anesthesia needed. Obese men and women are more likely to experience fertility problems than people whose weights are in the healthy range. Pregnant overweight or obese women have greater risks of developing diabetes (gestational diabetes), a form of severe hypertension during pregnancy, as well as giving birth to babies with birth defects and/or babies who do not survive.[11] Furthermore, being too fat can interfere with one's ability to perform daily activities that require walking, carrying, kneeling, and stooping.

Few obese individuals are free of physical health problems. Excess body weight can stress joints, especially weight-bearing joints in the knees and hips, so they wear out sooner. Obese people often have breathing problems because the excess fat interferes with lung expansion when they inhale.

When fat cells become too large, they lose their ability to respond to the hormone insulin, and the overfat person develops diabetes as a result. Fat tissue also contains cells called *macrophages*. Although these cells play a role in immune system processes that protect an individual from disease, they may multiply excessively and malfunction in people who

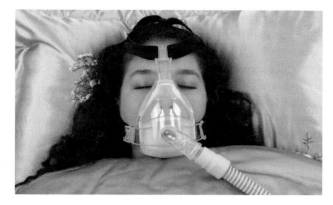

This person has sleep apnea and sleeps with a device that regulates her breathing.

have too much body fat. Macrophages found in fat tissue produce chemicals that cause inflammation, resulting in damage to the heart and blood vessels, which sets the stage for heart disease.[12]

An obese person does not have to become slim to reap some benefits of losing weight. By losing 10% of body weight and maintaining that loss, obese people can reduce their risks of obesity-related health problems such as heart disease and stroke.[13] Additionally, an obese person who loses weight can save thousands of dollars that would have been spent on treating medical conditions related to excess body fat.

Besides affecting physical health, excess body fat can have a negative impact on psychological health. Obese people, particularly obese women who seek weight loss treatment, often suffer from depression and low self-esteem.[11] An obese individual may develop these psychological problems after being discriminated against or having humiliating and embarrassing experiences while obtaining an education or seeking a job. Additionally, lean people often perceive obese individuals as physically unattractive, lacking willpower, and lazy. Not surprisingly, many overweight or obese individuals are dissatisfied and preoccupied with their body image.[14]

What are the factors that contribute to the development of excess body fat? Why are so many Americans too fat? Is it possible to control one's weight?

## The Caloric Cost of Living

### Energy for Basal (Vital) Metabolism

**Metabolism** refers to all chemical changes that take place in cells. Human cells use energy (calories) from

> **metabolism** All chemical reactions that take place in the body.
>
> **metabolic rate** The amount of energy the body requires to fuel cellular activities during a specified time.

food to perform vital activities such as building and repairing tissues, circulating and filtering blood, and producing and transporting substances. Nevertheless, cells release much of the calories from food as heat, which is necessary for maintaining one's body temperature. Every day the body expends the largest portion of calories (50% to 70%) to carry out these vital activities. The **metabolic rate** is the amount of energy required to fuel cellular activities within a specified time.

Metabolic rates vary; genetic factors probably play a major role in setting these rates. Hormones, especially thyroid hormone produced in the thyroid gland, regulate metabolism (**Figure 10.2**). In some people, the thyroid gland does not function properly, and as a result the organ produces too much or too little thyroid hormone. An individual who produces too much thyroid hormone has a higher than normal metabolic rate. This person feels warm, is nervous and shaky, has chronic diarrhea, and loses weight despite eating large amounts of food. People with overactive thyroid glands can take medication or have

### Figure 10.2

**The Thyroid Gland.** The thyroid gland produces hormones that control the metabolic rate.

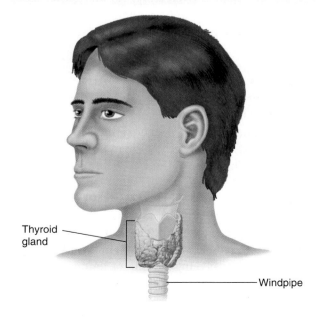

Thyroid gland

Windpipe

> **thermic effect of food (TEF)** The small amount of energy that the body uses to digest, absorb, and process the nutrients from foods.

surgery to reduce the amount of hormone produced by the organ. A person who suffers from lack of thyroid hormone has a lower than normal metabolic rate. This individual feels cold, has little energy, is constipated, and gains weight easily. People suffering from underactive thyroid glands can increase their metabolic rates by taking thyroid hormone pills. The vast majority of overfat people, however, have normal thyroid hormone levels and normal metabolic rates.

The proportion of muscle and fat tissue also influences the metabolic rate. Muscle cells use more energy than fat cells; therefore, people with greater amounts of muscle mass have higher metabolic rates than those with more fat tissue. *Testosterone* is a hormone that stimulates muscle mass development. Because men normally produce more testosterone than women do, they usually have more muscle and less fat. On average, men have higher metabolic rates than women do.

Age also influences the metabolic rate. Because they are growing rapidly, infants and children have higher metabolic rates than adults do. After 20 years of age, metabolic rates decline about 1% to 2% each decade. As a result of this gradual slowdown, aging people need less energy. If older people continue to eat the same amount of food as they did when younger, they gain weight. Although the declining metabolic rate is a contributing factor, many health experts think physical inactivity is more responsible for "middle-age spread" than is overeating. As one grows older, exercising regularly can help retain muscle mass and slow the decline in the metabolic rate.

## Energy for Physical Activity

In addition to the caloric cost of vital metabolic activities, the body expends energy to contract skeletal muscles. The amount of energy needed for physical activity depends on the type of activity, the time spent performing the activity (its duration), and the intensity at which it is performed. Although it is not related directly to physical activity, a person's body size influences the amount of physical effort needed to move. A person who weighs 120 pounds and another who weighs 175 pounds might spend the same amount of time playing a game of tennis. If both of them play tennis with the same intensity, the muscles of the heavier person require more energy to move than those of the lighter person.

According to the 2008 Physical Activity Guidelines for Americans, adults need 150 minutes of moderate-intensity aerobic activities each week.[15] Despite these recommendations, nearly one in four adults were not physically active, even during their leisure time, during 2008.[16] Chapter 11 identifies physical activities that are moderately intense.

People can increase the amount of energy expended during physical activity by increasing its duration or intensity. Furthermore, the metabolic rate often remains elevated for several hours after one discontinues vigorous physical activity. This elevation may result from an increase in the metabolic activity of muscle cells that occurs after physical exertion. Therefore, individuals who engage in regular vigorous activity may be able to raise their resting metabolic rates.

Some health experts classify physical activities as sports types of exercise, movement for daily living, or spontaneous muscular movements. *Sports types of exercise* are physical activities that are planned and carried out for the purpose of improving health and well-being. Swimming, brisk walking, and lifting weights are sports types of exercises. *Movement for daily living* includes various unstructured physical activities such as housework, gardening, walking, and leisure-time physical activities that are not associated with sports, eating, or sleeping.[17] Each day, the typical American expends more energy for physical activities associated with daily living than for sports types of exercise. *Spontaneous muscular movement* includes fidgeting and maintaining balance and body posture. Movements for daily living and spontaneous muscular movements are sometimes referred to as *nonexercise activity thermogenesis (NEAT)*. As a result of NEAT, people can reduce the risk of gaining body fat by being restless and busy because they will metabolize far more energy each day than people who spend much of their day engaging in sedentary activities such as lying down or sitting still. Nevertheless, more research is needed to determine the role of NEAT in weight maintenance.

**Table 10.3** lists some common physical activities and the number of calories people expend per minute of performing each activity. Note that the number of calories used for an activity varies according to body weight. For most people, the total number of calories expended daily for physical activity is less than the number expended for basal metabolism. To assess your daily energy expenditure, visit www.mypyramidtracker.gov and click on "Assess Your Physical Activity."

## Energy for the Thermic Effect of Food

Together, metabolic and physical activity energy needs constitute more than 90% of a person's energy expenditure. After eating a meal, the body requires a small amount of energy to digest, absorb, and process the nutrients from food. This use of energy, the **thermic effect of food (TEF)**, accounts for a very small portion, less than 10%, of one's total energy expenditures.

How many calories does your body need daily? To estimate your daily caloric expenditures, you can add the number of calories needed for basal metabolism, physical activity, and TEF. The assessment activity in the Student Workbook section at the end of this text

can help you estimate the number of calories you expend in a day.

## The Basics of Energy Balance

In general, people maintain, gain, or lose body weight according to the basic principles of energy balance, as illustrated in **Figure 10.3**. When the caloric intake from food equals the number of calories expended for energy needs, no change in body weight occurs. When caloric intake is less than caloric expenditures, the body loses weight as cells burn stored fat. If caloric intake is more than caloric expenditures, the body conserves much of the excess calories as fat, and weight gain occurs. Each pound of body fat represents about 3,500 calories of potential energy; therefore, consuming as little as 100 extra calories per day for a year can result in a 10-pound weight gain.

### Table 10.3

## Approximate Energy Costs of Various Physical Activities

| Physical Activity | Calories per Pound of Body Weight per Minute | |
| --- | --- | --- |
| | Range for Women | Range for Men |
| **Sedentary** | up to 0.017 | up to 0.017 |
| Sitting quietly, playing a musical instrument | | |
| **Light** | 0.017 to 0.033 | 0.017 to 0.035 |
| Playing pool, bowling, golf, volleyball, walking (3 mph) | | |
| **Moderate** | 0.033 to 0.050 | 0.035 to 0.052 |
| Badminton, canoeing, gymnastics, hockey, cycling, swimming, dancing, tennis, skiing | | |
| **Vigorous/Heavy** | 0.050+ | 0.052+ |
| Basketball, climbing, cross-country running, rowing | | |

To estimate the number of calories you expend while performing a particular physical activity, multiply the calories per pound per minute by your weight. Use the figures in the left-hand column if you are a woman, and in the right-hand column if you are a man. Then, multiply that number by the number of minutes spent performing the activity. For example, if you are a woman who weighs 120 lb, and you spent 40 min cycling: 0.033 × 120 = 3.96 calories per minute; 3.96 × 40 minutes = about 158 calories spent. (The rates of caloric expenditure per minute are given as ranges. For example, if you cycled intensely, use a rate at the high end of the range.)

*Source:* Adapted from Durnin, J. V. G. A., & Passmore, R. (1967). *Energy, work, and leisure.* London, England: Heinemann.

**Figure 10.3**

**Energy Balance.** (a) When energy expenditure equals energy intake, the body maintains its weight; (b) when energy expenditure is greater than energy intake, the body loses weight; (c) when energy expenditure is less than energy intake, the body gains weight.

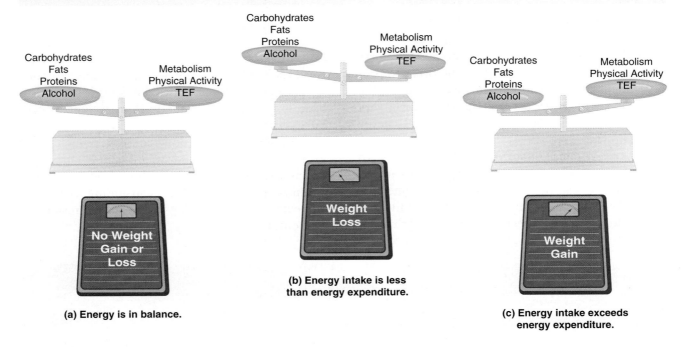

(a) Energy is in balance.

(b) Energy intake is less than energy expenditure.

(c) Energy intake exceeds energy expenditure.

## Body Composition

### How Much Fat Is Normal?

When you step on a scale, you can determine your body weight as a number of pounds or kilograms. That weight, however, does not specify how much water, muscle, or fat is in your body. Fat-free body weight consists of water, proteins, and minerals found in the bones, muscles, and organs (*lean tissues*). About 60% of a healthy adult's weight is water; 6% to 22% is protein, and 3% is minerals. Most of the remaining weight is fat.

Many health experts use the percentage of body fat to determine if a person is overfat. The average healthy young woman has more body fat than the average healthy young man because the fat is needed for hormonal and reproductive purposes. Although people tend to gain fat as they age, the increase does not necessarily cause health problems. **Table 10.4** indicates percentages of body fat that are healthy, overweight, and obese.

About one-half of an average healthy person's body fat is located in a layer under the skin (*subcutaneous*

*fat*). Small amounts of fat are stored in muscles, which rely on the fat for energy. Besides subcutaneous and muscle fat, regions of the abdomen, thighs, hips, and buttocks store considerable amounts of fat.

**Table 10.4**

**Classifying Adult Weight by Percentage of Body Fat**

| Classification | Body Fat (%) | |
| --- | --- | --- |
| | Men | Women |
| Healthy | 13–20 | 23–30 |
| Overweight | 21–24 | 31–36 |
| Obese | ≥ 25 | ≥ 37 |

*Source:* Adapted from Institute of Medicine, Food and Nutrition Board. (2005). *Dietary Reference Intakes for energy, carbohydrate, fiber, fat, fatty acids, cholesterol, protein, and amino acids (macronutrients)*. Washington, DC: National Academies Press. Table 5.5, p. 126.

Every year Americans spend money on useless treatments to eliminate "cellulite." Many people think cellulite is an abnormal type of fat that appears as lumpy, dimpled skin on the buttocks and thighs. Cellulite fat, however, does not exist. There is no difference between the fat cells in so-called cellulite and those in subcutaneous fat.[18] Strands of connective tissue hold subcutaneous fat in place. If these strands hold the fat in an irregular pattern, the fat tissue can extend into layers of skin, giving the skin a lumpy appearance. Women are more likely than men to have irregular connective tissue under their skin. The best way to improve the appearance of thighs and buttocks is to exercise and lose excess weight.

**Fat Cells** Obesity can begin at any age. However, the number and size of fat cells increase dramatically when this condition occurs during childhood and other periods of rapid growth.[19] People who become overweight in adulthood usually have normal numbers of fat cells, but their fat cells are larger than normal. The number of fat cells, however, can increase when extreme obesity occurs during the adult years.

Once fat cells form, there is little evidence that they can disappear with short-term weight reduction efforts. Under these conditions, most fat cells shrink as they release stored fat to meet the energy needs of other tissues. After shrinking, fat cells may send chemical signals to the nervous system that stimulate the urge to eat, making it difficult for people to maintain their reduced body weights.

## Estimating Body Fat

A variety of methods is used to determine one's percentage of body fat, including hydrostatic weighing, bioelectrical impedance, dual-energy x-ray absorptiometry, air-displacement plethysmography, and skinfold thicknesses. The following sections discuss these techniques.

**Hydrostatic Weighing** Hydrostatic weighing (underwater weighing) is one of the most reliable methods to estimate an individual's percentage of body fat (**Figure 10.4**). Body fat is less dense than lean tissues or water; therefore, extra fat makes the body more buoyant. Because the equipment needed to perform hydrostatic weighing is not widely available, the method is not a practical or convenient way to determine a person's percentage of body fat.

**Bioelectrical Impedance** Bioelectrical impedance uses electrical currents to estimate the percentage of body fat. Water and certain mineral elements conduct electrical currents, whereas fat is a poor con-

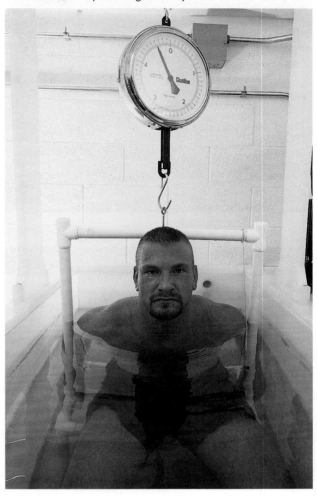

### Figure 10.4

**Hydrostatic (Underwater) Weighing.** Hydrostatic weighing is one of the most reliable methods to estimate an individual's percentage of body fat.

ductor of electricity. The equipment shown in **Figure 10.5** safely measures the body's electrical conductivity to determine the percentage of body fat. When subjects have normal amounts of body water, bioelectrical impedance provides reliable estimates of their percentage of body fat.

**Dual-Energy X-ray Absorptiometry** Dual-energy x-ray absorptiometry (DEXA or DXA) is often used in clinical studies to measure body fat as well as bone density, which is useful for diagnosing osteoporosis (**Figure 10.6**). Although the technique is very accurate for measuring body composition, the equipment is very expensive and requires trained x-ray technicians to use it.

## Figure 10.5

**Bioelectrical Impedance.** This woman is having her percentage of body fat determined by the bioelectrical impedance method.

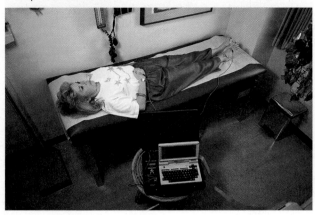

## Figure 10.6

**Dual-Energy X-ray Absorptiometry.** DEXA is often used in clinical studies to measure body fat as well as bone density.

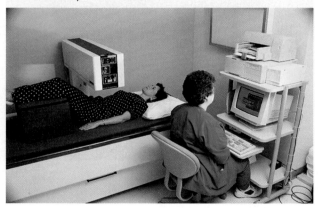

## Figure 10.7

**Air-Displacement Plethysmography.** The technique uses a special chamber to measure a person's body volume.

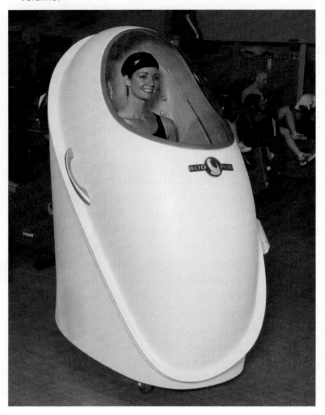

**Air-Displacement Plethysmography** The air-displacement plethysmography technique uses a special chamber (BOD POD) to measure a person's body volume (**Figure 10.7**). The BOD POD determines the volume of air that a body displaces while sitting in the device. After information about the air displacement has been obtained, the person's fat mass can be calculated. Air-displacement plethysmography is a quick and reliable way to measure fat mass and involves no exposure to radiation as does DEXA.[20]

**Skinfold Thicknesses** Several years ago, advertisements for a breakfast cereal asked people to "pinch an inch" as a method of determining their amount of body fat. If people could pinch a fold of abdominal skin that was more than an inch wide, they were too fat. This crude technique of measuring skinfold thicknesses relied on the principle that one-half of an average person's fat is located beneath the skin.

Using skinfold thicknesses to assess body composition is not as accurate as the underwater weighing and bioelectrical impedance techniques, but it is more practical and less costly. Instead of using fingers to pinch a section of skin and its underlying layer of fat, a trained person uses special calipers to measure skinfold thickness more precisely (**Figure 10.8**). Skinfold measurements should be taken at three or more body sites; averaging these measurements accounts for individual differences in body fat distribution.

The reliability of using skinfolds to estimate the percentage of body fat depends on the accuracy of the calipers, the number of skinfolds measured, and the skill of the person performing the measurements. Although measuring skinfolds is a popular technique,

**Figure 10.8**

**Skinfold Thickness Measurements.** A trained person uses special calipers to measure skinfold thickness at three or more body sites. This person is having her triceps skinfold measured.

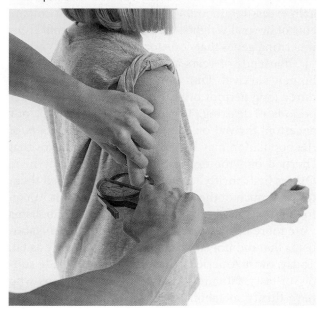

some health experts challenge the value of skinfold thicknesses to determine the degree of body fat in obese individuals. Unlike average persons, obese individuals have less than half of their body fat under their skin, and they store considerable amounts of fat in their abdomens.

**Waist Circumference** The distribution rather than the percentage of body fat may be a more important risk factor for the health conditions that are associated with excess body fat. Men and women who have large body fat deposits centrally located deep within their abdomens tend to have higher blood cholesterol levels and a greater risk of developing diabetes, hypertension, and heart disease than individuals with the same amount of fat located below the waist.[21] Why? Certain obese abdominal fat cells (*visceral fat*) may be more likely to release inflammatory compounds into the blood than subcutaneous fat cells found in the hips and thighs. Excessive amounts of these substances in the blood increase the risk of cardiovascular disease and type 2 diabetes.[22] More research is needed, however, to determine the link between abdominal fat and these chronic diseases.

As both men and women grow older, they usually add body fat in their abdominal regions, which often increases their waist circumference to unhealthy levels. **Figure 10.9** shows a man with central obesity ("apple-shaped") and a woman whose excess body fat is located primarily below the waistline ("pear-shaped").

The only equipment you need to determine your waist circumference is a flexible but nonstretchable tape measure. **Figure 10.10** illustrates where to place the tape measure. To measure your waistline, place the tape around your body just below the ribcage and at the top of the hipbone. What is your waist circumference? Men who have waistlines greater than 40 inches and women with waist circumferences greater than 35 inches have increased risks of developing the health problems associated with being too fat.[23]

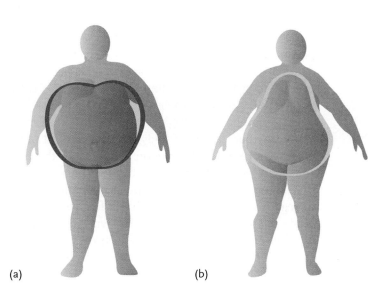

(a)  (b)

**Figure 10.9**

**Typical Fat Distribution in Obese Persons.** Men and women who have large body fat deposits centrally located deep within their abdomens tend to have a higher risk of chronic health problems than do individuals with the same amount of fat located below the waist. (a) Obese males typically have central fat deposits ("apple-shaped bodies"). (b) Obese females often have excess body fat below the waist ("pear-shaped bodies").

## Figure 10.10

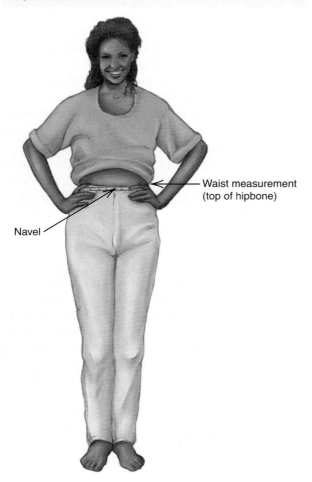

**Measuring Waist Circumference.** To determine one's waist circumference, measure the waist directly above the hipbone.

Waist measurement (top of hipbone)

Navel

# What Causes Obesity?

In most cases, there is no single cause for obesity. According to the principles of energy balance, the body gains fat when it has an excess of food energy; the body loses weight when energy intake does not meet its needs. However, biological, environmental, social, and emotional factors contribute to weight gain by influencing food intake. The following section examines these factors.

## Biological Influences

Genes control the development of many physical characteristics, including height, fat distribution, and body frame size. Genes may also code for weight gain by determining the production of hormones that regulate one's metabolic rate and interest in eating tasty foods. As a result, cases of obesity are more likely to occur in certain families. When one or both parents are obese, they are more likely to have offspring who gain excessive amounts of body fat than do two parents of normal weights. Could a person benefit from inheriting genes that code for gaining weight easily?

Thousands of years ago, "fat" genes were vital to human survival. Our early ancestors probably endured long periods of fasting, interrupted by shorter periods of feasting. When food was plentiful, our ancestors thrived on the bounty. Some members of the population may have inherited metabolisms that "burned off" the excess food energy as body heat. Others had "thrifty" metabolisms that enabled them to store much of the excess energy as body fat. When food was scarce, individuals with thrifty metabolisms were more likely to survive than those with metabolisms that did not store as much excess energy as fat. Today, most Americans have access to a steady supply of tasty, fattening food. Therefore, persons who have thrifty metabolisms find it difficult to control their weight in such environments. The Diversity in Health essay "The Plight of the Pima" discusses the harmful effects that genetic and environmental factors have had on the Pima Indian population of southern Arizona.

**The Set Point Theory** Although body weight usually fluctuates slightly from day to day, most people report that their weight remains fairly stable for months, even years. This observation led some medical experts to propose that the level of body fat is genetically preset. Once the level of body fat reaches this **set point**, the metabolic rate and other internal mechanisms maintain the degree of fatness, like a thermostat can be set to maintain the temperature of a room. Lean persons may have lower set points than do obese individuals. For example, when lean people deliberately overeat to gain weight, they usually lose the extra weight after resuming their normal eating habits.

Although having a high set point may result in an unhealthy percentage of body fat, that amount of fat may be normal for the person. As a result, the person's fat cells may resist efforts to lose storage fat. Furthermore, an obese person who loses weight is likely to regain some or all of it within a few years. Why? Some scientists think "slimmed down" fat cells send messages to the brain that are interpreted as hunger. As a result, the person overeats and his or her fat cells expand again.

# Diversity in Health

## The Plight of the Pima

After the July rains, the Sonora Desert of southwestern Arizona becomes transformed for a brief time into a natural fast-food restaurant. For hundreds of years, the Pima Indians residing in this harsh environment harvested the seasonal bounty of mesquite pods, acorns, wolfberries, prickly pears, tepary beans, and cholla blossoms to supplement their regular diet of hunted animals and cultivated maize (corn) and lima beans. The Pima were slim, but they flourished while enduring this cycle of feast and famine.

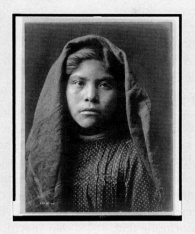

By the 1930s, the Arizona Pima had discontinued eating most of their ancient fare and adopted Western foods that provided generous amounts of lard (pork fat), refined starches, and sweets. Within a couple of decades, an alarming number of U.S. Pima had become obese and developed type 2 diabetes. According to one study, about 64% of U.S. Pima males and 75% of U.S. Pima females were obese. Among the U.S. Pima, about one-third of the men and almost half of the women had type 2 diabetes. Rates of obesity and diabetes are much higher in the U.S. Pima population than in the Mexican Pima Indians. U.S. Pima have the highest known incidence of type 2 diabetes in the world. Why are the U.S. Pima so severely affected by obesity and type 2 diabetes?

Medical experts suspect certain biological and environmental factors influence the development of obesity and diabetes in this population. Experts think the Pima have thrifty metabolisms that allow them to survive their harsh desert environment with its natural cycles of feast and famine. Although their current dietary habits have made the need for such metabolisms obsolete, the Pima are still genetically programmed to conserve a major share of their food intake as fat. Additionally, most Arizona Pima lead more sedentary lives than their ancestors did or relatives living in Mexico do. The typical Mexican Pima Indian has fewer labor-saving devices and performs more physical work than the typical Arizona Pima.

The Arizona Pima's abandonment of ancient dietary practices may contribute to their current health problems. Besides being lower in fat, traditional Pima foods provide more complex carbohydrates than typical modern menus do.

Furthermore, the ancestral diet supplied substances that may have protected the Pima from diabetes. Many desert plants contain significant amounts of amylose, a digestible carbohydrate, as well as gums and mucilages, two forms of soluble fiber. Eating foods rich in these substances slows digestion and delays the absorption of glucose from the small intestine. This delay prevents sharp increases in blood levels of insulin, the hormone that signals cells to remove glucose (blood sugar) from the blood. Under normal circumstances, the body can prevent sharp increases or decreases of blood glucose. However, individuals who suffer from type 2 diabetes are unable to avoid dramatic fluctuations in blood glucose or insulin levels, which can damage the body.

Today medical experts are studying the U.S. Pima to determine what steps can be taken to reduce their prevalence of obesity and diabetes. Some scientists think tribal members should return to their former dietary practices; many of these ancestral foods are still available. By eating desert plant foods rich in amylose and soluble fibers, the Pima may reduce their risk of developing type 2 diabetes. If the U.S. Pima are to survive as a population, they may need to recover their traditional "roots."

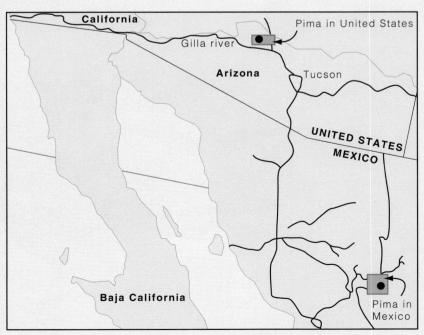

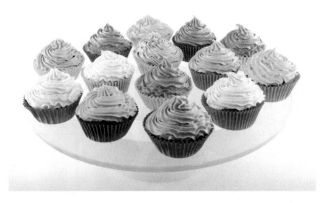

**hunger** The physiological drive to seek and eat food.

**appetite** The psychological desire to eat foods that are appealing.

**satiety** The feeling that enough food has been eaten to relieve hunger and turn off appetite.

**Appetite Regulation** Nearly everyone knows what it feels like to be hungry. **Hunger** is the physiologic drive to seek and eat food. **Appetite** is the psychological desire to eat specific foods, which is not the same as being hungry. **Satiety** is the feeling that enough food has been eaten to relieve hunger and turn off appetite.

The digestive system, brain, and fat cells play important roles in controlling hunger and satiety. While a person is eating, the intestinal tract releases several chemicals that signal the brain to eat less food. Additionally, the sensation of stomach fullness results in termination of eating. *Leptin*, a hormone produced by fat cells, and *insulin*, the pancreatic hormone that lowers blood sugar levels, affect the *hypothalamus*, a region of the brain that regulates eating behavior (**Figure 10.11**). Leptin and insulin play important roles in regulating eating behavior, but in obese people, these hormones seem to lose their effectiveness.[24]

**Composition of the Diet** An excess of calories from carbohydrate, protein, fat, and alcohol can result in weight gain. Foods that are rich sources of simple carbohydrates (sugars) contribute to overconsumption of calories. Sugar-sweetened soft drinks ("liquid candy") are convenient to purchase from vending machines and convenient stores. However, high-fat diets are associated with overeating and gaining body fat.[25] An ounce of fat supplies more than twice the number of calories as an ounce of carbohydrate or protein. Furthermore, the body stores more fat when the excess of calories is supplied by dietary fat rather than carbohydrate or protein.[26]

No specific calorie-restricted diet enhances long-term weight loss and maintenance. However, overweight people often lose weight when following a low-fat, high-complex carbohydrate diet because the food plan includes generous servings of fruits, vegetables, beans, and whole-grain cereals. These nutrient-dense, high-fiber foods are quite filling, and dieters may fail to eat enough to meet their total permissible number of calories.

Carbohydrate-rich foods often taste better when they are fried or when fats such as butter, sour cream,

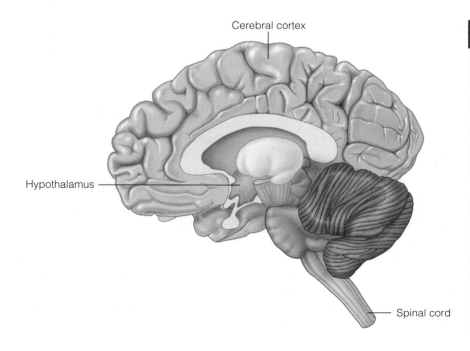

Cerebral cortex

Hypothalamus

Spinal cord

### Figure 10.11

**Hypothalamus.** Research indicates that regions of the hypothalamus in the brain control hunger and satiety.

or gravy are added to them. Most desserts and snack foods contain refined carbohydrates and fat; mixtures of sugar and fat are almost irresistible. Thus, the typical American diet promotes overeating because it provides an interesting, tasty, and enjoyable variety of fatty, sweet foods.

Obese people often claim that they gain weight by eating small amounts of food. Underreporting caloric intake, however, is common, especially by obese individuals.[25] Many people are unaware of or they underestimate the number of calories that are in their snacks and meals. Calorie and fat-counting guides are helpful if you are trying to control your weight. Keeping a record of everything you eat and drink each day can also be useful for identifying problem foods and poor eating habits. By eating more fruits and vegetables and fewer sugary and fatty foods, you can control your caloric intake.

## Environmental, Social, and Psychological Influences

A variety of environmental, social, and psychological factors promotes overeating in the United States. Since the early 1900s, typical portions of many popular foods have increased.[27] When the Hershey chocolate bar was introduced in 1906, it weighed a little over half an ounce; today a regular-sized Hershey bar weighs 1.6 ounces. Compared with original bakery bagels, an average bakery bagel now weighs three times as much and provides three times the amount of energy. Fast-food hamburgers and standard servings of french fries and soft drinks are often considerably larger than those served when these popular restaurants first opened in the 1950s and 1960s. Many fast-food and family-style restaurants promote their "super-size" portions as being bargains. Such food production practices encourage overeating and excess caloric intake.

Advertisers know the value of making foods look appealing. To stimulate sales, for example, fast-food restaurants show hamburgers topped with crisp lettuce and bacon extending beyond the bun. Actors in food ads appear to be happy and satisfied with their food choices.

Today, it is easier to obtain meals and snacks when you are not at home than in the past. Many fast-food restaurants, convenience stores, and supermarkets are open 24 hours. Supermarkets often have a deli section that offers cooked or fried chicken, baked macaroni and cheese, a variety of potato salads, and other ready-to-eat foods. You do not even have to

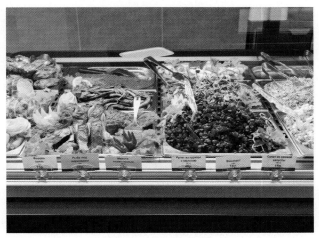

Deli sections of supermarkets usually offer a variety of appealing prepared foods.

leave home to buy food; pizza, Chinese, and other food can be delivered to your front door.

Many people respond to certain social situations by overeating. For example, you may be "stuffed" after eating a Thanksgiving dinner, but when you see pumpkin pie topped with whipped cream, you can find "room" in your stomach for dessert. Additionally, events that mark important milestones of life usually include big meals and special foods. Imagine a birthday party or wedding celebration that does not include a frosted layer cake!

Work and home environments often do not provide opportunities for Americans to be physically active. Modern technology enables machines, instead of our muscles, to do much of our work. As a result, we tend to spend more time sitting than walking around during the day. At home, many people spend their leisure time engaged in sedentary activities such as watching television or using a computer. Physically inactive people are likely to gain weight unless they restrict their food intake.

Psychological state can influence eating behavior. Some people eat long after satisfying their hunger because they are excited, anxious, or bored. Many distressed and depressed individuals seek comfort from eating, especially foods that are fatty and sugary. The following personal reflection written by an overweight young woman illustrates how emotions can affect eating behavior:

*I gained 20 pounds between the ages of 16 and 18. At the time I was in an abusive relationship with my boyfriend. I felt like dirt and the only thing that made me feel good was food. I was totally devastated when he was killed in a car accident when I was 18. I ate even more. I went to a nutritionist for a diet. I tried to stay on it but failed. Looking back, every time I gained weight it was due to stress. When I am stressed, I need to get out of the house, take my mind off things.*

In developed nations, eating disorders such as bulimia nervosa and binge eating affect considerable numbers of people, especially girls and women. These conditions are associated with serious psychological disturbances; therefore, they are discussed in Chapter 2.

## Weight Management

According to a survey conducted in 2003, about 56% of overweight or obese adult Americans were trying to lose weight.[28] Improving one's appearance and health were among the reasons subjects gave for deciding to reduce their excess weight. The majority of the people who wanted to lose weight used calorie reduction as their primary method.

Dissatisfaction with body size is common, particularly among young women. In a 2009 survey of American high school students, about 60% of females and 30% of males reported that they were attempting to lose weight at the time of the survey.[29]

Even though they may have gained the weight gradually, overweight or obese individuals who want to lose weight often seek methods that promise quick and dramatic results. These people are likely to believe advertisements for weight loss methods or products that guarantee pounds will "melt fast without sweating or dieting." As a result, most people lose more than just body fat by using various weight loss

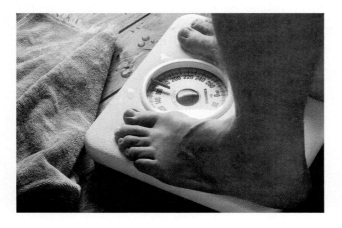

products and services. Each year, Americans spend billions of dollars on various weight control efforts. These efforts include joining weight loss programs or spas and buying special foods, books, pills, and gadgets. Do these products and services enable people to lose weight? How can you judge the value of a weight loss method? The following sections answer these questions.

## Weight Reduction Diets

As mentioned earlier, the body loses weight when its caloric intake is less than its energy needs. In this situation, the body relies primarily on stored fat for energy. To lose weight, overweight individuals should eat fewer calories than they need or expend more calories. Most reliable weight reduction regimens incorporate both of these features by combining a low-calorie diet with a plan that increases physical activity.

**Fad Diets** Some of the more popular weight loss diets of the last three decades have included a variety of recommendations such as fasting, counting calories, not counting calories, avoiding certain food combinations, eating plenty of protein and little carbohydrate, or eating only a few foods (**Table 10.5**). Such diets are often referred to as **fad diets** because they remain popular for a period of time and then quickly lose their widespread appeal. The low-carbohydrate "Atkins diet," for example, gained many followers when it was first introduced in 1973, but dieters soon lost interest in its restrictive food choices. When the Atkins diet was reintroduced about 25 years later, its renewed popularity resulted in the marketing of a wide array of "low-carb" foods. By the fall of 2004, however, most American dieters had lost their enthusiasm for the low-carbohydrate diet fad.

Fad diets usually have a few common features— gimmicks and caloric restriction. A gimmick is a promotional feature that makes a fad weight loss diet appear to be new, unique, and more effective than other diet plans. Some fad diets, including the Atkins diet, use carbohydrate restriction as a gimmick. Other fad diets use gimmicks such as prescribed food combinations based on your blood type, dietary supplements that "melt fat while you sleep," and "secret" food ingredients that allow you to eat all your favorite foods or retain fat in desirable places (the breasts of women, for example) while shedding it from the hips, abdomen, and thighs. Although such claims are untrue and not based on scientific evidence, they attract people who are seeking quick and easy ways to lose their excess fat.

## Table 10.5

## Some Fad Diets

| Diet | Approach | Possible Problems |
|---|---|---|
| Dr. Atkins Diet Revolution<br>Enter the Zone<br>The Doctor's Quick Weight Loss Diet<br>Protein Power<br>Calories Don't Count<br>The Complete Scarsdale Medical Diet<br>Sugar Busters | Restrict carbohydrate intake while increasing protein and fat intake | High animal fat intake may contribute to heart disease. Although initial weight loss can be impressive, long-term results are similar to other calorie-reduced plans. |
| Pritikin Diet<br>Macrobiotic Diet (certain types)<br>The Rice Diet<br>Eat More, Weigh Less<br>T-Factor Diet<br>Stop the Insanity<br>The Pasta Diet<br>The McDougall Plan<br>The Maximum Metabolism Diet | Limit food choices; very low fat | Boredom with limited food choices; feeling of deprivation because favorite foods are limited or prohibited.<br><br>High fiber intake results in increased intestinal gas and may interfere with mineral absorption; dieter often feels deprived and hungry. |
| Cabbage Soup Diet<br>The New Beverly Hills Diet<br>Dr. Berger's Immune Power Diet<br>Bloomingdale's Diet<br>Eat to Win<br>Two-Day Diet<br>Spirulina Diet<br>Vinegar Diet<br>Grapefruit Diet | Promote certain nutrients, substances, foods, or food combinations as having special "fat-burning" or weight loss abilities | Boredom with limited food choices; may result in nutritional deficiencies if followed for long periods. |

Source: Byrd-Bredbenner, C., et al. (2009). *Wardlaw's perspectives in nutrition* (8th ed.). Boston, MA: McGraw-Hill.

Overweight people can lose weight while following fad diets because the diet plans that accompany the gimmicks usually provide fewer calories than the level of energy supplied by typical American diets. Regardless of the type of diet they used to lose excess fat, the majority of formerly overweight people find it difficult to maintain their new body weights.

***Very Low-Calorie Diets*** Very low-calorie diets may provide fewer than 800 calories per day and be nutritionally inadequate because they limit food choices. Diets that provide 400 or fewer calories daily are often called fasts. Fasts are essentially starvation regimens. Some fasts permit only fruit juices and nutrient supplements. Fasting accelerates the loss of fat and lean body tissue, creating unhealthy metabolic by-products. Healthy individuals should not fast for more than a day without medical supervision.

Initially, obese people typically lose substantial amounts of weight while following a low-calorie diet or fast. When caloric intake is very low, the body burns fat as well as lean tissue for energy. Because fat and lean tissue store water, using these tissues for energy creates a surplus of water in the body. The kidneys eliminate the excess water, causing a dramatic loss of weight that often encourages dieters during the early phase of their weight reduction efforts. Within a few weeks, however, the body regains its normal water balance, and the rate of weight loss slows.

Very low-calorie diets or fasts trigger energy-conserving mechanisms in the body that are designed to help people survive starvation. The metabolic rate decreases with caloric restriction, especially when individuals consume fewer than 800 calories a day. Thus, dieters must cut their caloric intakes even further to continue losing weight, which often makes adhering to their diets even more difficult.

Despite their efforts, most individuals experience a decline in their rate of weight loss after several weeks of following a calorie-reduced diet. Some of this slowdown occurs because the body expends fewer calories to maintain the new weight. As the body adjusts to the reduced caloric intake, it metabolizes less fat and lean tissue for energy, slowing the rate of weight loss. Additionally, dieters who follow restrictive diet plans for more than a few weeks often become bored with the regimens and gradually return to their old eating habits.

Most people who have lost weight regain some or all of it—and often, even more weight—after a period of caloric restriction. Frustrated dieters often blame themselves for lack of self-control. Episodes of losing and regaining weight are referred to as "yo-yo" dieting or weight cycling. Results of studies do not provide consistent evidence that weight cycling is associated with increased disease or death.[30] Although more research is needed, obesity appears to pose more health risks than does weight cycling. Rather than endure

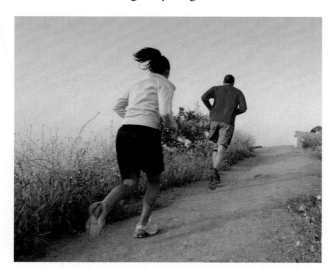

Exercise may result in a healthy increase in muscle mass.

periodic fad dieting, overfat people should consider other, more successful methods of losing weight—changing eating and exercise patterns for life.

## Physical Activity

Many American adults are less active physically than when they were younger, partly because they have occupations that require little physical effort. Men who had trim, athletic builds during adolescence often develop bulging waistlines by the time they are 40 years old. As they reach middle age, women often blame "gravity" or pregnancy for the expanding dimensions of their waists, hips, and thighs. Can adopting more physically active lifestyles reverse these changes?

*I gained 20 pounds before my wedding. My husband bought me a stepper for a wedding present (that's what I wanted), and I use it with an exercise video. Now, I exercise more than ever, but I haven't lost much weight.*

This student has discovered that exercising to lose body fat often does not produce the desired change in body weight. Physical activity alone is not as effective as low-calorie diets for treating obesity because most overweight individuals cannot perform enough exercise to create a significant deficit of calories. This does not mean that overweight people should abandon physical activity as a means of losing excess body fat. Exercise retains lean tissue and builds muscle mass, which may stabilize or even increase one's body weight. Thus, what appears to be a lack of progress while restricting food intake and exercising may be the result of a healthy increase in muscle mass.

In addition to tracking weekly changes in body weight, physically active overweight individuals can keep weekly records of waist circumferences. People who become more physically active while dieting often report that their clothing fits better, or they can wear smaller sizes, even though they have not lost much weight. Besides improving physical appearance, exercise reduces elevated blood pressures and lipid levels. Furthermore, individuals who exercise for at least 250 minutes per week may be more likely to maintain their weight loss than those who are less active.[31]

Most overweight individuals can safely increase their physical activity by walking, bicycling, or swimming for at least 30 minutes, preferably on a daily basis. Regardless of the activity, it should be enjoyable and practical to perform on a year-round basis. Before beginning a vigorous physical activity program,

**Figure 10.12**

**Gastric Bypass Surgery.** Gastric bypass is a type of surgical procedure used to treat severe obesity. After surgery, the obese person experiences discomfort after overeating and is less likely to overeat.

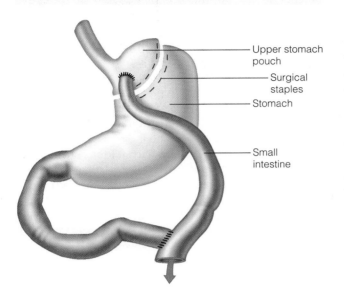

- Upper stomach pouch
- Surgical staples
- Stomach
- Small intestine

inactive people over 40 years of age should obtain the approval of their personal physicians.

## Surgical Procedures

Severely obese individuals generally experience little success following low-calorie diet plans and exercising to lose weight. *Bariatric surgeries*, particularly *gastric bypass* procedures, may be used to treat extremely obese individuals. **Figure 10.12** illustrates the appearance of the stomach and small intestine after one type of gastric bypass surgery. A surgeon drastically reduces the capacity of the stomach by creating a small pouch in the upper part of the stomach for food to enter. After having this procedure, the obese person loses weight rapidly because he or she can no longer eat large portions of food without vomiting or uncomfortable feelings of fullness. On average, people who have had gastric bypasses can lose about 60% of their presurgery weight, improving their overall health.[32]

*Liposuction*, a surgical procedure that involves vacuuming subcutaneous fat out of the body, is the most common type of cosmetic surgery in the United States. Before removing the fat, the area is injected with an anesthetic-containing fluid or treated with ultrasound (*ultrasound-assisted lipoplasty*). This technique has cosmetic value when used to remove

**Figure 10.13**

**Liposuction.** Liposuction is a medical procedure in which a special instrument is inserted into body fat through an incision made in the skin, and the fat is vacuumed from the body.

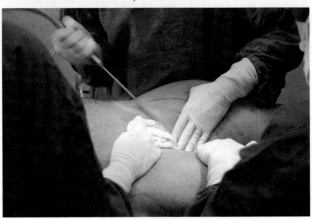

small areas of fat that create unsightly bulges such as "saddlebag thighs" or double chins (**Figure 10.13**). Liposuction can be hazardous; infections, blood clots, disfigurement, and even death can result. For most overfat individuals, liposuction is not an acceptable weight loss method.

## Medications

Overweight people who are trying to follow low-calorie diets often lose control over their appetites and as a result overeat. For decades, medical researchers have been testing various compounds to determine whether they can help people adhere to their diet plans more easily or lose weight faster.

Orlistat (Xenical) is the only FDA-approved prescription drug for weight loss. Orlistat does not suppress appetite but interferes with fat digestion. As a result, some of the fat in foods is not digested and is eliminated in feces. Fat-soluble vitamins are generally found in fats and oils, so a person taking orlistat will not absorb as many of these nutrients from foods, and therefore should take a vitamin supplement. An over-the-counter version of orlistat (Alli) became available in 2007.

## Alternative Therapies

Overfat people may turn to alternative therapies to lose weight, especially if they have had no success with conventional medical weight loss practices that include calorie restriction and increased physical ac-

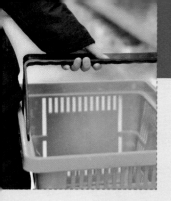

# Consumer Health

## Dietary Supplements: Weight Loss Aids

Anyone who has tried to lose weight knows it can be a frustrating effort. Hunger seems to be a constant companion. For years, overweight people have taken various pills and dietary supplements sold over the counter to promote weight loss and prevent hunger. **Table 10.A** includes several of the more popular supplements that people take to lose weight and provides information concerning the scientific support for health-related claims associated with the product.

Consumers need to be wary of weight loss products that are marketed at Internet websites. Such products often include misleading or untruthful claims such as the following:

"Eat all you want without gaining weight."

"Lose weight by blocking starch."

"Clinically tested fat inhibitor instantly prevents weight gain."

"Prevents carbs from being converted into fat."

"Burns fat without increasing your metabolic rate."

Claims about a supplement's effect on the structure or function of the body must be supported by scientific evidence, and not be misleading or dishonest.

Taking certain weight loss products may be dangerous. In 2011, the Food and Drug Administration determined that "Slim Xtreme Herbal Slimming Capsules," which were available at various online websites, contained an undeclared drug ingredient (*sibutramine*). The agency warned consumers to stop using the capsules and discard them because the product posed a threat to health. Sibutramine is known to increase blood pressure in some people and could be harmful for patients with heart disease and stroke.

Individuals should not use any dietary supplement for weight loss without the advice and monitoring of their physician. If you experience any side effects while taking such products, report the problem to the FDA's Med-Watch hotline by calling 1-800-332-1088 or the agency's online reporting site at https://www.accessdata.fda.gov/scripts/medwatch/medwatch-online.htm.

### Table 10.A

### Dietary Supplements: Weight Loss

| Dietary Supplement | Claims | Scientific Findings |
|---|---|---|
| Garcinia | Reduces body fat | The evidence to support the claim is weak. |
| Bitter orange | Enhances weight loss | Bitter orange can increase heart rate and blood pressure; therefore, its use is risky. |
| Blue-green algae (spirulina) | Promotes weight loss, boosts immune system functioning, and treats asthma, depression, and several other common disorders | No evidence to support claims. Algae may be contaminated with toxins that are in their environment. |
| Chitosan (chitin) | Enhances weight loss, reduces blood lipid levels | No evidence to support weight loss claim. Chitosan may reduce cholesterol levels, but the effect is minimal. |
| Chromium picolinate | Increases metabolic rate, facilitates weight loss | May result in slight reduction in body weight, but the loss is not impressive. |
| Glucomannan | Enhances weight loss | Some evidence to support claim, but more research is needed. |
| Yerba maté | Enhances weight loss | Results of one study suggest that a combination of yerba maté, guarana, and damiana may assist weight loss, but more research is needed. |
| Hoodia | Suppresses appetite | No human studies support claims of hoodia's effectiveness or safety. |

Sources: Swartzberg, J. E., Margen, S., et al. (2001). *The complete home wellness handbook.* New York, NY: Health Letter Associates; Pittler, M. H., & Ernst, E. (2004). Dietary supplements for body-weight reduction: A systematic review. *American Journal of Clinical Nutrition, 79*(4):529–536; and Hollarnder, J. M., & Mechanick, J. I. (2008). Complementary and alternative medicine and the management of the metabolic syndrome. *Journal of the American Dietetic Association, 108*(3):495–509.

# Analyzing Health-Related Information

This advertisement promotes a weight loss product. Read the ad and evaluate it using the model for analyzing health-related information. The main points of the model are noted here; the model is explained fully in Chapter 1.

1. Which statements are verifiable facts, and which are unverified statements or value claims?
2. What are the credentials of the person who makes the health-related claims? Does this person have the appropriate background and education in the topic area? What can you do to check the person's credentials?
3. What might be the motives and biases of the person making the claims?
4. What is the main point of the ad? Which information is relevant to the product? Which information is irrelevant?
5. Is the source reliable? What evidence supports your conclusion that the source is reliable or unreliable? Does the source of information present the pros and cons of the topic or the benefits and risks of the product?
6. Does the source of information attack the credibility of conventional scientists or medical authorities?

Based on your analysis, do you think that this ad is a reliable source of health-related information? Summarize your reasons for coming to this conclusion.

---

## FINALLY!

Pond scum, grapefruit pills, cabbage soup, stimulants, prepackaged foods, cellulite creams—you name the diet or diet product—you probably have tried it and have been disappointed. The fat didn't budge, and what's worse, you may have gained even more weight as a result of your efforts. You are not alone. There are millions of victims of diet failure—people, like you, who wasted their money and hope on diets and diet products that promised so much and delivered so little.

*a weight-loss product that lives up to your expectations!*

New and improved FLAB-BE-GONE speeds up your cells' natural fat-burning potential by 68%.

**Now you can stop dieting and get the slim, trim figure that you've always wanted.**

HOW? Take FLAB-BE-GONE, the revolutionary new method of weight loss that uses your cells' own fat-burning ability to shed unwanted pounds of ugly fat from your body. FLAB-BE-GONE enables you to lose weight effortlessly, while you sleep or watch TV. There's no need for exercise that makes you sweat and damages your joints. You don't have to count calories, grams of carbs or fat, or starve yourself. Just take two FLAB-BE-GONE tablets with meals or snacks. Want an ice cream sundae? Go ahead, eat it. Just take FLAB-BE-GONE with it! Within hours, watch as those pounds of fat and cellulite melt off your body!

**Can you believe it? Yes, it's true.**
The unique formulation of FLAB-BE-GONE makes it possible to lose up to 10 pounds overnight. Guaranteed!
If you don't lose weight after 1 week of using FLAB-BE-GONE as directed, we will refund your money. You can't lose!

For a month's supply, send $59.95 to:

**LOSE UP TO: 10 inches off your waistline**
**6 inches off your hips**
**8 inches off your thighs.**

Warning: We must ask you to consult your physician before taking this product. If your weight drops too quickly while taking FLAB-BE-GONE, simply reduce the dose.

---

tivity. Acupressure, a therapy that is based on ancient Chinese medicine, is a popular alternative therapy for weight, but there is a lack of scientific evidence to support its long-term effectiveness.[33]

Dietary supplements such as those containing chitosan, green tea, chromium picolinate, and hoodia are promoted for weight loss. Medical experts, however, do not recommend these products because reports of their safety and effectiveness are not based on well-designed clinical studies. Manufacturers of weight loss products often recommend that dieters also follow a calorie-reduced diet and an exercise regimen. Therefore, any significant weight loss can be attributable to the calorie-restricted diet and increased physical activity—not the product. People who have lost weight with the help of "diet drugs" usually regain it when they discontinue using the products and following the diet and exercise plan. The Consumer Health feature "Dietary Supplements: Weight Loss Aids" provides information about some popular over-the-counter weight loss products. The

Analyzing Health-Related Information feature in this chapter includes an advertisement for a dietary supplement that is marketed for weight loss.

## Strategies for Successful Weight Loss

Overweight individuals can lose body fat and maintain their new weight by following sensible and safe weight loss plans, which have four major characteristics:

1. They are medically and nutritionally sound.
2. They include practical ways to engage in regular physical activity.
3. They are adaptable to one's psychological and social needs.
4. They can be followed for a lifetime.

Nutritionally sound weight reduction diets emphasize nutrient-dense foods, and they are nutritionally well balanced and adequate. Without being overly

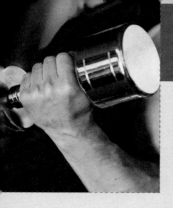

# Managing Your Health

## General Features of Reliable Weight Reduction Plans

Use the following features to judge the quality of weight loss programs.

**The diet plan is medically sound if it:**
- Provides recommendations that are safe and supported by scientific evidence
- Suggests receiving a physician's approval prior to initiating the plan
- Encourages gradual weight loss

**The diet is nutritionally sound if it:**
- Meets nutritional needs
- Includes foods from each food group
- Encourages eating smaller portions of nutritious foods
- Encourages self-control over problem foods such as sweets
- Considers individual food preferences
- Includes reasonable amounts of fiber and complex carbohydrates
- Reduces caloric intake to no lower than 1,000 calories per day
- Recommends losing 0.5 lb to 2 lb per week
- Avoids requiring special or costly supplements and foods
- Avoids claims about the superiority of the plan
- Avoids guarantees concerning weight loss

**The diet plan considers physical fitness needs if it**
- Recommends an exercise plan that is tailored to the individual's needs, time constraints, interests, and capabilities
- Includes practical suggestions for altering sedentary behaviors
- Encourages daily aerobic activities that last at least half an hour
- Avoids promoting costly exercise equipment, joining exercise clubs, or buying special gadgets to shed pounds
- Recommends physical activities that are safe and enjoyable
- Considers special health concerns of the individual

**The diet plan meets psychological and social needs if it:**
- Provides practical suggestions for modifying food-related attitudes and behaviors
- Educates about the need to set realistic weight loss goals
- Includes techniques to monitor progress (such as weekly recording of waist circumference)
- Builds self-esteem
- Includes tips to control eating in social situations
- Includes foods that family and friends eat
- Provides strategies for coping with setbacks, difficult situations, and nonsupportive people
- Offers opportunities for group support

*Source:* Adapted from Dwyer, J. T. (1992). Treatment of obesity: Conventional programs and fad diets. In P. Björntorp & B. N. Brodoff (Eds.), *Obesity* (pp. 662–676). Philadelphia, PA: Lippincott.

---

restrictive, such diets supply fewer calories than overweight people need. No special foods are necessary; the recommendations of the U.S. *Dietary Guidelines* and MyPlate (www.choosemyplate.gov) form the basis of nutritious calorie-reduced daily menus.

Reasonable and reliable diet plans recommend ways to increase physical activity such as by adding 30 to 90 minutes of walking, swimming, or bicycling to one's routine on most days of the week. Additionally, weight loss plans should meet the psychological and social needs of overweight persons. A reliable plan, for example, helps a person set an achievable weight loss goal, recognize faulty eating habits, build self-esteem and body shape satisfaction, and obtain family or group support. You can use the criteria listed in the Managing Your Health tips titled "General

Features of Reliable Weight Reduction Plans" to judge the effectiveness of most weight reduction methods.

Effective weight loss plans usually emphasize behavior modification. Behavior modification involves learning to identify behaviors that contribute to one's inability to lose weight, such as eating too much fatty food and not engaging in enough physical activity. Additionally, the overweight person learns to modify inappropriate behaviors so that weight loss and its maintenance are possible. **Table 10.6** lists key behaviors, such as not watching television while eating, that can help overweight people achieve their weight loss goals. By identifying and modifying behaviors that resulted in weight gain, an overweight person can develop a weight loss and maintenance plan that works best for him or her.

## Table 10.6

### Examples of Behavior Modification for Weight Management

| Behavior | Actions to Modify Behavior |
|---|---|
| Identify faulty eating behaviors and eliminate or ignore improper eating cues. | • Keep daily food records to identify problem foods.<br>• Use a shopping list and do not buy problem foods.<br>• Eat fruit or a meal before shopping for food.<br>• Discard problem foods.<br>• While at home, restrict eating to the kitchen or dining room.<br>• Do not eat while watching TV, reading, or talking on the phone.<br>• Avoid places with vending machines.<br>• Avoid fast-food restaurants that do not sell low-fat foods. |
| Reduce caloric intake. | • Serve meals on smaller plates.<br>• Prepare smaller amounts of foods to reduce the likelihood of "seconds."<br>• Avoid buffet-style or all-you-can-eat restaurants.<br>• Eat a low-fat, high-fiber snack such as a piece of fruit or vegetable before a meal.<br>• Keep fruit and vegetables on hand to snack on when hungry.<br>• Ask for salad dressing "on the side" at restaurants.<br>• Prepare low-calorie lunches and snacks to take to work or school.<br>• Substitute fresh fruit or yogurt for rich desserts.<br>• Read nutrition labels to identify high-calorie foods.<br>• Learn to leave some food on your plate. |
| Stay focused on weight loss goal. | • Set reasonable incremental goals, such as losing 5 pounds in 5 weeks.<br>• Place a picture of yourself on the refrigerator, pantry door, or bedroom mirror.<br>• Measure your waistline once a week.<br>• Place exercise equipment and walking shoes where you can see them.<br>• Buy new pants that are one size smaller and hang them where you can see them.<br>• Ask your friends and family to support your efforts. Give them examples of how they can help. |
| Practice appropriate behaviors. | • Find ways to move around while at work, school, or home. For example, take the stairs instead of the elevator.<br>• If you relapse, tell yourself that this is normal. Do not label yourself a failure. Ask yourself what you can learn from the experience so it is less likely to affect your eating again. Minor occasional indulgences will not affect your weight. Continue to focus on your weight loss goal.<br>• Set aside at least 30 minutes each day to engage in an enjoyable physical activity. Gradually increase the duration of the activity to 45 to 60 minutes daily. |
| Use nonfood rewards for behaviors. | • Praise yourself frequently for exercising or taking smaller servings of high-calorie appropriate foods.<br>• Buy a desired item such as a new CD, DVD, or an item of clothing.<br>• Take a walk or ride a bike through a park. |

To avoid regaining weight, successful dieters must make lifestyle changes they can follow throughout their lifetimes, such as exercising regularly and controlling caloric intake. Small incremental changes that are implemented gradually are easier to adopt than extreme exercise regimens and overly restrictive diets. Most fad diets do not focus on behavior modification. However, even reliable weight loss programs that promote behavior modification do not offer guarantees for long-term success. The process of changing behaviors takes education, practice, time, and perseverance.

The majority of people who have lost weight through nonsurgical methods experience relapse, regaining some or all of the weight within 4 years.[33] Relapses occur when overweight persons fail to modify eating behaviors and physical activity patterns permanently and have unrealistic weight loss expectations. Individuals who lose weight while following fad diets are prone to relapse when they return to their usual food habits.

Presently, there is no safe or effective treatment that "cures" being overweight. Therefore, one should strive to prevent excessive weight gain by making permanent lifestyle changes that include reducing the size of food portions, especially fatty foods, and increasing physical activity.

## Weight Gain

Although it may seem that nearly everyone is on a diet to lose weight, some people are underweight and trying to gain weight. Many health experts think underweight individuals should avoid gaining body fat unless their condition is the result of chronic illness. Nevertheless, thin individuals are often just as dissatisfied with their body sizes as overweight people.

To gain lean tissue, underweight persons need to consume at least 700 to 1,000 more calories per day than they usually eat and perform muscle-building exercises. To obtain the extra calories, underweight people can eat more than three meals a day and snack on nutrient-dense foods such as dried fruit, whole-wheat muffins, granola bars, yogurt and fruit smoothies, peanut butter, and nuts. You can find other nutritious foods that are high in food energy by consulting food composition tables.

Because fatty foods are a source of considerable calories, physically active underweight individuals can eat as much as 35% of their caloric intake from these items. Because of the association with cardiovascular disease, people trying to gain weight should avoid eating excessive amounts of saturated fats. Avocados, olives, and nuts are high in unsaturated fat, which is healthier than saturated fat. For people trying to gain weight, the effort must be maintained over the long term, just as it is for people trying to lose weight.

If you are thinking about losing or gaining weight, complete the "Changing Health Habits" activity in the Student Workbook section at the end of this text. This activity can help you decide if you are ready to make the lifestyle changes needed to modify your weight and maintain a new, healthier weight for the rest of your life.

## Healthy Living Practices

- ☐ If you want to lose weight, modify your lifestyle. For example, eat less fatty sugary foods by replacing them with more nutrient-dense foods.

- ☐ To lose or control your body weight, engage in vigorous physical activity such as jogging, brisk walking, cycling, or swimming for at least 30 minutes, preferably every day.

- ☐ To judge whether a weight loss plan or program is sensible and safe, determine whether it is medically and nutritionally sound, includes a plan to increase regular physical activity, is adaptable to your psychological and social needs, and can be followed for a lifetime.

- ☐ If you want to gain weight, add at least 700 to 1,000 calories to your usual daily intake and exercise to build muscle mass. To boost the caloric content of meals and snacks, eat more nutrient-dense foods such as dried fruit, whole-wheat muffins, granola bars, peanut butter, and nuts.

## Across THE LIFE SPAN

### WEIGHT MANAGEMENT

The amount of weight a woman gains during pregnancy affects the health of her baby. Women who begin pregnancy at a healthy weight should gain about 25 to 35 pounds during the following 9 months.[34] This weight gain includes not only the fetus's weight, but also the weight of the pregnant woman's additional body fluids, fat stores, and breast and uterine tissues. Women who are underweight when they become pregnant can expect to gain more weight; those who are overweight may gain less than average. **Table 10.7** indicates suggested ranges of weight gain for pregnant women based on their prepregnancy BMIs.

In 2006, 21% of pregnant women gained more than 40 lb during their pregnancies.[35] Some pregnant women restrict their food intake to limit their weight gain because they do not want to struggle with losing the extra pounds after the baby arrives. However, caloric restriction during pregnancy may be hazard-

| Table 10.7 | | |
|---|---|---|
| **Suggested Weight Gain During Pregnancy** | | |
| Weight Classification (prior to pregnancy) | BMI | Range of Weight Gain (pounds) |
| Underweight | < 18.5 | 28–40 |
| Healthy | 18.5–24.9 | 25–35 |
| Overweight | 25.0–29.9 | 15–25 |
| Obese | 30.0 and up | 11–20 |

*Source:* Data from March of Dimes (2009). Weight gain during pregnancy. Available: http://www.marchofdimes.com/pregnancy/yourbody_weightgain.html. Retrieved on September 14, 2011.

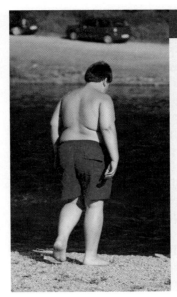

**Figure 10.14**

**Childhood Obesity.** The percentage of obese children is increasing in the United States.

ous to the developing fetus. The time to lose weight is *before* or *after* pregnancy and not during this period. Nevertheless, within 2 years of giving birth, many women remain several pounds heavier than those who have not been pregnant.

Infancy is a period characterized by rapid gains in both weight and height. According to the rule of thumb, a healthy baby doubles its birth weight by the time it is 6 months of age and triples its birth weight by its first birthday. A 7-pound newborn, for example, should weigh about 14 pounds at 6 months of age and 21 pounds when it is 12 months of age.

Many babies who are overweight at their first birthday slim down by the time they enter school. However, rapid weight gain during the first 2 years of life is associated with increased blood pressure, BMI, and waist circumference in adulthood.[36] Women who smoke cigarettes or gain too much weight during their pregnancies are more likely to have overweight or obese infants and young children.[35] On the other hand, babies who are breastfed, particularly for the recommended length of time, are less likely to develop obesity in adulthood. As mentioned in the beginning of this chapter, the percentage of overweight school-age children is increasing in the United States (**Figure 10.14**). Children and adolescents need adequate amounts of energy for physical development and activity, but they often eat more calories than recommended by dietitians. Besides dietary factors, preoccupation with sedentary activities such as play-

ing computer games and watching television contributes to the increase of childhood obesity.[37]

No one can predict whether an obese child will become an obese adult. However, obese children and adolescents are more likely to remain obese into adulthood.[36] Thus, preventing childhood obesity has become a national health priority. What are the consequences of childhood obesity?

According to the Centers for Disease Control and Prevention,[38] obese children are more likely to have the following disorders:

- High blood pressure and high cholesterol (risk factors for heart disease and stroke)
- Type 2 diabetes
- Breathing problems, such as sleep apnea and asthma
- Joint problems
- Fatty liver disease, gallstones, and heartburn
- Poor self-esteem

Childhood and adolescent obesity often becomes a problem that affects the entire family. Obese children may develop eating disorders and low self-esteem when parents, other adults, or peers treat them negatively. An effective program that helps obese children lose weight should not interfere with their normal physical development and should not encourage the development of eating disorders. Successful treatment involves teaching children and their parents how to make appropriate dietary modifications, in-

Weight Management    **335**

crease physical activity, and resolve conflicts that may involve eating habits.

By 65 years of age, most people have experienced a decline in their lean mass and an increase in their fat mass. This change occurs to a lesser extent in individuals who maintain a high degree of physical activity as they grow old. Even modest increases in physical activity, such as walking, swimming, or light exercise, can benefit most elderly people.

Contrary to conventional wisdom, many older adults enjoy good health and live longer by being overweight and even obese.[39] The extra fat may serve as an energy source if older adults lose their appetites during illness. Furthermore, the body fat may protect the elderly from serious internal injuries if they fall.

Obese older adults who have chronic health problems that are associated with excess body fat can follow the same recommendations for losing weight as do younger individuals: Select nutrient-dense foods, reduce intakes of fatty and sugary foods, and become more physically active.

## Healthy Living Practices

- ☐ Weight gain is necessary during pregnancy, so if you are pregnant, follow recommendations concerning weight gain and do not try to lose weight at this time.
- ☐ Encourage your children to be physically active.
- ☐ To avoid becoming too fat as you age, select nutrient-dense, low-fat foods and maintain moderate to high degrees of physical activity.

# CHAPTER REVIEW

## Summary

Recent health surveys indicate that more Americans are overweight or obese than in previous decades. More than 65% of the adult U.S. population is too fat. Excess body fat is associated with low self-esteem and increased risks of chronic health conditions such as osteoarthritis, sleep apnea, gallbladder disease, gout, hypertension, diabetes, certain cancers, and heart disease.

The body uses the energy in foods to power vital metabolic activity, to move skeletal muscles, and to process nutrients after meals. According to the principles of energy balance, the body requires a certain number of calories to maintain its weight. When one consumes more calories than needed, weight gain occurs; when one ingests fewer calories than needed, weight loss occurs. Because each pound of body fat represents about 3,500 calories, consuming 500 fewer calories a day than needed should result in a weight loss of about 1 lb per week.

Methods of determining the percentage of body fat include measuring subcutaneous fat (skinfold thicknesses), hydrostatic weighing, and bioelectrical impedance. To determine whether they are overfat, many people rely on waist circumference measurements and body mass indices (BMIs). Risks of chronic health problems and death increase as the waist circumference and BMI increase.

Obesity is not simply the result of a lack of willpower. The development of obesity is a complex process involving interactions among biological, psychological, social, and environmental factors. These factors include genetics, responses to social situations, food availability and composition, and levels of physical activity.

Obesity is a chronic disease. Most people who have lost weight will regain much or all of it within a few years. To lose weight and maintain the loss, overweight individuals need to decrease their caloric intake by eating less food and increase their caloric expenditures by increasing their levels of physical activity. A reliable weight loss regimen should include a well-balanced, nutritionally adequate but calorie-reduced diet and an exercise regimen that can be followed for life.

To increase her chances of having healthy babies, a healthy woman needs to gain about 25 to 35 pounds during pregnancy. While pregnant, women should not consume low-calorie diets because caloric restriction may harm the fetus. Children and adolescents need adequate amounts of energy for physical development and activity. In the United States, the percentage of children and teenagers who are obese is growing. Experts think that this increase is primarily the result of sedentary lifestyles and poor eating habits. Obese children are at risk of being obese when they are adults. Many older adults benefit from having some extra body fat.

## Applying What You Have Learned

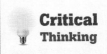
Critical Thinking

1. Develop a day's menu, including meals and snacks, for a nutritionally adequate weight loss plan. Your plan should include foods from all major food groups. **Application**
2. You see an advertisement for a special drink that is supposed to eliminate excess body fat while you sleep. According to the ad, this product helps you lose weight "fast" by increasing your metabolic rate; there is no need to eat less food or exercise more often. Explain why you think this ad is a source of reliable or unreliable health-related information. **Synthesis**

3. A man has been maintaining his weight by consuming 2,500 calories a day. If he does not alter his physical activity level, how many calories should he consume daily to lose 4 lb in a month? **Application**

4. Compare your present weight to your weight of 2 years ago. If you have gained or lost weight over

the past couple of years, explain how you reached your present weight by evaluating your lifestyle. What factors might account for the weight change? If you have not gained or lost weight during this period, explain why this situation has occurred. **Evaluation**

| **Key** | **Application**<br>using information in a<br>new situation. | **Synthesis**<br>putting together<br>information from different<br>sources. | **Evaluation**<br>making informed<br>decisions. |
|---|---|---|---|

# Reflecting on Your Health

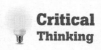

**Critical Thinking**

1. "Fat people could lose weight if they would just push themselves away from the dinner table." After reading this chapter, what have you learned about obesity and weight control that might cause you to react differently to this statement than you might have prior to reading this chapter?

2. As mentioned in this chapter, normal-weight people often have negative feelings toward obese individuals. What were your feelings about obese people before you read this chapter? After reading this chapter, have your feelings about obese persons changed? If so, describe how your feelings changed.

3. How would you respond if a close friend or relative told you that you needed to lose weight? If

someone you know is trying to lose weight, what would you do to help with his or her weight loss efforts?

4. The U.S. National Transportation Safety Board (NTSB) proposed reducing the weight limit of each airline passenger and his or her luggage because of concern that the excess load could result in plane crashes. Explain your reaction to this proposal.

5. How does the media influence your satisfaction with your body size and shape? Do you think the media should encourage people to be more satisfied with their body sizes and shapes? If you think the media should take such steps, how could this affect people's health?

# References

1. Centers for Disease Control and Prevention. Office of Surveillance, Epidemiology, and Laboratory Services. (n.d.). Behavioral Risk Factor Surveillance System: Prevalence and trends data. Overweight and obesity (BMI)—2009. Retrieved on May 21, 2011, from http://apps.nccd.cdc.gov/BRFSS/page.asp?yr=2009&state=All&cat=OB#OB

2. Yanovski, S. Z., & Yanovski, J. A. (2002). Obesity. *New England Journal of Medicine, 346*(8):591–601.

3. Mokdad, A. H., et al. (2005). Correction: Actual causes of death in the United States, 2000. *Journal of the American Medical Association, 293*(3):293–294.

4. Centers for Disease Control and Prevention. (2011, April). Overweight and obesity, data and statistics, obesity rates among all children in the United States. Retrieved on May 19, 2011, from http://www.cdc.gov/obesity/childhood/data.html

5. Ogden, C. L., et al. (2008). High body mass index for age among U.S. children and adolescents, 2003–2006. *Journal of the American Medical Association, 299*(20):2401–2405.

6. U.S. Department of Health and Human Services, National Center for Health Statistics, Public Health Service. (2000). *Healthy People 2010*. Washington, DC: Government Printing Office.

7. World Health Organization. (2011, March). *Obesity and overweight*. Geneva, Switzerland. Retrieved on May 19, 2011, from http://www.who.int/mediacentre/factsheets/fs311/en/index.html

8. Olver, I. N., & Grogan, P. B. (2008). Cancer adds further urgency to prioritising obesity control. *Medical Journal of Australia, 189*(4): 191–192.

9. Flegal, K. M., et al. (2005). Excess deaths associated with underweight, overweight, and obesity. *Journal of the American Medical Association, 293*(15):1861–1867.

10. Calle, E. E., et al. (2003). Overweight, obesity, and mortality from cancer in a prospective studied cohort of U.S. adults. *New England Journal of Medicine, 348*(17):1625–1638.

11. Kulie, T., et al. (2011). Obesity and women's health: An evidence-based review. *Journal of the American Board of Family Medicine, 24*(1):75–85.

12. Zhang, H., et al. (2010). Emerging role of adipokines as mediators in atherosclerosis. *World Journal of Cardiology, 2*(11):370–376.

13. Wee, C. C., et al. (2004). Assessing the value of weight loss among primary care patients. *Journal of General Internal Medicine, 19*(12): 1206–1211.

14. Kim, K. Y., et al. (2007). The impacts of obesity on psychological well-being: A cross-sectional study about depressive mood and quality of life. *Journal of Preventive Medicine and Public Health, 40*(2):191–195.

15. Centers for Disease Control and Prevention. (2011, March). How much physical activity do adults need? Retrieved on May 19, 2011, from http://www.cdc.gov/physicalactivity/everyone/guidelines/adults.html

16. Centers for Disease Control and Prevention, National Center for Chronic Disease Prevention and Health Promotion. (2010, February). U.S. physical activity statistics. Retrieved on May 19, 2011, from http://www.cdc.gov/nccdphp/dnpa/physical/stats/index.htm

17. Levine, J. A. (2007). Nonexercise activity thermogenesis—liberating the life-force. *Journal of Internal Medicine, 262*(3):273–287.

18. Smalls, L. K., et al. (2005). Quantitative model of cellulite: Three-dimensional skin surface topography, biophysical characterization, and relationship to human perception. *Journal of Cosmetic Science, 56*(2):105–120.

19. Robertson, S. M., et al. (1999). Factors related to adiposity among children aged 3 to 7 years. *Journal of the American Dietetic Association, 99*(8):938–943.

20. Lee, S. Y., & Gallagher, D. (2008). Assessment methods in human body composition. *Current Opinion in Clinical Nutrition & Metabolic Care, 11*(5):566–572.

21. Leitzmann, M. F., et al. (2011). Waist circumference as compared with body-mass index in predicting mortality from specific causes. *PLoS ONE, 6*(4):e18582. doi:10.1371/journal.pone.0018582

22. Barnett, A. H. (2008). The importance of treating cardiometabolic risk factors in patients with type 2 diabetes. *Diabetes & Vascular Disease Research, 5*(1):9–14.

23. National Heart Lung and Blood Institute. (2000). *The practical guide: Identification, evaluation, and treatment of overweight and obesity in adults* (NIH Publication No. 00-4084). Retrieved on May 20, 2011, from http://www.nhlbi.nih.gov/guidelines/obesity/prctgd_b.pdf

24. Yamada, T., & Katagiri, H. (2007). Avenues of communication between the brain and tissues/organs involved in energy homeostasis. *Endocrinology Journal, 54*(4):497–505.

25. Goris, A. H., & Westerterp, K. R. (2008). Physical activity, fat intake and body fat. *Physiology & Behavior, 94*(2):164–168.

26. Little, T. L., et al. (2007). Modulation of high-fat diets of gastrointestinal function and hormones associated with the regulation of energy intake: Implications for the pathophysiology of obesity. *American Journal of Clinical Nutrition, 86*(3):531–541.

27. Young, L. R., & Nestle, M. (2003). Expanding portion sizes in the U.S. marketplace: Implications for nutrition counseling. *Journal of the American Dietetic Association, 103*(2):231–234.

28. Bish, C. L., et al. (2007). Health-related quality of life and weight loss practices among overweight and obese U.S. adults, 2003 Behavioral Risk Factor Surveillance System. *Medscape General Medicine, 9*(2):35.

29. Eaton, D. K., et al. (2010). Youth risk behavior surveillance—United States, 2009. *Morbidity and Mortality Weekly Report, 59*(SS-5):1–141.

30. Field, A. E., et al. (2009). Weight cycling and mortality among middle-aged and older women. *Archives of Internal Medicine, 169*(9): 881–886.

31. Donnelly, J. E., et al. (2009). American College of Sports Medicine position stand: Appropriate physical activity intervention strategies for weight loss and prevention of weight regain for adults. *Medicine & Science in Sports & Exercise, 41*(2):459–471.

32. Shafipour, P., et al. (2009). What do I do with my morbidly obese patient? A detailed case study of bariatric surgery in Kaiser Permanente Southern California. *Permanente Journal, 13*(4):56–63.

33. Turk, M. W., et al. (2009). Randomized clinical trials of weight-loss maintenance: A review. *Journal of Cardiovascular Nursing, 24*(1):58–80.

34. March of Dimes. (2009). *Weight gain during pregnancy*. Retrieved on May 22, 2011, from http://www.marchofdimes.com/Pregnancy/yourbody_weightgain.html

35. Wojcicki, J. M., & Heyman, M. B. (2010). Let's move—Childhood obesity prevention from pregnancy and infancy onward. *New England Journal of Medicine, 362*(16):1457–1459.

36. Tzoulaki, I., et al. (2010). Relation of immediate postnatal growth with obesity and related metabolic risk factors in adulthood. *American Journal of Epidemiology, 171*(9):989–998.

37. Speiser, P. W., et al., on behalf of the Obesity Consensus Working Group. (2005). Consensus statement: Childhood obesity. *Journal of Clinical Endocrinology and Metabolism, 90*(3):1871–1887.

38. Centers for Disease Control and Prevention. (2011, April). *Overweight and obesity: Basics about childhood obesity*. Retrieved on May 23, 2011, from http://www.cdc.gov/obesity/childhood/basics.html

39. Corrada, M. M., et al. (2006). Association of body mass index and weight change with all-cause mortality in the elderly. *American Journal of Epidemiology, 163*(10):938–949.

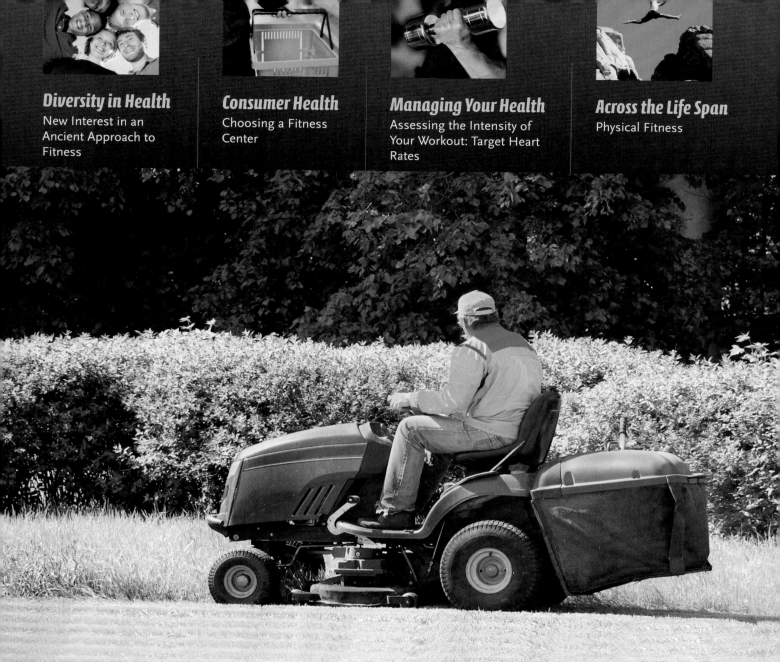

# Chapter Overview

The principles of physical fitness

The health-related components of fitness

Exercising for optimal health

Preventing and managing exercise injuries

Developing your own exercise program

# Student Workbook

Self-Assessment: Cardiorespiratory Fitness: The Rockport Fitness Walking Test | Push-Up Test for Muscular

Endurance | Sit-and-Reach Test for Flexibility Assessment | Check Your Physical Activity and Heart Disease IQ

Changing Health Habits: Do You Want to Be More Physically Active?

# Do You Know?

How to calculate your target heart rate?

How to bulk up safely?

If muscles can turn into fat?

## CHAPTER 11

# Physical Fitness

I f you look around your home, you will see many devices and products that make your life easier: electric can openers, microwave ovens, permanent-press clothes, dishwashers, garage-door openers, and remote controls. Outside of your home, there are more labor-saving machines. You can ride a lawn mower instead of push one, drive a car rather than walk to places, use elevators and escalators rather than climb stairs, and take moving walkways rather than walk through some of the larger airports. You can even make your leisure time less physically demanding by using a motorized cart to get around a golf course or a motorboat to get around a lake. Besides using labor-saving products, you can have other people perform your physical work. For example, you can pay a team of people to mow your grass, wash your car, or clean your house.

*"Most people can derive important health benefits by exercising regularly."*

A hundred years ago Americans often performed hard physical work at home and on the job. By the beginning of this century, a variety of machines, products, and services had become available that made our daily lives less physically demanding. Today, we generally have more leisure time than our great-grandparents did, but many of us spend it performing activities that do not contribute to our physical health.

Most people can derive important health benefits by exercising regularly and becoming more physically active. Healthy adults under age 65 years should perform moderate-intensity physical activity for 150 minutes

**tendons** Tough bands of tissue that connect many skeletal muscles to bones.

**joints** The places where two or more bones come together.

**ligaments** Tough bands of connective tissue that hold bones together at joints.

**physical activity** Movement that occurs when skeletal muscles contract.

**exercise** Physical activity that is usually planned and performed to improve or maintain one's physical condition.

per week.[1] Healthy adults can obtain similar health benefits by engaging in vigorous-intensity physical activity for 75 minutes a week. Moderate to vigorous activities should be performed in episodes that last at least 10 minutes, preferably spread throughout the week. Moderate-intensity physical activities include brisk walking, bicycling, housework, or other actions that cause small but noticeable increases in breathing or heart rates. Vigorous-intensity physical activities, such as running, performing aerobic exercise, or doing heavy yard work, cause relatively large increases in breathing or heart rates.

Each year, lack of regular physical activity (a *sedentary* lifestyle) contributes to thousands of American deaths, primarily from heart disease, stroke, and diabetes. In 2010, almost two-thirds of adult Americans reported that they were physically active.[2] Many adults, however, do not exercise during their leisure time.[3] A *physically fit* person has the physical strength, endurance, flexibility, and balance as well as energy to perform various daily living activities, including typical occupational responsibilities and recreational interests that require physical movement. This chapter discusses the basic principles of fitness, including the health benefits of exercise and a physically active lifestyle, and how to design a basic fitness program that you can follow for the rest of your life.

## Principles of Physical Fitness

### The Body in Motion

Physical movement involves the interrelated functioning of the muscular and skeletal systems. The functioning of the muscular system is so closely associated with the skeletal system that the two are often referred to as the musculoskeletal system.

The skeletal muscles provide shape, support, and movement for your body. Most skeletal muscles are attached to bones of the skeleton. *Figure 11.1* identifies the major skeletal muscle groups of the human body. A typical skeletal muscle consists of hundreds of muscle cells called muscle fibers. Movement occurs when the muscle fibers contract, shortening the length of the muscle. Skeletal muscles can contract voluntarily, which means the muscles contract when a nervous impulse from the brain signals them. Thus, a healthy person can choose when and how intensely to move a muscle.

**Tendons**, tough bands of fibrous tissue, connect skeletal muscles to bones or other muscles and play an important role in muscular movement. **Joints** are places where two or more bones come together. Most joints are movable; therefore, such joints permit the movement between bones. **Ligaments** are tough bands of connective tissue that hold bones together at the joints.

### The Circulatory and Respiratory Systems

Optimal functioning of the circulatory and respiratory systems (sometimes referred to as the cardiorespiratory system) is necessary to achieve a high degree of physical fitness. The circulatory system includes the heart, blood, and blood vessels. The lungs are the major structures of the respiratory system. As *Figure 11.2* illustrates, the functioning of the heart and lungs is interrelated.

The heart is a muscular pump that usually beats about 70 to 80 times each minute. Its job is to circulate blood throughout the body's vast network of blood vessels: the arteries, veins, and capillaries. Blood transports oxygen and nutrients to cells and carries waste products such as carbon dioxide away from them.

Cells need oxygen to release the energy stored in glucose and fats. As the heart pumps blood through microscopic blood vessels in the lungs, carbon dioxide leaves the blood and is exhaled. While in the lungs, hemoglobin in the red blood cells picks up oxygen from the inhaled air. The oxygen-rich blood returns to the heart, which pumps it to the rest of the body. As the blood moves through tiny capillaries in tissues, oxygen and nutrients move out of the bloodstream and into muscle fibers and other cells. Waste products move out of cells and into the blood. The blood then circulates through veins back to the heart. This cycle repeats itself with every heartbeat and breath.

## Figure 11.1

**Major Skeletal Muscles of the Human Body.** (a) Front view. (b) Back view.

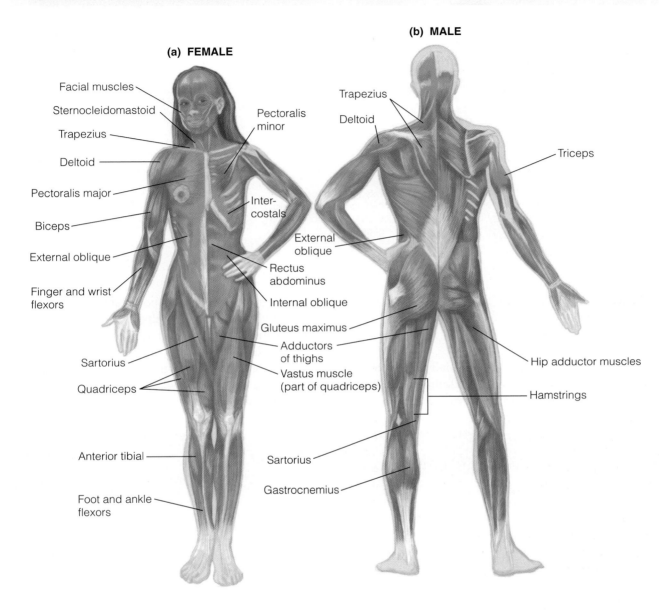

**(a) FEMALE**

- Facial muscles
- Sternocleidomastoid
- Trapezius
- Deltoid
- Pectoralis major
- Biceps
- External oblique
- Finger and wrist flexors
- Sartorius
- Quadriceps
- Anterior tibial
- Foot and ankle flexors

- Pectoralis minor
- Inter-costals
- External oblique
- Rectus abdominus
- Internal oblique
- Gluteus maximus
- Adductors of thighs
- Vastus muscle (part of quadriceps)
- Sartorius
- Gastrocnemius

**(b) MALE**

- Trapezius
- Deltoid
- Triceps
- Hip adductor muscles
- Hamstrings

# Defining Physical Activity and Exercise

**Physical activity** is movement that occurs when skeletal muscles contract; everyone engages in some physical activity as part of their daily living routines. These activities include shopping, housekeeping, and walking pets. **Exercise** is physical activity that is usu- ally planned and performed to improve or maintain one's physical condition. For example, doing biceps curls is an exercise that develops upper arm strength.

How does physical activity affect health? Before reading the following section, check your knowledge by taking the physical activity and heart disease quiz in the Student Workbook section at the end of this text.

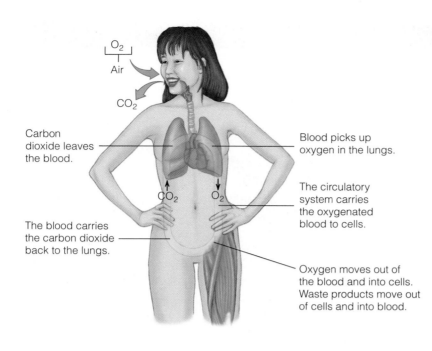

O₂

Air

CO₂

Carbon dioxide leaves the blood.

Blood picks up oxygen in the lungs.

CO₂     O₂

The circulatory system carries the oxygenated blood to cells.

The blood carries the carbon dioxide back to the lungs.

Oxygen moves out of the blood and into cells. Waste products move out of cells and into blood.

### Figure 11.2

**Cardiorespiratory System.** The functioning of the heart and lungs is interrelated. The heart pumps blood to the lungs, where the blood picks up oxygen. The oxygenated blood returns to the heart, which pumps it throughout the body

## Physical Activity and Health

Being physically active can substantially reduce your risks of serious chronic diseases including heart (coronary artery) disease, certain forms of cancer, type 2 diabetes, obesity, and hypertension (**Table 11.1**).[4] Regular physical activity helps maintain bone mass, muscle strength, and joint function. Furthermore, older adults can improve their balance and reduce their risk of falls by performing certain exercises regularly. Men and women who are physically fit have a lower risk of dying prematurely from all causes, in-

### Table 11.1

### Health Benefits of Physical Activity (Adults)

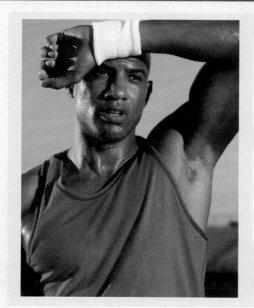

**Physical activity can lower the risk of:**

- Early death
- Heart disease
- Stroke
- High blood pressure
- Type 2 diabetes

- Metabolic syndrome
- Colon cancer
- Breast cancer
- Hip fracture

**A physically active lifestyle:**

- Prevents weight gain
- Aids weight loss, particularly when combined with reduced calorie intake
- Improves cardiorespiratory and muscular fitness

- Prevents falls
- Reduces depression
- Improves cognitive function (for older adults)
- Improves bone density

*Source:* U.S. Department of Health and Human Services. (2008). Chapter 2: Physical activity has many health benefits. In *Physical activity guidelines for Americans.* Retrieved May 25, 2011, from http://www.health.gov/paguidlines/guidelines/chapter2.aspx

cluding cardiovascular disease, than do people who are not physically fit. Regular physical activity improves health by reducing excess abdominal fat and elevated blood pressure, glucose, and triglyceride levels.

In addition to improving physical health, regular exercise and physical activity can enhance psychological health and sense of well-being. According to *Physical Activity and Health: A Report of the Surgeon General*, physical activity "reduces symptoms of anxiety and depression and fosters improvements in mood and feelings of well-being."[5] This does not mean that physical inactivity causes mental health problems or that exercising will cure these conditions. Additionally, regular physical activity can improve the quality of sleep, which benefits psychological health.[6]

Many people experience short-term psychological benefits during or immediately after exercising. Strenuous physical activity produces chemical changes in the body that can improve psychological health. For example, the central nervous system releases beta-endorphins during exercise. Beta-endorphins are pain-killing substances that may provide natural relaxing and mood-elevating effects. Also, exercise can divert a person's attention away from distressing thoughts and negative emotions, which relieves anxiety. Long-term psychological benefits of exercise may include boosting self-esteem.[7] Additionally, people who exercise with others can experience psychological benefits from the social interaction.

# The Health-Related Components of Physical Fitness

Cardiorespiratory fitness, muscular strength, muscular endurance, flexibility, and body composition are the health-related components of physical fitness. These physical characteristics provide support for the body, sustain its effective and efficient movement, and influence overall health and well-being.

## Cardiorespiratory Fitness

During intense physical activity, skeletal muscles need large quantities of oxygen to release enough energy to sustain movement. To supply more oxygen for working muscles, the heart and breathing rates increase as the intensity of physical activity increases. However, the lungs and heart have a maximum capacity to dis-

**cardiorespiratory fitness** The ability to perform muscular movements intensely and for long periods without tiring.

**aerobic** Refers to oxygen-requiring activities.

tribute an adequate supply of oxygen throughout the body within a certain time. Once the lungs and heart reach this maximum capacity, the skeletal muscles cannot obtain the additional oxygen needed to sustain their intense level of activity, and they become fatigued.

Individuals with high degrees of **cardiorespiratory fitness** (or endurance) can perform muscular work more intensely and longer without becoming fatigued than persons with low levels of cardiorespiratory fitness can. Young, healthy 20-year-old individuals can raise their heart rates to about 190 to 200 beats per minute while engaging in intense aerobic activities. As people grow older, their maximum heart rates decline. In addition to physical condition and age, other personal characteristics, including heredity, gender, and body composition, influence the maximum degree to which a person's lungs and heart can function.

During vigorous physical activity, the heart of a physically fit person pumps more blood with each beat. When the activity ceases, the fit person's heart and breathing rates rapidly return to normal. Even while resting, a fit individual's heart is efficient; each minute, it can pump the same amount of blood with fewer heartbeats than the heart of an unfit person can.

To develop cardiorespiratory fitness, you need to perform **aerobic** (oxygen-requiring) activities. An aerobic activity lasts longer than 2 minutes, increases heart and breathing rates, and involves vigorous movements of large muscles. Popular aerobic activities include running, jogging, race-walking, lap swimming, cycling, stair-stepping, aerobic dancing, cross-country skiing, and rope skipping. When you engage in vigorous physical activities, your heart and breathing rates increase considerably above resting values, and you may sweat excessively.

While performing aerobic activities, people can use their heart rates to determine whether the intensity of the activities is high enough to provide cardiorespiratory benefits. To be very effective, a physical activity should be vigorous enough to raise your heart rate to within a certain range, the target heart rate zone. After raising your heart rate to the target zone,

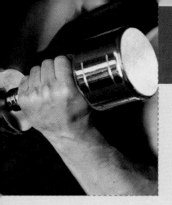

# Managing Your Health

## Assessing the Intensity of Your Workout: Target Heart Rates

To maximize the cardiorespiratory benefits of aerobic activity, you should work out at the level of intensity that raises your heart rate to within your target heart rate zone. To estimate your target heart rate zone, you need to take your pulse. **Figure 11.A** illustrates where you can feel your pulse using the carotid artery in your neck or radial artery in your wrist. Although locating the carotid artery pulse can be easier than the radial pulse, applying pressure to the carotid artery can reduce the heart rate, which interferes with obtaining a reliable measurement. For some people with cardiovascular disease, applying pressure to the carotid artery can be dangerous. Many medical experts advise using gentle pressure on your carotid artery to measure your pulse. Practice finding your radial pulse so that you can take it quickly while exercising.

To obtain the most accurate heart rate, measure your pulse while you are still engaging in the physical activity or within 10 seconds after discontinuing the muscular

### Figure 11.A

**Taking Your Pulse.** (a) Carotid site. (b) Radial site.

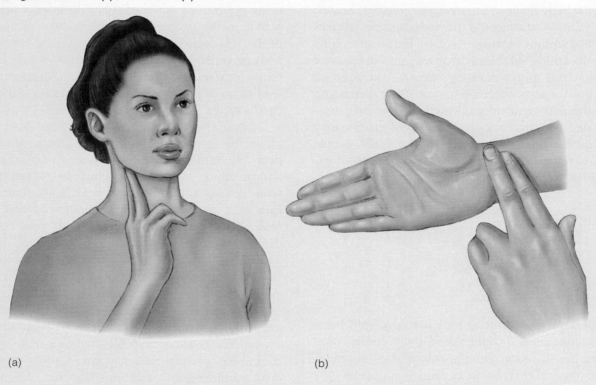

(a)

(b)

you should continue performing the aerobic activity, maintaining the level of intensity for at least 20 minutes. The above Managing Your Health box "Assessing the Intensity of Your Workout: Target Heart Rates" describes how to measure your heart rate and calculate your target heart rate zone.

You do not have to jog 6 miles daily to reap the health benefits of a physically active lifestyle; most people can improve their health by performing a minimum of 30 minutes of moderately intense physical activity 5 days a week.[1] People can even benefit from intermittent episodes of aerobic activity that

movement. This timing is necessary because your pulse declines rapidly when you stop exercising. Count your pulse for 10 seconds, and then multiply that number by 6 to obtain your heart rate per minute.

To estimate your target heart rate zone, obtain your *age-predicted maximum heart rate* by subtracting your age from 220. For example, if you are 20 years old and healthy, your age-predicted maximum heart rate is 200 beats per minute. Recently, a team of heart experts proposed a different formula for healthy women.[8] According to their formula, a woman should multiply her age in years by 0.88, and then subtract that figure from 206. For example, a 20-year-old woman would multiply her age (20) by 0.88, which equals 17.6. By subtracting 17.6 from 206, she would determine her maximum heart rate to be about 188 beats per minute. Exercising at your age-predicted maximum heart rate is undesirable and uncomfortable; this extreme level of intensity is unnecessary for achieving cardiorespiratory fitness. Healthy people should exercise with enough intensity to raise their heart rates to within 65% to 90% of their age-predicted maximum heart rates. This interval is the *target heart rate zone* (**Figure 11.B**). People in excellent physical condition may calculate their target heart rates at the 85% to 90% intensity level. Most experts do not recommend that individuals raise their heart rates more than 90% of their age-predicted maximum levels.

If you are sedentary and just starting an exercise program, strive for a maximum heart rate at the low end of your target zone. As your physical condition improves, you will need to recalculate your target heart rate so that it is in "the zone."

While exercising, if you can raise your heart rate to a value in your target zone and maintain this rate for 30 to 60 minutes, you are giving your heart and lungs a beneficial aerobic workout. During aerobic activity, you should measure your pulse about every 10 minutes without stopping the activity. If your heart rate is higher than the maximum value of your target heart rate zone, it is possible that you underestimated your zone, or you may be overexerting yourself at your present level of fitness.

## Figure 11.B

**Target Heart Rate Zones.** The space between the blue lines represents pulse rates within the 65% and 90% intensity ranges for men. The space between the red lines represents the 65% and 90% intensity ranges for women.

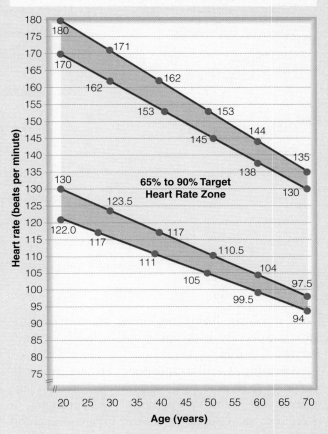

You may need to reduce your muscular workload. On the other hand, if your heart rate during aerobic exercise is less than the target range, you may not be working hard enough to achieve cardiorespiratory benefits.

last 10 minutes and accumulate to at least 30 minutes in one day.[1] Most sedentary and overweight people can integrate more physical activity into their daily routines, for example, by climbing stairs instead of taking elevators and walking to nearby places instead of driving. By exercising more vigorously, however, people can achieve even greater health benefits. **Table 11.2** lists some physical activities classified as light, moderate, and intense.

If you have heart disease or other serious chronic conditions, are unfit, or are 40 years of age or older (male) or 50 years of age or older (female), consult

## Table 11.2

### Physical Activities: Intensity Levels

| Light Activity (less than 3 calories/kg/hr) | Moderate Activity (3 to 6 calories/kg/hr) | Intense/Vigorous Activity (more than 6 calories/kg/hr) |
|---|---|---|
| Walking slowly (1 to 2 mph) | Walking briskly (3 to 4 mph) | Walking briskly uphill with a load |
| Cycling, stationary bike | Cycling for pleasure or transportation | Cycling, fast or racing |
| Swimming, slow treading | Swimming, moderate effort | Swimming, fast treading, or crawl |
| Conditioning exercises: light stretching | Conditioning exercises: general calisthenics | Conditioning exercises: ski or stair-climbing machine |
| — | Racket sports: table tennis | Racket sports: racketball, singles tennis |
| Golf, using power cart | Golf, pulling cart or carrying clubs | — |
| Bowling | — | — |
| Fishing, sitting | Fishing, standing and casting | — |
| Boating (power boat) | Canoeing leisurely (2 to 3.9 mph) | Canoeing rapidly (≥4 mph) |
| Carpet sweeping | General housecleaning | Moving furniture |
| Carpentry | Housepainting | — |

Source: Adapted from Pate, R. R., et al. (1995). Physical activity and public health. *Journal of the American Medical Association, 273*:402–407.

your physician before beginning an exercise program, especially if the program includes vigorous aerobic activities.

**Assessing Cardiorespiratory Fitness** You can judge your level of cardiorespiratory fitness by answering the following questions. While engaging in strenuous exercise, can you carry on a conversation with others, or are you panting for air and unable to talk? How long does it take you to catch your breath or for your heart to stop racing after you stop the activity? If you are unable to talk while exercising and it takes you a long time to recover your normal breathing and heart rates when you finish the physical activity, you probably have a relatively low degree of cardiorespiratory fitness. The first assessment activity for this chapter involves a simple test that you can perform to determine your level of cardiorespiratory fitness (see the Student Workbook section at the end of the book).

Many formerly out-of-shape people discover that their resting heart rates have declined after a few months of regular aerobic exercise. Observing such a decline in resting heart rate not long after beginning a regular aerobic exercise program is usually an indication that cardiorespiratory fitness has improved.

To track your aerobic fitness progress, record your resting heart rates before and after initiating an exercise regimen. Determine your resting heart rate by measuring your pulse when you first wake up, before getting out of bed, on 3 consecutive days. Calculate your average resting heart rate over this 3-day period, and record it and the date. After a few months of engaging in a vigorous exercise program, repeat the procedure to determine your resting heart rate and compare the before and after measurements.

## Muscular Strength

Muscular strength is an important aspect of muscular fitness. **Muscular strength** is the ability of muscles to apply maximum force against an object that is resisting this force. Many individuals perform specific resistance exercises to increase muscular strength because they want to lift heavy objects with ease or improve their appearance (**Figure 11.3**). Other people are interested in developing larger, stronger muscles because they want to compete in sporting events that require strength. How do the strength and size of a muscle increase?

To develop a high degree of strength, muscles need to be overloaded by moving heavy objects repeatedly,

## Figure 11.3

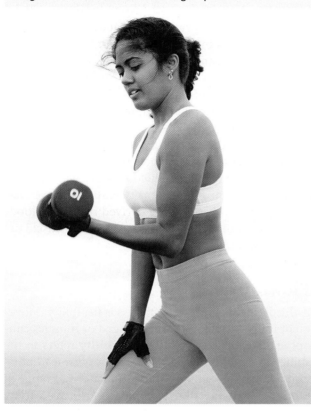

**Muscular Strength.** Many individuals perform specific exercises to improve their appearance or to develop larger, more well-defined muscle groups.

**muscular strength** The ability to apply maximum force against an object that is resisting this force.

**hypertrophy** A condition in which muscles become larger and stronger.

**atrophy** A condition in which muscles lose size and strength.

**detraining** A condition characterized by atrophied and weak muscles, which occurs when skeletal muscles are not used regularly.

**isotonic** A type of exercise in which the individual exerts muscular force against a movable but constant source of resistance.

**isometric** A type of exercise in which the individual exerts muscular force against a fixed, immovable object.

particularly objects that become progressively heavier over time. For example, using a weight-lifting machine regularly can increase the size and strength of the biceps muscle in the upper arm. This response is called the *training effect*. Under these conditions, the individual fibers of the biceps muscle can enlarge, or **hypertrophy**, making the entire muscle stronger and larger. Once muscle cells enlarge, they require a regular program of resistance exercise to maintain their size and strength.

The saying "Use it or lose it" generally applies to skeletal muscles. Muscular **atrophy**, a condition of a muscle that has lost size and strength, results from a few weeks of **detraining**. If you have ever had a broken arm or leg, you may recall that after the cast was removed, the muscles of the recovered limb were atrophied and weak. When you first used the limb, the weakened muscles ached for a brief time, but within days they became stronger. Eventually, using these muscles enabled them to regain their full strength and original size.

**Exercising for Muscular Strength** A safe and effective way to increase muscle strength and size is to perform repetitive exercises that overload a particular muscle group, such as lifting weights. A repetition is the completion of a particular exercise, for example, lifting a handheld weight and returning to the resting position. A set involves performing the same resistance exercise movement usually 8 to 12 times. Healthy people can begin to train their major muscle groups by performing a single set of exercises for each group of muscles.[9] Over time, the individual should develop enough muscular strength to perform multiple sets (generally three) during his or her resistance workout.[10] For best results, a person should do the resistance workout three times a week.

Two forms of exercise that increase muscular strength are isotonic and isometric exercises. When performing **isotonic** exercises, a person exerts muscular force against a movable but constant source of resistance. During isotonic exercise, the muscle shortens and bulges. Isotonic exercises include lifting barbells, performing push-ups, or using weight machines (**Figure 11.4**). Instead of describing the exercises as isotonic, some fitness experts prefer to use the term *dynamic constant external resistance* because it reflects the nature of these movements more accurately. An exercise is dynamic if the skeleton moves during the activity.

In an **isometric** exercise an individual exerts muscular force against a fixed, immovable object of resistance. For example, applying a constant amount of force while pushing against an immovable door frame is an isometric exercise. During isometric contraction, the muscle does not shorten, so it does not bulge. Although isometric exercises can increase muscular strength, they do not increase muscular en-

**muscular endurance** A muscle's ability to contract repeatedly without becoming fatigued.

**flexibility** The ability to move a muscle to any position in its normal range of motion.

### Figure 11.4

**Isotonic Contraction.** While performing isotonic exercise, the muscle contracts, shortening in length.

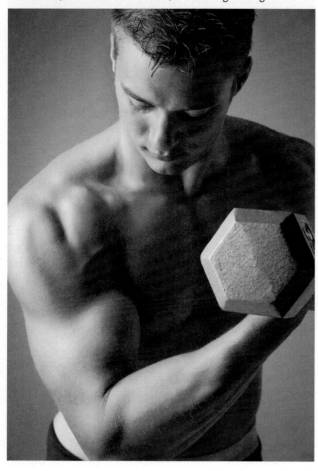

durance or flexibility effectively. Furthermore, muscles can apply excessive pressure on certain arteries during isometric contractions, raising blood pressure. Therefore, many physicians do not recommend isometric exercises for people older than 35 years or those suffering from cardiovascular disease.

## Muscular Endurance

Muscular endurance is another important aspect of muscular fitness. **Muscular endurance** is the ability of a muscle to contract repeatedly without becoming fatigued easily. For example, many people perform

"crunches" to strengthen their abdominal muscles. A sedentary person may experience muscular fatigue after the third crunch and not be able to do another one. If this person, however, continues to perform crunches regularly and increases the number performed during each exercise session, he or she will develop muscular endurance in the abdominal muscles. As a result, this person can do numerous crunches with ease. You can assess your muscular endurance by taking the push-up test in the Student Workbook section at the end of this book.

To achieve muscular endurance, you need to train skeletal muscles by contracting them repeatedly. Furthermore, the ability to sustain muscular contractions over a relatively long period requires a constant source of energy. Glucose is skeletal muscles' preferred fuel for high-intensity endurance exercise. Muscles metabolize glucose derived from the bloodstream or from glycogen that is stored in muscle tissue. Additionally, muscle fibers can use fatty acids and amino acids for energy.

## Flexibility

A third aspect of muscular fitness is flexibility. Movement is limited if joints are damaged or muscles cannot extend themselves fully. **Flexibility** refers to the ability to extend muscles, enabling a person to position a movable joint anywhere in its normal range of motion. Flexibility allows people to perform a variety of skeletal movements with ease, including bending, gliding, rotating, and twisting. Many daily tasks require the ability to extend muscles and move joints easily: reaching for an item stored on a high shelf, stretching to pull up a back zipper, or bending to pick up a tennis ball. Having fully extendable muscles and flexible joints enables you to care for yourself and to participate in enjoyable activities. You can assess your flexibility by taking the sit-and-reach test in the Student Workbook.

People can develop flexibility by performing yoga, Pilates, or stretching exercises such as those shown in *Figure 11.5*. *Static stretching* involves slowly and fully extending the muscle and nearby joints throughout their natural ranges of motion. When performing a static stretch, gently extend the muscle until you feel tension; if you feel discomfort, relax the stretch slightly. While stretching, breathe normally; do not hold your breath. You should be comfortable holding this position for 15 to 30 seconds. Although sources of fitness information often recommend static stretching for 15 to 30 seconds, a review of scientific literature indicates that a variety of stretching techniques,

**Figure 11.5**

**Stretching to Improve Flexibility.** Flexible muscles enable one to make a variety of skeletal movements occur with ease. People can develop flexibility by performing stretching exercises such as the (a) low back stretch, (b) calf stretch, (c) modified hurdle, (d) lunge stretch, (e) supine hamstring stretch, and (f) groin stretch.

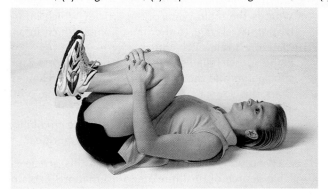

(a)

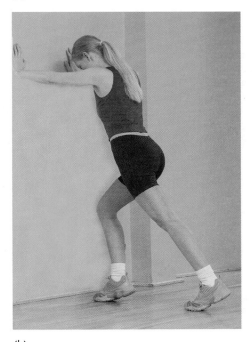

(b)

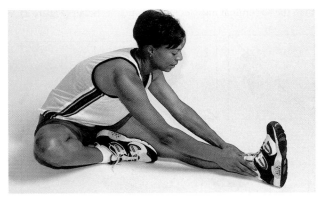

(c)

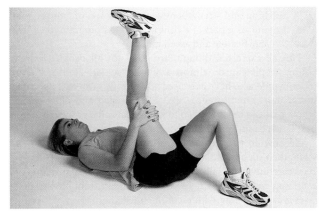

(d)

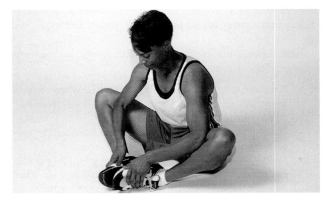

(e)

(f)

The Health-Related Components of Physical Fitness    **351**

# Analyzing Health-Related Information

The accompanying article describes safe alternatives to outdated exercises. Read the article and evaluate it using the model for analyzing health-related information. The main points of the model are noted here; the model is explained fully in Chapter 1.

1. Which statements are verifiable facts, and which are unverified statements or value claims?
2. What are the credentials of the person who wrote the article? Does this person have the appropriate background and education in the topic area? What can you do to check the person's credentials?
3. What might be the motives and biases of the person who wrote the article?
4. What is the main point of the article? Which information is relevant to the main point? Which information is irrelevant?
5. Is the source reliable? What evidence supports your conclusion that the source is reliable or unreliable? Does the source of information present the pros and cons of the topic?
6. Does the source of information attack the credibility of conventional scientists or medical authorities?

Based on your analysis, do you think this article is a reliable source of health-related information? Explain why you would or would not use the information. Summarize your reasons for coming to this conclusion.

## Safe Alternatives for Outdated Exercises

Bryant Stamford, PhD

Stretching and strengthening exercises are, of course, good for you. As a part of a complete fitness program, they help you stay flexible and avoid injury.

Not all exercises, though, are good for all people. Healthy young people can do almost any exercise with little risk. And older people who have exercised all their lives can exercise safely under most circumstances. But middle-aged and older people who have been inactive need to know that some of the old stand-bys—such as sit-ups and toe touches—can result in injury.

So how do you get the important benefits of stretching and strengthening but avoid the injuries? You need to choose exercises carefully, especially if you are getting up in years and haven't exercised regularly. To help you, potentially troublesome exercises are cited below, with recommended alternatives.

If you aren't very flexible or have had back problems, it's best to consult a doctor before starting an exercise program. You may be more susceptible to injury because of a number of factors, including past injuries, fitness, body type, flexibility, technique, and age.

Regardless of the exercises you select, apply the following principles for maximum safety:

- Use strict technique. Stop using an exercise when physical limitation prevents you from performing it well. Also stop when you are tired.
- Use a slow, deliberate approach. Never bounce: The momentum can make a safe exercise dangerous.
- Hold stretches at least 6 seconds initially, building gradually to 30 seconds, then to 2 minutes. Holding a stretched position is more effective than doing many repetitions.
- Reject the "no pain, no gain" philosophy. Pain means something is wrong, so stop immediately.

Many popular exercises stress the lower back. High on the list is the standing toe touch, which stretches the hamstring muscles at the back of your thighs. This is a bad exercise even if done slowly, but it's even worse if you bounce. A safer option is the one-legged stretch (**Figure 1**).

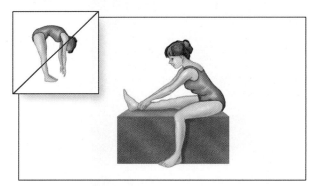

Figure 1: One-legged stretch.

Sit-ups are popular, supposedly for stomach toning. But full sit-ups stress the lower back, and they work the hip muscles more than the abdominal muscles. The "crunch" is better (**Figure 2**).

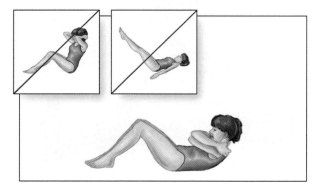

Figure 2: The crunch.

The donkey kick can also be dangerous, especially to your neck and lower back. It involves being on all fours and lifting one leg as high as possible in a kicking fashion. An alternative to the donkey kick is the rear-thigh lift (**Figure 3**).

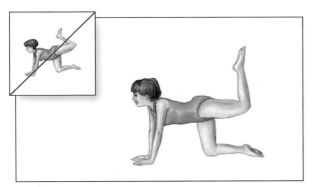

Figure 3: Rear-thigh lift.

Exercises that involve twisting can be especially dangerous. Windmills, in which you bend over and try to touch one hand to the opposite foot, are very stressful on the lower back. But in some sports—like golf—twisting plays a major part. Therefore, when recovering from a low-back injury, perform mild, pain-free twisting movements under professional supervision.

Some exercises can harm the neck. Head rolls, in which you roll your head in a complete circle, are very stressful to the upper spine. Do neck stretches instead (**Figure 4**).

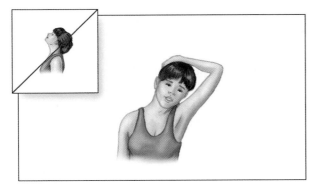

Figure 4: Neck stretch.

People do the yoga plow to stretch upper and lower back muscles by lying on their back and bringing their feet up and over until they touch the floor beyond their head. Unfortunately, this forces the discs in the neck to bulge, risking injury. For the same reason, avoid the "bicycle," in which you lie on your back, raise your hips, and "pedal" your feet. An excellent alternative is the fold-up stretch (**Figure 5**).

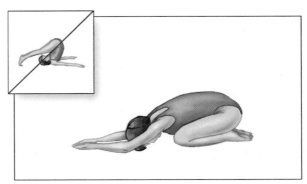

Figure 5: Fold-up stretch.

Full squats or deep knee bends can damage your knees, especially when you bounce out of the squat. Partial squats done slowly and under control are safer.

Jumping jacks involve considerable forces on your legs, particularly the knees. If you land on your toes, the Achilles tendons at the back of your heels bear a major load and could rupture if your legs aren't in the best of shape. Gently running in place provides a lower-impact way to warm up.

**Less Risky Business**

No matter what your age or physical condition, choosing safer exercise options will lower your risk of injury. And remember that whatever the exercise, good technique is essential.

*Remember:* This information is not intended as a substitute for medical treatment. Before starting an exercise program, consult a physician.

*Source:* Stamford, B. (1995). Safer alternatives to outdated exercises. *The Physician and Sportsmedicine, 23*(6):87–88. Reproduced with permission from The McGraw-Hill Companies. All rights reserved.

*This article was written when Dr. Stamford was director of the Health Promotion and Wellness Center and Professor of Allied Health in the School of Medicine at the University of Louisville, Kentucky.*

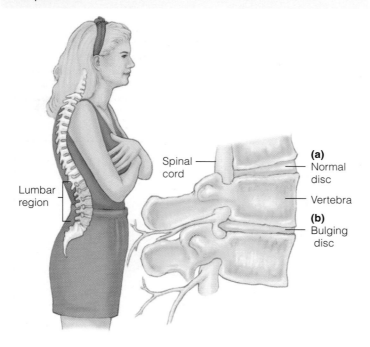

**Figure 11.6**

**Spinal Discs.** (a) Normal disc position. (b) Bulging disc pressing on spinal cord.

Spinal cord

Lumbar region

**(a)** Normal disc

Vertebra

**(b)** Bulging disc

durations, and positions are effective means of increasing hamstring muscle flexibility.[11]

Most fitness experts do not recommend *ballistic stretching* activities that involve bouncing. Additionally, you should not use unnatural stretching motions that injure muscles and tendons or extend joints beyond their normal ranges of motion. If pain occurs while stretching, discontinue the activity immediately. The Analyzing Health-Related Information activity in this chapter describes safe alternatives to outdated stretching exercises.

**Low Back Pain** The majority of Americans encounter low back pain during their lives.[12] As its name implies, low back pain occurs in the lumbar region of the spine (the lower back, above the hips), and it can be disabling (**Figure 11.6**). People with this condition are unable to perform activities essential to daily living comfortably, if at all. Furthermore, low back pain is responsible for a significant percentage of worker absenteeism and workers' medical compensation claims.

Weak abdominal, back, and leg muscles as well as worn lumbar *spinal discs* often contribute to the development of low back pain. The spinal discs are flexible pads that separate the bones of the spine

and act as shock absorbers, protecting the bones from striking each other. As people age, their spinal discs become worn and sometimes bulge out of their normal position. Pounding, twisting, and lifting place physical stress on the lumbar spine and are likely responsible for displacing or damaging some discs. Such movements include jogging on a sidewalk, swinging a golf club, carrying a heavy backpack, and picking up a heavy box or a child. Additionally, people who have poor posture, sit for hours in awkward positions, wear high-heeled shoes, or have too much body fat are susceptible to low back pain, especially if they have weak abdominal muscles.

Although medical experts agree that exercising to strengthen the abdominal, hip, upper leg, and back muscles can prevent or treat many cases of low back pain, they do not agree on which exercises to recommend. Some physicians recommend aerobic exercises; others promote various stretching activities. **Figure 11.7** shows various exercises designed to strengthen the weak muscles that contribute to low back pain and improve the flexibility of the spinal joints.

You can reduce your risk of developing low back pain by changing some behaviors; for example, lose excess body fat, exercise regularly, and wear shoes with low or no heels. Additionally, you can often prevent low back pain by following the lifting and sitting practices recommended in **Figure 11.8**.

Over-the-counter pain medicines and heat treatments can often relieve low back pain. After the discomfort subsides, people should perform exercises that strengthen the lower back, hip, and abdominal muscles. If the pain is intense or persists, however, the person should obtain a complete medical evaluation to determine the source of the pain. In some cases, surgery may be necessary.

## Body Composition

As mentioned in Chapter 10, a healthy body contains large quantities of water and smaller amounts of fat and lean tissues (bones, muscles, and organs). Body composition, the percentages of body weight contributed by lean tissue and fat mass, is a major factor in health. Although a small amount of body fat (about 4% in men and 10% in women) is essen-

## Figure 11.7

**Exercises to Prevent Low Back Pain.**

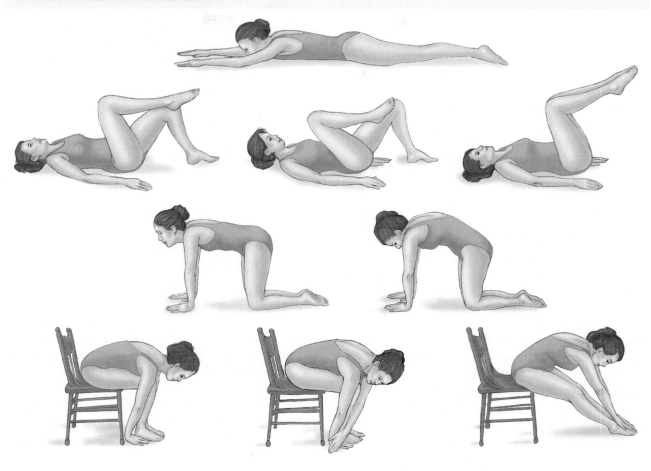

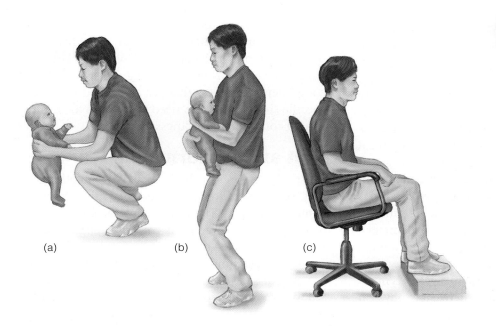

## Figure 11.8

**Practices to Protect Your Lower Back.** (a) To bend safely, bend your knees, not your back. (b) When lifting a child or heavy object, hold it close to your body, at chest level, and do not make twisting motions. (c) To protect your lower back while sitting, rest your lower back against the chair's back and avoid bending forward. Use an adjustable seat and prop up your feet so that you sit with your hips slightly lower than your knees.

The Health-Related Components of Physical Fitness    **355**

tial, too much fat contributes to a variety of chronic diseases, including cardiovascular disease, hypertension, and diabetes. Regular exercise builds and maintains muscle mass and helps keep the amount of body fat at healthy levels.

The cells that comprise lean tissues, particularly muscle cells, are more metabolically active than fat cells are. Therefore, muscle cells burn more calories than fat cells do. By exercising and increasing muscle mass, you can increase your metabolic rate.[13]

Aging muscle cells eventually wear out and die. Unfortunately, the body does not replace these cells. As a result, people usually lose muscle mass and gain fat as they age. Many people think that unused or dying muscle cells can "turn into" fat cells. Muscle cells, however, do not transform themselves into fat cells. A muscle cell is very different from a fat cell; each type of cell has specific structures and functions. Nevertheless, you can preserve more of your muscle mass as you get older if you continue to follow a regular exercise program.

Although regular physical activity can help a person maintain muscle mass while losing weight, "spot" exercising, such as performing 100 crunches daily to shrink the abdominal area, does not reduce the amount of fat stored there. During physical activity, fat deposits throughout the body release fatty acids into the bloodstream to supply energy for the vigorously moving muscles. Exercising a specific muscle group, however, can improve physical fitness and appearance by increasing the strength of the exercised muscles and improving their ability to hold in the underlying fat mass.

Engaging in moderate- to vigorous-intensity aerobic activities for at least 60 minutes nearly every day, while not exceeding your calorie needs, can be an effective method of "burning" body fat for energy. Performing at least 60 minutes of moderate-intensity physical activity each day may help you avoid gaining body fat. If you have lost weight, you may need as much as 90 minutes of moderate-intensity physical activity daily to prevent regaining the body fat.

Walking 2 miles at a brisk pace expends about 200 calories, which is about the number of calories in four chocolate chip cookies (2.25-inch diameter) or one plain cake doughnut (3.25-inch diameter). This may seem to be a small amount of energy, but a person who consumes 200 more calories a day than necessary can gain more than 20 lb in a year. As mentioned in the previous chapter, increasing physical activity and eating a sensible calorie-restricted diet is the most effective way to control weight.

## Healthy Living Practices

☐ Engaging in intense aerobic activity regularly can improve your cardiorespiratory fitness and burn excess body fat.

☐ Engaging in regular resistance exercises, such as lifting weights, can increase the size and strength of your muscles.

☐ Stretching muscles can improve their flexibility.

# Athletic Performance

## The Sports-Related Components of Fitness

Although genetic factors contribute to cardiorespiratory fitness, training is essential for athletes to develop their inborn physical capabilities and compete successfully in sports. The sports-related components of fitness include *speed*, *power*, *coordination*, *agility*, *balance*, and *reaction time*. Speed is the rate of movement; power is the ability to concentrate a considerable amount of force, usually from a particular group of muscles, when performing work. Coordination is the ability to perform a series of complicated muscular movements in a continuous manner. Agility enables a person to make quick precise movements, such as changing direction, with ease. Balance enables one to maintain a poised upright body position. Reaction time is the time it takes a person to adjust his or her body position to a changing environment. Although athletes often focus on improving the sports-related components of fitness that are associated with their specific sports, they also need to develop the health-related components of fitness.

## Diet and Performance

Most athletes are on the lookout for something—a diet, supplement, or drug—that may give them the competitive edge. The best advice for all athletes is to drink adequate amounts of water and choose a well-balanced diet composed of a variety of foods. By eating more servings of fruits and vegetables, athletes can obtain safe quantities of vitamins and minerals without taking supplements. There is no scientific evidence that protein-rich diets build bigger muscles, so eating large servings of meat or taking protein supplements is unnecessary. High protein intakes may cause dehydration and accelerate the loss of calcium from bones. Furthermore, protein-rich foods often contain a lot of fat, especially saturated fat.

Carbohydrate is the preferred fuel of the body, and a diet that supplies plenty of complex carbohydrates from starchy foods is recommended. Starchy foods usually contain more vitamins and minerals than sugary foods do. Some athletes practice "carbohydrate loading" to maximize the amount of carbohydrate stored in their muscles. A few days before an event, for example, the athlete gradually increases the amount of carbohydrate eaten to about 70% of calories and gradually decreases the amount of time working out. Two to 4 hours before the competitive event, the athlete eats a light meal composed of starchy foods such as bagels, pasta, or breads and cereals. Not all athletes find that carbohydrate loading helps their performance. Thus, one should test the effects of the diet when not preparing for competition.

## Ergogenic Aids

**Ergogenic** (work-producing) **aids** include a variety of products such as dietary supplements, stimulant drugs, and mechanical devices that supposedly enhance physical development or performance. Some of these aids are beneficial and harmless, but others are dangerous and illegal. *Chromium picolinate*, for example, is a popular dietary supplement that some people use to build lean body mass. Although results of some studies indicate chromium picolinate may provide some health benefits, more research is needed. Furthermore, information about the long-term safety of chromium picolinate supplementation is lacking.

Another popular ergogenic aid is *creatine*, a compound that is naturally in muscle tissue. According to research, creatine can be effective in increasing strength, especially for short bouts of high-intensity physical activities such as sprinting and jumping.[14] Although creatine supplementation appears to be safe, more research is needed to determine the safety of taking creatine supplements over the long term. *Table 11.3* lists some dietary supplements, claims about their ergogenic effects, and information concerning whether scientific studies support these claims. In many instances, more research is needed to support or refute claims. For information about other dietary supplements, see Tables 1.5, 9.10, and 10.A.

For more than four decades, the outstanding physical accomplishments of many athletes have

**ergogenic aids** Products or devices that enhance physical development or performance.

been tainted by reports of athletes relying on "doping," the use of foreign substances to enhance performance. For example, Danish cyclist Knud Enemark Jensen crashed his bike and fractured his skull while competing in the 1960 Summer Olympics. The young man died a few hours later. The autopsy of the cyclist's body revealed he had used amphetamines, a class of stimulant drugs. By the late 1960s, the International Olympic Committee (IOC) and some other sports federations had established lists of banned substances and required their athletes to be tested for these chemicals. In January 2008, a judge sentenced track star Marion Jones to several months in jail after she admitted lying to federal investigators about her use of performance-enhancing drugs and her involvement in a check-fraud scheme (**Figure 11.9**). As

### Figure 11.9

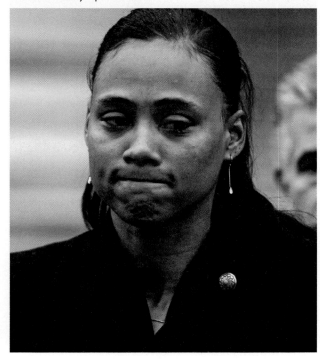

**Fallen Star.** In January 2008, a judge sentenced Marion Jones to spend several months in jail after she admitted lying to federal investigators about her use of performance-enhancing drugs and involvement in a check-fraud scheme. Because of her admission, the International Olympic Committee disqualified Jones from the five track events in which she won medals at the 2000 Summer Olympic Games.

## Table 11.3

## Dietary Supplements as Ergogenic Aids

| Aid | Claim | Current Scientific Findings |
|---|---|---|
| Caffeine | Improves strength<br><br>Enhances fat metabolism | Increases alertness, but at high doses causes nervousness; raises free fatty acid levels during exercise; might provide modest improvement of performance. |
| Creatine | Enhances release of energy during exercise | May enhance performance during short bouts of intense exercise; more research is needed. |
| Carnitine | Enhances fat metabolism | No significant improvement in performance, but more research is needed. |
| Wheat-germ oil | Increases oxygen uptake by cells, improving stamina | Results of well-designed studies do not support ergogenic claims. |
| Lecithin and choline | Increases production of a neurotransmitter, resulting in more muscular strength | Results of well-designed studies do not support ergogenic claims. |
| Omega-3 fatty acids | Makes blood flow better, stimulates muscle growth | Results of well-designed studies do not support ergogenic claims; large doses may increase the risk of stroke. |
| Amino acids, brewer's yeast, enzymes, and DNA supplements | General performance-enhancing effects | Results of well-designed studies do not support ergogenic claims; large doses of amino acids can inhibit amino acid absorption and increase water requirement. |
| $CoQ_{10}$ (coenzyme Q or ubiquinone) | Improves heart function | Results of well-designed studies do not show consistent improvement in performance; more research is needed. Long-term safety is unknown. |
| Bee pollen | Shortens recovery time | Results of well-designed studies do not support ergogenic claims; may cause allergic responses in some individuals. |
| CLA (conjugated linoleic acid) | Increases lean body mass | Results of well-designed studies do not support ergogenic claims. Long-term safety is unknown. |

a result of her admission, the IOC disqualified Jones from the five track events in which she won medals at the 2000 Summer Olympic Games. Shortly before being disqualified, Jones returned her Olympic medals to the Committee.

Athletes in other sports also use banned substances to improve their physical abilities. According to the 2007 Mitchell Report, doping is widespread among professional baseball players.[15] The report includes the names of several Major League Baseball players who allegedly purchased illegal substances, particularly *anabolic steroids*, to enhance their performance. In the report, former U.S. Senator George Mitchell recommends that the players and the management of

Major League Baseball teams work together to rid the sport of doping.

**Anabolic Steroids** Both men and women may lift weights during their workout sessions to build stronger, more well-defined muscles. Men, however, are capable of developing larger muscles and having greater overall strength because their testosterone levels are higher than those of women. Testosterone is an anabolic (tissue-building) hormone.

**Anabolic steroids** are a group of synthetic and natural substances that are chemically related to testosterone and may have muscle-building properties. Although certain anabolic steroids are classified as controlled substances, they can be prescribed by physicians for legitimate medical uses. These drugs, however, are often illegally obtained and abused by athletes and others who want to enhance their physical performance or muscle development or both. In the United States, it is difficult to estimate the prevalence of anabolic steroid abuse because people are often unwilling to admit to taking the substances.

Medical experts are especially concerned about anabolic steroid use among adolescents because of the long-term serious health consequences. In 2010, 2% of American high school seniors reported using steroids at some point in their lives.[16]

Why is there so much concern over the abuse of anabolic steroids? Athletes who abuse these drugs to improve their physical strength can have an unfair competitive advantage over athletes who choose not to use them. Additionally, anabolic steroids can have serious irreversible effects on the body (**Figure 11.10**). Male anabolic steroid abusers often experience shrunken testicles and infertility. Women who abuse these drugs may become bald, grow facial hair, and experience menstrual irregularities. Anabolic steroid abuse increases the risks of developing heart and kidney diseases, certain cancers, and liver tumors. In some cases, damage to the liver or kidneys is so severe that death occurs. Additionally, anabolic steroids can affect personality. People who abuse anabolic steroids may act more aggressive, hostile, and irritable than usual. Regular resistance exercise is the

**Healthy Living Practices**

☐ Do not use anabolic steroids to build your muscles; they can be very harmful.

only safe way to increase the size and strength of a muscle.

## Exercising for Health

People often engage in a particular type of exercise because of its healthful benefits. Aerobic activities increase cardiorespiratory fitness and muscular endurance. Additionally, performing high-impact aerobic activities, including basketball and jogging, can build stronger bones. Although isometric and isotonic exercises develop muscular strength, these activities may not increase cardiorespiratory fitness significantly. Many people combine aerobic and muscle-strengthening activities in their daily workouts to improve their overall physical condition; others perform isotonic and aerobic workouts on alternate days. For example, one day's workout session would be devoted to weightlifting; the following day's session would involve race-walking.

The frequency, duration, and intensity of exercise also influence the degree of health benefits a person derives from it. Exercise *frequency* is the number of times an individual exercises, usually reported as the number of days or exercise sessions in a week. People who exercise at least three times a week generally experience more rapid improvements to their overall fitness than do people who exercise less often.

The *duration* of exercise refers to the total time the person is physically active during each exercise session. For example, people who jog for 40 minutes, 3 days a week experience more cardiorespiratory benefits than do those who jog for 10 minutes, 3 days a week.[17,18] Sedentary people can develop cardiorespiratory fitness if they engage in an aerobic exercise program that gradually increases the duration of the activity, usually over several weeks.

A relatively easy way to assess and increase your physical activity level is to measure the number of steps you take in a day. You will need to purchase a pedometer; inexpensive ones sell for under $30 (**Figure 11.11**). Before you begin a typical day's activities, place the pedometer on your belt or waistband. Then, check the pedometer before going to bed and record the number of steps you took that day. If you have a sedentary lifestyle, you probably will have

## Figure 11.10

**Possible Effects of Anabolic Steroids on the Body.** To increase their muscle mass, some men and women abuse anabolic steroids or other chemicals that are promoted for their muscle-building properties. These drugs can have serious irreversible effects on the body.

**Anabolic steroids may cause:**

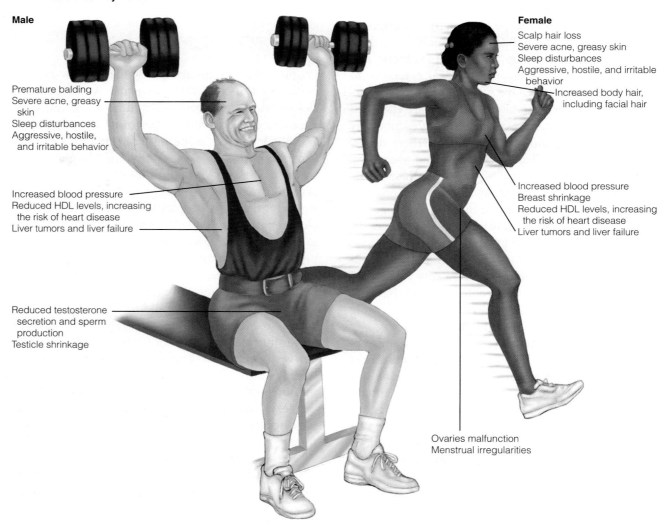

**Male**

Premature balding
Severe acne, greasy skin
Sleep disturbances
Aggressive, hostile, and irritable behavior

Increased blood pressure
Reduced HDL levels, increasing the risk of heart disease
Liver tumors and liver failure

Reduced testosterone secretion and sperm production
Testicle shrinkage

**Female**

Scalp hair loss
Severe acne, greasy skin
Sleep disturbances
Aggressive, hostile, and irritable behavior
Increased body hair, including facial hair

Increased blood pressure
Breast shrinkage
Reduced HDL levels, increasing the risk of heart disease
Liver tumors and liver failure

Ovaries malfunction
Menstrual irregularities

---

taken fewer than 3,000 steps. Gradually increase the number of steps you take by making a conscious effort to be more active. A brisk walking routine, for example, can increase the number of steps you take daily and increase your cardiorespiratory fitness level. Your goal should be to record at least 8,000 steps each day.

The *intensity* of an exercise reflects the amount of physical exertion a person uses while performing the activity. Fitness experts use several methods to estimate the intensity of exercise, including the rate of oxygen consumption during exercise, heart rate, and

personal perceptions of physical exertion. For the average person, playing nine holes of golf while using a power golf cart or bowling for 30 minutes are light activities; playing tennis or walking briskly for a half-hour are moderate activities; and jogging for 6 miles or playing racquetball for 30 minutes are intense activities (see Table 11.2).

The frequency, duration, and intensity of aerobic physical activities influence fitness. For example, you can exercise intensely for 20 minutes or moderately for 30 minutes and achieve similar cardiorespiratory benefits.

**Figure 11.11**

**Examples of Pedometers.** A pedometer is a relatively easy way to assess your physical activity level.

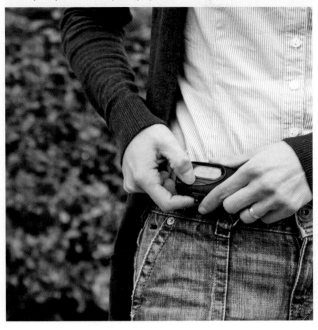

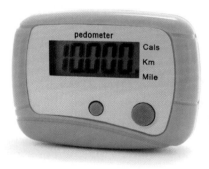

## The Exercise Session

People should *warm up* before and *cool down* ("warm down") after intense exercise. Warming up reduces the physical stress that vigorous exercise can place on the body. The person's skeletal muscles become warm and extend easily, joints become more flexible, and heart and breathing rates increase gradually. Warming up can reduce the extent of muscle soreness after exercise[19] and may reduce the likelihood of injuries.[20] More research is needed to support these findings. Cooling down facilitates the circulation of blood, especially in the leg muscles, enabling the body to recover from intense physical activity.

To warm up the entire body before engaging in a vigorous physical activity, you can walk at an easy pace, and then gradually increase your speed until you have walked for 5 to 10 minutes. At this point, your muscles should be warm enough to perform stretching exercises such as those shown in Figure 11.5. Stretching muscles before the warm-up session is usually not recommended because extending "cold" muscles may injure them. Stretching, however, does not protect against sports injuries.[21,22]

After stretching, many persons perform active, task-specific activities to warm up specific muscles. For example, a jogger would jog slowly for a few minutes, gradually increasing the pace until reaching his or her usual training speed.

Warming up before exercising is essential for people with heart disease. Abnormal functioning of the heart may occur when sedentary, middle-aged people begin to exercise suddenly without warming up. Warm-up activities increase the blood flow to the heart gradually, reducing the risk of heart attack during physical exertion.

After exercising vigorously, people should cool down by gradually reducing the intensity of their activity and by stretching. Many types of strenuous exercise increase the blood supply to the leg muscles; suddenly stopping these intense muscular movements can cause blood to accumulate in the leg veins, which can reduce the blood flow to the brain, causing dizziness, faintness, or loss of consciousness. Cooling down by engaging in 5 to 10 minutes of light exercise gradually decreases the blood flow to the leg muscles. **Figure 11.12** illustrates a 50-minute workout session that consists of 10 minutes of warm-up activities, 30 minutes of jogging, and 10 minutes of cool-down exercises.

## Exercise Danger Signs

Exercise improves the functioning of the heart and reduces the risk of heart disease. Sudden and intense physical exertion, however, can strain the heart, especially the heart of an unfit individual or someone with cardiovascular disease.

To reduce the risk of overtaxing your cardiovascular system during vigorous exercise, warm up first, and then exercise at a reduced intensity level for about 10 to 15 minutes. Keep records of your activity level and any discomfort that you experience. Discontinue the activity and consult a physician if any of the following signs or symptoms of heart disease occur during or after exercising:

**Figure 11.12**

**A Suggested Workout Session.** A reasonable 50-minute workout session may consist of 10 minutes of warm-up activities, 30 minutes of jogging, and 10 minutes of cool-down exercises.

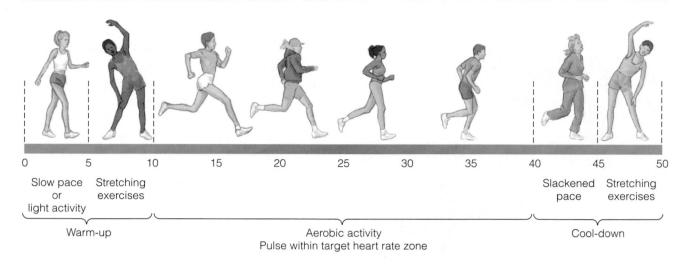

| 0 | 5 | 10 | 15 | 20 | 25 | 30 | 35 | 40 | 45 | 50 |

Slow pace or light activity    Stretching exercises        Slackened pace    Stretching exercises

Warm-up        Aerobic activity Pulse within target heart rate zone        Cool-down

- Heart abnormalities, such as irregular rhythms, a feeling that your heart is pounding in your throat, or fluttering in your chest
- Pain or pressure in your chest, throat, or arms
- Shortness of breath, dizziness, sudden loss of coordination, cold sweating, or fainting

## Preventing and Managing Common Exercise Injuries

Everyone should be concerned about personal safety while exercising. People should check their exercise equipment for defects and wear the proper clothing, shoes, and protective gear for the activity. Additionally, people should use some common sense about when and where they exercise. Bicyclists and joggers, for example, should obey traffic signals and avoid busy roads that have narrow or rocky shoulders. Engaging in physical activity outdoors at night is especially dangerous; people should wear clothing with reflective strips to become more visible.

Although engaging in regular physical activity is essential for optimal health, some activities are likely to result in musculoskeletal injuries. Suddenly raising the intensity level or duration of a physical activity may damage muscles or supportive tissues or aggravate existing injuries. Physically active people can use some general precautions to minimize their risk of musculoskeletal injury. Sudden, awkward movements are likely to injure muscles, tendons, and joints; therefore, people should avoid physical activities that involve exaggerated twisting.

## Strains and Sprains

Almost everyone who is physically active has experienced muscle soreness or musculoskeletal injuries such as *strains* and *sprains*. Although there are no clear clinical definitions for strain or sprain, a **strain** generally refers to the damage that a muscle or tendon sustains when overextended rapidly. A **sprain** usually refers to a damaged ligament. Although these two types of injuries often occur together, a sprain tends to be more serious than a strain is. The sprained ligament may be partially or completely torn, and the nearby muscle, joint, or bones may be damaged; therefore, severe sprains generally require immediate medical attention.

*RICE*, the acronym for rest, ice, compression, and elevation, is often effective for treating strains and sprains:

- *Rest* can reduce the pain, but light exercise or activity that uses the injured muscles is usually recommended, as long as the discomfort is tolerable.

- *Ice* treatments should be limited to 20-minute sessions and can be repeated every 2 hours (while the injured person is awake) for 2 to 3 days. Do not place ice directly on the skin.

- *Compression*, an external source of pressure, can prevent swelling. Apply a pressure bandage on the injury to produce compression. Make sure the bandage is not tight enough to interfere with circulation.

- *Elevation* also reduces swelling. When an injured limb is elevated, gravity helps the veins of the limb return blood to the heart, reducing the amount of blood and other fluids that accumulates in the damaged tissue.

With RICE and over-the-counter pain medicines, muscle soreness usually disappears within a day or two. If an injured area does not improve with RICE and the pain persists or worsens, consult a physician.

## Dislocation

Healthy joints control the ability of muscles to move bones. Joints are susceptible to *dislocation*, that is, becoming displaced by force. Dislocation can result when joints and their supportive tissues are torn or worn after engaging in certain strenuous physical activities. When a joint becomes damaged, the injury reduces its normal range of motion, and movement

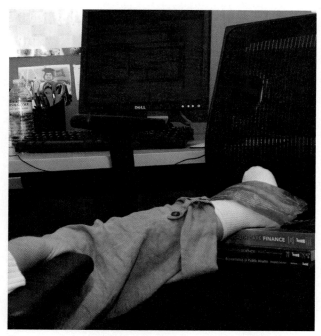

Elevation and ice treatments can reduce swelling of a sprain or strain.

**strain** Generally refers to an injured muscle or tendon.

**sprain** Generally refers to an injured ligament.

**hyperthermia** A condition that occurs when body temperature rises above the normal range.

**heat cramps** In a dehydrated and hot person, the signs and symptoms of heat cramps include muscular tightening and pain in the limbs or abdomen.

**heat exhaustion** The extreme fatigue that results from exercise or work in hot temperatures.

**heatstroke** A life-threatening condition that can occur when people exercise or work in hot temperatures.

often becomes painful. Although involvement in certain sports, such as American football, increases the risk that the participants will damage their joints, any physically active person can experience joint injuries. A later section of this chapter describes steps for designing personal fitness programs that can reduce the risk of such injuries.

## Temperature-Related Injuries

When exercising in sunny weather, the body gains heat from the environment and from its active muscles. To cool itself, the body perspires heavily, transferring heat to the environment. *Dehydration* (lack of body water) can occur if a person does not replace the fluid lost by perspiration. Signs of dehydration include weight loss immediately after exercising and reduced urine production.[23] The muscles of a person suffering from dehydration are less able to work efficiently. It is essential that people replace the water lost in sweat by consuming adequate amounts of fluids, especially plain water. Soups, fruits, vegetables, and nonalcoholic drinks contribute water to the diet also.

**Hyperthermia Hyperthermia**, higher than normal body temperature, can result from dehydration. If a person becomes hot and dehydrated, heat cramps, heat exhaustion, or heatstroke may occur. The signs and symptoms of **heat cramps** include muscular tightening and pain in the limbs or abdomen. The affected individual usually recovers after stopping the activity, resting in a shady area, stretching the cramped muscles, and drinking several ounces of water. After recovering, this person should not exercise for the remainder of the day.

**Heat exhaustion** and **heatstroke** are more serious conditions than heat cramps. People suffering from heat exhaustion have pale and clammy skin; sweat profusely; and feel nauseated, tired, and weak. They need to move to a cooler area and drink plenty

**hypothermia** A condition that occurs when the body's core temperature drops below 95°F.

of cool water. If heat exhaustion is not recognized and treated, heatstroke can develop. The signs and symptoms of heatstroke include hot, dry, reddened skin; rapid pulse; fever; and loss of consciousness. Heatstroke is a life-threatening emergency; victims should be removed from the heat and receive immediate medical attention.

When the weather is hot and humid, avoid exerting yourself outdoors during the hottest time of the day. If you must be outdoors when it is hot, follow a few precautions to reduce the likelihood of heat-related injury. Several hours before exercising or performing intense physical activity, especially in warm conditions, slowly drink water or other acceptable fluids and eat salty foods or snacks to achieve adequate hydration.[23] Alcoholic beverages are not acceptable fluids for hydration because alcohol is a *diuretic*. A diuretic increases urine production; therefore, people lose some body water when they drink alcohol-containing beverages. Although caffeine is also a diuretic, drinking caffeinated beverages does not stimulate excess urine production by the body.[23]

During and after engaging in activities that make you perspire heavily, consume enough fluids to replace the amount of weight lost by sweating. Drinking too much fluid before, during, or after physical activities should be avoided because the practice may cause *overhydration*, a potentially deadly condition. A rule of thumb is to drink about 1.5 L (approximately 6.25 cups) of water or other acceptable beverage for every kilogram (2.2 lb) of body weight lost during the activity.[23] When the weather first becomes hot, individuals should begin working or exercising outdoors at a reduced intensity, and then gradually increase the intensity over a 2-week period to become *acclimatized*, that is, physically adjusted to the extreme temperature change. Wearing light-colored, loose clothing in sunny, hot, and humid weather helps people stay comfortable because light colors reflect sunlight and loose clothing allows perspiration to evaporate more easily. When environmental temperature and humidity are very high, most individuals should consider reducing the intensity and duration of their outdoor workouts to reduce the risk of heat-related illness.

People who perspire excessively can lose considerable amounts of sodium chloride in their sweat. Most of these individuals can drink more water and fruit juices and consume foods to replace the lost nutri-

ents. While engaging in strenuous exercise that lasts an hour or more, people can also consume sports drinks for fluid replacement.[24] In addition to water, these drinks contain sodium chloride and energy-supplying carbohydrate. Most physically active people do not need to take salt (sodium chloride) tablets.[25]

**Frostbite and Hypothermia** Participating in outdoor activities during the winter months increases the risk of cold injury. Exposed to cold temperatures, the body reduces its blood flow to the skin, conserving body heat. The chilled person shivers and feels tingling, numbness, or burning in exposed skin or body parts. *Frostbite* occurs when ice crystals form in the deeper tissues of the skin, damaging them. Blood flow to the affected area slows, causing clots to form. Unable to obtain oxygen and nutrients, the tissue dies. The damage may be so extensive that the frostbitten areas must be amputated. A person's fingers, toes, nose, ears, and face are most susceptible to frostbite, but any exposed skin can become frostbitten. Frostbite requires immediate and proper medical treatment. Avoid rubbing frostbitten skin because it can further damage cold tissues. To prevent frostbite, people need to wear gloves or mittens, thick socks, hats that can be pulled down over the ears, and scarves when outdoors in cold weather.

**Hypothermia** occurs when the body's core temperature drops below 95°F.[26] (A rectal thermometer is used to measure core body temperature.) As body temperature declines, the person shivers, feels tired, displays poor judgment, acts disoriented, and eventually loses consciousness. Death can occur when the core temperature falls below 82°F, and breathing and circulation are too weak to support life.

As in cases of frostbite, hypothermia requires prompt medical treatment. It is important to shelter people suffering from hypothermia from the cold and remove their wet clothing. Covering them in dry

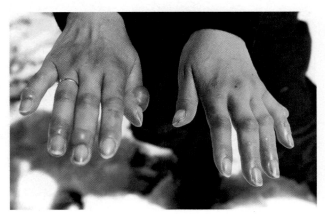

Frostbite

blankets keeps them warm until they can be taken to a hospital. To protect against hypothermia, wear a hat and layers of warm, dry clothing when you are in cold environments.

## Healthy Living Practices

- ☐ If you have musculoskeletal injuries as a result of exercise, use RICE as treatment. If pain and swelling persist, contact your personal physician.
- ☐ If you develop heat cramps or heat exhaustion while working or exercising, stop the activity immediately, get out of the heat, and drink plenty of water.
- ☐ If you plan to exercise or work in hot conditions, wear loose, light clothing and take an ample supply of water, fruit juices, or sports drinks with you.
- ☐ When you exercise or work in cold conditions, protect yourself against hypothermia and frostbite by wearing layers of warm, dry clothing, a hat or ski mask, gloves or mittens, and thick socks.
- ☐ Avoid drinking beverages that contain alcohol to replace body water that is lost by sweating.

# Developing a Personal Fitness Program

A basic personal physical fitness program should include activities that enhance cardiorespiratory fitness, muscular strength and endurance, and flexibility. To develop an effective program, determine your needs, interests, and limitations. Answering the following questions can help you accomplish this step:

- How can I schedule my day's activities so that I have time to exercise?
- Which physical activities am I most likely to enjoy and practice regularly for the rest of my life?
- Do I want to develop or enhance specific sports-related skills?
- Would I rather work out alone or with others?
- Where will I exercise?
- Do I have physical limitations that require special equipment or rule out certain activities?

The "Changing Health Habits" activity for this chapter can help you determine whether you are ready to improve your level of physical fitness (see the Student Workbook section at the end of this text).

After completing the first step, make a list of your general fitness goals. One of them should be to enhance the health-related components of fitness, for example, improving your cardiorespiratory fitness or flexibility. Other goals may be changing your appearance or building agility. Although your list may include several goals, choose one or two to work on at a time.

At this point, you need to choose enjoyable physical activities that will help you meet your fitness goals. As mentioned earlier, aerobic exercise is necessary for achieving cardiorespiratory fitness. Resistance training is important for increasing lean body mass and maintaining muscular strength and endurance. Warm-up and cool-down stretching exercises can improve range of motion. Faculty who conduct personal fitness classes in the physical education department at your college can answer your questions concerning the need for special equipment or how to perform activities safely.

If you are overweight or have been sedentary, give your body time to adapt to the fitness program. For the first 2 weeks, do not try to exercise at a high intensity level or for more than 15 minutes. Some people keep an exercise log or diary to track their progress. Stop when you experience signs of exercise intolerance, such as pain or breathlessness, and note this in your log. A common problem encountered by enthusiastic but out-of-shape people is trying to do too much too soon.

When you do not experience fatigue or discomfort as a result of the activity, you are ready to move on to the improvement stage of the program. By gradually increasing the intensity and duration of your physical activity, you can progressively overload your muscles and achieve your fitness goals. For example, add 5 minutes to the time of your aerobic workout session each week, until you are exercising for 45 to 90 minutes most days of the week. If you are walking at 2 mph, gradually increase the pace until you are able to walk between 3 and 4 mph without effort. To acquire the fitness benefits of aerobic exercise, a person must engage in the activity for at least 30 minutes at a time. However, engaging in aerobic exercise more often, for longer periods, and at higher intensity levels develops much higher degrees of fitness.

You can enhance muscular size and strength with a weightlifting program that gradually overcomes the resistance of progressively heavier weights. As your muscles adapt to the workload, you should be able to develop strength by adding resistance while performing fewer repetitions. After each bout of heavy training, muscles engaged in resistance exercises need about 48 hours to recover, to repair themselves, and to grow. Thus, experts often recommend alternating the days of the week in which you perform cardiorespiratory and strength training activities. **Table 11.4** shows a sample aerobic and weight resistance program that includes stretching exercises. By the end of 6 months, you should be ready to move on to the maintenance stage of the program.

## Table 11.4

### A Sample 4–Week Combined Workout Program

| Week 1 | Warm-Up* (min) | Workout | Cool-Down* (min) | Week 3 | Warm-Up* (min) | Workout | Cool-Down* (min) |
|---|---|---|---|---|---|---|---|
| Monday | 5 to 10 | Brisk walking 15 min. | 5 to 10 | Monday | 5 to 10 | Brisk walking 25 min. | 5 to 10 |
| Tuesday | 5 to 10 | Resistance training, beginning load Reps: 5, Sets: 4 | 5 to 10 | Tuesday | 5 to 10 | Resistance training, beginning load Reps: 5, Sets: 4 | 5 to 10 |
| Wednesday | 5 to 10 | Brisk walking 15 min. | 5 to 10 | Wednesday | 5 to 10 | Brisk walking 25 min. | 5 to 10 |
| Thursday | 5 to 10 | Resistance training, beginning load Reps: 5, Sets: 4 | 5 to 10 | Thursday | 5 to 10 | Resistance training, beginning load Reps: 5, Sets: 4 | 5 to 10 |
| Friday | 5 to 10 | Brisk walking 15 min. | 5 to 10 | Friday | 5 to 10 | Brisk walking 25 min. | 5 to 10 |
| Saturday | 5 to 10 | Resistance training, beginning load Reps: 5, Sets: 4 | 5 to 10 | Saturday | 5 to 10 | Resistance training, beginning load Reps: 5, Sets: 4 | 5 to 10 |
| Sunday | 5 to 10 | Brisk walking 15 min. | 5 to 10 | Sunday | 5 to 10 | Brisk walking 25 min. | 5 to 10 |

| Week 2 | Warm-Up* (min) | Workout | Cool-Down* (min) | Week 4 | Warm-Up* (min) | Workout | Cool-Down* (min) |
|---|---|---|---|---|---|---|---|
| Monday | 5 to 10 | Brisk walking 20 min. | 5 to 10 | Monday | 5 to 10 | Brisk walking 30 min. | 5 to 10 |
| Tuesday | 5 to 10 | Resistance training, beginning load Reps: 5, Sets: 4 | 5 to 10 | Tuesday | 5 to 10 | Resistance training, beginning load Reps: 10, Sets: 4 | 5 to 10 |
| Wednesday | 5 to 10 | Brisk walking 20 min. | 5 to 10 | Wednesday | 5 to 10 | Brisk walking 30 min. | 5 to 10 |
| Thursday | 5 to 10 | Resistance training, beginning load Reps: 5, Sets: 4 | 5 to 10 | Thursday | 5 to 10 | Resistance training, beginning load Reps: 10, Sets: 4 | 5 to 10 |
| Friday | 5 to 10 | Brisk walking 20 min. | 5 to 10 | Friday | 5 to 10 | Brisk walking 30 min. | 5 to 10 |
| Saturday | 5 to 10 | Resistance training, beginning load Reps: 5, Sets: 4 | 5 to 10 | Saturday | 5 to 10 | Resistance training, beginning load Reps: 10, Sets: 4 | 5 to 10 |
| Sunday | 5 to 10 | Brisk walking 20 min. | 5 to 10 | Sunday | 5 to 10 | Brisk walking 30 min. | 5 to 10 |

*Slow walking and stretching.

A major feature of the maintenance stage of your fitness program is sustaining your fitness level and interest. Adding new activities prevents boredom with the workout program and develops different muscle groups or skills. **Cross-training**, incorporating a variety of aerobic activities into a fitness program, is an excellent way to maintain enthusiasm and interest. Working out in different environments can also add interest. Walking in parks or hiking on trails, for example, can be more interesting than walking around indoor tracks. By working out with friends or family members, you can enhance your physical as well as social health.

Once people achieve high degrees of physical fitness, they need to continue exercising to maintain the healthful benefits gained during their training program. Sometimes physically fit individuals discontinue intensive regular exercise regimens for a variety of reasons, such as experiencing injuries or losing motivation. Detraining can occur within a couple of weeks after exercise sessions are discontinued. Even if they have to reduce the frequency of their exercise sessions, people can usually maintain their high level of physical fitness as long as they do not stop working out.

## Healthy Living Practices

- ☐ Perform isometric or isotonic exercises to increase your muscular strength, and also engage in aerobic exercises to enhance your cardiorespiratory fitness.

- ☐ You can enhance your muscular strength, muscular endurance, and flexibility by increasing the frequency, duration, and intensity of your exercise sessions.

- ☐ If you have heart disease or other serious chronic conditions, are unfit, or are older than 40 years (males) or 50 years (females), obtain your physician's approval before beginning an exercise program, especially if the program includes vigorous aerobic activities.

## Active for a Lifetime

People are more likely to engage in physical activity regularly if they enjoy it, recognize the health benefits, and make it a priority. Some sedentary people dislike vigorous exercise because they do not feel competent performing the activity; others may associate the activity with sweating, strain, and pain. Adults who enjoy being active make exercise and physical movement integral parts of their daily routines.

Many people find it easier to be physically active while in college than when they are out of school and working full time. Most college and university campuses have physical education departments that offer a variety of sports and fitness courses; some of these departments have well-equipped fitness centers. Additionally, the staff of the physical education department may conduct intramural athletic programs that are open to students, and at certain times, they may open the college's gyms and athletic fields to all students. While in school, students should take advantage of the fitness opportunities available on their college or university campus.

After leaving college, individuals can continue to build or maintain their fitness level by exercising at home or by joining fitness centers or clubs. Although large resistance exercise machines are highly effective for building muscular strength, their expense and size make them unlikely to be found in most homes. However, you can buy barbells and smaller handheld weights at most department or sporting goods stores for use at home. To improve cardiorespiratory fitness, rowing machines, stationary bikes, and cross-country skiing machines can be purchased for home fitness centers. Before buying any large piece of fitness equipment, you should visit a gym or fitness club to test the machine and discuss its value with qualified fitness experts. For additional information, check popular consumer magazines that occasionally rate exercise equipment.

Building or maintaining physical fitness does not require a long-term commitment with a gym or fitness club, but many people enjoy the social aspects of exercising at these facilities. The quality and cost of gyms and fitness clubs vary, so you may want to consider the points listed in the Consumer Health feature "Choosing a Fitness Center" before joining one.

Unless you have a job that requires physical exertion or you work at a company that provides a work-site fitness center for its employees, you need to find ways to be more physically active at work. If your office building has stairways, climb the stairs rather than ride the elevators. Instead of eating lunches in restaurants, bring your lunches from home to eat at your desk, and use the remaining time to go outside

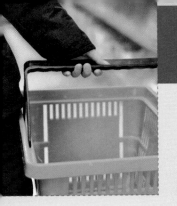

# Consumer Health

## Choosing a Fitness Center

Every year millions of Americans join health clubs, gyms, and exercise and fitness centers. Thousands of these people complain about their membership to states' attorneys general, Better Business Bureaus, and other consumer protection groups. The following tips can help you avoid becoming another dissatisfied health and fitness center consumer:

- Determine whether you can afford to join the center.
- Inspect the center for cleanliness, type and quality of equipment, and especially staff qualifications. Ask if staff are certified as aerobics instructors, weight trainers, or athletic trainers. Are they trained in cardiopulmonary resuscitation (CPR) and first aid?
- Ask current members if they are satisfied with the center's facilities and why or why not.

- Ask your local Better Business Bureau about the number and nature of complaints against the organization.
- Ask for a trial period to use the facilities before joining.
- Never sign a contract under pressure at the center. Many centers use confusing and misleading advertising, including prizes or special short-term offers, to spark your interest. Once you are in the facility, aggressive sales staff engage in high-pressure sales tactics to convince you to sign a contract.
- Before signing, take a few days to read the contract carefully. Make certain that you understand the details concerning payment options, membership restrictions, cancelation terms, and the membership period. If a staff member makes additional promises, have the individual record it in writing, on the contract.

---

and walk. You might consider buying two pairs of athletic shoes—one for your office and one for home. You may like walking with others better than walking alone; ask someone to walk with you. Colleagues, spouses, or friends can provide the valuable social support you may need to maintain your motivation to exercise at work or home. In addition to increasing your physical activity at work, you can move around more at home. Child care, housework, and gardening chores often require contracting large muscle groups, which expends energy and strengthens the muscles. How many times a week do you go up and down steps, walk a pet, or go shopping? What lifestyle changes can you make to increase your physical activity?

Like many people, you may want to be more active, but you cannot seem to find the time to exercise. It is important to remember that you do not have to spend hours each day engaging in strenuous exercises to improve your health. Even 10 to 20 minutes of vigorous aerobic activity can boost your fitness level. Determine how you spend your leisure time. Each day, how much time do you spend engaging in sedentary activities such as watching TV, communicating with others in a chat room, or playing computer games? Can you set aside at least 30 minutes each day to engage in some moderately intense physical activities? **Figure 11.13** illustrates physical activity recommendations for healthy lifestyles. To track your physical activity, visit http://www.choosemyplate.gov /supertracker-tools.html.

Many aerobic and resistance activities do not require extensive time, complex skills, or special and costly equipment. For example, people can exercise by dancing to music or videos, or by performing tai chi in the privacy of their homes. The main objective is to select physical activities that you enjoy and can perform regularly for the rest of your life.

As mentioned earlier, if you are unfit or older than 40 years (males) or 50 years (females), consult a physician before beginning a physical fitness program, especially one that includes vigorous-intensity activities. This precautionary measure can determine whether you have serious health problems. If you have a chronic condition, consult your physician for an exercise prescription. Most adults can begin a regular walking program to get into shape; after a few weeks, they can add more intense forms of physical activity to boost their cardiorespiratory fitness.

**Figure 11.13**

**The Activity Pyramid.** This physical activity pyramid includes recommendations for healthy lifestyles.

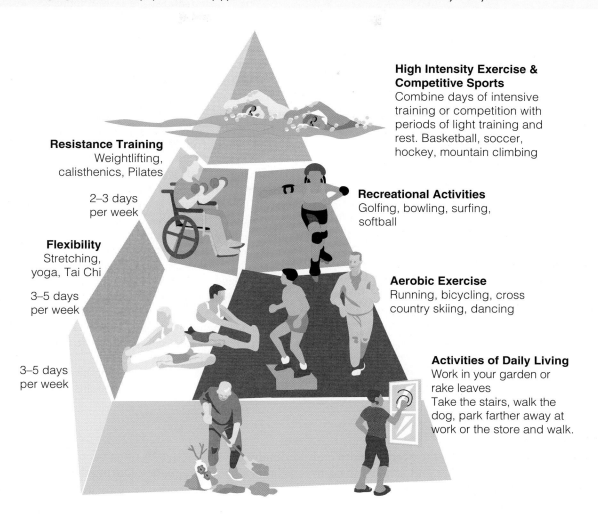

**High Intensity Exercise & Competitive Sports**
Combine days of intensive training or competition with periods of light training and rest. Basketball, soccer, hockey, mountain climbing

**Resistance Training**
Weightlifting, calisthenics, Pilates

2–3 days per week

**Recreational Activities**
Golfing, bowling, surfing, softball

**Flexibility**
Stretching, yoga, Tai Chi

3–5 days per week

**Aerobic Exercise**
Running, bicycling, cross country skiing, dancing

3–5 days per week

**Activities of Daily Living**
Work in your garden or rake leaves
Take the stairs, walk the dog, park farther away at work or the store and walk.

## Healthy Living Practices

- ☐ To become physically fit or to maintain a high degree of fitness, design a personal fitness program that includes activities that you enjoy and can perform regularly while you are in college and throughout your lifetime.

- ☐ If you have a sedentary lifestyle, find ways to become more physically active at work and home, such as walking some of the way to work, using the stairs instead of elevators, doing housework, and walking during your leisure time.

## Across THE LIFE SPAN

### PHYSICAL FITNESS

The health habits that a person adopts in childhood, including physical and sports activities, are likely to be practiced and enjoyed for a lifetime. Children who are physically active have better measures of all health-related fitness components than those who are sedentary. Because sedentary lifestyles are associated with heart disease in adults, many pediatricians are concerned that children may begin to develop this disease, especially if they do not engage in physical

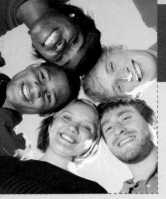

# Diversity in Health

## New Interest in an Ancient Approach to Fitness

In motion
all parts of the body must be
light,
nimble,
and strung together.

> *From T'ai chi ch'uan*
> *by Chang San-feng (1279–1386)*

To people outside of China, it may seem difficult to believe that the graceful dancelike movements of t'ai chi ch'uan (tie-jee-chwahn), commonly called "tai chi," are a form of exercise. Unlike Western physical activities that often require rapid, forceful, and extensive motions, tai chi involves gentle gliding muscular movements that do not overextend body parts. According to its promoters, tai chi promotes good health, physical fitness, and longevity.

The exact origins of traditional tai chi are unknown. For more than 2,000 years, the Chinese have practiced *qigong* (*ch'i-kung*), a series of simple exercises that focus on breathing, maintaining certain body postures, and relaxing. These features are also emphasized in tai chi. In fact, the word *chi* means "breath energy." Thus, the ancient practice of qigong may have set the stage for the development of tai chi.

In addition to qigong, the Chinese martial arts probably contributed to the development of tai chi ch'uan. *Ch'uan* means "the joy of fighting with bare fists." Originally tai chi ch'uan may have been used for self-defense or boxing. However, a major principle of tai chi ch'uan is to overcome brute force and harshness with softness, gentleness, and smoothness.

Chang San-feng, the thirteenth-century Taoist priest whose writing appears here, is usually credited with creating tai chi. Taoism is an ancient Chinese religion and philosophy that emphasizes living in harmony with nature. To Taoists, the harmonious functioning of the body is important if one is to achieve good health and live a long life. Today, tai chi is growing in popularity with Western exercise enthusiasts who are interested in achieving its potential health benefits (**Figure 11.C**). Promoters of tai chi claim that the physical exercises improve digestion and circulation, as well as increase alertness. People who practice tai chi often report that the exercises reduce stress (see Chapter 3).

While performing the specific sequential exercises, the upper part of the body remains loose; the knees

---

activities regularly. To improve the overall health and well-being of children, parents and schools need to find ways to encourage youngsters who are physically unfit to increase their fitness levels.

Another major concern of health and fitness experts is the proportion of American children and adolescents who spend a considerable amount of time engaged in sedentary activities, such as playing computer games or viewing television. In 2009, about 33% of American high school students attended physical education (PE) classes 5 days a week.[27] More research is needed to determine the long-term effects of childhood and adolescent activity habits on their future health.

Regular exercise is just as important during pregnancy as in the other times of a woman's life. Healthy, physically fit women can continue engaging in a program of mild to moderate physical activity throughout their pregnancies.[28] However, performing strenuous exercise (e.g., jogging) five or more times per week may increase the risk of having a low-birth-weight baby.[29] The ability to engage comfortably and safely in

many physical activities often becomes limited in the latter stage of pregnancy. During this time, a woman's weight usually increases dramatically, especially in the center and front part of her body. As a result, she often feels awkward while engaging in many physical activities, and her risk of injury increases.

A pregnant woman should avoid activities if they pose a risk to her health and that of her developing fetus. Physical activities that might result in falls or injuries to the abdominal area and exhaustive exercises such as contact sports, heavy weightlifting, or training and participating in competitive events are generally not recommended for pregnant women. Additionally, exercising while lying down may interfere with blood flow to the uterus and is not recommended. It is important for pregnant women to be well hydrated before, during, and after exercise and to avoid overheating. Physicians do not recommend that pregnant women exercise in hot, humid conditions or use hot tubs and saunas because these activities can raise the woman's body temperature, endangering the fetus.

are slightly bent but firmly supporting the weight of the body. Movements flow from one to another. Opposing arms and legs move in harmony; for example, as one arm gracefully arches upward, the other moves down in the same fashion. According to those who teach tai chi, if one body part does not follow another, the body is not in harmony. The series of vertical and horizontal movements continues until the sequence of exercises has been completed.

An important aspect of tai chi is mental concentration. As individuals engage in these exercises, they focus their attention on the sensations associated with the sequential movements; such attention requires silence.

As with other physical activities, practicing tai chi every day improves flexibility, muscular strength, and balance. Since tai chi does not require rapid, forceful muscular movements, it is a beneficial form of physical activity for elderly people or anyone who cannot engage in aerobic exercises.

A specially trained instructor is necessary to teach the proper posture, sequences of coordinated movements, and breathing technique of tai chi. Therefore, if you are interested in learning the exercises, check with the physical education department at your college or university to see if it offers tai chi instruction. Fitness centers in your community, such as the YMCA, might also offer tai chi classes.

## Figure 11.C

**Tai Chi.** Practicing tai chi improves flexibility, muscular strength, and balance.

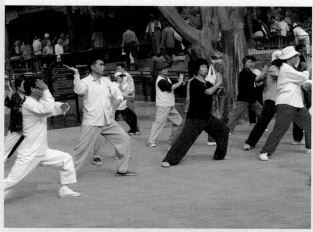

*Sources:* Lie, F. T. (1988). *T'ai chi ch'uan: The Chinese way.* New York, NY: Sterling; Lo, B. P. J., Inn, M., Amacker, R., & Foe, S. (Trans. and Eds.). (1979). *The essence of t'ai chi ch'uan.* Richmond, CA: North Atlantic Books.

It is a good idea for pregnant women to discuss their exercise plans with their physicians. Nearly all pregnant women can safely walk, swim, or ride a stationary bicycle (**Figure 11.14**). Healthy pregnant women should engage in at least 30 minutes of moderate-intensity exercise daily on most or all days of the week.[28] Those who are obese or severely underweight, are sedentary, or have histories of health problems should consult their physicians before following an exercise program.

As people age, they experience numerous changes that indicate a decline in their physical conditions. For example, the maximum age-predicted heart rates of older adults are lower during exercise, and their hearts pump less blood with each beat. Compared to when they were young adults, most aged persons have more body fat. Although exercise training of older adults does not prevent these physical changes, it can limit the extent of the decline.

Most Americans become less active as they age. In 2008, only about 33% of people 65 years of age and older were physically active during their leisure

## Figure 11.14

**Exercising During Pregnancy.** Nearly all pregnant women can safely stretch, walk, swim, or ride a stationary bicycle.

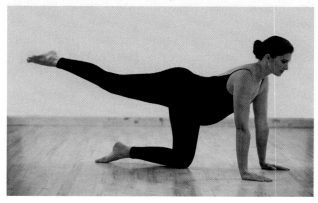

time.[30] It is important for people to continue exercising as they age (**Figure 11.15**). Physically fit aged persons usually have healthier hearts and body compositions than unfit persons of the same age. Even by

**Figure 11.15**

**Exercise Is for Everyone.** It is important for people to continue exercising as they age.

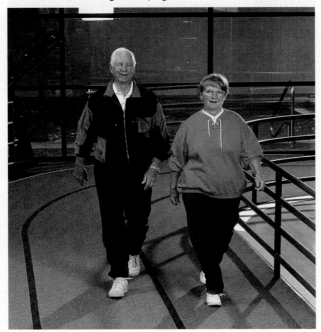

minor fall that would not injure a healthy 23-year-old person can have dire consequences for a frail 85-year-old one. An elderly person who falls is more likely to suffer a disabling bone fracture or die from the injury than a younger person is. Aged people who survive falls often experience some degree of immobility and pain that limits their ability to care for themselves and interact socially. By participating in exercise classes that improve balance and muscular strength, older adults can reduce their risk of falls.[32] The Diversity in Health essay in this chapter describes the benefits of tai chi, a form of martial arts that helps some elderly people become healthier.

It is never too late to become physically fit. By increasing physical activity, even very old people can gain healthful benefits such as improved muscular strength and endurance, flexibility, and psychological well-being. To achieve these benefits, participation in strenuous formal exercise programs is not necessary; most elderly people can improve their overall health by engaging in light to moderate physical activities regularly such as walking, gardening, or mall-walking every day.

performing light physical activities regularly, older adults can reduce their risk of heart disease, colon cancer, diabetes, obesity, and hypertension.[31] Additionally, physical activity helps maintain or improve the flexibility of joints as well as the strength and endurance of muscles. Regular exercise improves the mood of elderly people and increases their ability to live independently.[31] Older adults can enjoy the social aspects of exercising by joining mall-walking, dancing, or fitness classes that are designed for older adults.

People lose their ability to maintain their balance as they age, which increases their risk of falling. A

 **Healthy Living Practices**

☐ If you have children, consider limiting the amount of time they spend watching television or playing computer games. Encourage your children to be physically active.

☐ If you are pregnant, consult your physician to determine which physical activities are safe to perform during this time.

☐ As you age, exercise regularly and be physically active.

# CHAPTER REVIEW

## Summary

Regardless of age and physical condition, nearly everyone can achieve numerous health benefits by engaging in physical activity and exercise. Performing regular, vigorous exercise and physical activity can build, maintain, and preserve skeletal muscles; improve the circulation and functioning of the heart; and regulate the amount of body fat. Additionally, weight-bearing exercises such as walking, dancing, and jogging strengthen bones, which can prevent or delay the development of osteoporosis. Healthy adults younger than 65 years should perform moderate-intensity physical activity for 30 minutes a day, 5 days a week.

Besides improving physical health, exercise can have short-term and long-term psychological benefits. Physical activity can reduce symptoms of anxiety and depression and improve mood and well-being.

The health-related components of physical fitness are cardiorespiratory fitness, muscular strength, muscular endurance, flexibility, and body composition. Many fitness experts consider cardiorespiratory fitness the most important health-related element of physical fitness.

Regular aerobic exercise enhances cardiorespiratory fitness, increasing the stroke volume of the heart and reducing the resting heart rate. Examples of popular aerobic activities include running, jogging, race-walking, lap swimming, cycling, stair-stepping, aerobic dancing, cross-country skiing, and rope skipping.

To develop muscular strength, muscles need to be overloaded by repeatedly moving objects that become progressively heavier. When muscles are overloaded, they hypertrophy; when muscles are not used, they atrophy or detrain. Detraining can occur within a couple of weeks after people discontinue their exercise training regimen. Thus, people must maintain their exercise programs to avoid detraining.

Immediate first aid for most musculoskeletal injuries includes RICE, the combination of rest, ice, compression, and elevation. Hypothermia and hyperthermia are serious temperature-related injuries that can occur when the body is unable to maintain its temperature in the normal range. Exercising in hot weather can produce heat cramps, heat exhaustion, or heatstroke. If untreated, heat cramps or heat exhaustion can lead to heatstroke, which can be fatal. Maintaining adequate hydration and avoiding overexertion in hot and humid conditions can reduce the risk of heat-related illnesses. To avoid frostbite or hypothermia, people should dress warmly while outdoors in cold and windy conditions, keeping their skin well covered.

When planning an effective overall fitness regimen, people need to consider the type, frequency, duration, and intensity of their exercise activities. Additionally, individuals should design personal fitness programs that provide health benefits, satisfy their needs and interests, and can be followed for a lifetime. Before beginning fitness regimens that include aerobic activities, people with heart disease or other serious chronic conditions and people who are out of shape or older than 40 years should obtain the approval of their physicians.

Regular physical activity is just as important for youngsters as for adults. Performing certain activities may be risky during pregnancy; therefore, pregnant women should discuss their physical activity with their physicians. In most cases, it is never too late for people to begin fitness programs. By engaging in light to moderate physical activities regularly, such as walking or gardening every day, older adults can improve their overall health.

# Applying What You Have Learned

**Critical Thinking**

1. Calculate your target heart rate zone. **Application**
2. For 3 days, record the amount of time you spend engaging in various physical activities, such as walking to class, playing racquetball, or riding a bike. Use Table 11.2 to classify your physical activities as being light, moderate, or intense. **Analysis**

3. Plan an exercise program that you can follow for a lifetime. **Synthesis**
4. Use the step test in the assessment activity to evaluate your current level of cardiorespiratory fitness. **Evaluation**

**Key**

| **Application**<br>using information in a new situation. | **Analysis**<br>breaking down information into component parts. | **Synthesis**<br>putting together information from different sources. | **Evaluation**<br>making informed decisions. |

# Reflecting on Your Health

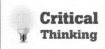

**Critical Thinking**

1. Are you satisfied with your level of physical fitness? Why or why not? If you are dissatisfied, what ideas did you get from reading this chapter that will help you improve your fitness? If you are satisfied, how will you maintain your fitness?
2. What benefits would you derive from adopting a more physically active lifestyle? What factors interfere with and what factors reinforce your efforts to become more physically fit?
3. Before reading this chapter, how did you feel about ergogenic aids such as dietary supplements or anabolic steroids to enhance athletic performance? Based on what you have read in

this chapter, has your attitude changed? Why or why not?
4. If you have children or are thinking about having children, how would you encourage them to maintain a balance between the time they spend engaging in sedentary activities such as watching TV and in activities that develop physical fitness?
5. Which labor-saving devices would you be willing to stop using so that you could use your muscles to do the work? Why did you choose these devices or machines? Describe practical steps you can take to increase your physical activity level.

# References

1. U.S. Department of Health and Human Services. (2008). *Physical activity guidelines for Americans*. Retrieved on May 24, 2011, from http://www.health.gov/PAGuidelines/factsheetprof.aspx

2. Centers for Disease Control and Prevention. (2010). *State indicator report on physical activity, 2010*. Retrieved on May 24, 2011, from http://www.cdc.gov/physicalactivity/downloads/PA_State_Indicator_Report_2010.pdf

3. Centers for Disease Control and Prevention. (2010). *U.S. physical activity statistics*. Retrieved on May 24, 2011, from http://apps.nccd.cdc.gov/PASurveillance/StateSumV.asp

4. U.S. Department of Health and Human Services. (2008). Chapter 2: Physical activity has many health benefits. In *Physical activity guidelines for Americans*. Retrieved on May 25, 2011, from http://www.health.gov/paguidelines/guidelines/chapter2.aspx

5. U.S. Department of Health and Human Services. (1996). *Physical activity and health: A report of the Surgeon General*. Atlanta, GA: Centers for Disease Control and Prevention, National Center for Chronic Disease Prevention and Health Promotion.

6. Youngstedt, S. D. (2005). Effects of exercise on sleep. *Clinics in Sports Medicine, 24*(2):355–365.

7. Elavsky, S., et al. (2005). Physical activity enhances long-term quality of life in older adults: Efficacy, esteem, and affective influences. *Annals of Behavioral Medicine, 30*(2):138–145.

8. Gulati, M., et al. (2010). Heart rate response to exercise stress testing in asymptomatic women: The St. James Women Take Heart Project. *Circulation, 122*(2):130–137.

9. Feigenbaum, M. S., & Pollock, M. L. (1999). Prescription of resistance training for health and disease. *Medicine & Science in Sports & Exercise, 31*(1):38–45.

10. Willardson, J. M. (2006). A brief review: Factors affecting the length of the rest interval between resistance exercise sets. *Journal of Strength and Conditioning Research, 20*(4):978–984.

11. Decoster, L. C., et al. (2005). The effects of hamstring stretching on range of motion: A systematic literature review. *Journal of Orthopedic Sports Physical Therapy, 35*(6):377–387.

12. Speed, C. (2004). Low back pain. *British Medical Journal, 328*(7448): 1119–1121.

13. Binzen, C. A., et al. (2001). Postexercise oxygen consumption and substrate use after resistance training in women. *Medicine & Science in Sports & Exercise, 33*:932–938.

14. Schoch, R. D., et al. (2006). The regulation and expression of the creatine transporter: A brief review of creatine supplementation in humans and animals. *Journal of International Society of Sports Nutrition, 3*:60–66.

15. Mitchell, G. J. (2007). *Report to the commissioner of baseball of an independent investigation into the illegal use of steroids and other performance enhancing substances by players of Major League Baseball*. Retrieved on May 25, 2011, from http://files.mlb.com/mitchrpt.pdf

16. National Institute on Drug Abuse. (2010, August). *NIDA infofacts: High school and youth trends*. Retrieved on May 25, 2011, from http://www.nida.nih.gov/infofacts/hsyouthtrends.html

17. Yu, S., et al. (2003). What level of physical activity protects against premature cardiovascular death? The Caerphilly study. *Heart, 89* (5):502–506.

18. Sundquist, K., et al. (2005). The long-term effect of physical activity on incidence of coronary heart disease: A 12-year follow-up study. *Preventive Medicine, 41*(1):219–225.

19. Law, R. Y., & Herbert, R. D. (2007). Warm-up reduces delayed onset muscle soreness but cool-down does not: A randomised controlled trial. *Australian Journal of Physiotherapy, 53*(2):91–95.

20. Fradkin, A. J., et al. (2006). Does warming up prevent injury in sport? The evidence from randomised controlled trials. *Journal of Science and Medicine in Sport, 9*(3):214–220.

21. Thacker, S. B., et al. (2004). The impact of stretching on sports injury risk: A systematic review of the literature. *Medicine & Science in Sports & Exercise, 36*(3):371–378.

22. Hart, L. (2005). Effect of stretching on sport injury risk: A review. *Clinical Journal of Sport Medicine, 15*(2):113.

23. American College of Sports Medicine, Sawka, M. N., et al. (2007). American College of Sports Medicine position stand: Exercise and fluid replacement. *Medicine & Science in Sports & Exercise, 39*(2):377–390.

24. Coyle, E. F. (2004). Fluid and fuel intake during exercise. *Journal of Sports Sciences, 22*(1):39–55.

25. Williams, M. H. (2007). *Nutrition for health, fitness, and sport* (8th ed.). New York, NY: WCB McGraw-Hill.

26. National Library of Medicine, National Institutes of Health. (2011, May 18). Hypothermia. Retrieved on May 25, 2011, from http://www.nlm.nih.gov/medlineplus/hypothermia.html

27. Centers for Disease Control and Prevention. (2008). Youth risk behavior surveillance: United States, 2007. *Morbidity and Mortality Weekly Report, 57*(SS04):1–131.

28. American College of Obstetricians and Gynecologists. (2002; reaffirmed 2009). ACOG committee opinion: Exercise during pregnancy and the postpartum period. *International Journal of Gynaecology and Obstetrics, 77*(1):79–81.

29. Campbell, M. K., & Mottola, M. F. (2001). Recreational exercise and occupational activity during pregnancy and birth weight: A case-control study. *American Journal of Obstetrics and Gynecology, 184*(3):403–408.

30. Centers for Disease Control and Prevention. (2010, January). *U.S. physical activity statistics*. Retrieved on May 25, 2011, from http://apps.nccd.cdc.gov/PASurveillance/DemoCompareV.asp?ErrorMsg=3&Year=&State=&CI=&Cat=#result

31. Agency for Healthcare Research and Quality, Centers for Disease Control and Prevention, U.S. Department of Health and Human Services. (2002). *Physical activity and older Americans: Benefits and strategies*. Retrieved on May 25, 2011, from http://www.ahrq.gov/ppip/activity.htm

32. Liu, H., & Frank, A. (2010). Tai chi as a balance improvement exercise for older adults: A systematic review. *Journal of Geriatric Physical Therapy, 33*(3):103–109.

**Diversity in Health**
The Italian Gene: A Hope for Reversing Atherosclerosis?

**Consumer Health**
Vitamin Pills for a Healthier Heart?

**Managing Your Health**
Heart Attack and Stroke (Brain Attack) Symptoms: What to Do in an Emergency

**Across the Life Span**
Cardiovascular Health

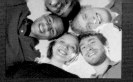
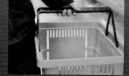
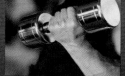
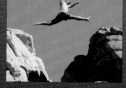

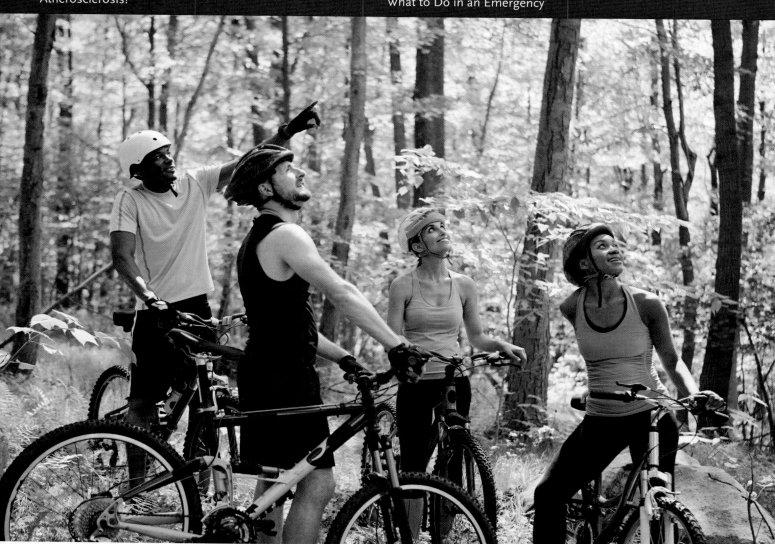

# Chapter Overview

How the cardiovascular system works

Symptoms of and treatments for cardiovascular disease

Risk factors for cardiovascular disease

How to maintain your cardiovascular health

# Student Workbook

Self-Assessment: What Is Your Risk of Developing Heart Disease or Having a Heart Attack?

Changing Health Habits: Reducing Your Risk of Cardiovascular Disease

# Do You Know?

What to do to keep your heart and blood vessels healthy?

What to do if you or someone you know is having a heart attack?

If you are likely to have a heart attack or stroke?

## CHAPTER 12

# Cardiovascular Health

**D**o you think that you are immune from cardiovascular disease—dysfunction of the heart and blood vessels—because you are young? If so, think again! Even though cardiovascular disease (CVD) does not normally occur in young adults, unhealthy lifestyle patterns practiced and ingrained during this stage of life predispose a person to cardiovascular disease. Metabolic processes leading to cardiovascular disease *can* begin in childhood and accelerate at adolescence.[1]

In one large multicenter study, medical researchers examined the relationship of the risk factors for cardiovascular disease (such as smoking, obesity, poor diet, and lack of exercise) to the development of fatty deposits in the arteries, which is one process that occurs in the development of this condition.[2] They studied nearly 3,000 persons aged 15 to 34 years who died from accidents, homicides, and suicides. The results of the study revealed that young persons with risk factors for CVD began developing fatty streaks within their arteries in their teenage years. By age 25, young persons with risk factors also had developed raised lesions in the major blood vessels of the heart. The results of this and other studies show that reducing the likelihood of developing cardiovascular disease later in life involves controlling risk factors early in life.[3] Behaviors in adolescence and young adulthood *do* matter: They can influence your health for years to come and can affect your life span.

> "*... reducing the likelihood of developing cardiovascular disease later in life involves controlling risk factors early in life.*"

**arteries** Blood vessels that carry blood away from the heart.

**capillaries** (KAP-ih-LAIR-eez) Microscopic blood vessels that permeate tissues, connecting small arteries to small veins.

**veins** Blood vessels that return blood to the heart.

**coronary arteries** Blood vessels that arise from the base of the aorta and bring freshly oxygenated blood to the heart muscle.

Research results also show that college students are aware of cardiovascular risk factors, but many do not put this knowledge into practice. In other words, their understandings of heart-healthy behaviors and their lifestyles do not match.[4]

One reason for this disconnect may be rooted in emotions and psychology; how people feel about what they know has an effect on their actions. For example, if you know smoking causes many types of cancers, but you love to smoke, it may affect how you feel about that knowledge. You may decide that cancer couldn't happen to you or that the risk is worth the pleasure you get from your cigarettes.

Another reason for the disconnect between knowledge and actions may have to do with misconceptions, and college students hold many misconceptions about heart disease.[4] For example, many college students think that heart disease is a significant health concern only for men, when it is the leading cause of death in both genders. College-aged women holding this misconception may think that practicing heart-healthy behaviors is not important for them. Many college students also think that whites are the ethnic group most affected by heart disease, when blacks and Pacific Islanders have higher death rates from heart disease than whites do. Thus, some blacks and Pacific Islanders may not perceive themselves at high risk for heart disease and may ignore adopting behaviors that would lower their risk.

The "Changing Health Habits" feature "Reducing Your Risk of Cardiovascular Disease" in the Student Workbook pages at the end of this text can help you develop motivation to implement heart-healthy lifestyle changes. But first, this chapter explores the cardiovascular system and how it works. It then describes the causes of cardiovascular diseases and hypertension—noninfectious diseases in which hereditary, environmental, and lifestyle factors interact to create an individual's risk level for developing any one of them. It also describes the interrelatedness of these diseases and how the development of one affects the development of another. Last, it explores the factors critical to maintaining cardiovascular health, to help you preserve the fitness of your heart and blood vessels throughout your lifetime.

## The Cardiovascular System and How It Works

You may have heard the cardiovascular system also referred to as the circulatory system. These terms are often used interchangeably. The term *cardiovascular* refers to the heart (*cardio-*) and blood vessels (*vascular*). The term *circulatory* refers to the circulation of the blood. In practical use, both terms describe a body system that pumps blood enclosed in blood vessels to all parts of the body.

Blood is a somewhat viscous fluid made up of cells suspended in a liquid. Blood performs many functions:

- It contains red blood cells and fluid (plasma) that transport the respiratory gases (oxygen and carbon dioxide), nutrients, hormones, enzymes, and waste products.

- It helps regulate body temperature by distributing the heat generated by chemical reactions in the body.

- It contains blood clotting factors (including pieces of cells called *platelets*) that protect the blood supply from excessive losses and help in tissue repair.

- It contains white blood cells (including the lymphocytes of the immune system) that help protect the body from infection (see Chapter 14).

The blood is pumped by the heart, a muscular, fist-sized organ that lies in the chest cavity about midway between the shoulders and the waist, and slightly to the left of the midline (**Figure 12.1**). The heart consists of four chambers: two upper chambers called *atria* and two lower chambers called *ventricles*. The upper chambers receive blood and then push it into the lower chambers, which pump blood to the lungs and the rest of the body.

Blood flows within a vast network of blood vessels. **Arteries** carry blood away from the heart. They have muscular, elastic walls that bulge slightly when the left ventricle contracts and pushes blood through

**Figure 12.1**

**The Major Arteries of the Body.** The heart is located to the left of the midline in the chest cavity. The arteries take blood away from the heart and are shown in red. Veins return blood to the heart and are shown in blue.

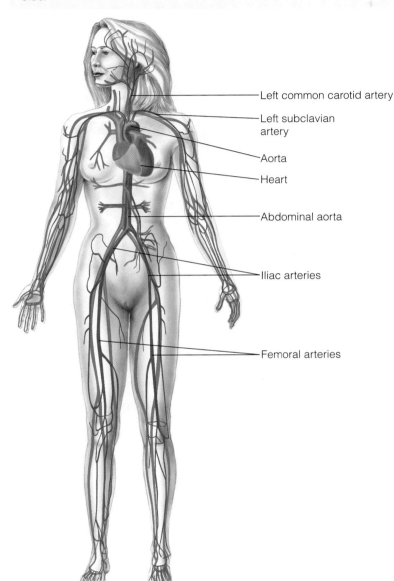

- Left common carotid artery
- Left subclavian artery
- Aorta
- Heart
- Abdominal aorta
- Iliac arteries
- Femoral arteries

them, and they recoil at the end of the beat. Arteries branch into smaller vessels called *arterioles*. When these vessels become so small that they allow the passage of only one blood cell at a time, they are called **capillaries**.

The capillaries permeate tissues. These tiny blood vessels have walls that are only one cell thick. The thinness of capillary walls allows substances such as nutrients and oxygen to move out of the blood, and other substances such as waste products and carbon dioxide to move into the blood. Capillaries join to form larger vessels called *venules*, which in turn join to form still larger vessels, the veins.

**Veins** return blood to the heart. By the time the blood reaches the veins, it has lost most of the force (pressure) of its push from the heart. Therefore, veins have thinner walls than do arteries; they contain less muscle and elastic tissue. In addition, veins have one-way valves along their length, which help prevent the backflow of blood. Blood returning to the heart from the head, neck, and shoulders is helped along by the force of gravity. Blood returning to the heart from the arms, legs, and torso combats the force of gravity but is pushed along as the skeletal muscles squeeze the veins in these areas.

If the walls of the veins in the arms, legs, and torso are weak, or if the valves are stretched or damaged, blood may not be returned to the heart efficiently. Blood may collect in the veins and may flow backward. This situation puts additional pressure on the walls of the veins and contributes to a condition called *venous disease*. Venous disease includes varicose veins (distended or stretched veins), deep vein thrombosis (blood clots in the deep veins), and chronic venous insufficiency (swollen legs). **Figure 12.2** shows varicose veins.

The incidence of both moderate and severe venous disease increases with age. Although women are twice as likely as men to have moderate venous disease, men are more likely to have severe disease. Non-Hispanic whites are much more likely to have severe venous disease compared to Hispanics, African Americans, and Asians, in that order. Other risk factors for venous disease include family history of the disease, obesity, having borne more than one child, and consistently standing for prolonged periods.[5]

**Coronary arteries** arise from the base of the aorta and bring freshly oxygenated blood to the heart muscle itself. (Although blood flows in and out of the heart's chambers, the heart muscle is not nourished

**coronary artery disease (CAD)** A condition in which the coronary vessels are blocked partially or completely by fatty deposits, blood clots, or both. Also commonly called coronary heart disease (CHD).

**angina pectoris** (an-JEYE-nah PECK-tor-iss) Chest pain caused by insufficient oxygen in a portion of the heart.

**cardiovascular disease (CVD)** (KAR-dee-oh-VAS-ku-lar) Disorders of the heart and blood vessels.

### Figure 12.2

**Close-up of Varicose Veins on a Man's Leg.**

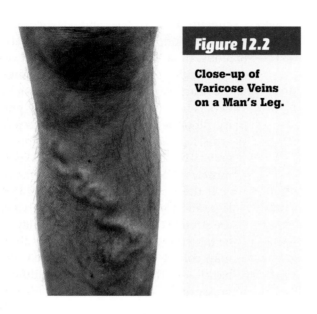

### Figure 12.3

**Leading Causes of Death, United States, 2007.** This graph shows that cardiovascular disease is the number one cause of death for both men and women (all races, all ages).
*Source:* Xu, J., et al. (2010, May). Deaths: Final Data for 2007. *National Vital Statistics Reports, 58*(19). Retrieved on April 5, 2011, from http://www.cdc.gov/nchs/data/nvsr/nvsr58/nvsr58_19.pdf

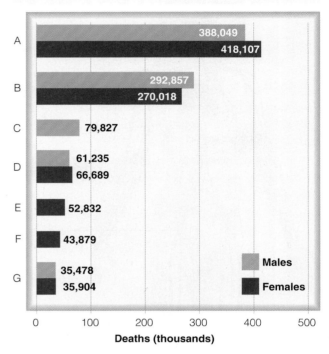

**A** Total cardiovascular (including cerebrovascular) diseases
**B** Cancer
**C** Accidents
**D** Chronic lower respiratory diseases
**E** Alzheimer's disease
**F** Accidents
**G** Diabetes mellitus

by the blood while it is in the chambers.) There are two main coronary arteries: the left and the right coronary arteries (see Figure 12.8 later in this chapter). Both of these arteries branch into multiple vessels that supply the entire heart with blood.

## Cardiovascular Diseases

A person with blocked coronary arteries is said to have **coronary artery disease (CAD)**, one type of cardiovascular disease. (Coronary artery disease is also commonly called coronary heart disease [CHD].) Coronary artery disease may result in a heart attack in which a portion of the heart muscle dies, or in **angina pectoris** (chest pain).

Coronary artery disease is only one type of **cardiovascular disease (CVD)**, or dysfunction of the heart and blood vessels. Other major cardiovascular diseases are hypertension (chronic high blood pressure), stroke (blood vessel disease of the brain), and rheumatic heart disease (a complication of strep

throat). Atherosclerosis (blood vessel disease) is an important cardiovascular disease process that is an underlying cause of CAD and stroke. Other cardiovascular diseases are described throughout this chapter. More than 82 million Americans (more than 1 in 3) are estimated to have one or more forms of CVD.[6] As **Figure 12.3** shows, cardiovascular disease kills more people in the United States than does any other disease.

Of the cardiovascular diseases, coronary artery disease is the number one killer, accounting for about half of all CVD deaths each year. Stroke is the next biggest CVD killer.[6] Coronary artery disease and stroke result from the development of yet another cardiovascular disease: atherosclerosis.

## Atherosclerosis

In many CAD cases, the blood supply to portions of the heart is reduced because the coronary arteries are blocked by fatty deposits. These fatty deposits, or **plaques**, develop as part of a disease of the arteries called **atherosclerosis**. (Arterial plaque is not the same as dental plaque.) An *atheroma* is a deteriorated, thickened area on the inner lining of a large or medium-sized artery. *Sclerosis* refers to loss of elasticity, or hardening of these arteries. *Atherosclerosis* is one form of arteriosclerosis (hardening of the arteries).

Atherosclerosis may begin with an injury to the lining of a blood vessel. Factors such as high blood pressure, for example, can damage this lining, or the immune system may play a role. Lipids, especially cholesterol, accumulate at injury sites and cling to the interior of blood vessel walls. These plaques thicken blood vessel walls, which narrows the interiors of arteries (**Figure 12.4**) and interferes with arterial cells' ability to obtain nutrients. Eventually, the wall beneath a plaque degenerates. Scar tissue forms and calcium is often deposited there, "hardening" the artery. Blood clots sometimes develop there, too, and may be the ultimate cause of a heart attack or stroke.

Although the incidence of atherosclerosis increases with age, not all elderly people have extensive plaques. Conversely, *some young people do* (see this chapter's opening section).

Atherosclerosis occurs most often in the aorta and in the coronary, femoral, iliac, internal carotid, and cerebral arteries. Most of these vessels are labeled on Figure 12.1. As you can see, these arteries supply blood to the heart, torso, legs, and head. The cerebral arteries, not shown in the diagram, branch from

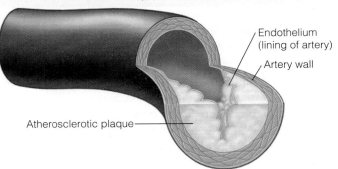

### Figure 12.4

**A Plaque in an Artery.** A plaque is formed by a buildup of fatty material on an artery wall. This illustration shows the interior of an affected artery that has been narrowed by plaque.

Endothelium (lining of artery)

Artery wall

Atherosclerotic plaque

**plaques** (plaks) Fatty deposits in artery walls.

**atherosclerosis** (ATH-er-oh-skle-ROW-sis) Disease of large and medium-sized arteries in which the inner lining has areas that are deteriorated, thickened, and inelastic.

**peripheral vascular disease** Any blockage of vessels other than those to the heart.

**thrombus** (THROM-bus) A stationary blood clot.

**coronary thrombosis** (throm-BOW-sis) The development of a stationary blood clot that blocks blood flow in an artery that brings blood to the heart muscle.

the carotid arteries and other vessels to supply large portions of the brain with blood. Atherosclerosis is most serious when it develops in the vessels that supply the heart, which can lead to heart attacks, and in the vessels that supply the brain, which can result in strokes.

Heart attacks can also be caused by *coronary microvascular dysfunction*. Heart disease in women is often to the result of this dysfunction, alone or in addition to plaques that block blood flow in the large coronary arteries. In coronary microvascular dysfunction, the small blood vessels of the heart do not dilate (widen) properly to supply sufficient blood to the heart muscle. Because of differences in the sizes of vessels that may be blocked or that do not function properly in their hearts, men and women often experience different symptoms when suffering heart attacks (see the section titled "Heart Attack" later in this chapter).[7]

Any blockage of vessels other than those to the heart is often referred to as **peripheral vascular disease**. This disease affects the organs and tissues that blocked vessels serve. One result of peripheral vascular disease, for example, can be erectile dysfunction (impotence) in men (see Chapter 6).

## Coronary Artery Disease

In CAD, coronary vessels may become partially or completely blocked by one or more of the following: fatty deposits, which narrow blood vessels (see the previous section titled "Atherosclerosis"); a blood clot that develops at the site of fatty deposits; or a floating blood clot that lodges in a vessel. A stationary blood clot, called a **thrombus**, can block a vessel already narrowed by fatty deposits. Blood clots frequently form in vessels in which blood flow is slowed by fatty deposits. The development of a thrombus that blocks a coronary artery is called **coronary thrombosis**.

**embolus** (EM-bow-lus) A floating blood clot.

**coronary embolism** (EM-bow-lizm) A floating blood clot that lodges in an artery that brings blood to the heart muscle, blocking blood flow.

**ischemia** (is-KI-me-ah) Insufficient blood in part of the heart.

**angioplasty** (AN-jee-oh-PLAS-tee) The reconstruction of damaged blood vessels.

**stent** A springlike mesh device that is implanted within an artery to cover compressed plaque, support the artery, and smooth the artery wall.

**atherectomy** (ATH-er-EK-toe-me) The removal of plaque from the interior of an artery.

**coronary artery bypass graft (CABG) surgery** A surgical procedure in which healthy blood vessels are used to redirect blood flow around blocked vessels of the heart.

A thrombus may dislodge from the place in which it forms and become a floating blood clot, or **embolus**. An embolus can block a coronary artery downstream from where it was formed, producing a **coronary embolism**. In the early stages of CAD, coronary arteries may also become narrowed by muscle spasms of these vessels, frequently triggered by exposure to cold, physical exertion, or anxiety. Usually such muscle spasms are short lived and do not damage the heart muscle.

**Angina Pectoris** Spasms, partial blockage, or complete blockage of one or more of the coronary vessels can cause insufficient blood to reach part of the heart, which is called **ischemia**. When this happens, the heart does not receive sufficient oxygen and a person experiences angina pectoris, or chest pain. Angina is felt beneath the breastbone and extends to the left shoulder and down the left arm. (Pain in the arm may help you distinguish between angina and heartburn or other gastric distress.) Angina pain may also be felt in the jaw and neck and, infrequently, in the back. The pain is described as aching, squeezing, burning, heaviness, or pressure. Some people experience *silent* (painless) *angina*, which consists of strange feelings at angina sites without pain. Silent angina can be diagnosed by exercise testing or by wearing a portable device that monitors the electrical activity of the heart during a 24-hour period.

Angina attacks may come and go, brought on by physical exertion or by mental or emotional stress, but they are signs of serious coronary artery disease. Angina should not be ignored; a person experiencing angina attacks should seek medical attention im-

mediately. Rest and drugs that dilate, or widen, the blood vessels (such as nitroglycerin) relieve attacks of angina. Other drugs used to treat angina include those to reduce blood pressure or those that slow the heart rate. Both types of drugs reduce the workload of the heart and its need for oxygen.

**Diagnosis** To diagnose whether chest pain is heart-related and to find out how well the heart handles work, a physician may begin testing the heart with a *stress test*. During this test, the patient walks on a treadmill while hooked up to equipment that monitors the heart. The physician notes the patient's heart rate and electrical activity along with breathing and blood pressure as the conditions of the stress test change. The physician may also suggest an *echocardiogram*, in which the chambers of the beating heart are visualized using ultrasound (sound waves) at the same time as the heart's electrical activity is measured. In this way a physician can examine the structure of the heart and its pumping function.

If the physician suspects that one or more blood vessels of the heart are blocked, he or she may suggest a *coronary angiography* to visualize the coronary blood vessels. This test can determine the degree and location of vessel blockage to help assess whether further treatment is necessary to reduce symptoms and avoid a heart attack.

An *angiogram* is an x-ray image of blood vessels after they have been injected with a fluid called a *contrast medium*. The contrast medium used in angiography is composed primarily of iodine because it absorbs x-rays, making visible the interiors of blood vessels. To perform coronary angiography, physicians first thread a thin plastic tube called a *catheter* through an artery in the arm or the groin until it reaches the coronary arteries. After injecting the contrast medium into the catheter, they take high-speed x-ray movies of blood flowing through the arteries. *Figure 12.5* shows frames of such a movie and indicates where physicians are able to detect irregularities and narrowing of the coronary arteries.

Other tests such as magnetic resonance imaging (MRI) are also performed at many medical centers to create images of the heart and its vessels for various diagnostic purposes. MRI uses magnetic fields and radio waves to visualize structures.

**Unclogging Arteries** If a patient has atherosclerosis in many coronary vessels, a physician may recommend coronary artery bypass graft surgery. If only one of a patient's coronary arteries is narrowed significantly, a physician may recommend widening the interior of the artery with a type of **angioplasty**, the

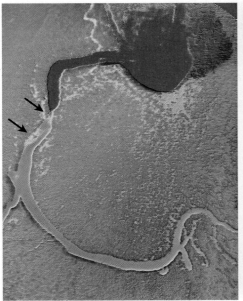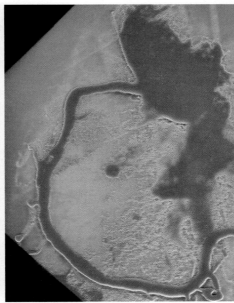

## Figure 12.5

**Coronary Angiogram.** The arrows on the left angiogram point out some of the irregularities and areas of narrowing of this coronary artery. This same vessel is shown in the right image, taken minutes after balloon angioplasty.

reconstruction of damaged blood vessels. In balloon angioplasty, the physician threads a catheter through an artery in the arm or the groin until it reaches the coronary arteries, as done when performing an angiogram. However, instead of injecting dye into the catheter, the physician threads a second, balloon-tipped catheter through the first. When the second catheter reaches the area of blockage, the balloon is inflated, breaking up the plaque while compressing it against the arterial wall (**Figure 12.6**). This balloon technique also stretches the artery somewhat. In almost all balloon angioplasties, a stent is also used.

A **stent** is a springlike mesh device (**Figure 12.7**) that is mounted on an angioplasty balloon and implanted within an artery to cover the compressed plaque, support the artery, and smooth the artery wall. The first stents were made of bare metal. After a time, tissue frequently grew around the stent, increas-

ing the risk of the artery reclogging. Newer types of stents are coated with drugs that inhibit reclogging, but improvements are still needed.[8] Biodegradable stents are in development that support the artery as it heals from angioplasty, and then the stent dissolves.[9]

**Atherectomy** refers to methods that remove plaque from the interior of an artery. The procedure is performed like balloon angioplasty, but the second catheter contains a rotating cutting device (burr tip) or a laser instead of a balloon tip.

One technique that is used frequently to treat coronary artery disease is bypass surgery. In the United States in 2007 an estimated 408,000 of these procedures were performed.[6]

The phrase *bypass surgery* usually means **coronary artery bypass graft (CABG) surgery**. The coronary arteries are blood vessels that supply oxygen-rich blood to the heart muscle. When these vessels

## Figure 12.6

**Balloon Angioplasty.** In balloon angioplasty, a thin tube containing a balloon is threaded through an artery until it reaches the area of plaque that is narrowing the vessel. The balloon is inflated, compressing the plaque against the artery wall and stretching the artery.

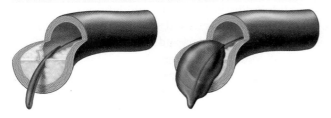

## Figure 12.7

**An Arterial Stent.** This springlike mesh device is implanted in an artery after balloon angioplasty to cover the compressed plaque, smooth the artery wall, and support the vessel.

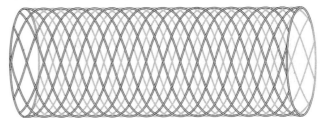

**heart attack** Myocardial infarction (MI); an area of heart muscle that dies because it does not receive enough oxygen as a result of insufficient blood supply.

**arrhythmias** (uh-RITH-me-uhs) Abnormal heartbeats.

**heart failure** Ineffective pumping of the heart, which results in the overfilling of the veins that bring blood to the heart.

**sudden cardiac arrest** Cessation of the heartbeat.

become blocked, blood flow is slowed and the heart muscle does not get enough oxygen.

People who have chronic angina, blockage in the vessels that supply the left side of the heart (the side that pumps blood to the body), or blockage in multiple coronary arteries are often candidates for bypass surgery. To perform this operation, surgeons first open the chest cavity. Using a blood vessel taken from another part of the patient's body (usually the leg), they graft one end of the new vessel to the aorta, the major artery that carries blood away from the heart and to the body. Heart surgeons graft the other end of the new vessel to the damaged coronary artery, past the area of blockage (**Figure 12.8**). The grafted vessel thus bypasses the blocked portion of the diseased vessel.

A therapy aimed at increasing blood flow to the heart muscle is transmyocardial laser revascularization (TMLR), which has been used for more than two decades. In TMLR, surgeons use a laser to bore narrow channels from the heart chamber into the heart muscle. Although TMLR does not help a heart patient live longer, it reduces the frequency of recurrent heart pain and increases the quality of life. In addition, TMLR is being used in conjunction with CABG. Together, these procedures appear to provide results superior to CABG alone or to TMLR alone.[10]

**Heart Attack** Victims of coronary artery disease are often unaware that the arteries supplying their heart with blood have become blocked. They may have no signs or symptoms of CAD or may not notice any. For this reason, one-third to one-half of persons with CAD are stricken suddenly and unexpectedly with a **heart attack**, which healthcare practitioners call a *myocardial infarction (MI)*. *Myocardial* simply means heart (*cardium*) muscle (*myo-*). An infarction is an area of heart muscle that dies because it does not receive enough oxygen because of insufficient blood. As heart muscle dies, it may trigger abnormal electrical activity that causes the ventricles to beat irregularly. Abnormal heartbeats are called **arrhythmias**. Heart failure, cardiac arrest, and death may occur during ventricular arrhythmia.

## Figure 12.8

**Vessel Position in a Coronary Artery Bypass Graft.** In a coronary artery bypass graft, blood vessels taken from another part of the body are grafted to the aorta, the large artery emerging from the heart. The other ends of these vessels are grafted to the coronary arteries (those that serve the heart) beyond the area of blockage.

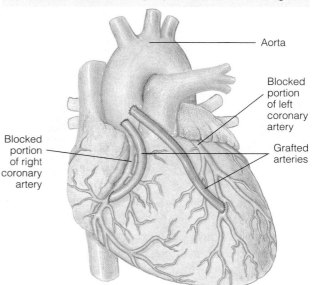

Aorta

Blocked portion of left coronary artery

Grafted arteries

Blocked portion of right coronary artery

**Heart failure** is sometimes called *congestive* heart failure because the veins bringing blood to the heart become congested, or overfilled, with blood when the heart cannot pump effectively. Heart failure (ineffective pumping) may be the result of all forms of cardiac disease, including CAD, structural heart defects, and rheumatic heart disease, and may also be a chronic condition, resulting in shortness of breath, retention of fluid, congestion of the lungs, and fatigue. A person experiencing severe cardiac failure may be a candidate for a heart transplant or the implantation of a left ventricular assist device (which has replaced the artificial heart) while waiting for a donor heart. The pump is implanted in the abdomen and is connected to the main pumping chamber of the heart, the left ventricle. The power source for the pump is located outside of the patient's body on a rolling cart or is a portable battery that hangs by a strap from the shoulder (**Figure 12.9**).

**Sudden cardiac arrest** (sudden cardiac death) may also occur as a result of a heart attack. During cardiac arrest, the heart suddenly stops beating. Getting immediate medical care is crucial in such a situation because the heart must be *defibrillated* (given electric shock) within a few minutes of its stopping to cause it to begin beating again and avoid heart, lung,

**Figure 12.9**

**The Left Ventricular Assist Device (LVAD).** Billy Bean has an LVAD implanted in his body. A tube from the LVAD exits his body at the abdomen and connects to a power source that Billy keeps on a rolling cart (not shown).

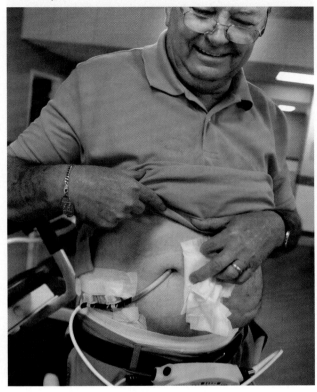

**Figure 12.10**

**A Heart Attack Prematurely Ended the Life of Former All-Star Third Baseman Ken Caminiti.** Caminiti fought drug and alcohol problems for much of his adult life. The drugs he took are thought to have weakened his heart; he died of a heart attack at age 41 in October 2004.

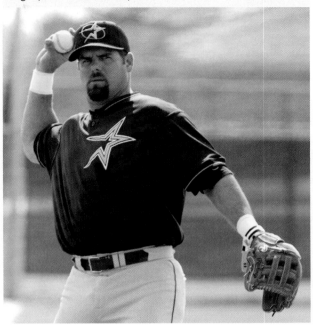

kidney, and brain damage and to avoid death. Sudden cardiac death is the result of an unresuscitated cardiac arrest.

From 250,000 to 350,000 persons in the United States die each year from sudden cardiac arrest. In the United States, the average age for a man to have his first heart attack (but not necessarily die from it) is 66 years, and for women it is 70 years. Most of the time the underlying cause of a heart attack and cardiac arrest is coronary artery disease, although medical researchers now realize that heart attacks in women often may be caused by *coronary microvascular dysfunction* (see the section titled "Atherosclerosis"). Other causes of heart attacks include conditions such as an inflammation of the heart caused by infection, rheumatic fever, or medications; heart muscle disorders having unknown causes; congenital heart defects; and drug abuse (**Figure 12.10**). (Rheumatic fever is a disorder that sometimes occurs as a result of strep throat. It affects the heart.) One of these conditions is often the reason a young, physically fit per-

son such as an athlete dies suddenly on the basketball court, track, or skating rink.

Learn the warning signs of a heart attack and what to do if you or someone you are with experiences them (see the Managing Your Health feature). You can distinguish a heart attack from angina by the severity of the pain: Heart attack pain is much more severe and lasts longer than that of angina. The pain of a heart attack is usually described as pressure (heaviness), burning, aching, and tightness, which is felt in the same locations as angina pain. The person suffering a heart attack may also experience shortness of breath, profuse sweating, weakness, anxiety, or nausea. Women may have these symptoms or may have more subtle symptoms: discomfort spread over a wide chest area, exhaustion, depression, and shortness of breath. In addition, women are more likely than men to have nausea, vomiting, back or jaw pain, and shortness of breath with chest pain.

If you experience some or all of these signs and symptoms or are with someone who does, obtain emergency medical care *immediately*. Many heart attack victims die because they do not seek medical attention quickly, denying that they are having a

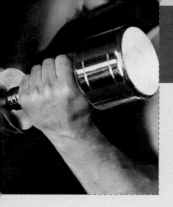

# Managing Your Health

## Heart Attack and Stroke (Brain Attack) Symptoms: What to Do in an Emergency

IF YOU NOTICE ONE OR MORE OF THESE SIGNS IN ANOTHER PERSON (OR IF YOU HAVE THEM YOURSELF), DON'T WAIT. CALL 9-1-1 OR YOUR EMERGENCY MEDICAL SERVICES AND GET TO A HOSPITAL RIGHT AWAY!

### Common or "classic" signs of heart attack:

- Uncomfortable pressure, fullness, squeezing, or pain in the center of the chest that lasts more than a few minutes or goes away and comes back
- Pain that spreads to the shoulders, neck, or arms
- Chest discomfort with light-headedness, fainting, sweating, nausea, or shortness of breath

### Less common warning signs of heart attack:

- Atypical chest, stomach, or abdominal pain
- Nausea or dizziness (without chest pain)
- Shortness of breath and difficulty breathing (without chest pain)
- Unexplained anxiety, weakness, or fatigue
- Palpitations, cold sweat, or paleness

Not all of these signs occur in every heart attack. Sometimes they go away and return. If some occur, get help fast.

### Some or all of these signs accompany a stroke:

- Weakness, numbness, or paralysis on one side of the body
- Loss or dimming of vision, particularly in one eye
- Loss of speech, or difficulty speaking or understanding speech
- Sudden, severe headache
- Sudden dizziness, unsteadiness, or episodes of falling

### Be prepared:

- Keep a list of emergency rescue service numbers next to the telephone and in your pocket, wallet, or purse.
- Find out which area hospitals have 24-hour emergency cardiovascular care.
- Know (in advance) which hospital or medical facility is nearest your home or office.

### Take action:

- If you have heart attack or stroke symptoms that last more than a few minutes, don't delay! Immediately call 9-1-1 or the emergency medical services (EMS) number so that an ambulance (ideally with Advanced Life Support) can quickly be sent for you.
- If ambulance service isn't available in your area, immediately have someone drive you to the nearest hospital emergency room (or another facility offering 24-hour life support).
- If you're with someone who may be having heart attack or stroke symptoms, immediately call 9-1-1 or EMS. Expect the person to protest—denial is common. Don't take "no" for an answer. Insist on taking prompt action.
- Give cardiopulmonary resuscitation (CPR; mouth-to-mouth breathing and chest compression) if it's needed and you're properly trained.

heart attack. However, if you call for help quickly, an emergency response team trained to provide prompt medical care can keep a heart attack victim alive and help reduce damage to the heart while transporting him or her to the hospital.

Most heart attacks are results of coronary artery thrombosis. Blood clots often form suddenly when the plaque in an artery breaks apart and blood platelets clump at that site (**Figure 12.11**). Therefore, in the emergency room, heart attack patients are quickly given clot-dissolving drugs intravenously.

Most patients who survive a heart attack do not experience complications after the attack if they receive appropriate medical treatment. Some may not even have detectable heart abnormalities if their heart attack involved only a small portion of the heart muscle. Unfortunately, some patients do experience life-threatening complications. If a substantial por-

## Figure 12.11

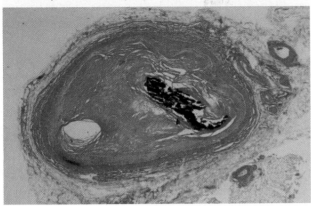

**An Occluded (Blocked) Vessel.** This coronary artery is totally blocked with plaque and a blood clot (dark area).

**stroke** A brain injury that occurs when arteries that supply the brain become blocked and prevent blood flow or become damaged and leak blood onto or into the brain.

**cerebral thrombosis** A stroke caused by a stationary blood clot.

**cerebral embolism** A stroke caused by a floating blood clot that becomes lodged in a cerebral artery, blocking blood flow.

**cerebral hemorrhage** (HEM-ah-rij) A stroke caused by a burst artery that supplies the brain.

**aneurysm** (AN-you-rizm) A swollen, weakened blood vessel.

**atrial fibrillation** (fih-brih-LAY-shun) A type of arrhythmia in which the upper chambers of the heart contract with no set pattern.

tion of the heart was involved, the heart attack victim may develop cardiogenic shock, in which the left ventricle of the heart does not pump sufficient blood to sustain the body. Although physicians can treat this condition with angioplasty or surgery, cardiogenic shock is fatal more than 50% of the time.[11]

After diagnosing a heart attack, the physician evaluates the health of the patient's heart. Using measurements of enzymes released from the heart and techniques to visualize the heart and blood vessels, such as an angiogram or MRI, the physician assesses cell damage and ventricular function (the ability of the heart to pump blood to the body) to select a patient's therapy. Such therapy may include surgical procedures, medications, and lifestyle changes.

## Stroke

A **stroke** (brain attack) occurs when arteries that supply the brain with blood become blocked, preventing blood flow. The primary cause of stroke is the same as that for heart attacks or angina pectoris: atherosclerosis—the buildup of plaque or a blood clot that blocks arteries bringing blood to the organ. Blood clots are a common cause of a stroke. If the stroke is caused by a stationary clot, the condition is called a **cerebral thrombosis**. If the blood clot was formed elsewhere and becomes lodged in a cerebral artery, blocking flow, it is called a **cerebral embolism**.

A stroke may also occur if an artery supplying the brain bursts. This situation is called a **cerebral hemorrhage** and may occur when atherosclerosis and high blood pressure are present. Cerebral hemorrhage may also occur from a head injury or from a burst **aneurysm** (a swollen, weakened blood vessel).

During a stroke, the brain cells normally supplied by the blocked or burst vessel do not receive oxygen. Brain cells, like heart cells, die when they do not receive the oxygen they need. A cerebral hemorrhage affects the brain in an additional way: Pressure builds in the brain as a result of blood that has leaked out of the burst vessel. When this blood clots, it can damage brain tissue, causing physical disability.

The signs and symptoms of a stroke vary (see Managing Your Health), depending on the location of the damage. In most cases, one side of the body becomes weak, numb, or paralyzed.

One group at highest risk for a stroke is people with **atrial fibrillation**. Atrial fibrillation is a type of arrhythmia. During atrial fibrillation, the upper chambers of the heart contract with no set pattern, which upsets the normal rhythm of the heartbeat. This arrhythmia can result in the formation of floating blood clots (emboli) that can travel to the brain, block a blood vessel, and result in a stroke.

More than 1 million Americans have atrial fibrillation. Its incidence increases with age because its primary underlying causes, hypertension and coronary artery disease, also increase with age.

Another group at high risk for strokes is persons with *stenosis* (narrowing) of one or both of the carotid arteries. The right and left carotid arteries branch off major vessels leaving the heart and bring blood up the neck to the brain (see Figure 12.1). Physicians diagnose carotid artery stenosis by using ultrasound (a technique that uses sound waves to visualize soft tissues of the body; see Chapter 5) or angiography.

Physicians often recommend *carotid endarterectomy* to reduce significantly the risk of stroke in patients with carotid artery stenosis. In this procedure, surgeons remove the inner lining of the partially blocked carotid artery along with the plaque. Also, physicians may prescribe long-term aspirin therapy or anticoagulant drugs for treatment of either carotid artery stenosis or atrial fibrillation.

In the hospital, physicians usually perform computed tomography (CT) scans (detailed x-rays of cross-sectional slices of body structures) or MRI scans of the brain of the stroke victim to confirm the diagnosis and determine the location and extent of injury (**Figure 12.12**). The standard therapy for stroke is a clot-dissolving drug called tissue plasminogen activator (tPA). If given within 3 hours of a stroke's onset, it raises the chances that no permanent brain damage will occur. Researchers are exploring ways to lengthen the window of time during which this drug can be administered.[12] Poststroke rehabilitation focuses on helping patients redevelop skills that may have been lost as a result of damage to part of the brain. These skills may involve movement, language, thinking, and memory. Mental health professionals work with stroke patients who may have had personality changes or who may have developed emotional disturbances, such as depression.

Just as heart attacks may be preceded by smaller angina attacks, major strokes may be preceded by minor strokes called **transient ischemic attacks**

### Figure 12.12

**CT Scan of a Stroke Victim.** The darkened area on the left side of the brain scan reveals dead tissue caused by a lack of oxygen during a stroke.

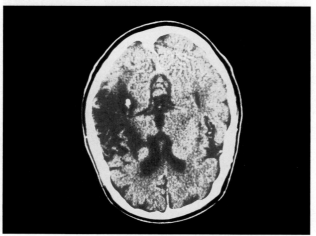

**(TIAs).** Ischemic attacks are similar to strokes, usually cause no permanent damage, and have signs that last only a short time. A TIA is a serious warning that a stroke may occur within weeks or months. Persons experiencing a TIA should see their physicians immediately. Often, blood-thinning drugs such as aspirin are prescribed to lessen the possibility of a stroke.

**The Incidence of Strokes Is Rising Among Young Americans** Stroke researchers reported at an American Stroke Association conference in early 2011 that the incidence of strokes rose 51% among men and 17% among women aged 15 through 34 years between 1994–1995 and 2006–2007. The incidence of strokes also rose 47% in males aged 35 to 44 years and 36% in females in the same age group. Researchers hypothesize that the obesity epidemic is a major factor in the increase in the stroke incidence in these age groups.

While the occurrence of strokes was rising in young adults, it was declining in older adults. The incidence of strokes dropped 25% among men and 28% in women aged 65 years and older between 1994–1995 and 2006–2007. Researchers suggest that this decline is caused in part by a better treatment of risk factors in older adults and better prevention efforts.[13]

### Healthy Living Practices

- ☐ Any person who experiences chest pain, especially pain beneath the breastbone that extends to the neck, shoulders, and/or arms, should seek medical attention immediately.

- ☐ Any person experiencing weakness, numbness, or paralysis on one side of the body; loss or dimming of vision; loss of speech, or difficulty speaking or understanding speech; a sudden, severe headache; or sudden dizziness or unsteadiness should seek medical attention immediately.

## Risk Factors for Cardiovascular Disease

Medical researchers have identified several risk factors for cardiovascular disease, traits that have been shown to be associated with the incidence of CVD. In general, people with more than one of these traits, which are listed in **Table 12.1**, have a greater prob-

## Table 12.1

### Risk Factors for Cardiovascular Disease

- Cigarette smoking
- Diabetes mellitus
- Blood cholesterol above 200 mg/dl
- A ratio of total cholesterol to high-density lipoprotein (HDL) cholesterol above 5:1 (optimum ratio is 3.5:1)
- High levels of low-density lipoprotein (LDL) cholesterol
- Physical inactivity
- Family history of cardiovascular disease
- Obesity
- Uncontrolled, persistent high blood pressure
- Heavy alcohol use
- Gender (women are at lower risk of heart attack until menopause)
- Age (risk increases with age)
- Anxiety disorders (increased risk of fatal heart attack in men)
- Elevated C-reactive protein*

\* Elevated C-reactive protein is an indicator of inflammation and is not specific to coronary artery disease.

**high-density lipoproteins (HDL)** (LIP-oh-PRO-teenz or LIE-poe-PRO-teenz) "Good" cholesterol that carries cholesterol from the cells and to the liver for removal from the body.

**low-density lipoproteins (LDL)** "Bad" cholesterol that carries cholesterol to the cells, including the cells that line the blood vessel walls.

## Family History

A family history of atherosclerosis, stroke, or coronary artery disease indicates a genetic predisposition to these conditions or reflects similar diets, stresses, and lifestyles among family members. A person with a family history of premature CAD is twice as likely to suffer a heart attack as a person with no family history. A history of premature atherosclerosis (heart attack or sudden death before 55 years of age in the father or other male first-degree relative, or before 65 years of age in the mother or other female first-degree relative) is more meaningful than having relatives who developed atherosclerosis in the elderly years. The genetic effect decreases at older ages. Unfortunately, you cannot change your family history, but you can monitor other factors to reduce your risk in other ways.

## Abnormal Blood Lipid Levels

Another major risk factor in the development of atherosclerosis, coronary artery disease, and stroke is abnormal blood lipid levels, including elevated blood cholesterol levels (also called serum cholesterol). The American Heart Association states that the desirable range of total blood cholesterol is less than 200 milligrams per deciliter (200 mg/dl). Only 55% of American adults have total blood cholesterol levels within this range. The borderline high range is 200 to 239 mg/dl, a category encompassing 29% of American adults. The high range is 240 mg/dl and higher, a category that includes 16% of adult Americans (**Table 12.2**).[14]

What is cholesterol? This substance is a *steroid*, a type of lipid. The most abundant steroid in the human body, cholesterol is used to make the sex hormones and composes part of the membranes of the body's cells. We take in cholesterol in most animal foods, such as egg yolks, fatty meats, and butter, but our bodies also make this chemical.

The blood levels of lipid-carrying molecules called lipoproteins are also critical to cardiovascular health. The major lipoproteins are **high-density lipoproteins (HDL)** and **low-density lipoproteins (LDL)**. HDL carries cholesterol from the cells and to the liver

ability of developing atherosclerosis and suffering a heart attack or stroke than do people with one or none of these risk factors. Many of these risk factors are modifiable. In other words, people can often reduce their risk of cardiovascular disease by changing one or more health-related behaviors.

The major risk factors for the development of CVD are male gender (comparable rates of a first major cardiovascular event occur 10 years later in women than in men), increasing age (the incidence of coronary artery disease rises in both men and women with each decade from age 40 to age 79 years), family history of cardiovascular disease, cigarette smoking, obesity, hypertension (chronic high blood pressure), abnormal blood lipid levels, and lack of physical activity. All these risk factors are important in the development of CAD. However, hypertension is the most important risk factor for stroke; abnormal blood lipid levels play only a small role in the development of this disease.

## Table 12.2

### Classification of Total, HDL, and LDL Cholesterol Levels and Triglyceride Levels (mg/dl)

| Total Cholesterol Levels | |
|---|---|
| Less than 200 mg/dl | Desirable level that puts you at lower risk for heart disease. A cholesterol level of 200 mg/dl or greater increases your risk. |
| 200–239 mg/dl | Borderline high. |
| 240 mg/dl and above | High blood cholesterol. A person with this level has more than twice the risk of heart disease compared with someone whose cholesterol is below 200 mg/dl. |
| **HDL Cholesterol Levels** | |
| Less than 40 mg/dl | A major risk factor for heart disease. |
| 40–59 mg/dl | The higher your HDL, the better. |
| 60 mg/dl and above | An HDL of 60 mg/dl and above is considered protective against heart disease. |
| **LDL Cholesterol Levels** | |
| Less than 100 mg/dl | Optimal. |
| 100–129 mg/dl | Near optimal/above optimal. |
| 130–159 mg/dl | Borderline high. |
| 160–189 mg/dl | High. |
| 190 mg/dl and above | Very high. |
| **Triglyceride Levels** | |
| Less than 150 mg/dl | Normal. |
| 150–199 mg/dl | Borderline high. |
| 200–499 mg/dl | High. |
| 500 mg/dl or above | Very high. |

*Source:* Reprinted with permission, Third Report of the NCEP Expert Panel on Detection, Evaluation, and Treatment of High Blood Cholesterol in Adults (*Circulation.* 2002;106:3237). © 2002 American Heart Association, Inc.

for removal from the body. LDL carries cholesterol to the cells, including the cells that line the blood vessel walls. You may have heard these molecules referred to as "good" cholesterol and "bad" cholesterol, respectively.

It is firmly established that the level of bad cholesterol, or LDL, is of major importance in the development of atherosclerosis and coronary artery disease. As the level of LDL rises, the risk of coronary artery disease and atherosclerosis rises because LDL is related to the formation and growth of plaques.

The level of good cholesterol, or HDL, is very important too. As the level of HDL rises, the risk of coronary artery disease and atherosclerosis falls. (Table 12.2 lists the classification levels for HDL and LDL.) High HDL levels are the key to why premenopausal women, in general, do not experience heart attacks at as young an age as men; the female sex hormone estrogen raises women's HDL levels by about 20%. As noted in Table 12.2, desirable levels of HDL cholesterol are above 40 mg/dl. Women are encouraged, however, to maintain an HDL cholesterol level above 50 mg/dl.[15]

A primary component of HDL is apolipoprotein A-I (apoA-I), which has been shown to reverse atherosclerosis and is therefore a potentially powerful treatment for vascular diseases. The Diversity in Health essay describes how a mutant form of this

# Diversity in Health

## The Italian Gene: A Hope for Reversing Atherosclerosis?

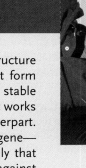

The University of Milan's Dr. Cesare Sirtori could hardly believe it: Thirty-eight members of one Italian family had no atherosclerosis. If that was not surprising enough, many of them smoked cigarettes and ate high amounts of fat in their diets. What was protecting them from developing plaques in their blood vessels? The answer to that question is a mutation in the gene that directs the production of a cholesterol-lowering protein.

We all have this cholesterol-lowering protein in our bodies: apolipoprotein A-I (apoA-I). ApoA-I is a primary component of high-density lipoprotein (HDL), so-called good cholesterol. HDL helps bring excess cholesterol to the liver for transport out of the body. (Researchers do not fully understand the exact mechanism of this action.) In women, estrogen increases the body's production of apoA-I and is thought to be one reason that premenopausal women have a greater protection than men of the same age from the development of atherosclerosis and heart attacks.

Apolipoprotein A-I (Milano) (apoA-IM) is a mutant apoA-I protein produced by the mutated Italian gene.

The change in the molecular structure of apoA-IM from the nonmutant form makes this HDL molecule more stable and alters its properties so that it works even better than its normal counterpart. Those who carry the apoA-IM gene—the members of the Italian family that Sirtori studied—are protected against vascular disease.

Researchers have been able to make apoA-IM in the laboratory. They have used this synthetic molecule in animal models to study its potential as a treatment to reverse atherosclerosis and cardiovascular disease. Results showed a rapid regression of atherosclerosis in the treated animals. Similar studies have been performed with humans and have shown similar results. Scientists are currently conducting larger clinical trials. If successful, scientists and generations of one Italian family will have made a medical breakthrough in slowing the death rate from the United States' number one killer.

*Sources:* Speidl, W. S., et al. (2010). Recombinant apolipoprotein A-I Milano rapidly reverses aortic valve stenosis and decreases leaflet inflammation in an experimental rabbit model. *European Heart Journal, 31*(16):2049–2057; Spillmann, F., et al. (2010). High-density lipoprotein-raising strategies: Update 2010. *Current Pharmaceutical Design, 16*(13):1517–1530.

---

cholesterol-lowering protein found in a certain Italian family (apoA-I [Milano]) protects them against vascular disease. ApoA-1 (Milano) has a more effective cholesterol-removing function than apoA-1 and may therefore prove to be a more effective treatment.[16]

Triglycerides, which are plasma lipids different from cholesterol, are also important in cardiovascular health. When the body does not immediately use all the energy-supplying nutrients consumed, it converts them to triglycerides and transports them to fat cells for storage. Excess triglycerides in the plasma are linked to CAD in some people. Additionally, researchers have linked high levels of triglycerides to an increased risk of stroke. A normal, fasting triglyceride level is less than 150 mg/dl (see Table 12.2).

## Cigarette Smoking

Smoking cigarettes significantly increases the risk of heart attack and stroke. Cigarette smokers are 2 to 4 times more likely than nonsmokers to develop CAD and over 10 times more likely to develop peripheral vascular disease.[14] In addition, smoking interacts with other risk factors, multiplying its negative health effects. Even more alarming is that cigarette smoking is directly responsible for the majority of heart disease in women under the age of 50 years.[17] These figures show that premenopausal women, who are generally protected from heart attacks by estrogen, raise their risk of heart disease significantly when they smoke.

Research results show that cigarette smokers tend to have reduced HDL levels, increased LDL levels, and increased levels of blood clotting factors. In addition, evidence suggests that compounds in cigarette smoke enter the bloodstream and may damage blood vessel linings directly, leading to the formation of plaques.[18] Chewing tobacco is a significant CVD risk factor also, but cigar and pipe smoking appear to be less important because cigar and pipe smokers are less likely than cigarette smokers to inhale the smoke.[19]

Passive smoking, breathing in other people's smoke, has also been identified as an important risk factor for cardiovascular disease. The AHA estimates that approximately 40,000 people die each year from heart and blood vessel disease caused by passive smoking.[19] Results of research show a harmful effect of passive smoking on the circulation of blood within the heart tissue itself.[20]

# High Blood Pressure

Blood pressure becomes elevated during periods of excitement or exertion; however, in healthy individuals it returns to normal levels when the activity stops. **Hypertension**, persistently high arterial blood pressure, is a major risk factor for heart attack and the most important risk factor for stroke. Data show that nearly one-third of Americans age 20 years and older are hypertensive.[21]

The cause of most cases of high blood pressure is unknown. It has been shown, however, that hypertension may have a genetic link; it runs in families. There are also racial genetic links in hypertension. African Americans and Latinos are more likely to have hypertension than whites and, as a result, suffer strokes at an earlier age and with greater severity. Nongenetic, modifiable factors that contribute to hypertension are obesity, lack of physical activity, cigarette smoking, stress, and long-term intake of excessive amounts of salt. Other identifiable causes of hypertension include increasing age, enzyme deficiencies, sleep apnea, drugs, chronic kidney disease, and thyroid or parathyroid disease.[22]

You may know your blood pressure reading, such as 120/75 mm Hg (millimeters of mercury). The first (higher) number is the **systolic pressure**, which is the pressure exerted by the blood on the artery walls when the left ventricle contracts and is able to move blood through the constricted artery (**Figure 12.13**). The second (lower) number is the **diastolic pressure**, which is the pressure exerted by the blood on the artery walls when the left ventricle relaxes. The units, mm Hg, refer to the force needed to push a column of mercury to a particular height, such as 120 mm or 75 mm. The normal blood pressure level for people older than 18 years is less than 120/80 mm Hg. *Prehypertension* is indicated by a systolic blood pressure between 120 and 139 mm Hg, or a diastolic pressure between 80 and 89 mm Hg. *Stage 1 hyper-*

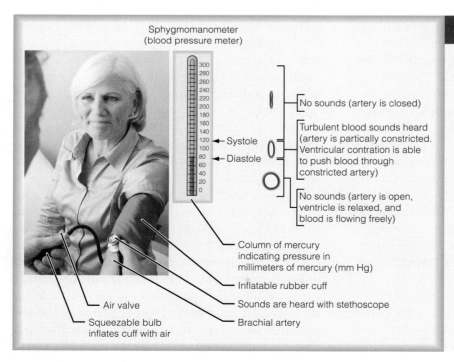

## Figure 12.13

**Blood Pressure.** The inflatable cuff, which is wrapped around the upper arm, squeezes the brachial artery tightly so that blood cannot pass. The systolic reading is taken when turbulent blood sounds can first be heard in this artery, indicating the strength of the pressure against the artery wall when the ventricle contracts and can push the blood through the constricted artery. If the blood pressure is high, it will force the blood vessel open sooner (at a higher reading) than if the blood pressure is low. The diastolic reading is taken when the turbulent blood sounds stop, indicating the strength of the pressure against the artery wall when the ventricle relaxes, the artery is no longer constricted, and the blood is flowing freely.

*tension* is indicated by a systolic reading between 140 and 159, or a diastolic reading of 90 to 99. *Stage 2 hypertension* is indicated by a systolic reading of 160 or more, or a diastolic reading of 100 or more.

Persistently high arterial blood pressure contributes to the development of atherosclerosis in two ways. First, high blood pressure may injure the lining of artery walls, triggering plaque formation. In addition, the increased pressure enhances the amount of lipid added to plaques, especially if serum LDL cholesterol levels are elevated.

## Physical Inactivity

Within the past two decades, physical inactivity has been shown to be a major risk factor for developing cardiovascular disease, although research results have linked physical activity and health for more than 60 years. Physically inactive people are about twice as likely as active people to develop coronary artery disease. This risk extends to people who sit for a large portion of the day rather than stand and move about, independent of exercising. Results of research studies show that sitting for extended periods raises the risk of dying from cardiovascular disease, and the longer one sits, the higher the mortality risk.[23]

The 1996 Surgeon General's report on physical activity and health recommends that persons of all ages obtain "a minimum of 30 minutes of physical activity of moderate intensity (e.g., brisk walking) on most, if not all, days of the week."[24] In 2011, the Centers for Disease Control and Prevention (CDC) suggests at least 150 minutes per week of physical activity of moderate intensity to lower the risk of heart disease and stroke.[25] However, as a group, Americans are relatively sedentary; more than 50% of American adults do not get enough physical activity to provide health benefits, and 25% are not active at all during leisure time.[26]

In addition to its direct cardiovascular benefits, routine exercise helps alleviate stress, reduce body weight, and control diabetes—other CVD risk factors. (Chapter 11 discusses the importance of a physically active lifestyle to health.)

## Obesity

Most medical researchers agree that obesity increases the risk of cardiovascular disease. If you are obese, you nearly double your risk of CAD. Being mildly overweight also increases your risk. Studies show a strong positive association between weight and heart disease in both men and women. Are you within the desirable weight range for your age and height? Do you have a body mass index (BMI) of less than 25? See Chapter 10 for an explanation of BMI and for a BMI graph.

## Diabetes Mellitus

Diabetes mellitus is a group of diseases in which glucose is not metabolized properly. Affected individuals are at a higher risk of developing cardiovascular disease because of their elevated blood glucose levels, which damage heart muscle, small coronary vessels, and major arteries. Therefore, atherosclerosis occurs more frequently and at an earlier age in diabetic patients, particularly women. Unfortunately, people with diabetes mellitus are about five times as likely to develop cardiovascular disease as are persons without this disease.

## Anxiety and Stress

As mentioned previously, stress can result in spasms of the coronary arteries, which can contribute to angina attacks. In addition, research studies link anxiety disorders (such as phobias and panic disorders; see Chapter 2) to an increased risk of fatal CAD and particularly to sudden, fatal heart attacks in men.[27] Persons with anxiety disorders are from two to six times as likely to die from a heart attack as persons without anxiety disorders.

## Elevated C-Reactive Protein

Results of research show that elevated blood levels of C-reactive protein (CRP) can be a positive risk factor for coronary artery disease.[28] C-reactive protein is produced by the liver during acute inflammation. Inflammation may be present at the site of plaques in CAD, but it may also be present in other diseases such as rheumatoid arthritis. Therefore, it is not a test specific to CAD. In addition, a low CRP value does not mean that inflammation is absent.

 **Healthy Living Practices**

☐ If any of your male first-degree relatives had a heart attack before age 55, or female first-degree relatives before age 65, you may be genetically predisposed to heart disease. See your physician for an evaluation and advice.

☐ If you are a healthy adult, you should have your serum cholesterol level and HDL level measured once every 5 years.

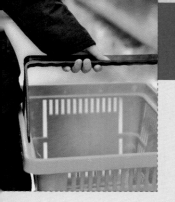

# Consumer Health

## Vitamin Pills for a Healthier Heart?

Vitamins A, C, E, $B_6$, $B_{12}$, folate, and the nonnutrient beta-carotene ... what do they have to do with cardiovascular health? Should you be rushing to the store for vitamin supplements to keep your blood vessels healthy?

Vitamins play many roles in cardiovascular health. For example, our bodies use vitamins $B_6$, $B_{12}$, and folate in the metabolism of amino acids, including the essential amino acid methionine. In the process of metabolizing methionine, cells produce homocysteine (ho-mo-SIS-teen), another amino acid. High blood levels of this amino acid can damage artery walls and encourage the formation of blood clots and plaques. However, if the cells have enough folate, $B_6$, and $B_{12}$, then methionine is metabolized normally and the blood level of homocysteine does not rise.

Methionine intake also affects homocysteine levels. In general, the more methionine people eat, the higher their blood levels of homocysteine. Diets rich in animal protein contain high amounts of methionine and may elevate blood homocysteine levels. Conversely, diets rich in plant protein may lower homocysteine levels because plant foods are relatively low in methionine yet rich in folate and vitamin $B_6$.

Other factors also influence homocysteine blood levels. Smoking cigarettes, drinking coffee, and a sedentary lifestyle are all associated with decreased $B_6$ activity, and therefore higher homocysteine levels. The use of oral contraceptives and hormone replacement therapy lowers homocysteine blood levels in women. Homocysteine levels also depend on age, gender, kidney function, genetics, and general health.

So, do you need to take vitamin pills to lower your blood homocysteine levels? The answer is not simple, and only your physician can advise you based on your health. If you show evidence of $B_6$ or $B_{12}$ deficiency (more likely in elderly than in younger populations) or evidence of folate deficiency (more likely in younger than in elderly populations), your physician may suggest testing. Also, if you are experiencing kidney failure, are on a special metabolic diet, have cancer, or have a strong family history of heart attack, stroke, or abnormal blood clotting, your physician may recommend that your homocysteine levels be checked. The determination of homocysteine

## Maintaining Cardiovascular Health

**Table 12.3** presents a summary of recommendations to help you maintain cardiovascular health and lower your risk of cardiovascular disease. As you can see, there are many factors to consider. You cannot control heredity, gender, and age. However, you can stop smoking, exercise regularly, lose weight, eat less fat, learn to relax, and reduce your salt intake. Results of research reveal that adopting a healthy lifestyle (at least 2½ cups of fruits and vegetables daily,[29] exercising regularly, maintaining a BMI of 18.5 to 29.9, and not smoking) is extremely important to cardiovascular health and a long life. When middle-aged adults (45 to 64 years) who were not following this healthy lifestyle changed their behavior to adopt these healthy habits, they reduced their risk of dying during the next 4 years by 40% and their risk of cardiovascular disease by 35% compared to those who did not change. Only 8% of middle-aged adults practice these healthy lifestyle behaviors.[30,31] Adopting a healthy lifestyle while you are young not only promotes immediate health but also increases the chances that you will continue these behaviors throughout your life, thereby increasing your chances of living a longer, heart-healthy life.

In addition to adopting healthy lifestyle behaviors, you can enhance your cardiovascular health by managing stress properly. Emotional stress contributes to hypertension and the incidence of angina attacks.

levels is complex, and interpretation of the finding is not simple.

So, what about vitamins A, C, E, and beta-carotene? (Beta-carotene is a yellow pigment in plants that the body converts to vitamin A.) As discussed in Chapter 9, vitamins E and C and beta-carotene are antioxidants, substances that can protect cells by preventing or reducing the formation of free radicals. Studies have consistently shown that the more antioxidants a population consumes in its food, the lower the rate of cardiovascular disease. But what about vitamin supplements? In general, vitamin supplements, including vitamins B, C, D, and E, and supplements of beta-carotene, calcium, and folic acid have not been found to lower the risk of cardiovascular diseases. In addition, the American Heart Association (AHA) does not recommend taking antioxidant vitamin supplements or other supplements such as selenium to prevent coronary artery disease. The AHA also notes that consuming soy protein products instead of dairy or other proteins does not show a direct cardiovascular health benefit.

So . . . should you take vitamin pills to reduce your risk of CVD? Only your physician can advise you properly because the answer depends on the status of various facets of your health, family history, and lifestyle. The best advice at this time is to get your vitamins in the food you eat—be sure to have at least 2½ cups of fruits and vegetables every day, including dark, leafy greens and members of the cabbage family. Consult your physician to determine whether you might also need to take vitamin pills because of possible vitamin deficiencies for a healthier heart and blood vessels.

*Sources:* American Heart Association Nutrition Committee. (2006). AHA scientific statement: Diet and lifestyle recommendations revision 2006. *Circulation, 114:*82–96; Clarke, R., et al. (2010). Effects of lowering homocysteine levels with B vitamins on cardiovascular disease, cancer, and cause-specific mortality: Meta-analysis of 8 randomized trials involving 37,485 individuals. *Archives of Internal Medicine, 170*(18):1622–1631; Cordero, Z., et al. (2010). Vitamin E and risk of cardiovascular diseases: A review of epidemiologic and clinical trial studies. *Critical Reviews in Food Science and Nutrition, 50*(5):420–440; Lichtenstein, A. H., et al. (2009). Nutrient supplements and cardiovascular disease: A heartbreaking story. *Journal of Lipid Research, 50*(Suppl):S429–433; Wang, L., et al. (2010). Systematic review: Vitamin D and calcium supplementation in prevention of cardiovascular events. *Annals of Internal Medicine, 152*(5):315–323.

Chapter 3, "Stress and Its Management," describes stress management skills and coping strategies that may help you lower your risk of stress-related hypertension and angina.

If you have diabetes mellitus, work with your primary diabetes physician, such as an endocrinologist, to develop a diabetes management plan that is specific for you; diabetics who conscientiously manage their disease and their blood sugar level lower their risk of cardiovascular disease.

Getting regular medical checkups (the frequency of which should be determined by your physician) can help you assess your CVD risk factors. Your physician may recommend other steps to lower CVD risks. The following sections describe actions that physicians often recommend for reducing CVD risk and maintaining cardiovascular health.

## Smoking Cessation

If you smoke, stop now. If you do not smoke, avoid breathing in secondhand (other people's) smoke. Approximately 150,000 cardiovascular deaths could be avoided each year if people did not smoke cigarettes.[14] Studies suggest that the smoker who quits cuts his or her elevated risk of CAD in half only 1 year after quitting. Within 15 years, the elevated risk of a former smoker declines to the level of a nonsmoker.[32] According to the National Stroke Association, the risk of stroke may revert to that of nonsmokers within 5 years after quitting. The more cigarettes a person

## Table 12.3

### How to Reduce Your Risk of Cardiovascular Disease

- Get regular medical checkups.

- Do not smoke cigarettes.

- Manage diabetes mellitus properly.

- Exercise regularly.

- Maintain an intake of dietary cholesterol of less than 300 mg per day, or less than 200 mg per day if you have high LDL levels.

- Maintain an intake of dietary fat of between 20% and 35% of daily calories.

- Maintain an intake of saturated fats of 7% or less* and trans fat of less than 1% of daily calories.

- Eat foods rich in soluble fiber, such as fruits, beans, and oats.

- Eat a diet rich in fruits, vegetables, and low-fat dairy products.

- Maintain an appropriate weight for your height.

- Limit alcohol consumption to 1 drink per day for women and 2 drinks per day for men.

- Maintain salt intake at approximately two-thirds teaspoon or 1,500 mg of sodium per day.*

- Reduce your stress level.

* This recommendation is from the American Heart Association. See: American Heart Association. (2011, January 31). American Heart Association supports the new USDA/HHS dietary guidelines and encourages adherence. AHA also expresses disappointment that sodium, saturated fat guidance is weak. Retrieved on October 4, 2011, from http://newsroom.heart.org/pr/aha/1243.aspx. Also see: U.S. Department of Agriculture and U.S. Department of Health and Human Services. (2010, December). *Dietary guidelines for Americans, 2010* (7th ed.). Washington, DC: U.S. Government Printing Office. Retrieved on April 11, 2011, from http://www.health.gov/dietaryguidelines/dga2010/DietaryGuidelines2010.pdf

smokes and the earlier a person started to smoke, the longer the recovery time. In addition, the risk of cardiovascular disease increases as the number of cigarettes smoked increases. Therefore, smoke fewer cigarettes if you cannot quit. Smoking "low-yield" (low tar and nicotine) cigarettes does not appear to reduce CVD risk.

## Weight Control

If your BMI is 25 or more, then losing weight will reduce your risk of cardiovascular disease. Chapter 10, "Body Weight and Its Management," presents background and suggestions for weight management. In addition, Chapter 9 provides key recommendations from *Dietary Guidelines for Americans, 2010*, and Chapter 10 includes a section on balancing calories to maintain weight. In general, a regular exercise program coupled with a low-calorie diet will reduce body fat. Weight reduction lowers total blood cholesterol levels, raises HDL levels, and lowers LDL levels. It also helps maintain proper blood glucose levels.

## Exercise

In the late 1980s, a review of 43 studies about the relationship between physical activity and the risk of CAD and atherosclerosis was conducted.[33] Two-thirds of these studies documented a substantial inverse relationship between physical activity and risk for these two related diseases: As the level of physical activity rose, the risk of CAD and atherosclerosis declined and vice versa. These findings have been upheld by more recent studies.[26] Research results also show that exercise is associated with a decreased risk of stroke.[34]

Exercise has been shown to lower blood pressure and boost HDL levels. The American Heart Association (AHA) recommends that healthy people perform any moderate- to vigorous-intensity aerobic activity, such as brisk walking, hiking, stair-climbing, jogging, bicycling, and swimming, for at least 30 minutes per day, five days per week.[35] (Aerobic activities are those that raise the heart rate for a sustained period of time.) The AHA notes that regular physical activity for longer periods or at greater intensity will likely provide greater health benefits. Even moderate-intensity activities, such as slow walking, gardening, housework, and recreational activities, can have some long-term health benefits when performed daily and can help lower the risk of cardiovascular disease.

## Lowering Blood Pressure

Nearly one of every three American adults has hypertension. In 90–95% of cases, hypertension can be controlled. Doing so reduces the risk of both stroke and heart attack. The American Heart Association recommends having your blood pressure checked every 2 years and more often if it is high.

To lower blood pressure, the AHA suggests decreasing sodium intake to a maximum of 1,500 mg per day, which is about two-thirds of a teaspoon of salt.[36] Nutritionists suggest checking the amount of sodium that you consume in prepackaged, processed foods and not salting your food. The sodium in salt causes the body to retain fluids and may contribute to hypertension in some people.

Dietary factors in addition to sodium affect blood pressure. The DASH diet (Dietary Approaches to Stop Hypertension) has been shown to lower blood pressure in diverse subgroups of the U.S. population. This diet is low in total and saturated fat compared to a more typical U.S. diet, and is rich in fruits, vegetables, and low-fat dairy foods. Researchers also studied decreased sodium intake with both the DASH diet and the typical U.S. diet. Data show highly significant decreases in blood pressure with either diet. Researchers conclude that the DASH diet plus reduced sodium intake is effective in controlling blood pressure.[37]

The blood pressure of overweight individuals often drops when they lose weight. If you are overweight and have high blood pressure, weight reduction is the most important action you can take to lower your blood pressure and risk of CVD. Regular aerobic exercise lowers blood pressure and will also help control weight. Reducing the intake of dietary saturated fat and cholesterol will promote overall cardiovascular health and will also help reduce caloric intake, which is important for weight control.

The heavy consumption of alcoholic beverages has also been shown to lead to high blood pressure, increasing the risk of heart attack, stroke, and death from CAD. Limiting consumption to 1 oz of alcohol (ethanol) per day (two drinks or fewer) for men and 0.5 oz (one drink) for women may help lower blood pressure and may reduce your risk of cardiovascular disease. One ounce of ethanol is equivalent to 2 oz of 100-proof whiskey, 8 to 10 oz of wine (the alcohol content in wines varies), or two 12-oz cans of beer.

If none of these lifestyle changes lowers the blood pressure sufficiently, hypertension can be treated with a wide array of antihypertensive drugs. These drugs are not suitable or appropriate for all hypertensive individuals but may be essential therapy for many.

## Reducing Blood Cholesterol

Decades of scientific research show that a high level of cholesterol in the blood is a major risk factor for cardiovascular disease. Eating saturated fats (found in foods such as red meat, cream, and whole milk), trans fats (found in many baked goods and french fries), and dietary cholesterol (found in foods such as meats, egg yolks, and dairy products) tends to raise blood cholesterol. Therefore, the American Heart Association recommends that healthy Americans older than age 2 years should limit their saturated fat intake (primarily animal fats and tropical oils) to less than 7% and their trans fat intake to less than 1%.[38] (Chapter 9 describes the types of fats in foods. Table 9.6 lists a variety of foods and their percentages of saturated fatty acids.) The AHA also recommends that Americans restrict dietary cholesterol intake to 300 mg per day. (One large egg, for example, has slightly more than 200 mg, and a quarter-pound cheeseburger has slightly more than 100 mg. Table 9.7 lists a variety of foods and their cholesterol content.)

Polyunsaturated fats (found in nuts, seeds, and certain plant oils, such as canola, safflower, and sesame oil) and monounsaturated fats (found in avocados and olive, canola, and peanut oil) tend to lower blood cholesterol levels. Additionally, omega-3 fatty acids, which are found in certain fish such as salmon, tuna, cod, and sole, appear to lower the risk of CAD and stroke. The American Heart Association suggests that individuals should adjust their total fat intake to meet their caloric needs. People who are overweight or obese should limit their overall fat intake to less than 30% of their daily intake of calories and replace saturated and trans fats in their diet with poly- and monounsaturated fats.[38]

Studies show that, on average, people can achieve a 10% reduction in cholesterol levels by following these dietary guidelines. Each 1% reduction in the blood cholesterol level reduces the risk of CAD by 2% to 3%, so a 10% reduction reduces your risk of CAD by 20% to 30%. If you are at high risk for cardiovascular disease, your physician will likely place you on a diet that has cholesterol and other fat intake recommendations different from those mentioned here, which are for the general population.

Eating whole grains and foods rich in soluble fiber (such as fruits, beans, oats, and barley) can help reduce your LDL and total cholesterol levels (**Figure 12.14**).[29] The American Heart Association notes that insoluble dietary fiber, found in many foods such as green leafy vegetables, fruit skins, seeds, and nuts, appears to decrease cardiovascular risk and slows progression of cardiovascular disease in high-risk individuals. The AHA suggests a total dietary fiber intake of 25 g from foods, not supplements, to ensure enough nutrients in the diet.[39] Currently, most Americans take in only half that amount.

If eating a heart-healthy diet and exercising regularly do not significantly reduce elevated blood

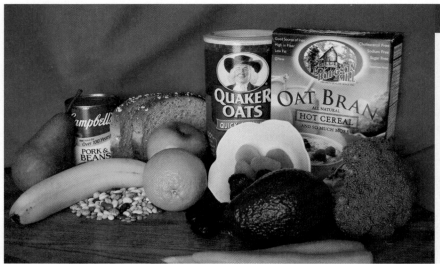

**Figure 12.14**

**Foods High in Soluble Fiber.** Soluble fiber helps lower LDL cholesterol. The foods shown here include whole wheat bread, oatmeal, broccoli, navel oranges, beans, avocado, and pitted prunes.

cholesterol levels, cholesterol-lowering medications called "statins" are available by prescription. Research results have shown that statins are safe, reduce CAD deaths, reduce total cholesterol and LDL cholesterol, and appear to reduce the risk of stroke.[40]

## Aspirin Therapy

A treatment to reduce the risk of cardiovascular disease that has gained attention in recent years is long-term use of aspirin in a dosage no greater than a baby aspirin (80 mg). The benefit of aspirin therapy increases with increasing cardiovascular risk; it reduces the risk for heart attack in men and strokes in women.[41] Aspirin can have damaging effects on the gastrointestinal system and reduces the blood's ability to clot; therefore, long-term aspirin therapy should be undertaken only on the advice of a physician.

## Hormone Replacement Therapy

Hormone replacement therapy (HRT) is the use of estrogen plus progestin in postmenopausal women, or the use of estrogen alone in postmenopausal women with prior hysterectomy (surgical removal of the uterus). Analysis of data from the Women's Health Initiative (WHI) 15-year research program, which addresses the most common causes of death, disability, and poor quality of life in postmenopausal women, suggests that cardiovascular risk is neither increased nor decreased in women who begin hormone therapy less than 10 years after menopause.[42–44] Cardiovascular risk increases in women beginning hormone therapy after that time. Women who are between 50 and 59 years of age when they begin post-

menopausal hormone therapy appear to have a lower risk of death from any cause than women who do not take postmenopausal hormones or who begin taking hormones later in life. Researchers caution, however, that HRT is not without risk and do not recommend postmenopausal hormone therapy for the prevention of heart attacks. Women nearing menopause should talk with their physicians to determine whether HRT is appropriate for them.

### Healthy Living Practices

☐ One of the most important things you can do to lower your risk of coronary artery disease and stroke is to reduce your modifiable risk factors, which include quitting smoking, maintaining a healthy body weight, and maintaining an active lifestyle that includes regular aerobic exercise.

☐ To lower your blood pressure, engage in regular aerobic exercise, lose weight if you are overweight, limit your alcohol consumption to 1 oz of ethanol per day for men and 0.5 oz per day for women, and limit your daily sodium intake to 1,500 mg.

☐ To reduce your total cholesterol level, raise your HDL level, and lower your LDL level, eat no more than 20% to 35% of your daily intake of calories from fat and no more than 7% from saturated fat and less than 1% from trans fat. Also, eat foods rich in soluble fiber, such as fruits, beans, and oats.

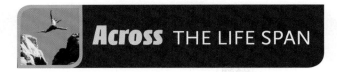

## CARDIOVASCULAR HEALTH

The American Heart Association estimates that approximately 1% of babies are born each year with a variety of heart and blood vessel structural and functional abnormalities.[45] Many congenital defects (those present at birth) can now be diagnosed before birth with the use of echocardiography, or ultrasound of the heart. Sound waves are directed through the heart of the fetus; as they pass through different types of tissues (such as heart muscle and blood), they are reflected, or echoed, producing an image of the movements of the heart structures. This technique can also be used with infants, children, and adults. Such early diagnostic techniques have helped surgeons correct infants' cardiovascular defects within the first few weeks of life. This approach helps avoid complications from cardiovascular defects in older children and adults. Presently, about 1 million Americans have congenital heart defects.

The Bogalusa Heart Study, a long-term study of the development of coronary artery disease, showed that cardiovascular disease caused by atherosclerosis is a process that begins in childhood.[46] Habits of diet and lifestyle develop at an early age and often continue into adulthood, affecting this disease process. Data from the Bogalusa Heart Study show that the average diet of children and adolescents consisted of 14% of their total daily calories from protein, 50% from carbohydrate, and 36% from fat.[47] The more recent School Nutrition Dietary Assessment Study found that most children and adolescents had nutritionally adequate diets, but 80% had diets too high in saturated fat and 92% had diets too high in sodium.[48] Such diets do not meet the recommendations of the American Heart Association and can lead to the development of atherosclerosis and obesity, both risk factors for coronary artery disease and stroke.

In the Bogalusa study, school breakfasts and lunches had a major impact on the diets of children, providing approximately half of the day's total caloric intake and about 49% of daily total fat intake—too high a proportion. Many school lunch programs have reduced their percentages of total fat, saturated fat, and sodium. In addition, several innovative "heart-healthy" school lunch programs such as Healthy Edge, Lunch Power, and Heart Smart have been developed in schools across the nation.

The results of studies show that older adults should be treated with lipid-lowering therapy when needed because it will help prevent the progression of CVD and other diseases common in this age group.[49] Treating hypertension in older adults is also recommended because it reduces the risk of cardiovascular events. However, treating hypertension in the very elderly (those older than 80 years) may have more risks than benefits.[50]

This article focuses on claims that manufacturers make on food labels. Explain why you think this article is a reliable or an unreliable source of information. Use the model for analyzing health information to guide your thinking; the main points of the model are noted here. The model is fully explained in Chapter 1.

1. Which statements are verifiable facts, and which are unverified statements or value claims?
2. What are the credentials of the source making these health-related claims? Does the source have the appropriate background and education in the topic area? What can you do to check the credentials of this source?
3. What might be the motives and biases of the source making the claims?

4. What is the main point of the article? Which information is relevant to the issue, main point, product, or service? Which information is irrelevant?
5. Is the source reliable? What evidence supports your conclusion that the source is reliable or unreliable? Does the source of information present the pros and cons of the topic or the benefits and risks of the product?
6. Does the source of information attack the credibility of conventional scientists or medical authorities?

Based on your analysis, do you think that this article is a reliable source of health-related information? Summarize your reasons for coming to this conclusion.

## Trans Fat Now Listed with Saturated Fat and Cholesterol on the Nutrition Facts Label

### Trans Fat Coming to a Label Near You!

The Food and Drug Administration (FDA) now requires food manufacturers to list trans fat (i.e., trans fatty acids) on Nutrition Facts and some Supplement Facts panels. Scientific evidence shows that consumption of saturated fat, trans fat, and dietary cholesterol raises low-density lipoprotein (LDL or "bad") cholesterol levels that increase the risk of coronary heart disease (CHD). According to the National Heart, Lung, and Blood Institute of the National Institutes of Health, over 12.5 million Americans suffer from CHD, and more than 500,000 die each year. This makes CHD one of the leading causes of death in the United States today.

FDA has required that saturated fat and dietary cholesterol be listed on the food label since 1993. By adding trans fat on the Nutrition Facts panel (required as of January 1, 2006), consumers now know for the first time how much of all three—saturated fat, trans fat, and cholesterol—are in the foods they choose. Identifying saturated fat, trans fat, and cholesterol on the food label gives consumers information to make heart-healthy food choices that help them reduce their risk of CHD. This revised label, which includes information on trans fat as well as saturated fat and cholesterol, will be of particular interest to people concerned about high blood cholesterol and heart disease.

## Nutrition Facts

Serving Size 1 cup (228g)
Servings Per Container 2

| Amount Per Serving | |
|---|---|
| **Calories** 250 | Calories from Fat 110 |

| | % Daily Value* |
|---|---|
| **Total Fat** 12g | |
| Saturated Fat 3g | |
| *Trans* Fat 1.5g | |
| **Cholesterol** 30mg | 10% |
| **Sodium** 470mg | 20% |
| **Total Carbohydrate** 31g | 10% |
| Dietary Fiber 0g | 0% |
| Sugars 5g | |
| **Protein** 5g | |

Appearing on product labels as of January 2006

| | |
|---|---|
| Vitamin A | 4% |
| Vitamin C | 2% |
| Calcium | 20% |
| Iron | 4% |

\* Percent Daily Values are based on a 2,000 calorie diet. Your Daily Values may be higher or lower depending on your calorie needs:

| | Calories: | 2,000 | 2,500 |
|---|---|---|---|
| Total Fat | Less than | 65g | 80g |
| Sat Fat | Less than | 20g | 25g |
| Cholesterol | Less than | 300mg | 300mg |
| Sodium | Less than | 2,400mg | 2,400mg |
| Total Carbohydrate | | 300g | 375g |
| Dietary Fiber | | 25g | 30g |

**Nutrition Label.**

*Source:* Food and Drug Administration. (2011, June 24). Retrieved on October 11, 2011, from http://www.fda.gov/Food/LabelingNutrition/ConsumerInformation/ucm109832.htm

However, all Americans should be aware of the risk posed by consuming too much saturated fat, trans fat, and cholesterol. But what is trans fat, and how can you limit the amount of this fat in your diet?

## What Is Trans Fat? Where will I find trans fat?

Vegetable shortenings, some margarines, crackers, cookies, snack foods, and other foods made with or fried in partially hydrogenated oils.

Unlike other fats, the majority of trans fat is formed when liquid oils are made into solid fats like shortening and hard margarine. However, a small amount of trans fat is found naturally, primarily in some animal-based foods. Essentially, trans fat is made when hydrogen is added to vegetable oil—a process called hydrogenation. Hydrogenation increases the shelf life and flavor stability of foods containing these fats.

Trans fat, like saturated fat and dietary cholesterol, raises the LDL (or "bad") cholesterol that increases your risk for CHD. On average, Americans consume four to five times as much saturated fat as trans fat in their diet.

Although saturated fat is the main dietary culprit that raises LDL, trans fat and dietary cholesterol also contribute significantly. Trans fat can often be found in processed foods made with partially hydrogenated vegetable oils such as vegetable shortenings, some margarines (especially margarines that are harder), crackers, candies, cookies, snack foods, fried foods, and baked goods.

## Are All Fats the Same?

Simply put: no. Fat is a major source of energy for the body and aids in the absorption of vitamins A, D, E, and K, and carotenoids. Both animal- and plant-derived food products contain fat, and when eaten in moderation, fat is important for proper growth, development, and maintenance of good health. As a food ingredient, fat provides taste, consistency, and stability and helps us feel full. In addition, parents should be aware that fats are an especially important source of calories and nutrients for infants and toddlers (up to 2 years of age), who have the highest energy needs per unit of body weight of any age group.

Saturated and trans fats raise LDL (or "bad") cholesterol levels in the blood, thereby increasing the risk of heart disease. Dietary cholesterol also contributes to heart disease. Unsaturated fats, such as monounsaturated and polyunsaturated, do not raise LDL cholesterol and are beneficial when consumed in moderation. Therefore, it is advisable to choose foods low in saturated fat, trans fat, and cholesterol as part of a healthful diet.

## What Can I Do About Saturated Fat, Trans Fat, and Cholesterol?

When comparing foods, look at the Nutrition Facts panel, and choose the food with the lower amounts of saturated fat, trans fat, and cholesterol. Health experts recommend that you keep your intake of these nutrients as low as possible while consuming a nutritionally adequate diet. However, these experts recognize that eliminating these three components entirely from your diet is not practical because they are unavoidable in ordinary diets.

## Where Can I Find Trans Fat on the Food Label?

Take a look at the Nutrition Facts panel accompanying this article. Consumers can find trans fat listed on the Nutrition Facts panel directly under the line for saturated fat.

## Why Do Some Products Not Declare Trans Fat on Their Labels?

There may be two reasons why you are not seeing trans fat on a product's label.

First, products entering interstate commerce on or after January 1, 2006, must be labeled with trans fat. As this is happening, FDA realizes that it will take some time for food products to move through the distribution chain to a store shelf. Thus, it may take a few months for products that are listing trans fat on their label to show up on a store shelf. However, you will see many products with trans fat listed since companies have already begun to declare trans fat on their products' labels.

Second, FDA has granted enforcement discretion to some firms to use old label stock that do not declare trans fat after the effective date of January 1, 2006. In these cases, food firms followed the required process described in FDA's Guidance for Industry and FDA: Requesting an Extension to Use Existing Label Stock After the Trans Fat Labeling Effective Date of January 1, 2006 (Revised). For each request, FDA is considering whether the declared label value for trans fat is 0.5 g or less per serving. This information is important because lower amounts of trans fat would have less impact on public health than higher amounts of trans fat. Thus, trans fat information in the Nutrition Facts panel will be missing on some products (that contain lower amounts of trans fat) throughout the next year.

If trans fat is not declared on the label and you are curious about the trans fat content of a product, contact the manufacturer listed on the label.

## How Do Your Choices Stack Up?

With the addition of trans fat to the Nutrition Facts panel, you can review your food choices and see how they stack

*(Continues)*

up. The following labels illustrate total fat, saturated fat, trans fat, and cholesterol content per serving for selected food products.

Don't assume similar products are the same. Be sure to check the Nutrition Facts panel (NFP) when comparing products because even similar foods can vary in calories, ingredients, nutrients, and the size and number of servings in the package. When buying the same brand product, also check the NFP frequently because ingredients can change at any time and any change could affect the NFP information.

Look at the highlighted items on the sample labels. Combine the grams (g) of saturated fat and trans fat and look for the lowest combined amount. Also, look for the lowest percent (%) Daily Value for cholesterol. Check all three nutrients to make the best choice for a healthful diet.

Note: The following label examples do not represent a single product or an entire product category. In general, the nutrient values were combined for several products and the average values were used for these label examples.

## How Can I Use the Label to Make Heart-Healthy Food Choices?

The Nutrition Facts panel can help you choose foods lower in saturated fat, trans fat, and cholesterol. To lower your intake of saturated fat, trans fat, and cholesterol, compare similar foods and choose the food with the lower combined saturated and trans fats and the lower amount of cholesterol.

*Source:* Food and Drug Administration. (2011, June 24). *Trans* fat now listed with saturated fat and cholesterol on the Nutrition Facts label. Retrieved October 11, 2011, from http://www.fda.gov/Food/LabelingNutrition/ConsumerInformation/ucm109832.htm.

## Compare Spreads!*

Keep an eye on saturated fat, trans fat, and cholesterol!

### Butter**

**Nutrition Facts**

Serving Size 1 Tbsp (14g)
Servings Per Container 32

**Amount Per Serving**

**Calories** 100          Calories from Fat 100

% Daily Value*

**Total Fat** 11g          17%

  Saturated Fat 7g ←          35%

  *Trans* Fat 0g ←

**Cholesterol** 30mg          → 10%

| Saturated Fat : | 7 g |
| + *Trans* Fat : | 0 g |
| Combined Amt. : | 7 g |
| Cholesterol : | 10 % DV |

### Margarine, stick†

**Nutrition Facts**

Serving Size 1 Tbsp (14g)
Servings Per Container 32

**Amount Per Serving**

**Calories** 100          Calories from Fat 100

% Daily Value*

**Total Fat** 11g          17%

  Saturated Fat 2g ←          10%

  *Trans* Fat 3g ←

**Cholesterol** 0mg          → 0%

| Saturated Fat : | 2 g |
| + *Trans* Fat : | 3 g |
| Combined Amt. : | 5 g |
| Cholesterol : | 0 % DV |

### Margarine, tub†

**Nutrition Facts**

Serving Size 1 Tbsp (14g)
Servings Per Container 32

**Amount Per Serving**

**Calories** 60          Calories from Fat 60

% Daily Value*

**Total Fat** 7g          11%

  Saturated Fat 1g ←          5%

  *Trans* Fat 0.5g ←

**Cholesterol** 0mg          → 0%

| Saturated Fat : | 1 g |
| + *Trans* Fat : | 0.5 g |
| Combined Amt. : | 1.5 g |
| Cholesterol : | 0 % DV |

*Nutrient values rounded based on FDA's nutrition labeling regulations. Calorie and cholesterol content estimated.

**Butter values from FDA Table of Trans Values, 1/30/95.

†Values derived from 2002 USDA National Nutrient Database for Standard Reference, Release 15.

## Compare Desserts!*

Keep an eye on saturated fat, trans fat, and cholesterol!

### Granola Bar±

**Nutrition Facts**

Serving Size 1 bar (33g)
Servings Per Container 10

Amount Per Serving

**Calories** 140     Calories from Fat 45

% Daily Value*

**Total Fat** 5g     8%

Saturated Fat 1g ←     5%

Trans Fat 0g ←

**Cholesterol** 0mg → 0%

Saturated Fat :     1 g
+ Trans Fat :     0 g
Combined Amt. :     1 g
Cholesterol : 0 % DV

### Sandwich Cookies±

**Nutrition Facts**

Serving Size 2 cookies (28g)
Servings Per Container 19

Amount Per Serving

**Calories** 130     Calories from Fat 45

% Daily Value*

**Total Fat** 5g     8%

Saturated Fat 1g ←     5%

Trans Fat 1.5g ←

**Cholesterol** 0mg → 0%

Saturated Fat :     1 g
+ Trans Fat :     1.5 g
Combined Amt. :     2.5g
Cholesterol : 0 % DV

### Cake, Iced and Filled±

**Nutrition Facts**

Serving Size 2 cakes (66g)
Servings Per Container 6

Amount Per Serving

**Calories** 280     Calories from Fat 140

% Daily Value*

**Total Fat** 16g     25%

Saturated Fat 3.5g ←     18%

Trans Fat 4.5g ←

**Cholesterol** 10mg → 3%

Saturated Fat :     3.5g
+ Trans Fat :     4.5g
Combined Amt. :     8 g
Cholesterol : 3 % DV

*Nutrient values rounded based on FDA's nutrition labeling regulations.

±Values for total fat, saturated fat, and trans fat were based on the means of analytical data for several food samples from Subramaniam, S., et al., "Trans, saturated, and unsaturated fat in foods in the United States prior to mandatory trans-fat labeling," *Lipids* 39:11–18, 2004. Other information and values were derived from food labels in the marketplace.

## Compare Snacks!*

Keep an eye on saturated fat, trans fat, and cholesterol!

### Frozen Potatoes± (e.g., French Fries)

**Nutrition Facts**

Serving Size 3 oz (84g/ about 12 pieces)
Servings Per Container 11

Amount Per Serving

**Calories** 160     Calories from Fat 50

% Daily Value*

**Total Fat** 6g     9%

Saturated Fat 1g ←     5%

Trans Fat 1.5g ←

**Cholesterol** 0mg → 0%

Saturated Fat :     1 g
+ Trans Fat :     1.5g
Combined Amt. :     2.5g
Cholesterol : 0 % DV

### Potato Chips±

**Nutrition Facts**

Serving Size 1 oz (28g/ about 20 chips)
Servings Per Container 12

Amount Per Serving

**Calories** 150     Calories from Fat 90

% Daily Value*

**Total Fat** 10g     15%

Saturated Fat 2g ←     10%

Trans Fat 0g ←

**Cholesterol** 0mg → 0%

Saturated Fat :     2 g
+ Trans Fat :     0 g
Combined Amt. :     2 g
Cholesterol : 0 % DV

### Mini-Sandwich Crackers±

**Nutrition Facts**

Serving Size 14 pieces (31g)
Servings Per Container 10

Amount Per Serving

**Calories** 160     Calories from Fat 70

% Daily Value*

**Total Fat** 8g     12%

Saturated Fat 2g ←     10%

Trans Fat 2g ←

**Cholesterol** < 5mg → 1%

Saturated Fat :     2 g
+ Trans Fat :     2 g
Combined Amt. :     4 g
Cholesterol : 1 % DV

*Nutrient values rounded based on FDA's nutrition labeling regulations.

±Values for total fat, saturated fat, and trans fat were based on the means of analytical data for several food samples from Subramaniam, S., et al., "Trans, saturated, and unsaturated fat in foods in the United States prior to mandatory trans-fat labeling," *Lipids* 39:11–18, 2004. Other information and values were derived from food labels in the marketplace.

# CHAPTER REVIEW

## Summary

The leading cause of death in the United States is a noninfectious disease: coronary artery disease (CAD). In CAD, the arteries that supply blood to the heart become blocked, restricting blood flow. CAD is only one disease of the cardiovascular system; hypertension, stroke, and rheumatic heart disease are three other prominent cardiovascular diseases. Atherosclerosis is an important cardiovascular disease process that is an underlying cause of CAD and stroke.

The cardiovascular system includes the heart and blood vessels. The heart, a muscular, fist-sized organ, pumps blood to the body. The blood performs many functions, such as bringing nutrients and oxygen to the tissues and removing wastes, including the waste gas carbon dioxide. Blood vessels called arteries bring blood away from the heart; veins return blood to the heart. Microscopic vessels called capillaries join the two and allow the exchange of nutrients, gases, and wastes at the tissues.

Fatty deposits develop in arteries as part of a disease called atherosclerosis. Atherosclerosis occurs most frequently in the arteries supplying blood to the heart, brain, and legs. In coronary artery disease, the coronary arteries, which supply the heart muscle with blood, become blocked by fatty deposits, a blood clot, or both. When the heart is deprived of the blood (and therefore the oxygen) that it needs, chest pain (angina pectoris) or a heart attack results. A physician usually performs diagnostic tests to assess the degree and location of blockage. Medication can help widen blood vessels and reduce symptoms.

During a heart attack, part of the heart muscle dies. As the muscle dies, it may trigger electrical activity that causes the ventricles to stop beating properly, possibly resulting in heart failure, cardiac arrest, and death. A heart attack victim needs immediate medical care.

A stroke occurs when arteries that supply blood to the brain become blocked by fatty deposits or by a blood clot. A stroke may cause a loss or dimming of vision, difficulty in speaking or understanding speech, headache, dizziness, unsteadiness, and even death.

The major risk factors for developing cardiovascular disease are family history, abnormal blood lipid levels, cigarette smoking, high blood pressure, physical inactivity, obesity, diabetes mellitus, and stress. Behaviors that may lower the risk of cardiovascular disease are stopping smoking, controlling weight, exercising, lowering the blood pressure, maintaining favorable blood lipid levels, managing diabetes mellitus to stabilize the blood glucose level, and coping effectively with stress.

Infants may be born with a wide variety of heart and blood vessel structural and functional abnormalities. Many of these congenital defects can now be diagnosed before birth and treated during the first few weeks of life.

Cardiovascular disease caused by atherosclerosis may begin in childhood. American children are still consuming diets that promote cardiovascular disease. Healthy school meal programs can help change this fact, and education can promote healthy lifestyles.

Data suggest that physicians should treat abnormal lipid levels and high blood pressure in older adults.

# Applying What You Have Learned

**Critical Thinking**

1. If a family member experienced a transient ischemic attack, how would you recognize it? What would you do? What long-term action might this family member take to avoid the onset of a stroke? **Analysis**

2. Analyze your lifestyle to determine which modifiable risk factors are raising your probability of developing cardiovascular disease. List these risk factors. **Analysis**

3. Using the list you developed by answering question 2, describe how you could modify your behavior to lower your risk of developing cardiovascular disease. **Synthesis**

4. List all of your risk factors for developing cardiovascular disease, both those you can change and those you cannot. Using the information from answer 3, evaluate your course of action. Which changes do you realistically expect to make and which do you expect not to make? Give rationales for your answers. If you follow this plan, do you think that you will substantially reduce your risk of developing CVD? Why or why not? **Evaluation**

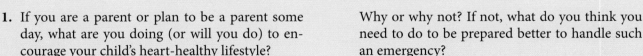

**Analysis**
breaking down information into component parts.

**Synthesis**
putting together information from different sources.

**Evaluation**
making informed decisions.

**Key**

# Reflecting on Your Health

**Critical Thinking**

1. If you are a parent or plan to be a parent some day, what are you doing (or will you do) to encourage your child's heart-healthy lifestyle?

2. If you are a cigarette smoker, do you think your risk for cardiovascular disease is affected by your habit? After learning about the effects of smoking on cardiovascular health, are you willing to quit? If not, discuss the reasons behind your answer and explain why you are willing to risk your health to continue smoking. If you are a nonsmoker, list the situations in which you regularly breathe second-hand smoke. Reflect on what you believe to be your increased risk of cardiovascular disease because of your exposure. What can you do to lessen your exposure?

3. Do you feel confident that you would be able to recognize when another person is having a stroke, TIA, or heart attack and help him or her?

Why or why not? If not, what do you think you need to do to be prepared better to handle such an emergency?

4. Rate your lifestyle on a scale of 1 to 10, with 1 being an extremely heart-unhealthy lifestyle and 10 being an extremely heart-healthy lifestyle. Why did you rate your lifestyle as you did? Based on what you read in this chapter, what changes can you make to move closer to a 10 if you're not already there?

5. Do you think medical researchers are able to assess accurately the factors that are detrimental or helpful to cardiovascular health? Why do you feel this way? How do you think your attitudes concerning medical research affect your behavior? Have your attitudes about medical research and cardiovascular health changed since reading this chapter? Why or why not?

# References

1. Tailor, A. M., et al. (2010). An update on the prevalence of the metabolic syndrome in children and adolescents. *International Journal of Pediatric Obesity, 5*(3):202–213.

2. Zieske, A. W., et al. (2002). Natural history and risk factors of atherosclerosis in children and youth: The PDAY study. *Pediatric Pathology and Molecular Medicine, 21*:213–237.

3. Roberts, C. K., et al. (2007). Effect of a short-term diet and exercise intervention in youth on atherosclerotic risk factors. *Atherosclerosis, 191*:98–106.

4. Collins, K. M., et al. (2004). Heart disease awareness among college students. *Journal of Community Health, 29*(5):405–420.

5. Kostas, T. I., et al. (2010). Chronic venous disease progression and modification of predisposing factors. *Journal of Vascular Surgery, 51*(4):900–907.

6. American Heart Association. (2011). Heart disease and stroke statistics—2011 update. *Circulation, 123*:e1–e192. Retrieved on April 5, 2011, from http://circ.ahajournals.org/cgi/reprint/CIR.0b013e3182009701

7. Leuzzi, C., & Modena, M. G. (2010). Coronary artery disease: Clinical presentation, diagnosis and prognosis in women. *Nutrition, Metabolism, and Cardiovascular Diseases, 20*(6):426–435.

8. Wessely, R. (2010). New drug-eluting stent concepts. *Nature Reviews Cardiology, 7*(4):194–203.

9. Garg, S., & Serruys, P. (2009). Biodegradable stents and non-biodegradable stents. *Minerva Cardioangiologica, 57*(5):537–565.

10. Pratali, S., et al. (2010). Transmyocardial laser revascularization 12 years later. *Interactive Cardiovascular and Thoracic Surgery, 11*(4):480–481.

11. National Institutes of Health. (2010). Cardiogenic shock. Retrieved April 6, 2011, from http://www.nlm.nih.gov/medlineplus/ency/article/000185.htm

12. Elijovich, L., & Chong, J. Y. (2010). Current and future use of intravenous thrombolysis for acute ischemic stroke. *Current Atherosclerosis Reports, 12*(5):316–321.

13. Associated Press. (2011, February 10). Strokes are rising fast among young, middle-aged. Retrieved on April 6, 2011, from http://www.npr.org/templates/story/story.php?storyId=133624707

14. American Heart Association. (2009). *Heart disease and stroke statistics—2009 update.* Dallas, TX: Author. Retrieved on April 7, 2011, from http://circ.ahajournals.org/content/119/3/e21.extract

15. Mosca, L., et al. (2007). Evidence-based guidelines for cardiovascular disease prevention in women: 2007 update. *Circulation, 115*:1481–1501.

16. Spillmann, F., et al. (2010). High-density lipoprotein-raising strategies: Update 2010. *Current Pharmaceutical Design, 16*(13):1517–1530.

17. U.S. Department of Health and Human Services. (2001). *Women and smoking: A report of the Surgeon General.* Atlanta, GA: U.S. Department of Health and Human Services, Centers for Disease Control and Prevention, National Center for Chronic Disease Prevention and Health Promotion. Retrieved on April 7, 2011, from http://www.surgeongeneral.gov/library/womenandtobacco/index.html

18. U.S. Department of Health and Human Services. (2010). *How tobacco smoke causes disease: The biology and behavioral basis for smoking-attributable disease: A report of the Surgeon General.* Atlanta, GA: Author. Retrieved on April 3, 2011, from http://www.surgeongeneral.gov/library/tobaccosmoke/report/full_report.pdf

19. American Heart Association. *Cigarette smoking and cardiovascular diseases: AHA scientific position.* Retrieved on October 4, 2011, from http://www.youngchoices.org/index.php?option=com_content&view=article&id=63:cigarette-smoking-and-cardiovascular-diseases-&catid=40:tobacco-information&Itemid=75

20. U.S. Department of Health and Human Services. (2006). *The health consequences of involuntary exposure to tobacco smoke: A report of the Surgeon General.* Atlanta, GA: Centers for Disease Control and Prevention, National Center for Chronic Disease Prevention and Health Promotion, Office on Smoking and Health. Retrieved on April 7, 2011, from http://www.surgeongeneral.gov/library/secondhandsmoke/report/fullreport.pdf

21. National Center for Health Statistics. (2011). *Health, United States, 2010.* Hyattsville, MD: Author. Retrieved on April 7, 2011, from http://www.cdc.gov/nchs/data/hus/hus10.pdf

22. Mayo Clinic Staff. (2011). High blood pressure (hypertension): Risk factors. Retrieved on April 7, 2011, from http://www.mayoclinic.com/health/high-blood-pressure/DS00100/DSECTION=risk-factors

23. Katzmarzyk, P. T., et al. (2009). Sitting time and mortality from all causes, cardiovascular disease, and cancer. *Medicine & Science in Sports & Exercise, 41*(5):998–1005

24. U.S. Department of Health and Human Services. (1996). *Physical activity and health: A report of the Surgeon General.* Atlanta, GA: U.S. Department of Health and Human Services, Centers for Disease Control and Prevention, National Center for Chronic Disease Prevention and Health Promotion. Retrieved on April 7, 2011, from http://www.cdc.gov/NCCDPHP/sgr/pdf/sgrfull.pdf

25. Centers for Disease Control and Prevention. (2011). Physical activity for everyone. Retrieved on April 7, 2011, from http://www.cdc.gov/physicalactivity/everyone/health/index.html#ReduceCardiovascularDisease

26. U.S. Department of Health and Human Services. (2008). *Physical activity and good nutrition: Essential elements to prevent chronic diseases and obesity 2008.* Atlanta, GA: Centers for Disease Control and Prevention, National Center for Chronic Disease Prevention and Health Promotion. Retrieved on April 7, 2011, from http://www.cdc.gov/nccdphp/publications/aag/pdf/dnpa.pdf

27. Katerndahl, D. A. (2008). The association between panic disorder and coronary artery disease among primary care patients presenting with chest pain: An updated literature review. *Primary Care Companion to the Journal of Clinical Psychiatry, 10*:276–285.

28. Zakynthinos, E., & Pappa, N. (2009). Inflammatory biomarkers in coronary artery disease. *Journal of Cardiology, 53*(3):317–333.

29. U.S. Department of Agriculture and U.S. Department of Health and Human Services. (2010, December). *Dietary Guidelines for Americans, 2010* (7th ed.). Washington, DC: U.S. Government Printing

Office. Retrieved on April 11, 2011, from http://www.health.gov/dietaryguidelines/dga2010/DietaryGuidelines2010.pdf

30. King, D. E., et al. (2007). Turning back the clock: Adopting a healthy lifestyle in middle age. *American Journal of Medicine, 120*:598–603.

31. King, D. E., et al. (2009). Adherence to healthy lifestyle habits in U.S. adults, 1988–2006. *American Journal of Medicine, 122*(6):528–534.

32. American Heart Association. Smoke-free living: Benefits and milestones. Retrieved on October 11, 2011, from http://www.heart.org/HEARTORG/GettingHealthy/QuitSmoking/QuittingSmoking/Why-Quit-Smoking_UCM_307847_Article.jsp

33. Powell, K., et al. (1987). Physical activity and the incidence of coronary heart disease. *Annual Review of Public Health, 8*:253–287.

34. Galimanis, A., et al. (2009). Lifestyle and stroke risk: A review. *Current Opinion in Neurology, 22*:60–68.

35. American Heart Association. (2011, January 19). American Heart Association Guidelines. Retrieved on April 11, 2011, from http://www.heart.org/HEARTORG/GettingHealthy/PhysicalActivity/GettingActive/American-Heart-Association-Guidelines_UCM_307976_Article.jsp

36. American Heart Association. (2011, January 31). American Heart Association supports the new USDA/HHS dietary guidelines and encourages adherence. AHA also expresses disappointment that sodium, saturated fat guidance is weak. Retrieved on April 11, 2011, from http://newsroom.heart.org/pr/aha/1243.aspx

37. Appel, L. J., et al. (2006). Dietary approaches to prevent and treat hypertension: A scientific statement from the American Heart Association. *Hypertension, 47*:291–308.

38. American Heart Association. Know your fats. Retrieved on October 11, 2011, from http://www.heart.org/HEARTORG/Conditions/Cholesterol/PreventionTreatmentofHighCholesterol/Know-Your-Fats_UCM_305628_Article.jsp

39. American Heart Association. (2011, January 24). Whole grains and fiber. Retrieved on April 12, 2011, from http://www.heart.org/HEARTORG/GettingHealthy/NutritionCenter/HealthyDietGoals/Whole-Grains-and-Fiber_UCM_303249_Article.jsp

40. Taylor, F., et al. (2011). Statins for the primary prevention of cardiovascular disease. *Cochrane Database of Systematic Reviews, 19*(1): CD004816.

41. Wolff, T., et al. (2009). Aspirin for the primary prevention of cardiovascular events: An update of the evidence for the U.S. Preventive Services Task Force. *Annals of Internal Medicine, 150*(6):405–410.

42. Writing Group for the Women's Health Initiative Investigators. (2011). Health outcomes after stopping conjugated equine estrogens among postmenopausal women with prior hysterectomy. *Journal of the American Medical Association, 305*(13):1305–1314.

43. Writing Group for the Women's Health Initiative Investigators. (2008). Health risks and benefits 3 years after stopping randomized treatment with estrogen and progestin. *Journal of the American Medical Association, 299*(9):1036–1045.

44. Women's Health Initiative Participant Website. (2007, April). Postmenopausal hormone therapy and risk of cardiovascular disease by age and years since menopause. Retrieved on April 13, 2011, from http://www.whi.org/findings/ht/cvd.php

45. American Heart Association. About congenital cardiovascular defects. Retrieved on October 4, 2011, http://www.heart.org/HEARTORG/Conditions/CongenitalHeartDefects/AboutCongenitalHeartDefects/About-Congenital-Heart-Defects_UCM_001217_Article.jsp

46. Tulane University School of Medicine, Center for Cardiovascular Health. The Bogalusa Heart Study. Retrieved on April 13, 2011, from http://tulane.edu/som/cardiohealth/index.cfm

47. Nicklas, T. A., et al. (2001). Trends in nutrient intake of 10-year-old children over two decades (1973–1994): The Bogalusa Heart Study. *American Journal of Epidemiology, 153*:969–977.

48. Clark, M. A., & Fox, M. K. (2009). Nutritional quality of the diets of U.S. public school children and the role of the school meal programs. *Journal of the American Dietetic Association, 109*(2 Suppl): S44–56.

49. Pohlel, K., Grow, P., Helmy, T., & Wenger, N. K. (2006). Treating dyslipidemia in the elderly. *Current Opinion in Lipidology, 17*:54–57.

50. Pinto, E. (2007). Blood pressure and aging. *Postgraduate Medical Journal, 83*:109–114.

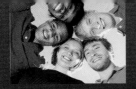

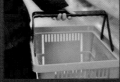

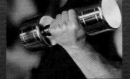

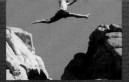

## Diversity in Health

Stomach Cancer: Variation in Mortality Among Countries

## Consumer Health

Alternative Cancer Therapies

## Managing Your Health

Screening Guidelines for the Early Detection of Cancer in Average-Risk Asymptomatic People | Breast Self-Examination | Testicular Self-Examination | Reducing Your Risk for Cancer | Cancer's Seven Warning Signs

## Across the Life Span

Cancer

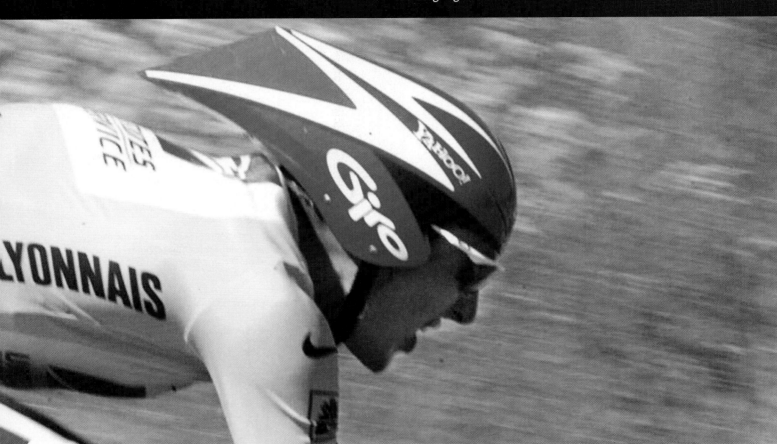

## Chapter Overview

What is cancer?

How cancers develop and spread

How physicians detect cancer

How cancer is treated

Which cancers are the most prevalent in the United States

How you can reduce your risk for cancer

## Student Workbook

Self-Assessment: What Are Your Cancer Risks?

Changing Health Habits: Modifying Behavior to Reduce Cancer Risk

## Do You Know?

What the most prevalent cancer is for your age group?

What you can do to lower your risk of cancer?

Which cancers are on the rise?

## CHAPTER 13

# Cancer

"By winning the Tour, you stick in the minds and hearts of the cycling public. You can win every classic and the world championship, but the Tour is everything. It's a global event."[1]

These words were uttered to newspaper reporters by Lance Armstrong, the second American to win the Tour de France and the only person to win the Tour seven times. Armstrong officially retired from competitive cycling in February 2011, but on that clear sunny day in July 1999, he won more than this most rigorous and prestigious 3-week cycling race. He showed the world that he had truly won his battle with testicular cancer—a battle that had nearly cost him not only his career but also his life. His cancer, diagnosed in 1996, had spread to his lungs and brain, but aggressive chemotherapy helped his body win the war against this dreaded disease.

> "Many cancers can be cured, especially those detected early."

For years, questions about Armstrong's use of performance-enhancing drugs cast a shadow of doubt over his wins. Armstrong vigorously denied the accusations. In 2012, he ended his battle to defend his titles with the U.S. Anti-Doping Agency.

Armstrong won the Tour de France each year from 1999 through 2005. Then at age 37, after a 4-year hiatus from biking competition, Armstrong entered the 2009 Tour to promote his cancer-support foundation Lives-

**metastasize** (meh-TAS-tah-size) The ability of cancer cells to spread from where they develop to another part of the body.

**malignant (mah-LIG-nant) tumors** Masses of cancer cells that invade body tissues and interfere with the normal functioning of tissues and organs.

**mutations** (myou-TAY-shunz) Changes in genes or chromosomes; damaged genes.

**oncogenes** (ONG-ko-geenz) Tumor genes that manufacture altered proteins that speed cell growth and decrease the level of cell differentiation.

**tumor-suppressor genes** Pieces of hereditary material that slow cell growth; anti-oncogenes.

Cells are the building blocks of all organisms; they are the smallest unit of living material. In any multi-celled organism such as humans, cells divide and differentiate as an individual grows and develops, and when its tissues need repair. The timing and events of cell division, growth, and differentiation are highly controlled by regulatory proteins. Cells make regulatory proteins in response to the instructions of the hereditary material, or genes. Normal cells are programmed to grow and divide, and to stop growing and dividing at appropriate times.

Unlike normal cells, cancer cells do not stop growing and dividing at appropriate times. Additionally, cancer cells do not differentiate normally and tend to spread. These cells may form masses called **malignant tumors** that invade body tissues and interfere with the normal functioning of tissues and organs. Tumors often cause pain as they invade nerves or press on nerves. Why do cancer cells behave differently from noncancer cells? The answer lies in the genetic material in the cell.

## How Cancers Develop and Spread

Cancer develops only in cells that have **mutations**, that is, damaged genes. Mutations can be inherited or can occur from exposure to low-dose radiation, drugs, or toxic chemicals. Infection with certain viruses can also cause changes in genes. Excluding inheritance, then, cancer is determined largely by environmental factors, including components of lifestyle. Lifestyle factors play a major role in cancer prevention.

### Genes and Cancer Development

**Oncogenes** are "on" switches that speed cell growth. Successive mutations to the hereditary material of particular body cells produce oncogenes. **Tumor-suppressor genes** are "off" switches that slow cell growth. If tumor-suppressor genes mutate or are lost from the hereditary makeup of a cell, they will no longer restrict cell growth.

The activation of oncogenes and deactivation of tumor-suppressor genes (and, therefore, the development of cancer) is a multistage process. In other words, successive genetic changes must take place for a normal cell to change into a cancer cell. These changes take place over time as various environmen-

trong. He finished third on the Tour. At the time of Armstrong's retirement in 2011, International Cycling Union President Pat McQuaid referred to Armstrong as "the global icon for cycling."[2]

Although it is still the nation's second biggest killer (cardiovascular disease is the first), cancer is not an automatic death sentence. Armstrong and other cancer survivors, such as former Major League Baseball pitcher Dave Dravecky, pro football Hall of Famer Len Dawson, and American figure skater and gold-medal Olympian Peggy Fleming are living testimony to that fact. Many cancers can be cured, especially those detected early. Even cancers in advanced stages, as was Armstrong's, may respond to therapies available today.

Cancer researchers are making discoveries daily that help win the war against cancer. A tremendous body of research is available that provides guidelines to help people avoid cancer, and people can take many actions to lessen their risk of developing certain cancers. This chapter discusses such preventive measures.

## What Is Cancer?

People often talk about cancer as if it were a single disease. However, cancer is many diseases. Lung cancer, for example, is a very different disease from leukemia (cancer of the blood) or skin cancer. Although different, all cancers have common characteristics: Their cells exhibit abnormal growth, division, and differentiation. Differentiation is the process by which cells develop into certain types, such as liver cells or muscle cells. In addition, cancer cells have the potential to **metastasize**, or spread from where they develop to another part of the body.

tal factors affect cells and cause mutations. Therefore, the chances of developing cancer generally increase with age and with exposure to cancer-causing substances, or **carcinogens**. Of course, many factors determine an individual's risk for developing cancers. These factors, discussed throughout this chapter, modify this generalization.

Cells that begin to grow abnormally, although not yet cancer cells, may form growths called **benign tumors**. Surrounded by a fibrous capsule, benign tumors remain in one location; they do not invade surrounding tissues. Usually these growths are not life threatening unless their presence interferes with a vital function. For example, a benign brain tumor may be life threatening if it compresses blood vessels serv-

**carcinogens** (kar-SIN-oh-jenz) Cancer-causing substances.

**benign (be-NINE) tumors** Encapsulated masses of abnormal cells that remain in one location and do not invade surrounding tissues.

**carcinomas** KAR-si-NO-mahz) Cancers that arise from epithelial tissues.

**sarcomas** sar-KO-mahz) Cancers that arise from connective or muscle tissue.

**leukemias** (lew-KEY-me-ahz) Cancers of the blood and related cells.

## Figure 13.1

**A Comparison of Dysplastic and Normal Cells.**
(a) Dysplastic cells. These cells (stained differently from those in [b]) are irregular in size and the appearance of their nuclei. (b) Normal cells. These cells are all approximately the same size and have nuclei that look similar.

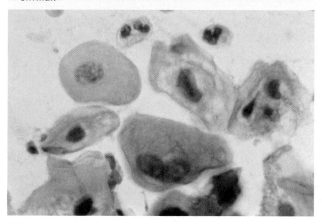

(a)

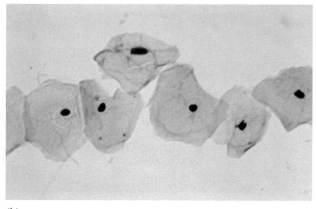

(b)

ing a vital center in the brain. In most cases benign tumors can be removed completely by surgery.

Some benign tumor cells exhibit traits that are characteristic of the development of cancer cells. These cells are said to exhibit dysplasia. Notice that the dysplastic cells in **Figure 13.1a** vary in size, shape, and the appearance of their nuclei. They are not differentiating properly into a specific type of cell. The normal cells, however, are somewhat regular in these same characteristics (**Figure 13.1b**). Dysplastic cells have the potential to develop into cancer cells.

## Metastasis

One of the characteristics of cancer cells is their ability to spread, or metastasize, from where they initially developed to other places in the body. Cells with the ability to metastasize are *malignant*. As a cancer develops, metastasis does not take place immediately. As cancer cells grow and divide, they often form a malignant tumor. At this stage the cancer is in situ (in place) because it has not invaded other tissues. However, these localized cancer cells begin to secrete chemicals that destroy the substances that hold the surrounding tissues together. When this occurs, cancer cells enter blood and lymph vessels and travel to other parts of the body. Cancerous cells can move out of the blood vessels at a distant location, enter the tissues there, and divide to form new masses of malignant cells. **Figure 13.2** shows this process of cancer cell division and metastasis. Once metastasis occurs, the cancer becomes much more difficult to control.

Cancers are named according to the type of tissue from which they develop. **Carcinomas** (which comprise most adult cancers) arise from epithelial tissue, which lines and covers internal and external body surfaces. Lung, oral, stomach, skin, breast, colon, and ovarian cancers are carcinomas. **Sarcomas** are cancers that arise from connective or muscle tissue. **Leukemias** are cancers of the blood and related cells.

**Lymphomas** are cancers of the lymphatic system, the network of vessels and nodes that transports and filters tissue fluid. Cancers of the nervous system have a variety of names.

**Figure 13.3** shows death rates (the number of persons dying per year per 100,000 people) of various cancers in the United States. Overall cancer death rates have decreased since the early 1990s.[3] Continued declines for overall cancer death rates and for many of the top cancers (see Figure 13.3) reflect progress in the prevention, early detection, and treatment of cancer.

## Cancer Detection and Staging

**Cancer screening** is an examination to detect malignancies in a person who has no symptoms. The American Cancer Society (ACS) recommends the screening procedures listed in the Managing Your Health box that follows.

Cancer screening or detection methods vary depending on the location of the possible cancer. Superficial cancers, such as cancers of the skin and oral cavity, can be detected by visual examination, or a biopsy can be performed. A **biopsy** is the removal of a small piece of tissue from a suspect area. It can be cut from the body with a scalpel or removed with a needle.

Some cancers in internal areas can be detected by collecting cells for microscopic examination. This process is possible, for example, for detecting cancer of the cervix and of the esophagus. Even mucus

---

### Figure 13.2

**How Cancer Cells Multiply and Spread.** Cancer cells secrete chemicals that destroy the substances holding tissues together. As these tissues break down, cancer cells move from their original site, enter the blood and lymph, and travel to other parts of the body.

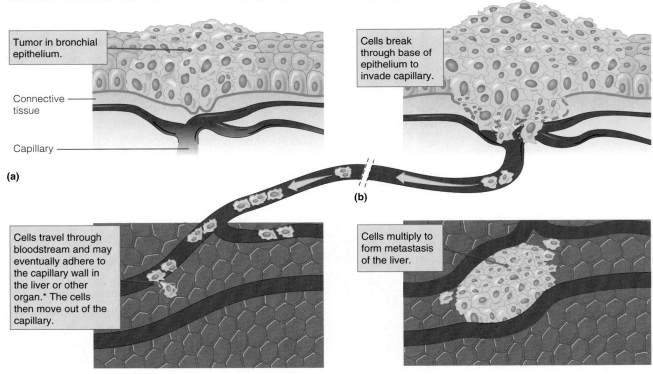

Tumor in bronchial epithelium.

Connective tissue

Capillary

**(a)**

Cells break through base of epithelium to invade capillary.

**(b)**

Cells travel through bloodstream and may eventually adhere to the capillary wall in the liver or other organ.* The cells then move out of the capillary.

Cells multiply to form metastasis of the liver.

*Less than 1 in 1,000 survive to form metastases.

**(c)**

**(d)**

**Figure 13.3**

**Cancer Death Rates, 1930–2007.** (a) Male. (b) Female.

*Source:* American Cancer Society. *Cancer Facts and Figures 2011.* Atlanta: American Cancer Society, Inc.

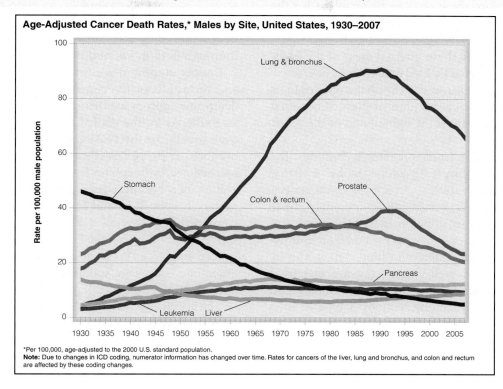

(a)

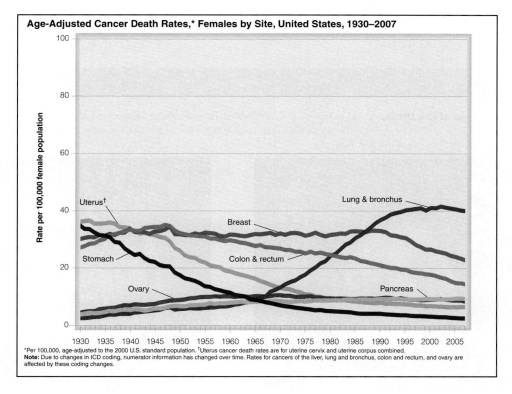

(b)

**cancer staging** A description of the extent of the growth and metastasis of a cancer to determine appropriate therapy and prognosis.

coughed up from the lungs can be analyzed for the presence of cancer. Some cancers, such as colon cancer and stomach cancer, can be detected by fiber-optic examination. To see these internal areas of the body, the physician inserts a flexible tube called a fiberscope into the area to be examined. The fiberscope contains bundles of specially coated glass or plastic fibers that transmit an image from the lighted end of the scope to an eyepiece.

X-rays are used in some screening techniques. The computed tomography (CT) colonography, or *virtual colonoscopy*, can be used to screen for colon cancer. This technique uses special x-ray equipment to create two- and three-dimensional images of the interior of the colon. Other cancers that grow embedded in tissues, such as breast cancer and lung cancer, can be detected by x-rays as well. Chest x-rays are often used for lung cancer screening, and mammograms, used for breast cancer screening, employ a type of low-dose x-ray.

PET scans and MRI can also be used to detect deeply embedded cancers, such as brain cancer. PET scans, or positron emission tomography, use small amounts of radioactive positrons (positively charged particles) to visualize body structures. MRI, or mag-netic resonance imaging, uses magnetic fields and radio waves for visualization. MRI is sometimes used in breast cancer screening (**Figure 13.4**).

Ultrasound, an imaging technique that uses sound waves, is used occasionally to detect cancerous growths. (See Chapter 5 Managing Your Health "Genetic Counseling and Prenatal Diagnosis" for a more thorough description of ultrasound.)

**Cancer staging** describes the extent of the growth and metastasis of the cancer so that physicians can determine appropriate therapy and provide a prognosis (outlook) for the patient. To stage a cancer, physicians usually use the TNM system first. T describes the original tumor, N describes whether the cancer has reached nearby lymph nodes, and M describes whether the cancer has metastasized (spread) to distant body parts. Once the T, N, and M are determined, they are combined for an overall stage. These overall stages are I, II, III, and IV, with stage I cancer being the least advanced and stage IV cancer being the most advanced. Sometimes stages are subdivided (such as stage IIB), and sometimes other staging systems are used.

The 5-year survival rate is the percentage of persons who are alive 5 years after their cancer is diagnosed, whether they are disease-free, under treatment, or in remission (having a partial or complete disappearance of the signs and symptoms of the cancer). The overall 5-year survival rate for all cancers diagnosed between 1999 and 2005 was 68%, up from 50% in the

## Figure 13.4

**PET and MRI Scans of the Brain.** In (a), a PET scan of the brain, the round blue area on the side of the brain is a benign tumor. In (b), an MRI of the brain, the round blue area toward the back of the brain is a cancerous tumor. The round structures at the front of the brain are the eyes.

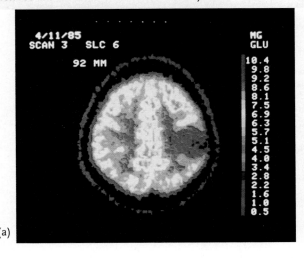

(a)

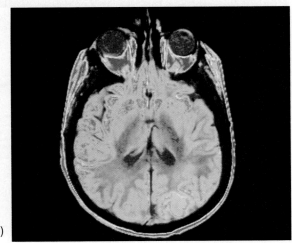

(b)

1970s.[3] **Table 13.1** shows the 5-year survival rate for cancers discussed in this chapter.

# Cancer Treatment

The principal forms of cancer treatment are surgery, radiation, and chemotherapy. Newer modes of treatment are biomodulation (immunotherapy), photodynamic therapy, antiangiogenesis therapy, and bone marrow and peripheral blood stem cell transplants. In the past, physicians referred to a cancer as "cured" if the patient survived for 5 years with no sign of the cancer returning. This is no longer the case, however, because some cancers grow after extended periods and others recur after they seem to have been eliminated. Today, the term *cure* means that all traces of a localized tumor have been removed from the body and the former cancer patient has the same life expectancy as a person who never had cancer.

## Surgery

During surgery, physicians remove a localized cancer by cutting it away from noncancerous tissue. Microscopic extensions of cancerous tissue may not be easy to detect during surgical procedures, so a physician usually removes tissue beyond the obvious cancer to increase the probability that all the cancerous tissue is removed. Although surgery is often a life-saving treatment, one drawback is that removal of healthy tissue with unhealthy tissue may impair the body's functioning or cause disfigurement. The other drawback is that surgery is futile if the cancer has spread to multiple sites in the body.

## Table 13.1

### Five-Year Survival Rates* (%) by Stage at Diagnosis, 1999–2006

| | All Stages | Local | Regional | Distant | | All Stages | Local | Regional | Distant |
|---|---|---|---|---|---|---|---|---|---|
| Breast (female) | 89 | 98 | 84 | 23 | Ovary | 46 | 94 | 73 | 28 |
| Colon & rectum | 65 | 90 | 70 | 12 | Pancreas | 6 | 23 | 9 | 2 |
| Esophagus | 17 | 37 | 19 | 3 | Prostate | 99 | 100 | 100 | 30 |
| Kidney† | 69 | 90 | 63 | 11 | Stomach | 26 | 63 | 27 | 3 |
| Larynx | 61 | 78 | 42 | 33 | Testis | 95 | 99 | 96 | 72 |
| Liver‡ | 14 | 26 | 9 | 3 | Thyroid | 97 | 100 | 97 | 58 |
| Lung & bronchus | 16 | 53 | 24 | 4 | Urinary bladder | 79 | 73 | 36 | 6 |
| Melanoma of the skin | 91 | 98 | 62 | 16 | Uterine cervix | 70 | 91 | 58 | 17 |
| Oral cavity & pharynx | 61 | 83 | 55 | 32 | Uterine corpus | 83 | 96 | 68 | 17 |

*Rates are adjusted for normal life expectancy and are based on cases diagnosed in the SEER (Surveillance, Epidemiology, and End Results Program) 17 areas from 1999–2006, followed through 2007.

†Includes renal pelvis. ‡Includes intrahepatic bile duct.

**Local:** an invasive malignant cancer confined entirely to the organ of origin. **Regional:** a malignant cancer that 1) has extended beyond the limits of the organ of origin directly into surrounding organs or tissues; 2) involves regional lymph nodes by way of lymphatic system; or 3) has both regional extension and involvement of regional lymph nodes. **Distant:** a malignant cancer that has spread to parts of the body remote from the primary tumor either by direct extension or by discontinuous metastasis to distant organs, tissues, or via the lymphatic system to distant lymph nodes.

*Source:* American Cancer Society. *Cancer Facts and Figures 2011.* Atlanta: American Cancer Society, Inc.

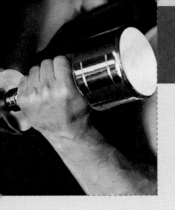

# Managing Your Health

## Screening Guidelines for the Early Detection of Cancer in Average-Risk Asymptomatic People

| Cancer Site | Population | Test or Procedure | Frequency |
|---|---|---|---|
| Breast | Women, age 20+ | Breast self-examination | Beginning in their early 20s, women should be told about the benefits and limitations of breast self-examination (BSE). The importance of prompt reporting of any new breast symptoms to a health professional should be emphasized. Women who choose to do BSE should receive instruction and have their technique reviewed on the occasion of a periodic health examination. It is acceptable for women to choose not to do BSE or to do BSE irregularly. |
| | | Clinical breast examination | For women in their 20s and 30s, it is recommended that clinical breast examination (CBE) be part of a periodic health examination, preferably at least every 3 years. Asymptomatic women aged 40 and over should continue to receive a clinical breast examination as part of a periodic health examination, preferably annually. |
| | | Mammography | Begin annual mammography at age 40.* |
| Colorectal[†] | Men and women, age 50+ | *Tests that find polyps and cancer:* | |
| | | Flexible sigmoidoscopy,[§] or | Every 5 years, starting at age 50 |
| | | Colonoscopy, or | Every 10 years, starting at age 50 |
| | | Double-contrast barium enema (DCBE),[§] or | Every 5 years, starting at age 50 |
| | | CT colonography (virtual colonoscopy)[§] | Every 5 years, starting at age 50 |
| | | *Tests that mainly find cancer:* | |
| | | Fecal occult blood test (FOBT) with at least 50% test sensitivity for cancer, or fecal immunochemical test (FIT) with at least 50% test sensitivity for cancer[§,‡] or | Annual, starting at age 50 |

| Cancer Site | Population | Test or Procedure | Frequency |
|---|---|---|---|
| | | Stool DNA test (sDNA)[§] | Interval uncertain, starting at age 50 |
| Prostate | Men, age 50+ | Prostate-specific antigen test (PSA) with or without digital rectal exam (DRE). | Asymptomatic men who have at least a 10-year life expectancy should have an opportunity to make an informed decision with their healthcare provider about screening for prostate cancer after receiving information about the uncertainties, risks, and potential benefits associated with screening. Men at average risk should receive this information beginning at age 50. Men at higher risk, including African American men and men with a first degree relative (father or brother) diagnosed with prostate cancer before age 65, should receive this information beginning at age 45. Men at appreciably higher risk (multiple family members diagnosed with prostate cancer before age 65) should receive this information beginning at age 40. |
| Cervix | Women, age 18+ | Pap test | Cervical cancer screening should begin approximately 3 years after a woman begins having vaginal intercourse, but no later than 21 years of age. Screening should be done every year with conventional Pap tests or every 2 years using liquid-based Pap tests. At or after age 30, women who have had three normal test results in a row may get screened every 2 to 3 years with cervical cytology (either conventional or liquid-based Pap test) alone, or every 3 years with an HPV DNA test plus cervical cytology. Women 70 years of age and older who have had three or more normal Pap tests and no abnormal Pap tests in the past 10 years and women who have had a total hysterectomy may choose to stop cervical cancer screening. |
| Endometrial | Women, at menopause | At the time of menopause, women at average risk should be informed about risks and symptoms of endometrial cancer and strongly encouraged to report any unexpected bleeding or spotting to their physicians. | |
| Cancer-related checkup | Men and women, age 20+ | On the occasion of a periodic health examination, the cancer-related checkup should include examination for cancers of the thyroid, testicles, ovaries, lymph nodes, oral cavity, and skin, as well as health counseling about tobacco, sun exposure, diet and nutrition, risk factors, sexual practices, and environmental and occupational exposures. | |

*Beginning at age 40, annual clinical breast examination should be performed prior to mammography.

†Individuals with a personal or family history of colorectal cancer or adenomas, inflammatory bowel disease, or high-risk genetic syndromes should continue to follow the most recent recommendations for individuals at increased or high risk.

‡For FOBT or FIT used as a screening test, the take-home multiple sample method should be used. A FOBT or FIT done during a digital rectal exam in the doctor's office is not adequate for screening.

§Colonoscopy should be done if test results are positive.

¶Information should be provided to men about the benefits and limitations of testing so that an informed decision about testing can be made with the clinician's assistance.

*Source:* American Cancer Society. *Cancer Prevention & Early Detection Cancer Facts and Figures 2010.* Atlanta: American Cancer Society, Inc.

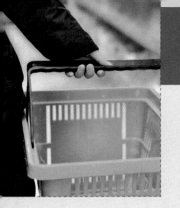

# Consumer Health

## Alternative Cancer Therapies

Modern medicine has its limitations; not every condition can be prevented, managed, or cured. It is not surprising, therefore, that some individuals who are diagnosed with incurable conditions seek help from anyone who offers a cure. Cancer patients who seek alternative therapies also hope to find a "soft-er" treatment with fewer side effects. Many want to use a holistic approach or take charge of their health when conventional medicine offers no more options. When faced with a potentially life-threatening illness such as cancer, most people feel the need to do everything possible to survive.

Most users of alternative cancer therapies expect their treatments to boost their immune system or slow the progression of or cure their cancer. However, the effectiveness of most alternative therapies in cancer treatment has not been established in scientific studies. Additionally, cancer patients erroneously perceive alternative therapies as safe because they are "natural," but therapies such as herbal and vitamin supplements may interact in dangerous ways with drugs or therapies being used in conventional cancer treatment. Many have serious side effects of their own. And if cancer patients delay conventional treatment in favor of unconventional treatment, they may diminish their chances of survival, spend money needlessly, and lower their quality of life.

Herbal therapies, plant extracts, and therapeutic vitamins are the most common alternative therapies in cancer treatment today, and up to 45% of cancer patients use some form of alternative treatment. A few of the more popular of these therapies are discussed on the next page. The greatest danger with the use of substances not controlled by the Food and Drug Administration (FDA) in cancer treatment is the risk of contamination, misidentification, or substitution with a harmful substance because of lack of quality control.

If you or someone you know is thinking about using alternative therapies for cancer treatment, remember that it is important to evaluate all evidence about these methods carefully and make decisions with a cancer physician (oncologist). At the least, informing the physician about other therapies being used can help avoid adverse drug interactions. Also, in evaluating therapies, remember that any remedy used by a large number of people will, by chance, be used by a long-term survivor. In many cases, the patient used conventional treatments as well as alternative ones. However, the alternative method often gets the credit even though there is no evidence to show that it played a role in the patient's long-term survival.

### Figure 13.A

**Plant Extracts Are a Common Type of Alternative Cancer Therapy.** (a) *Astragalus membranaceus.* An extract of this plant is used to produce Huang ch'i.

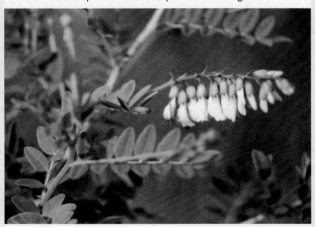

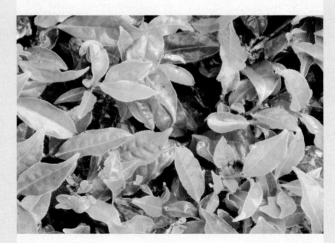

(b) *Camellia sinensis.* Green tea is made from the dried leaves and leaf buds of this shrub.

*Sources:* Cabanillas, F. (2010). Vitamin C and cancer: What can we conclude 1,609 patients and 33 years later? *Puerto Rico Health Sciences Journal, 29*(3):215–217; Ulbricht, C., et al. (2009). Essiac: Systematic review by the Natural Standard Research Collaboration. *Journal of the Society for Integrative Oncology, 7*:73–80; Yang, A. K., et al. (2010). Herbal interactions with anticancer drugs: Mechanistic and clinical considerations. *Current Medicinal Chemistry, 17*(16):1635–1678; Yang, C. S., & Wang, X. (2010). Green tea and cancer prevention. *Nutrition and Cancer, 62*(7):931–937.

| Alternative Therapy | What Is It? | Claims and Research Studies | Possible Side Effects |
|---|---|---|---|
| Huang ch'i | Extract from the plant *Astragalus membranaceus* (**Figure 13-Aa**) | *Claims:* Stimulation of the immune system.<br><br>*Studies:* Results of a University of Texas study show that it may boost immune system function. It may also reduce the side effects of chemotherapy. | Can trigger low blood pressure.<br><br>May induce dizziness and fatigue. Too much may suppress the immune system. |
| Essiac | Herbal tea. Mixture of four herbs: burdock root, Indian rhubarb, sheep sorrel, and slippery elm | *Claims:* Strengthens immune system, improves appetite, relieves pain, may reduce tumor size.<br><br>*Studies:* Results are inconclusive. Some studies show no activity in reducing the size of animal tumors, while others show some inhibition of tumor cell growth and enhancement of the immune response. Essiac has no significant effect on health-related quality of life or mood states in women with breast cancer. | Nausea, vomiting, diarrhea |
| Green tea | Tea made from the steamed and then dried leaves and leaf buds of the shrub *Camellia sinensis* (**Figure 13-Ab**). (Black tea is prepared from the fermented leaves of this plant.) | *Claims:* Results of a variety of studies suggest that regular consumption moderately decreases the risk of cancer, especially cancers of the upper digestive tract. Therefore, use as a treatment is being studied.<br><br>*Studies:* Extracts of green tea have shown inhibitory effects against the formation and development of tumors in animals. | High caffeine content may cause nervousness, insomnia, and irregularities in heart rate. Moderate consumption appears safe. |
| Vitamins A (or beta-carotene), C, and E | Vitamin "cocktail" taken in megadoses | *Claims:* Combination of these vitamins improves general well-being, strengthens the immune system, and may delay the development and progression of serious disease.<br><br>*Studies:* Some animal studies have shown the ability of vitamin A and beta-carotene to enhance the immune response, to retard tumor growth, and to decrease the size of established tumors. In laboratory experiments, vitamin C has been shown to inhibit tumor growth, kill tumor cells, and may enhance the effects of some cancer drugs. Human studies are inconclusive. Very little research has been conducted on the role of vitamin E in cancer treatment. At this time, there is not enough evidence for physicians to recommend that cancer patients take vitamin supplements. Beta-carotene supplements increase the risk of lung and prostate cancer in smokers. | Vitamin A: Headache, irritability, drowsiness, dizziness, itchiness. Megadoses may cause liver damage. Taking beta-carotene, which is transformed into vitamin A in the body, is safer than taking vitamin A.<br><br>Vitamin C: Generally well tolerated. Megadoses may cause stomach irritation, heartburn, nausea, vomiting, drowsiness, headaches, rash, and abnormalities in iron metabolism.<br><br>Vitamin E: Toxicity in adults appears to be low. High levels can adversely affect the absorption of vitamins A and K. Long-term megadoses may cause nausea, diarrhea, and blurred vision. |

## Radiation

Radiation is also used to treat localized cancers, either alone or in conjunction with surgery. Radiation is energy or particles emitted from the nucleus of an atom. The energy of any high-dose radiation interferes with the molecular structures of cells, killing them. Healthy cells recover more quickly and easily from radiation treatment than do cancer cells, so the healthy tissue surrounding a cancer usually survives while the cancer dies. For this reason, a physician may recommend radiation over surgery in particular instances. Preserving healthy tissue surrounding a cancer is extremely important, especially with cancers such as laryngeal cancer (cancer of the voice box), in which it may mean the difference between a patient's retaining or losing the ability to speak. Physicians also choose radiation over surgery for treatment of cancers that respond well to radiation therapy, such as cervical cancer, prostate cancer, and Hodgkin's disease. Additionally, physicians often use radiation treatment with elderly patients because their chances of recovering from it may be higher than that of recovering from surgery.

High-dose x-ray and gamma-ray irradiation are widely used today. Patients may undergo one of two methods of radiation treatment. One method is to focus a beam of radiation on the cancerous tissue from an outside source. The machine delivering the beam of radiation rotates around the patient while continually targeting the tumor so that various areas of healthy tissue receive minimal doses of radiation but the tumor receives high doses. Another method is to implant tiny radioactive "beads" in the cancerous tissue for a specific time and then remove them. With either approach, cancer patients usually undergo numerous treatments over a 5- to 8-week period.

**Figure 13.5** shows a highly effective treatment against cancer called *proton therapy*. In this treatment, a patient's cancer is bombarded with a stream of positively charged subatomic particles called protons.

At high doses, proton irradiation kills cells, as does any type of high-dose radiation. Proton radiation, however, can be focused more precisely on the cancer than can other forms of radiation. Therefore, a higher dose of radiation can be used with less radiation affecting surrounding cells. Nonetheless, proton therapy is still not in widespread use because it is about three times as costly as traditional radiation therapies, and few treatment facilities in the United States offer proton irradiation.

### Figure 13.5

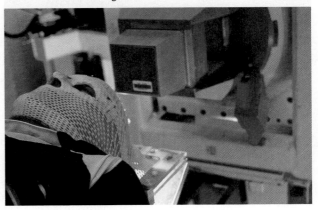

**Proton Therapy.** This patient at the James M. Slates, M.D. Proton Treatment Center at Loma Linda University is ready to receive proton therapy to treat cancer of the brain. The mask immobilizes the head to ensure that the beam will hit its target.

## Chemotherapy

Chemotherapy is the use of anticancer drugs to inhibit cancer cell reproduction or to destroy cancer cells. Chemotherapy is used most often when cancer has spread to various regions of the body. As with radiation therapy, chemotherapy may be used in conjunction with surgery. In certain cases, physicians combine all three approaches to cancer treatment.

Radiation and chemotherapy treatments also kill and damage healthy cells and may cause serious side effects such as severe nausea and hair loss. In addition, these treatments do not always destroy cancers completely because their doses are not high enough to do so. Doses sufficiently high to kill all cancer cells often cause too much damage to normal tissue. Also, certain tumors are drug resistant or develop drug resistance during therapy.

## Laser and Photodynamic Therapy

Lasers are high-intensity lights that can be focused with great precision. A few types of lasers are used in cancer treatment, and they shrink and destroy tumors. Lasers can be used not only to remove superficial cancers, such as some skin cancers, but they also can be used with an endoscope to deliver the laser light to interior body locations, such as the uterus, esophagus, and colon.

In photodynamic therapy, a chemical called a photosensitizer, which is administered to the patient, reacts with laser or other types of special light, killing tumor cells. The treatment is specific to tumors because they take up the photosensitizer better than do normal tissues, and physicians target the light at the tumors. Therefore, this type of treatment does not significantly damage normal tissues. Death of the tumor cells results from the interaction of the light and the chemical.[4] In addition, as the tumor cells become inflamed before dying, they trigger an immune response that not only acts on the treated cells but also on the same type of tumor cells that may be elsewhere in the body.[5]

## Targeted Therapies

The National Cancer Institute defines **targeted therapies** as "drugs or other substances that block the growth and spread of cancer by interfering with specific molecules involved in tumor growth and progression."[6] Targeted therapies are also called "molecularly targeted drugs" and "molecularly targeted therapies." Because these therapies target specific molecules in specific cancers, they are often more effective than general types of treatments and harm only the cancer, not surrounding tissues. One major limitation of targeted therapies, however, is that the cancer cells may develop mutations (changes) that no longer allow the therapy to work. Therefore, targeted therapies are often used alongside other targeted therapies and conventional treatments, such as surgery and radiation.

The two primary types of targeted therapies are small-molecule drugs and immunotherapy.

**Small-Molecule Drugs** Small-molecule drugs are tiny enough to pass through pores in the cell membrane and do their work from within the cancer cell. An array of small-molecule drugs for targeted cancer therapy has been developed and approved by the U.S. Food and Drug Administration (FDA) for use. Some are not yet approved but are in clinical trials.

Small-molecule drugs each do a specific job, such as blocking certain enzymes and growth factor receptors that cancer cells use as they grow and multiply, modifying the function of proteins that regulate cancer cell functions, and stopping cancerous tumors from developing new blood vessels.

**Immunotherapy** Some targeted therapies help the immune system destroy cancer cells. The umbrella term for these methods is *biomodulation* (biological response modification), or **immunotherapy**.

Key to the working of the immune system is its ability to recognize an intruder as foreign. The immune system does this by recognizing foreign antigens (certain foreign proteins) on intruders as nonself. However, tumor cells appear to contain antigens that evoke only a weak response from the immune system. As a result, the immune system has difficulty detecting and identifying malignant tumors, so it does a poor job destroying these abnormal cells.

Immunotherapies involve a variety of techniques that help boost the immune system response. For example, injecting tumor antigens into the patient's bloodstream can increase the numbers of tumor-fighting immune system cells in the body. This procedure is similar to the way in which a vaccine works to boost the body's immune response against an infectious disease. For this reason, such cancer-fighting products are called *cancer vaccines*. However, cancer vaccines are given to patients who already have cancer to help rid them of their disease, not to cancer-free persons to prevent cancer. Some medical facilities involved in cancer vaccine research are using a patient's own tumor cells to develop personalized cancer vaccines that hold promise for boosting immune system function higher than can vaccines developed from tumor antigens from other sources.[7]

Examples of other immunotherapies are drugs that decrease the suppressor mechanisms of the immune system, thus increasing the host's immune response. Another approach is to augment the patient's immune system by bone marrow transplants (tissue that produces immune system cells; see next subsection) or transfusions of particular immune system cells. Other immunotherapies are chemicals that act on tumor cells by making them more recognizable by the body or more susceptible to dying as a result of immune system processes.

## Bone Marrow and Peripheral Blood Stem Cell Transplants

Stem cells are undifferentiated cells whose daughter cells can develop into a variety of cell types. Bone marrow cells are stem cells that continually give rise to a variety of types of blood cells. Peripheral blood (blood in the bloodstream) can be used as a source of blood stem cells too, but donors must be treated with growth factors (hormone-like substances) a few days before

> **targeted therapies** Drugs or other substances that block the growth and spread of cancer by interfering with specific molecules involved in tumor growth and progression.
>
> **immunotherapy** Manipulation of the body's immune system to rid the body of cancer.

the donation, which causes their stem cells to grow and enter their bloodstream. Their harvested blood is processed by a machine that separates out the stem cells; the rest of the blood is returned to the donor.

Bone marrow and peripheral blood stem cell transplants are used in two primary ways in cancer treatment: (1) to resupply the bone marrow when it has been destroyed by chemotherapy or radiation, or (2) to supply healthy stem cells to a person who has cancer of the blood-forming tissue, such as leukemia. In the first situation, a patient's own stem cells are harvested before chemotherapy or radiation, and the stem cells are given back to the patient after the treatment. In the second instance, the stem cells come not from the patient but from a healthy donor whose tissue type best matches the patient. The healthy stem cells are transplanted into the patient, and these cells produce healthy blood cells.

Patients receive stem cell transplants (whether the stem cells are their own or those of a donor) in a process much like a blood transfusion. The stem cells take up residence in the bone marrow, grow, and send out new blood cells.

This section has discussed many types of cancer treatments. Although these useful and amazing treatments can be life-saving, prevention and early detection are still the best ways to live a healthy, long, cancer-free life.

## Prevalent Cancers in the United States

Over decades of research, scientists have learned what causes certain cancers. In some cases, scientists are unsure of the cause but know which factors are related to cancer development. These factors, when present, increase the chances that a person will develop a particular cancer, and thus are called risk factors. Although heredity influences cancer risk, it explains only a fraction of all cancers and variations in cancer risk. Behavioral factors such as cigarette smoking, dietary patterns, physical activity, and weight control, however, *substantially* affect the risk of developing cancer.[8]

This chapter organizes the discussion of cancers according to factors that appear to be significant in the development of particular cancers, most of which are prevalent in the United States. Advanced age is a significant risk factor for most cancers except certain childhood cancers, testicular cancer, cervical cancer, and, in part, breast cancer.

Before reading this section, take the self-assessment "What Are Your Cancer Risks?" found in the Student Workbook section at the end of this text.

## Cancers Caused by or Related to Tobacco

In 2004, U.S. Surgeon General Richard Carmona issued a report on smoking and health that listed tobacco smoking as a cause of various cancers.[9] **Table 13.2** lists these cancers. In 2010, U.S. Surgeon General Regina Benjamin expanded on the information in the 2004 report by issuing a new report on how tobacco smoke causes disease.[10] Thirty percent of all cancer deaths, including 87% of lung cancer deaths, can be attributed to tobacco use.[8]

This section explores the first seven cancers in Table 13.2 because they are all caused primarily by this preventable risk. Stomach cancer and cancer of the cervix are discussed in other sections of this chapter because their primary causes relate to factors other than tobacco use. Pancreatic cancer has a variety of risk factors.

**Lung Cancer** Looking at **Table 13.3**, you can see that lung cancer is the leading cause of cancer

| Table 13.2 |
| --- |
| **Cancers Caused by Cigarette Smoking** |
| Bladder |
| Esophagus |
| Kidney |
| Larynx (voice box) |
| Acute myeloid leukemia |
| Lung |
| Mouth and throat |
| Pancreas |
| Stomach |
| Cervix |

*Source:* U.S. Department of Health and Human Services. (2004). *The health consequences of smoking: A report of the Surgeon General.* Washington, DC: U.S. Government Printing Office.

## Table 13.3

## Leading Sites of New Cancer Cases and Deaths—2011 Estimates

| Estimated New Cases* | | Estimated Deaths | |
|---|---|---|---|
| **Male** | **Female** | **Male** | **Female** |
| Prostate | Breast | Lung & bronchus | Lung & bronchus |
| 240,890 (29%) | 230,480 (30%) | 85,600 (28%) | 71,340 (26%) |
| Lung & bronchus | Lung & bronchus | Prostate | Breast |
| 115,060 (14%) | 106,070 (14%) | 33,720 (11%) | 39,520 (15%) |
| Colon & rectum | Colon & rectum | Colon & rectum | Colon & rectum |
| 71,850 (9%) | 69,360 (9%) | 25,250 (8%) | 24,130 (9%) |
| Urinary bladder | Uterine corpus | Pancreas | Pancreas |
| 52,020 (6%) | 46,470 (6%) | 19,360 (6%) | 18,300 (7%) |
| Melanoma of the skin | Thyroid | Liver & intrahepatic bile duct | Ovary |
| 40,010 (5%) | 36,550 (5%) | 13,260 (4%) | 15,460 (6%) |
| Kidney & renal pelvis | Non-Hodgkin lymphoma | Leukemia | Non-Hodgkin lymphoma |
| 37,120 (5%) | 30,300 (4%) | 12,740 (4%) | 9,570 (4%) |
| Non-Hodgkin lymphoma | Melanoma of the skin | Esophagus | Leukemia |
| 36,060 (4%) | 30,220 (4%) | 11,910 (4%) | 9,040 (3%) |
| Oral cavity & pharynx | Kidney & renal pelvis | Urinary bladder | Uterine corpus |
| 27,710 (3%) | 23,800 (3%) | 10,670 (4%) | 8,120 (3%) |
| Leukemia | Ovary | Non-Hodgkin lymphoma | Liver & intrahepatic bile duct |
| 25,320 (3%) | 21,990 (3%) | 9,750 (3%) | 6,330 (2%) |
| Pancreas | Pancreas | Kidney & renal pelvis | Brain & other nervous system |
| 22,050 (3%) | 21,980 (3%) | 8,270 (3%) | 5,670 (2%) |
| All sites | All sites | All sites | All sites |
| 822,300 (100%) | 774,370 (100%) | 300,430 (100%) | 271,520 (100%) |

*Excludes basal and squamous cell skin cancers and in situ carcinoma except urinary bladder.

*Source:* American Cancer Society. *Cancer Facts and Figures 2011.* Atlanta: American Cancer Society, Inc.

deaths in both men and women in the United States. Death rates resulting from lung cancer have risen dramatically in men since the 1930s through the 1980s and in women since the 1960s through the early 1990s (see Figure 13.3). Estimates put tobacco use as the main cause of 90% of male lung cancers and 79% of female lung cancers; about 90% of lung cancer deaths overall can be attributed to smoking cigarettes.[11]

The increases in lung cancer death rates shown in Figure 13.3 are because of increases in the percentage of the population who smoked tobacco in the decades prior to the 1960s. Lung cancer, like most cancers, takes years to develop, so a rise in lung cancer death rates occurs decades after a rise in the percentage of the population who smoke.

Incidence rates of lung cancer (the number of people diagnosed per 100,000 population) have begun to stabilize in women and drop in men (see Figure 13.3). This stabilization and drop reflect the beginning of a predicted decline in incidence rates resulting from the steady decline in cigarette smoking in the U.S. population since 1964. In that year, U.S. Surgeon General Luther Terry issued a report that linked cigarette smoking to the development of lung cancer and other diseases.[12]

*Signs and Symptoms* In the early stages of disease, the signs and symptoms of lung cancer may be hard to detect. Cigarette smokers often have chronic cough, chronic bronchitis, or excess sputum (saliva and mucus) production (see Chapter 8). Tumors growing in the bronchioles (small airways in the lungs) also cause a cough and sputum production; they may also cause blood to appear in the sputum as they disrupt airway tissues. A lung cancer victim may also wheeze when breathing if the airways become substantially narrowed by tumor growth. In addition, the air sacs in that part of the lung may collapse and cease to function; infection may develop. The patient may experience pain in the chest, shoulder, and arm if the cancer spreads to the chest wall and affects certain nerves there.

Physicians use chest x-rays and other imaging techniques, including MRI and CT scans; analyses of the types of cells in the sputum; and fiber-optic examination of the bronchial passageways to assist in their diagnoses.

*Risk Factors and Prevention* Malignant growths develop in the lungs and airways in many persons as they inhale cancer-causing substances such as tobacco smoke over long periods of time. The risk of lung cancer rises proportionately with the number of cigarettes (or cigars or pipes) a person smokes per day, the number of years a person smokes, and how deeply he or she inhales. Persons who smoke low-tar cigarettes have a lower risk of lung cancer than those who smoke high-tar cigarettes.[9] (Smoking "low-yield" cigarettes does not lower cardiovascular disease risk; see Chapter 12.) Likewise, those who smoke filter-tipped cigarettes have a lower risk of lung cancer than those who smoke unfiltered cigarettes. However, results of research show that people who smoke filter-tipped or "low-yield" cigarettes are at increased risk for developing deep lung tumors because, when smoking, they inhale more deeply and forcefully than people who smoke non-filter-tipped or "regular-yield" cigarettes.[9]

If you are a smoker (of any age), giving up cigarette smoking will slowly lower your risk of developing lung cancer, several other cancers, and cardiovascular disease as well. Your risk of developing lung cancer will never return to that of a lifetime nonsmoker, but after 10 years it will be about half that of a person who continued to smoke.[9] (However, your risk of developing cardiovascular disease will lower considerably in only 1 year and return to that of a nonsmoker in 3 to 15 years, depending on how much and how long you smoked.)

Other lifestyle factors that appear to raise the risk of lung cancer are regular, high consumption of alcoholic beverages and obesity. Combined estrogen and progestin postmenopausal hormone therapy does not increase the incidence of lung cancer, but it does appear to increase the risk of death from lung cancer.[13] The relationships between various dietary factors and lung cancer is controversial;[11,14] more research is needed to determine clear associations.

Scientists have been unable to show that lung cancer is inherited. Nonetheless, correlational studies show that relatives of lung cancer patients have a higher risk of developing lung cancer if they smoke than do smokers with no relatives who have lung cancer. Scientists speculate that relatives of lung cancer patients may inherit a defect in their cells' ability to resist genetic damage by the carcinogens in cigarette smoke.

In the early 1970s, medical researchers began investigating the effects of passive smoking on the development of lung cancer. **Passive smoking** is the inhalation by nonsmokers of environmental tobacco smoke (ETS; secondhand smoke) present in the air from others who smoke. Environmental tobacco smoke has been associated with a 20–30% increase in lung cancer risk for persons who live with a smoker. The following are a few of the many conclusions regarding the effects of secondhand smoke in the 2006 Surgeon General's report *The Health Consequences of Involuntary Exposure to Tobacco Smoke*: "Secondhand smoke causes premature death and disease in children and in adults who do not smoke," "More than 50 carcinogens have been identified in sidestream and secondhand smoke," and "The evidence is sufficient to infer a causal relationship between secondhand smoke exposure and lung cancer among lifetime nonsmokers."[15]

Substances other than those in tobacco smoke have also been linked to lung cancer. Certain metals, for example, are carcinogenic and are listed in **Table 13.4**. Only people in certain occupations encounter most of these substances.

Two substances significantly associated with the development of lung cancer and often encountered in the environment are asbestos and radon. **Asbestos** is a fiber-like mineral found in rocks that resists damage by fire or other natural processes. Because of these properties, asbestos has been used in the manufacture of a variety of products and is used in the construction, shipbuilding, and railroad industries. People in these industries as well as those who mine asbestos are at risk of developing lung cancer if they inhale asbestos particles. Additionally, the effects of inhaling asbestos particles multiply the effects of smoking tobacco and therefore greatly increases risk. Chapter 16 discusses asbestos in greater detail.

> **asbestos** (as-BES-tose) A fiber-like mineral found in rocks that, when inhaled, can cause lung cancer or other lung conditions.

## Table 13.4

### Carcinogenic Metals Found in the Workplace

| Metal | Cancers | Present in | Human Carcinogen? | Workers Exposed |
|-------|---------|-----------|-------------------|-----------------|
| Arsenic | Skin, lung, bladder, kidney, liver | Wood preservatives, glass, pesticides | Yes | Smelting of ores containing arsenic, pesticide application, and wood preservation |
| Beryllium | Lung | Nuclear weapons, rocket fuel, ceramics, glass, plastic, fiberoptic products | Yes | Beryllium ore miners and alloy makers, phosphor manufacturers, ceramic workers, missile technicians, nuclear reactor workers, electric and electronic equipment workers, and jewelers |
| Cadmium | Lung | Metal coatings, plastic products, batteries, fungicides | Yes | Smelting of zinc and lead ores; producing, processing, and handling cadmium powders; welding or remelting of cadmium-coated steel; and working with solders that contain cadmium |
| Chromium | Lung | Automotive parts, floor covering, paper, cement, asphalt roofing, anticorrosive metal plating | Yes | Stainless steel production and welding, chromate production, chrome plating, ferrochrome alloys, chrome pigment, and tanning industries |
| Lead | Kidney, brain | Cotton dyes; metal coating; drier in paints, varnishes, and pigment inks; certain plastics; specialty glass | Probable carcinogen | Construction work that involves welding, cutting, brazing, or blasting on lead paint surfaces; most smelter workers, including lead smelters where lead is recovered from batteries; radiator repair shops |
| Nickel | Nasal cavity, lung | Steel, dental fillings, copper and brass, permanent magnets, storage batteries, glazes | Nickel metal: Probable carcinogen Nickel compounds: Yes | Battery makers, ceramic makers, electroplaters, enamellers, glass workers, jewelers, metal workers, nickel mine workers, refiners and smelters, paint-related workers and welders |

*Source:* National Cancer Institute. (2003). Cancer and the environment. Retrieved October 11, 2011, from http://www.cancer.gov/newscenter/Cancer-and-the-Environment.

**radon gas** A colorless, odorless, radioactive gas present in the rocks and soils in many areas in the United States that, when inhaled, can cause mutations in cells.

Exposure to radon gas also appears to multiply the carcinogenic effect of tobacco smoke. **Radon gas** is colorless and odorless, and is produced as the radioactive element uranium decays, emitting subatomic particles and energy. When inhaled, radon can cause mutations in cells because it is radioactive also. Radon is present in the rocks and soils in many areas in the United States (**Figure 13.6**). People who live in these regions may be exposed to radon gas if it leaks through cracks in basement walls and collects in their homes. Home radon detectors can ascertain the presence of this gas. If radon is present, specialists in radon abatement can advise a homeowner on procedures to prevent this gas from leaking into and accumulating in the house (**Figure 13.7**).

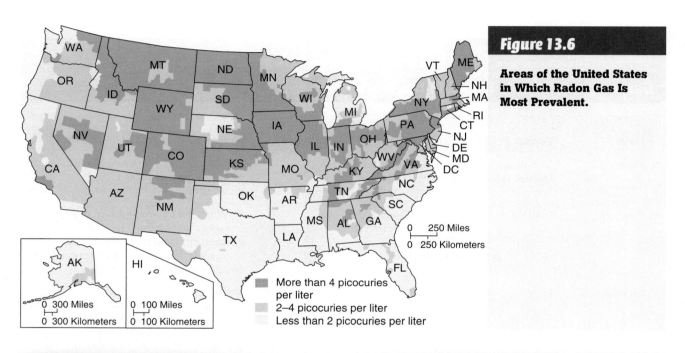

### Figure 13.6

**Areas of the United States in Which Radon Gas Is Most Prevalent.**

More than 4 picocuries per liter

2–4 picocuries per liter

Less than 2 picocuries per liter

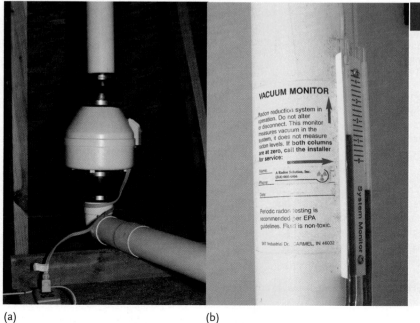

(a)  (b)

### Figure 13.7

**Radon Gas Abatement.** Although many types of radon gas abatement exist for homes, one of the most common and reliable is active subslab suction. This technique is used in homes with basements or built on slabs. One or more pipes is inserted through the floor slab into the crushed rock or soil below. The pipe travels up the wall to the attic, where the gas is vented. (a) The part of the pipe in the attic houses a radon exhaust fan. The fan draws the radon up the pipe while simultaneously creating a vacuum beneath the slab. The radon gas is vented to the outside. (b) Somewhere along its length, the pipe has a vacuum monitor so that the homeowner can see that the system is operating.

*Treatment* Physicians treat lung cancer primarily with surgery, radiation, and chemotherapy. Surgeons often remove the lobe of the cancerous lung. They may combine therapies if the cancer has spread, using radiation or chemotherapy with surgery, targeted therapies, and/or laser therapy.

**Cancers of the Larynx, Oral Cavity, and Esophagus** Although these cancers are not as prevalent as others, they have preventable causes: tobacco use, which includes the use of cigarettes, cigars, pipes, and smokeless (chewing) tobacco of all types; and excessive alcohol consumption. Heavy consumption of alcohol is often a causal factor in cancers of the esophagus and liver, but if a heavy drinker is also a smoker, the effects of both substances multiply the risk of developing cancer of the larynx, oral cavity, and esophagus.

Results of recent research show that an increasing percentage of oral cancers are associated with the human papillomavirus (HPV), which enters the mouth during oral sex with an infected person. The primary population developing HPV-related oral cancers is white men between the ages of 40 and 55 years.[16]

Cancers of the larynx, or voice box, are usually detected early if they involve the vocal cords because the voice quickly becomes hoarse. However, cancers of the larynx that do not involve the vocal cords are more difficult to discover early. Their symptoms may include a sore throat, difficulty in swallowing, or a visible lump in the neck.

The esophagus is the tube that carries food and drink from the mouth to the stomach. Difficulty swallowing is also a symptom of esophageal cancer. In addition, people who have recurrent heartburn or a burning sensation while swallowing should be checked for possible esophageal carcinoma.

In oral cancer, malignant or benign growths are often visible (**Figure 13.8**). Malignancies may appear as sores that bleed easily and do not heal, red or white patches that do not go away, or thickened areas of tissue. Oral cancer metastasizes relatively quickly; over half of cases are diagnosed in advanced stages. To detect oral cancer early, persons older than age 50 years should have complete oral examinations as part of their annual physical checkups. Dentists should routinely screen all of their patients for oral cancer.

**Cancers of the Kidney and Bladder** The kidneys and bladder are organs of the urinary system, yet tobacco smoking is a causal factor in cancers of these organs. These organs come in contact with inhaled carcinogens in tobacco smoke (or other inhaled carcinogens) after they enter the bloodstream

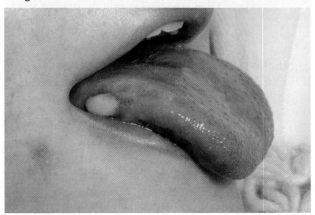

**Figure 13.8**

**Tongue Cancer.** This close-up of a cancer patient's mouth shows a malignant tumor on the edge of the tongue. This type of cancer spreads rapidly. The survival rate is low. Tongue cancer may be related to smoking cigarettes or to the use of smokeless tobacco.

at the lungs. The kidneys filter the carcinogens into the urine, which exposes the kidneys and bladder to these substances before urination.

Most signs and symptoms of kidney and bladder cancer are the same as those of several other conditions, so experiencing any of them is not a sure sign of cancer. One such sign of both cancers is blood in the urine. Frequent, urgent, or difficult urination is also a sign of bladder cancer. Additional signs and symptoms of kidney cancer include a fever of unknown origin, weight loss, and anemia (a decrease in the hemoglobin in the blood).

Most people who get bladder or kidney cancer are men older than 50 years of age who are heavy smokers. Cigarette smokers have 2 to 10 times the risk of developing bladder or kidney cancer as do nonsmokers. As with lung cancer, the risk increases with the number of cigarettes smoked per day and the number of years a person has been a smoker. People lessen their risk when they decrease the number of cigarettes they smoke or stop smoking. Obesity is another known risk factor for kidney cancer.[17]

**Cancer of the Pancreas** A long, slender gland, the pancreas lies near the stomach. As an accessory organ of the digestive system, the pancreas secretes digestive enzymes that enter the small intestine by means of a duct. As an endocrine gland, the pancreas secretes the hormones insulin and glucagon, which help regulate blood levels of glucose.

Pancreatic cancer is a particularly deadly form of cancer, striking men and women fairly equally. The

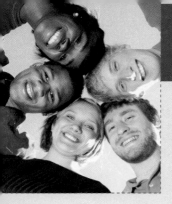

## Stomach Cancer: Variation in Mortality Among Countries

More Americans died of stomach cancer in 1930 than of any other type of cancer. In the United States, the death rate resulting from this cancer has fallen dramatically since then (see Figure 13.3). However, the International Agency for Research on Cancer at the World Health Organization reports that stomach cancer is still the number two cancer killer worldwide. (Lung cancer is number one.) Why has the death rate from this cancer fallen in the United States? Why is this cancer so prevalent in other parts of the world?

As scientists studied worldwide patterns of mortality from stomach cancer, they noticed high mortality rates in Central and South American countries such as Brazil, Chile, Colombia, Costa Rica, and Venezuela. They also noticed large differences in death rates from stomach cancer in some of these countries. In Colombia, for example, death rates from this disease differ dramatically in populations living in the mountains compared with populations living along the coast. A similar situation exists in central and eastern European countries. There are high mortality rates from stomach cancer in these countries; however, the death rates between countries and within countries in this part of the world vary. In addition, countries in Eastern Asia, which includes China, Taiwan, Japan, North Korea, South Korea, and Mongolia, have extremely high mortality rates from stomach cancer. Why are some countries' rates of death resulting from stomach cancer dramatically higher than others? (You can research incidence and mortality rates for various cancers in countries around the world at www-dep.iarc.fr/.)

Scientists have determined that differences in worldwide stomach cancer death rates are related to diet and environment rather than to race or country of origin. Likewise, the reduction in stomach cancer deaths in the United States is the result primarily of these factors.

Regarding diet, methods of food processing and preservation affect the incidence of stomach cancer. In the early 1900s in the United States, methods of food processing and preservation changed dramatically. By midcentury, refrigeration and freezing replaced salting, pickling, and smoking as the primary methods of food preservation. Scientists have since discovered that the regular consumption of highly salted foods (including pickled foods) increases the risk of developing stomach cancer. Foods that are smoke-cured, charbroiled, or grilled contain high quantities of polycyclic aromatic hydrocarbons (PAHs), which are carcinogenic and mutagenic. These compounds are also found in cigarette smoke and air pollution because they are the products of the incomplete combustion of fossil fuels such as charcoal and gasoline. Although many Americans enjoy eating grilled foods, their consumption of smoked, salted, and pickled foods has decreased since the early 1900s, reducing Americans' risk of developing and dying from stomach cancer. However, peoples of various cultures still use salting and smoking to preserve meats and pickling to preserve vegetables, thereby increasing their risk of stomach cancer.

Another dietary factor with an environmental link plays a role in the development of this disease. Ingesting nitrosamines, which are found in nitrite-cured foods (such as bacon, cold cuts, and some hot dogs) and in water supplies in some parts of the world (such as Colombia and South America), appears to increase the risk of stomach cancer. Nitrosamines are also found in cigarette smoke. Additionally, chemical reactions that occur in the stomach produce nitrosamines from other compounds. For example, substances in certain fish consumed in Japan and in fava beans consumed in Colombia are converted in the stomach to nitrosamines.

Eating fruits and vegetables appears to inhibit the reactions in the stomach that form nitrosamines. In addi-

---

fourth most common cause of cancer death in men and women (see Table 13.3), pancreatic cancer is often called a silent cancer because the early symptoms, which include nausea, vomiting, weakness, and discomfort in the abdomen, are vague and nonspecific. The more specific signs and symptoms of pancreatic cancer—jaundice (yellowing of the eyeballs and skin), pain, and weight loss—do not usually occur until the disease is advanced and then may be confused with many other diseases, such as gallbladder or liver disease.

The risk of pancreatic cancer increases after age 50; most cases occur in persons aged 65 to 79 years. The incidence of pancreatic cancer for smokers is more than twice as high as for nonsmokers. Other persons at risk for developing pancreatic cancer are chemists and those in occupations that involve close exposure to gasoline and dry cleaning agents. In-tion, they appear to protect the stomach from the effects of carcinogens. Populations who consume large quantities of fruit and vegetables generally have a low risk of stomach cancer.

In addition to dietary factors, infection with the bacterium *Helicobacter pylori* has been found to be associated with the development of stomach cancer. *H. pylori*, which also increases the risk of digestive system ulcers, is highly prevalent in Asian countries. Persons with *H. pylori* can be treated with antibiotics to eradicate the stomach infection. Although killing this microorganism is an effective treatment for ulcers, it results in only a slowing of the precancerous process and does not prevent all stomach cancers.

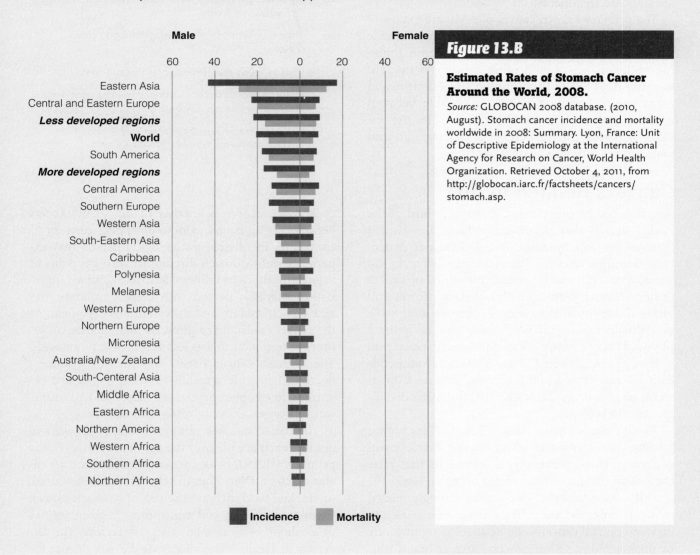

## Figure 13.B

**Estimated Rates of Stomach Cancer Around the World, 2008.**

*Source:* GLOBOCAN 2008 database. (2010, August). Stomach cancer incidence and mortality worldwide in 2008: Summary. Lyon, France: Unit of Descriptive Epidemiology at the International Agency for Research on Cancer, World Health Organization. Retrieved October 4, 2011, from http://globocan.iarc.fr/factsheets/cancers/stomach.asp.

haled carcinogens appear to reach the pancreas via the bloodstream. Risk also appears to increase with obesity, physical inactivity, chronic inflammation of the pancreas, diabetes, and cirrhosis of the liver. In addition, rates of pancreatic cancer appear to be higher in those who use smokeless tobacco.

Only 6% of people who have pancreatic cancer survive beyond 5 years.[3] Late detection and metastasis reduce survival. For the rare patients who discover their cancer in its early stages, surgery is a primary treatment that may lead to a cure and long-term relief of symptoms. In patients diagnosed in later stages of the disease, surgery, radiation, chemotherapy, and certain targeted cancer therapies may extend survival.

**Acute Myeloid Leukemia** Acute myeloid leukemia (AML) affects blood-producing cells in the bone marrow. In AML, white blood cells that combat bacterial infection (neutrophils) are primarily affected, but occasionally red blood cells or platelets are affected as well. These cells do not differentiate properly from stem cells in the bone marrow (see the section titled "Bone Marrow and Peripheral Blood Stem Cell Transplants" in this chapter), resulting in fewer than normal numbers of these cells in the bloodstream. AML is a serious disease and is likely fatal if not treated. Chemotherapy and stem cell transplantation are standard treatments.

The primary known causes of AML are exposure to benzene and ionizing radiation. Cigarette smoke contains benzene and substances that emit ionizing radiation, along with other substances thought to cause AML. Data from human and experimental animal studies show a causal relationship between smoking and acute myeloid leukemia. The risk for AML increases with the number of cigarettes smoked and with the duration of smoking.[9]

## Cancers Related to Diet

Research results suggest that about one-third of the cancer deaths that occur annually in the United States result from nutrition and physical activity factors, including obesity.[8] For Americans who do not use tobacco (to which another one-third of cancer deaths are attributed annually), dietary choices and physical activity are *the most important* modifiable determinants of cancer risk. Along with adopting a physically active lifestyle and maintaining a healthful weight, the American Cancer Society recommends eating a variety of healthful foods, with an emphasis on plant sources. **Table 13.5** lists the ACS's dietary recommendations.

As you can see from Table 13.5, diet has both a positive and a negative effect on the development of cancer. There are dietary components that raise the risk of certain cancers and others that lower the risk of certain cancers. One cancer strongly related to diet is stomach cancer. The other cancer related to diet—colorectal cancer—can be affected significantly by one's heredity. Other cancers, such as breast cancer, have risk factors related to diet but are related to other risk factors as well.

**Cancer of the Stomach** The incidence of and mortality from stomach cancer has declined dramatically over the past 75 years in the United States. In the early part of the twentieth century, stomach cancer, not lung cancer, was the number one cancer killer of Americans. (See the Diversity in Health essay titled "Stomach Cancer: Variation in Mortality Among Countries" for an explanation of this decline.)

### Table 13.5

### Dietary Recommendations for Reducing Cancer Risk

- Eat five or more servings of fruits and vegetables per day.

- Eat whole-grain foods rather than processed (refined) grain foods.

- Limit consumption of red meats and processed meats.

- Choose foods that help maintain a healthy weight.

- Drink no more than one alcoholic beverage per day (women) or two per day (men).

*Source:* Adapted from American Cancer Society. (2010). *Cancer facts and figures, 2010.* Atlanta, GA: Author.

Stomach cancer is another of the silent cancers because no signs and symptoms appear early in its course. As the disease progresses, a person may experience mild stomach discomfort with gas pains or vague sensations of fullness. Suspecting minor digestive problems, a person with these symptoms may take antacid tablets, and the symptoms disappear. As the cancer continues to grow, the malignancy causes more severe pain that is less responsive to antacids. The stomach cancer victim may then experience a decreased appetite, a feeling of fullness after just beginning to eat, pain on eating, nausea and vomiting, weight loss, excessive burping, and weakness.

The risk of stomach cancer increases with age and doubles each decade over the age of 55. However, the primary risk factors for cancer of the stomach are dietary factors. Diets high in salt-cured, nitrate-cured, or smoked food increase the risk of stomach cancer. Cigarette smoking and consuming large quantities of alcoholic beverages are also risk factors. The Diversity in Health essay discusses the risk factors for stomach cancer in greater detail.

Stomach cancer is easily diagnosed with barium studies. During this procedure, the patient swallows a milky fluid called barium sulfate. As this material reaches the stomach, a series of x-rays is taken that show the movement of this fluid through the stomach, while visualizing obstructions and other growths. Additionally, physicians often obtain stomach cells by the use of a fiber-optic tube, which can be fitted with instruments for such procedures. If a tumor is found, a biopsy is taken of the growth so that the cells can be studied and the diagnosis confirmed.

In the United States, stomach cancer is no longer a major killer; therefore, routine screening is not performed as it is in high-risk populations such as Japan. Thus, most stomach cancers are not diagnosed early in the United States. If found early, however, stomach cancer is treated with surgery to remove the tumor. Chemotherapy and radiation are also used to treat stomach cancer and may be used in conjunction with surgery.

**Cancer of the Colon and Rectum** The **colon**, or large intestine, is an organ of the digestive system that reabsorbs water and certain chemicals from waste materials (feces). Bacteria in the colon decompose materials that the human body cannot digest. The **rectum** is the lower part of the large intestine; it terminates at the anus.

Cancer of the colon and rectum, jointly referred to as *colorectal cancer*, is the third most deadly cancer in the United States (see Table 13.3). The signs and symptoms of colorectal cancer depend on the location of the tumor. A person may have no symptoms or few symptoms at first. Some persons first experience vague or crampy abdominal pain that may be mistaken for an ulcer. Other indications may be a change in bowel habits, such as constipation alternating with diarrhea. Blood may be visible in the stool (feces) or, on screening a person may have a positive occult (hidden) blood test. As the cancer worsens, a person with colorectal cancer may have a complete obstruction of the colon that requires emergency surgery.

The primary risk factors for developing colorectal cancer are advanced age, heredity, personal or family history of colorectal polyps (small growths) or inflammatory bowel disease, physical inactivity, obesity, smoking cigarettes, and heavy alcohol consumption. People with type 2 diabetes are at higher risk as well. A diet high in red or processed meat (hot dogs and some luncheon meats) and meat cooked at very high temperatures as in grilling and an inadequate intake of fruits and vegetables might raise colorectal cancer risk.[18]

Beginning at age 40, both men and women are at increased risk for developing colorectal cancer; this risk doubles with each decade after age 50 and peaks at about age 70. More than 90% of people diagnosed with colorectal cancer are older than age 50.[18] People who have hereditary conditions in which they tend to grow numerous (sometimes hundreds) of polyps in their gastrointestinal tracts have very high incidences

of colorectal malignancies. In addition, people who have a first-degree relative (parent or sibling) with colon cancer are three to five times more likely to develop colorectal cancer than are people with no such family history of this disease.

Aspirin has been found to have a protective effect against colorectal cancer when taken daily at a dose of at least 75 mg, about one baby aspirin, for 5 years or more.[19] In addition, exercising moderately and consistently reduces the risk of colon cancer. Consuming a diet that contains adequate amounts of fruits, vegetables, and whole grains; replaces red and processed meats with chicken and fish; and replaces most saturated fats with unsaturated fats can reduce the risk of colorectal cancer. Postmenopausal hormone replacement and calcium reduce colorectal cancer risk as well.[11,20]

Early detection of colorectal cancer usually results in a high chance of survival. Although colorectal cancer may have no easily recognizable early symptoms, tests are available to screen for this cancer. Common tests are the fecal occult blood test, digital rectal examination, sigmoidoscopy, and colonoscopy. Less common tests are the double-contrast barium enema, the CT colonography (virtual colonoscopy), and the stool DNA test (sDNA).

The **fecal occult blood test (FOBT)** detects hidden blood in the stool. The patient performs the simple test at home by smearing stool onto a piece of paper that has been sensitized to detect occult blood. Often, the test papers can be mailed to a laboratory or to the physician for interpretation. This test will not detect all colorectal cancers, however, because not all colorectal cancers bleed. Also, positive tests may indicate conditions other than colorectal cancer.

A stool DNA test for colorectal cancer screening was developed recently and is endorsed by the American Cancer Society. Using extremely sensitive laboratory methods, the sDNA test detects cells shed into the stool from precancerous or cancerous polyps, which have recognizable changes in their DNA. Research results show sDNA tests to be more effective than FOBT in detecting colorectal cancer.[21]

**digital rectal exam** A test in which a physician uses a gloved finger to feel the rectum or the prostate for abnormal growths.

**sigmoidoscopy** (SIG-moid-OS-ko-pee) A procedure in which a physician views the lower portion of the colon via a flexible fiber-optic tube.

**colonoscopy** (KO-lon-OS-ko-pee) A procedure in which a physician views the entire length of the colon using a flexible fiber-optic tube.

To perform the **digital rectal exam**, a physician uses a gloved finger to feel the rectum for abnormal growths. **Sigmoidoscopy** is a procedure in which the physician views the lower portion of the colon (the sigmoid [S-shaped] colon) with a flexible fiber-optic tube. During a similar procedure called a **colonoscopy**, the fiber-optic tube is threaded through the entire length of the colon. The sigmoidoscope or colonoscope can also be used to remove or biopsy polyps or other growths.

The double-contrast barium enema is an x-ray examination of the colon when it is filled with a barium solution. Additional x-rays are taken after the patient expels the solution. The barium provides a contrast medium that helps visualize polyps or other growths. Another method to visualize the entire length of the colon is the *virtual colonoscopy*. This test is a type of CT or MRI scan that produces both two- and three-dimensional images of the colon. Although expensive and not as sensitive as the colonoscopy, the virtual colonoscopy could become an option for patients who want a test that is less invasive than a colonoscopy.

See the Managing Your Health box titled "Screening Guidelines for the Early Detection of Cancer in Average-Risk Asymptomatic People" earlier in this chapter for information on early detection of colorectal cancer. When colorectal cancer is detected early, surgery is the primary treatment. Physicians often use chemotherapy and radiation therapy after surgery to kill any metastasized cancer that was not detected or removed by surgery. If surgery is not possible, a physician may treat the cancer with chemotherapy or radiation therapy alone. Targeted therapies may also be used.

## Cancers Related to Hormone Function

**Breast Cancer** From the mid-1950s until 1985 in the United States, breast cancer was the number one cancer killer of women. Lung cancer then usurped the top position because the death rate from lung cancer in women continued to rise while the death rate from breast cancer began to decline.

The incidence of breast cancer in women has remained stable for decades, but its incidence increased nearly 4% per year between 1980 and 1987 when mammography screening came into widespread use. More cancers in earlier stages were detected than previously, which showed up as in increase in the incidence rate. The incidence rate held steady from 1987 to 1994 but rose 1.6% from 1994 to 1999. The American Cancer Society suggests that this increase was because of rising rates of obesity and an increased use of postmenopausal combined estrogen plus progestin hormone replacement therapy (HRT). Combined HRT has since been shown to increase the risk of breast cancer, with the cancer risk rising with increasing length of use of HRT. From 1999 to 2006, incidence rates fell 2%, which may be the result of a decrease in mammography screening and a decrease in the use of HRT following the publication of the Women's Health Initiative study revealing the link between combined HRT and breast cancer in 2002.[22,23] Breast cancer is unusual in men; it accounts for 1% of U.S. cases.

*Signs and Symptoms* The signs and symptoms of breast cancer involve changes in the breast tissue, including lumps in the breast; dimpling, thickening, discoloration, irritation, or scaling of the breast skin; tenderness of the nipple or nipple discharge; and swelling or distortion of the breast. Pain is not usually a sign of breast cancer; most breast cancers are painless in their early development. Breast pain is usually caused by cyclic hormonal changes and related breast swelling.

*Risk Factors and Prevention* Approximately 5–10% of breast cancers are the result of the inheritance of mutations in the breast cancer susceptibility genes *BRCA1* and *BRCA2*.[24] In addition, women with first-degree relatives (mothers, sisters, daughters) who have breast cancer are at increased risk for developing the disease. Men are at very low risk for developing breast cancer. Genetic testing is available for people whose family history suggests that they carry breast cancer susceptibility genes.

Another major risk factor for the development of breast cancer in women is age. Breast cancer is rare in women younger than 20 years, but the incidence begins to climb throughout the 20s, rises dramatically during the 30s through the mid-70s, and then drops significantly (**Figure 13.9**). Researchers at the American Cancer Society estimated that 90% of new

# Managing Your Health

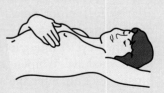

## Breast Self-Examination

Breast self-examination should be done once a month so you become familiar with the usual appearance and feel of your breasts. Familiarity makes it easier to notice any changes in the breast from month to month. Early discovery of a change from what is "normal" is the main idea behind BSE. The outlook is much better if you detect cancer in an early stage.

If you menstruate, the best time to do BSE is 2 or 3 days after your period ends, when your breasts are least likely to be tender or swollen. If you no longer menstruate, pick a day such as the first day of the month, to remind yourself it is time to do BSE.

Here is one way to do BSE:

1. Stand before a mirror. Inspect both breasts for anything unusual such as any discharge from the nipples or puckering, dimpling, or scaling of the skin.

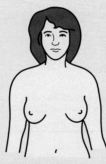

*The next two steps are designed to emphasize any change in the shape or contour of your breasts. As you do them, you should be able to feel your chest muscles tighten*

2. Watching closely in the mirror, clasp your hands behind your head and press your hands forward.

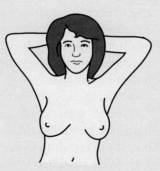

3. Next, press your hands firmly on your hips and bow slightly toward your mirror as you pull your shoulders and elbows forward.

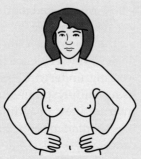

*Some women do the next part of the exam in the shower because fingers glide over soapy skin, making it easy to concentrate on the texture underneath.*

4. Raise your left arm. Use three or four fingers of your right hand to explore your left breast firmly, carefully, and thoroughly. Beginning at the outer edge, press the flat part of your fingers in small circles, moving the circles slowly around the breast. Gradually work toward the nipple. Be sure to cover the entire breast. Pay special attention to the area between the breast and the underarm, including the underarm itself. Feel for any unusual lump or mass under the skin.

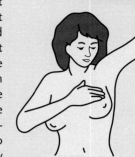

5. Gently squeeze the nipple and look for discharge. (If you have any discharge during the month—whether or not it is during BSE—see your doctor.) Repeat steps 4 and 5 on your right breast.

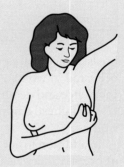

6. Steps 4 and 5 should be repeated lying down. Lie flat on your back with your left arm over your head and a pillow or folded towel under your left shoulder. This position flattens the breast and makes it easier to examine. Use the same circular motion described earlier. Repeat the exam on your right breast.

**Figure 13.9**

**Age-specific Female Breast Cancer Incidence (2004–2008) and Mortality (2003-2007) Rates.**
*Source:* American Cancer Society. *Breast Cancer Facts and Figures 2011-2012.* Atlanta: American Cancer Society, Inc.

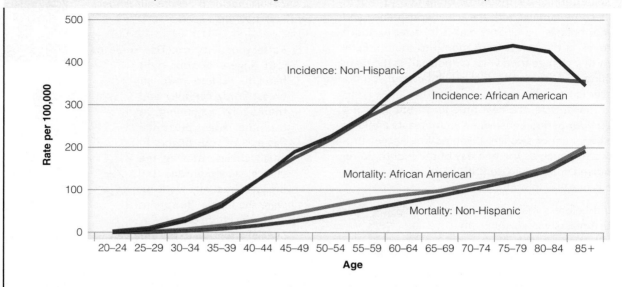

**Data sources:** *Incidence:* North American Association of Central Cancer Registries. Mortality: National Center for Health Statistics, Centers for Disease Control and Prevention, as provided by the Suveillance, Epidemiology, and End Results Program, National Cancer Institute. American Cancer Society, Surveillance Research, 2011.

breast cancer cases and 93% of breast cancer deaths occurred in women aged 45 years and older in 2009. Incidence and death rates from breast cancer are generally highest among white and African American women.[22]

In addition to age and heredity, a third major group of breast cancer risk factors are those that increase a woman's cumulative exposure to ovarian hormones, particularly estrogen. Evidence suggests that having a high number of menstrual cycles is a breast cancer risk factor. For example, early menarche (younger than age 12) and late menopause (older than age 55) are risk factors for breast cancer. Also, women who did not have a full-term pregnancy (therefore did not have their cycles interrupted) are at a higher risk than those who have. Women who did not have a full-term pregnancy until after age 30 are also at higher risk.[22]

Breast cancer risk is slightly elevated in women currently taking oral contraceptives and remains slightly elevated until about 10 years after use is discontinued. Recent use of hormone replacement therapy (HRT) that combines estrogen and progestin increases breast cancer risk as well. The longer HRT is taken, the greater the increase in risk.

Overweight and obesity are other risk factors for breast cancer because fat tissue produces estrogen. Therefore, overweight and obese women have higher circulating levels of estrogen than do nonoverweight and nonobese women. Postmenopausal obesity is thought to increase the risk of breast cancer three-fold;[11] overweight and obese women can lower their risk of breast cancer by exercising and losing weight. Regular exercise not only helps a person maintain a healthy weight but also appears to have an effect on hormones and energy balance in a way that lowers breast cancer risk.

Smoking cigarettes and drinking alcohol are also associated with breast cancer risk. Drinking more than one alcoholic drink per day raises the risk of breast cancer, so to lower risk, minimize alcohol intake. With smoking, women at greatest risk are those who have smoked for decades and who started smoking at a young age.[25]

The American Cancer Society notes that there is no scientific evidence linking breast cancer risk with wearing underwire bras, having breast implants, or using antiperspirants, as has been stated on many Internet sites. In addition, there is no evidence linking spontaneous or induced abortion with breast cancer.[22]

***Early Detection*** Three methods are generally used to detect breast cancer as early as possible: the breast self-examination, the breast clinical examination, and mammography. Breast self-examination (BSE) is considered optional by the American Cancer Society because research results do not show that monthly BSE saves lives. Research results also reveal that when women find changes or lumps in their breasts, it is usually not during structured breast self-examinations but during the normal course of dressing, bathing, or other similar activities.[22] However, women should become aware of how their breasts normally feel and report any breast change to a healthcare professional immediately. The Managing Your Health box titled "Breast Self-Examination" shows how to perform the BSE should you choose to do so. The breast clinical examination is performed by a healthcare professional. The ACS recommends that a clinical examination be performed every 3 years for women from ages 20 to 39 and every year thereafter.

Mammography is the process of taking x-rays of breast tissue to detect benign and malignant growths. As you can see in **Figure 13.10**, each breast is placed over a plate containing x-ray film, and the tissue is compressed. The ACS recommends that women aged 40 years and older have a mammogram every year. Women at high risk for breast cancer, such as those with a strong family history of the disease, should consult their physicians regarding the need for mammograms on a different schedule (e.g., at an earlier age, or more often).

If screening reveals a suspicious mass in the breast tissue, a physician usually performs a biopsy. To perform this procedure, a physician inserts a fine needle into the mass and withdraws cells. An individual trained to detect cancer studies the cells to determine if the growth is malignant. Fine-needle biopsy is relatively painless and is about 90% accurate.

*Treatment* Stage 0, I, or II breast cancer is usually treated with **lumpectomy**, surgical removal of the tumor, followed by breast irradiation. (Stage 0 in breast cancer is often a precancerous condition.) The surgeon also removes a layer of normal tissue surrounding the tumor so that it is less likely that cancer tissue is left in the breast. He or she also removes some lymph nodes under the nearby armpit to determine if the cancer has spread. About 6 weeks of radiation therapy typically follows lumpectomy. Clinical trials are under way to determine whether irradiating only the part of the breast with the excised tumor might be a better postsurgical approach than irradiating the entire breast, which is the current approach.

Accelerated partial-breast irradiation (APBI) might reduce the amount of radiation absorbed by normal breast tissue and increase the percentage of

**lumpectomy** (lum-PECK-toe-me) Surgical removal of a breast tumor, including a layer of surrounding tissue.

**total mastectomy** (mas-TEK-toe-me) Surgical removal of a breast and involved lymph nodes for the treatment of breast cancer.

**radical mastectomy** Surgical removal of a breast, underlying muscle, and underarm fat and lymph nodes as a treatment for breast cancer.

lumpectomy patients who choose radiation therapy. APBI would be a shorter course of treatment—only 1 to 2 weeks—but the doses of radiation would be higher than in whole-breast irradiation.[26]

Women with advanced breast cancer may need more aggressive surgery than a lumpectomy. **Total mastectomy** is removal of the entire breast and involved lymph nodes. A **radical mastectomy** is removal of the entire breast and underlying muscle as well as the

## Figure 13.10

**Mammography.** Each breast is placed on a platform, and the tissue is compressed while the x-ray is taken.

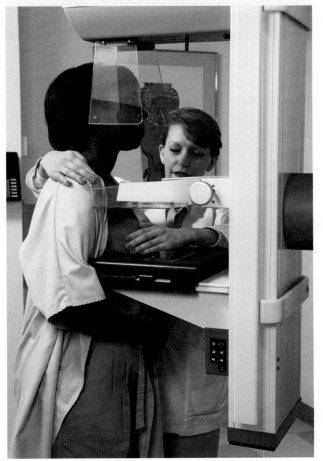

underarm lymph nodes and fat. In a *modified radical mastectomy*, underlying muscle is not removed.

Immunotherapy, hormonal therapy, and chemotherapy are also used in breast cancer treatment in addition to surgery and radiation. Herceptin (trastuzumab) is a drug used in targeted immunotherapy. Women with late-stage recurring cancer are often treated with this monoclonal antibody. Antibodies are receptor proteins that recognize foreign substances (antigens) in the body and bind to them. Monoclonal antibodies are made in the laboratory from a single type of antibody. In this case, Herceptin is an antibody that targets a particular breast tumor protein. After binding to this protein, the antibody works in various ways to shrink breast cancer tumors and stop tumor cells from multiplying. Women treated with both Herceptin and chemotherapy have been found to be less likely to experience a recurrence of their cancer than women treated with chemotherapy alone.[22]

The primary drug used in hormonal therapy is tamoxifen, an anti-estrogen. Anti-estrogens counteract the effects of estrogen on breast cancers that depend on estrogen for their growth. Tamoxifen has few serious side effects compared to other anticancer drugs, reduces the annual recurrence rate by 41%, and reduces the death rate by 33%.[22]

Chemotherapy is also used to treat breast cancer, sometimes in conjunction with tamoxifen. Compounds have been discovered that have demonstrated good antitumor activity in breast cancer treatment. Taxol was the first to be discovered. (Taxol is found in the bark of the Pacific yew tree [*Taxus brevifolia*].) Today a variety of drugs is used in breast cancer chemotherapy, with combinations of drugs providing more effective results than single drugs.[22]

**Endometrial Cancer** The endometrium is the lining of the uterus, the organ in which a fetus develops until birth (see Chapter 5). Endometrial cancer most often occurs in postmenopausal women; only 5% of endometrial cancers occur in women younger than 40 years.[27] The primary symptom of this cancer is abnormal uterine bleeding. Premenopausal women usually experience symptoms of irregular, heavy, or prolonged uterine bleeding during menstrual periods or bleeding between periods. Postmenopausal women experience uterine bleeding although they no longer have menstrual periods.

Most endometrial cancer is diagnosed at an early stage because of postmenopausal bleeding. The Pap test for cervical cancer does not detect cancer in the body of the uterus. (This test is discussed shortly.) However, if the physician suspects that a patient has endometrial cancer, he or she usually performs an endometrial biopsy, in which a sample of tissue is removed from the endometrium and examined microscopically.

Although the cause of endometrial cancer is unknown, it is associated with prolonged exposure to estrogen. Therefore, the risk factors for endometrial cancer are similar to those for breast cancer: early menarche, late menopause, not bearing children, and delaying pregnancy. Additionally, women who are more than 50 lbs overweight, especially postmenopausal women, have a 10-fold greater risk for developing endometrial cancer than women who are not overweight. As with breast cancer, exercising reduces risk.[3] Using oral contraceptives that combine estrogen and progesterone reduces risk as well, but estrogen replacement therapy without progesterone (unopposed ERT) is a risk factor.[13] Infertility and diabetes are possible risk factors for endometrial cancer as well.[3]

Many women diagnosed with endometrial cancer undergo total hysterectomy: removal of the uterus, fallopian tubes, and ovaries. Additionally, radiation, hormones, and/or chemotherapy are sometimes used after surgery. The outlook for survival after treatment for endometrial cancer is good: The 1-year and 5-year survival rates are 92% and 83%, respectively.[3]

## Cancers Related to Viral Infection: Cervical Cancer

Certain viruses are implicated in the development of a variety of cancers; **Table 13.6** lists these viruses and the cancers to which they are related. However, viruses alone do not appear to cause cancer. Scientists think that interactions between these viruses and other agents, or co-carcinogens, result in the development of cancer. For example, the high incidence of liver cancer in certain regions of Africa and Asia appears to be caused by interactions between the hepatitis B virus and aflatoxins. Aflatoxins are a group of carcinogens produced by a mold that grows on improperly stored peanuts and grains. Many people in these regions eat these moldy foods.

The virally related cancer most prevalent in the United States is cervical cancer. Since 1960, the incidence of cervical cancer has declined dramatically, primarily because of the widespread routine use of the **Papanicolaou test (Pap test)** to screen women

## Table 13.6

### Viruses and Cancers to Which They Are Related

| Virus | Cancer Type |
|---|---|
| Hepatitis B virus (HBV) | Primary liver cancer |
| Human T-cell lymphotropic/leukemia virus (HTLV) | Adult T-cell lymphoma/leukemia |
| Cytomegalovirus (CMV) | Kaposi's sarcoma |
| Human papillomavirus (HPV) | Cervical cancer, penile cancer, oropharyngeal cancer |
| Epstein-Barr virus (EBV) | Burkitt's lymphoma, nasopharyngeal cancer |

for cervical cancer. To perform the Pap test, a physician or other specially trained healthcare professional takes a sample of cells from the cervical canal. These cells are examined under a microscope. A newer method of collecting and analyzing samples is the liquid-based thin-layer slide preparation, which appears to be more sensitive than standard Pap tests. In addition, computer-automated readers improve the analysis of Pap tests.

Most women who are diagnosed with cervical cancer have no symptoms; their cancers are discovered at an early stage during their annual gynecologic examination and Pap test. If undiagnosed, the cancer may cause symptoms of abnormal vaginal bleeding (the most common symptom), pelvic pressure or pain, and/or a foul-smelling vaginal discharge.

Cervical cancer most often develops in young and middle-aged women, generally between the ages of 35 and 54 years, with a median age at diagnosis of 48. Fourteen percent of cervical cancer cases are diagnosed in women between the ages of 20 and 34 years.[28] If untreated, cervical cancer can invade surrounding tissues and metastasize. Having regular screening tests can reduce the risk of developing invasive cancer of the cervix.

A causal association exists between infection with human papillomavirus (HPV) and cervical cancer. HPV is transmitted by infected men to their female partners during sexual intercourse, and vice versa. Therefore, the greater the number of male sexual partners a woman has over time, the greater are her chances of becoming infected with HPV. If a woman is monogamous but her male sex partner is not, her risk rises because he is more likely to become infected than if he were monogamous. Also, women who had their first sexual intercourse before age 17 are at increased risk because they are more likely to have a greater number of sexual partners over time than those women who became sexually active at an older age. In addition, long-term use of oral contraceptives is associated with an increased risk of cervical cancer.[3]

At low risk for cervical cancer are women who are celibate, such as Roman Catholic nuns, or who are monogamous with a monogamous partner over many years. Sexually active women with multiple partners or with nonmonogamous partners can lower their risk by using male or female condoms to protect themselves against infection with HPV.

In 2006, the U.S. Food and Drug Administration (FDA) approved the first vaccine developed to prevent cervical cancer (Gardasil) and in 2009 approved a second (Cervarix). Gardasil is highly effective in preventing infection by four types of HPV. Two types (HPV-16 and HPV-18) cause approximately 70% of cervical cancers,[8] and the other two types (HPV-6 and HPV-11) cause about 90% of all genital warts (see Chapter 14). The FDA in 2009 expanded the approval of Gardasil for use in boys and young men to prevent genital warts. Cervarix acts against HPV-16 and HPV-18 only. The American Cancer Society recommends routine HPV vaccination for females aged 11 and 12 years, and for females aged 13 to 18 years "to catch up on missed vaccine or complete the vaccination series."[8]

HPV vaccines do not prevent infection with all types of HPV, so vaccinated women should still have regular Pap tests. In addition, neither vaccine protects nor treats women already infected with HPV, so it is important for girls and young women to be vaccinated before they become sexually active.

The American Cancer Society recommends that all women should have annual conventional Pap tests or biannual liquid-based Pap tests 3 years after their first vaginal intercourse but no later than age 21. The ACS suggests that after three consecutive normal Pap tests, women older than 30 years may have this test performed every 2 to 3 years or at the discretion of their physicians.

If the Pap test shows that cervical cancer may be present, a physician usually performs a *colposcopy*. Using a specially designed microscope, the physician examines the cervix. If the physician observes abnormal cervical tissue during this procedure, he or she usually performs a biopsy to confirm the diagnosis.

Physicians treat dysplasia or cervical cancers in situ with surgery, electrocoagulation, cryotherapy, and carbon dioxide ($CO_2$) laser surgery. Laser energy destroys the tissue. Cryotherapy is the use of extreme cold to destroy cells. Usually solid carbon dioxide or liquid nitrogen is applied briefly to the abnormal tissue with a sterile cotton-tipped applicator. A blister forms and the tissue dies. Electrocoagulation kills the tissue through intense heat by electric current.

With invasive cervical cancers, surgeons may perform a simple hysterectomy (removal of just the uterus) or a total hysterectomy (removal of the uterus and ovaries). With certain cervical cancers, radiation is the treatment of choice. Detected early, cervical cancer is highly survivable.

## Cancers Related to Ultraviolet Radiation: Skin Cancers

Lying on the beach or on a tanning bed to develop a tanned "healthy" look is anything but healthy! When skin tans it is a sign of skin damage. Certain skin cells produce a pigment called *melanin* to protect the skin from the damaging rays of the sun. Melanin is a built-in sun protector for dark-skinned people and is produced in response to sun damage in light-skinned people. In addition to causing the skin to wrinkle and age prematurely, the ultraviolet (UV) radiation in sunlight can result in the development of skin cancer. In fact, UV light exposure is the most important factor (other than heredity and age) that influences the development of skin cancer. In addition to tanning (UV rays) causing skin damage in general, sunburns during childhood and intense intermittent sun exposure increase the risk of melanoma and other skin cancers later in life.[8]

There are three types of ultraviolet radiation: UVA, UVB, and UVC. All three types are harmful and have the potential to cause skin cancer. Claims by tanning parlors that using only UVB rays will protect you from the effects of UV radiation are false. This type of ultraviolet radiation is associated with sunburn and skin cancer formation, as is UVA radiation. UVA radiation is also strongly associated with premature aging effects. Artificial UV sources, such as sun lamps and tanning beds, may also generate UVC rays. UVC radiation is a highly potent cancer-causing radiation. Although a danger from artificial sources, these rays are filtered out by the Earth's atmosphere and pose little danger from environmental sources.

There are three main types of skin cancer: basal cell carcinoma, squamous cell carcinoma, and malignant melanoma. Approximately 60% of skin cancers are basal cell carcinomas and approximately 30% are squamous cell carcinomas. Although malignant melanoma makes up less than 10% of skin cancers, this fast-growing, metastasizing cancer results in the most deaths. Malignant melanoma spreads quickly via the blood and lymph. Death is usually the result of either respiratory failure or brain or spinal cord complications. **Table 13.7** lists steps for preventing skin cancer.

**Basal cell carcinoma**, the most common cancer of the skin, often affects persons older than 40 years. A slow-growing cancer that rarely metastasizes, basal cell carcinoma frequently develops on portions of the skin exposed to the sun: the face, head, neck, and arms. Lesions may look like moles or chronic pimples with pearl-like borders. They often become crusty and scaly and may ulcerate and bleed (**Figure 13.11a**). Basal cell carcinoma tumors are usually removed by surgery and cryotherapy, freezing with liquid nitrogen. The cure rate for basal cell carcinoma is high.

### Table 13.7

### Steps to Reduce the Risk of Melanoma and Other Skin Cancers

- Do not use tanning beds.

- Avoid exposure to the sun (particularly sunbathing), especially between 10 a.m. and 4 p.m. when UV radiation is highest.

- When in the sun, wear sunglasses that block at least 99% of UVA and UVB radiation. Larger glasses and wraparounds provide the best protection.

- When in the sun, wear wide-brimmed hats and clothing that covers as much as possible of the arms, legs, and torso.

- Use sunscreens with a sun protection factor (SPF) of 15 or higher regularly on sun-exposed skin.

## Figure 13.11

**Skin Cancers.** (a) This basal cell carcinoma is a raised lesion with central depressions that bleed and crust over. (b) Squamous cell carcinoma looks like a red rounded mass or a flat sore as shown in the photo. (c) Lesions of malignant melanoma are usually characterized by irregular borders with red, white, blue, or blue-black spots. Some portions may be raised.

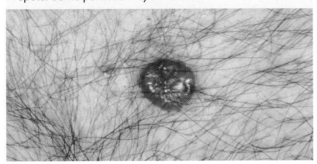

(a)

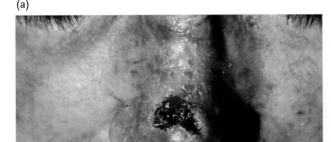

(b)

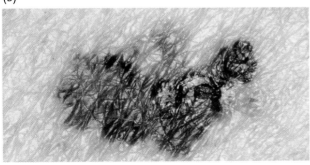

(c)

**Squamous cell carcinoma** is the second most common skin cancer in light-skinned persons; it develops in the same sun-exposed areas as does basal cell carcinoma. However, dark-skinned people can develop this type of cancer, not from sunlight exposure, but from exposure to noxious chemicals and high levels of x-rays, as well as from trauma (burns and chronic ulcers). The skin lesions of squamous cell carcinoma look flat, red, scaly, and may be slightly elevated (**Figure 13.11b**). These tumors are removed by the same methods as basal cell carcinoma.

**squamous (SKWAY-muss) cell carcinoma** A common form of skin cancer that develops from exposure to noxious chemicals and high levels of x-rays, as well as from trauma.

**malignant melanoma** (MEL-ah-NO-mah) A deadly form of skin cancer that develops most often in persons who have been exposed to the sun in short, intense sessions, have had severe sunburn and extensive sun exposure in childhood, or have first-degree relatives who had the disease.

Both basal and squamous cell carcinomas develop from prolonged, repeated exposures to the sun. At risk are persons who are outdoors much of the time, such as construction workers, farmers, and people who regularly sunbathe and use tanning beds.

**Malignant melanoma**, primarily a disease of whites, is a deadly skin cancer that affects men at a 50% higher rate than women. The incidence of melanoma has been rising over the last 30 years, most notably in young white women aged 15 to 39 years. Additionally, an increase has been seen in both sexes aged 65 years and older.[3]

The risk for developing malignant melanoma and other skin cancers is higher the closer a person lives to the equator because of the increasing intensity of UV rays. Additionally, fair-skinned people are at greater risk than those who have darker skin. At highest risk are persons with light blue eyes, very light hair, and skin that burns easily and freckles rather than tans. Malignant melanoma develops more often in persons who are exposed to the sun in short intense sessions, such as persons who work indoors and then vacation in a sunny climate. Severe sunburn and extensive sun exposure in childhood also increase the risk for developing malignant melanoma in adulthood. Additionally, first-degree relatives of people with melanoma have a two- to eightfold increase in their risk of developing this cancer. Individuals who have two or more relatives with a history of melanoma may be at substantially higher risk.

Malignant melanoma can develop on any skin surface as well as in the eye and on mucous membranes. In men, the trunk is the most common site; in women, the legs are a common site. If you are in a high-risk group for skin cancer, especially melanoma, examine your skin regularly. Early detection is key to curing this disease. Typically, melanoma tumors are asymmetrical, have irregular borders, multiple colors (such as blue, black, red, or gray), and have a diameter greater than a pencil eraser (**Figure 13.11c**). An easy way to remember these signs is ABCD: asymmetry,

This article focuses on the use of tanning beds and the link to malignant melanoma. Explain why you think this article is a reliable or an unreliable source of information. Use the model for analyzing health information to guide your thinking; the main points of the model are noted here. The model is fully explained in Chapter 1.

1. Which statements are verifiable facts, and which are unverified statements or value claims?
2. What are the credentials of the source making these health-related claims? Does the source have the appropriate background and education in the topic area? What can you do to check the credentials of this source?
3. What might be the motives and biases of the source making the claims?

4. What is the main point of the article? Which information is relevant to the issue, main point, product, or service? Which information is irrelevant?
5. Is the source reliable? What evidence supports your conclusion that the source is reliable or unreliable? Does the source of information present the pros and cons of the topic or the benefits and risks of the product?
6. Does the source of information attack the credibility of conventional scientists or medical authorities?

Based on your analysis, do you think that this article is a reliable source of health-related information? Summarize your reasons for coming to this conclusion.

## Study Links Tanning Bed Use to Increased Risk of Melanoma

People who use tanning beds are more likely to develop melanoma, the deadliest form of skin cancer, than never users, according to a new study from the University of Minnesota. The more regularly a person frequents tanning salons, the greater the risk, the study shows.

In July 2009, after a comprehensive review of the available research, the International Agency for Research on Cancer (IARC) elevated tanning devices to its highest cancer risk category—"carcinogenic to humans" (Group 1). Despite this risk, approximately 30 million Americans still visit indoor tanning salons each year. That may be at least in part because the tanning industry has pointed to limitations in previous studies and continues to tout the purported health benefits of tanning, including vitamin D production.

The new study, funded by the National Cancer Institute and the American Cancer Society, was designed to help answer more definitively whether tanning bed use is linked to skin cancer.

"Most reports were not able to adjust for sun exposure, confirm a dose-response, or examine specific tanning devices," said study author DeAnn Lazovich, PhD, professor of epidemiology, University of Minnesota School of Publishing and co-leader of the Masonic Cancer Center's Prevention and Etiology Research Program. "Our population-based, case-control study was conducted to address these limitations."

### What This Study Found

The researchers, led by Lazovich, collected detailed information on the tanning habits of more than 1,100 Minnesotans aged 25 to 59 who had been diagnosed with melanoma between July 2004 and December 2007, as well as a matched group of more than 1,100 people without melanoma.

border, color, and diameter. Medical researchers recently determined, however, that very rapidly growing melanomas do not necessarily show the ABCD signs. These melanomas, most often found in men and women older than age 65 years, may be red and raised with regular borders. They often itch and bleed.[29]

*Healthy People 2020* is a program to improve the health of all Americans by guiding individuals to make healthy choices and monitoring progress made. A *Healthy People 2020* objective is to reduce the death rate from malignant melanoma from 2.7 deaths per 100,000 population (baseline in 2007) to 2.4 deaths per 100,000. One way to achieve this objective is to increase to at least 80.1% the proportion of persons age 18 years or older who follow protective measures that may reduce the risk of skin cancer, such as limiting sun exposure and using sunscreens and protective clothing when exposed to sunlight. Baseline data from *Healthy People 2020* show that 72.8% of U.S. adults followed sun-protective measures in 2008. Another objective is to increase the proportion of high school students who follow sun-protective measures from 9.3% (baseline in 2009) to 11.2%.[30]

Reducing the proportion of adults and high school students who use tanning beds and lights is another

The researchers gathered data on tanning bed use, including years of use, age at which use began, and the specific devices used, as well as other factors such as age, sunscreen use, and family history of melanoma.

According to their findings, people who had ever used an indoor tanning device were about 75% more likely to have developed melanoma. Frequent users—defined as using a tanning device for at least 50 hours, at least 100 sessions, or at least 10 years—were 2.5 to 3 times more likely to develop melanoma than those who had never used them. The risk went up with increasing tanning bed use, the study showed, and was elevated regardless of the type of device.

"We found that it didn't matter the type of tanning device used; there was no safe tanning device," Lazovich said. "We also found—and this is new data—that the risk of getting melanoma is associated more with how much a person tans and not the age at which a person starts using tanning devices. Risk rises with frequency of use, regardless of age, gender, or device."

Lazovich and her team's findings are published in *Cancer Epidemiology, Biomarkers and Prevention*, a journal of the American Association for Cancer Research.

## Melanoma on the Rise

The number of new cases of melanoma in the United States has been increasing for at least 30 years. The American Cancer Society estimates that about 68,720 new melanomas will be diagnosed in the United States during 2009. Melanoma is 10 times more common in whites than in African Americans. It is slightly more common in men than in women.

More than 2 million skin cancers are diagnosed each year in the United States. That's more than cancers of the prostate, breast, lung, colon, uterus, ovaries, and pancreas combined.

Most skin cancers are caused by too much exposure to ultraviolet (UV) rays. Much of this exposure comes from the sun, but it also comes from manmade sources, such as tanning beds.

Because of the popularity of tanning among young people, both the World Health Organization and the International Commission on Non-ionizing Radiation Protection recommend that the use of indoor tanning should be restricted in anyone under the age of 18.

The American Cancer Society recommends people avoid tanning beds altogether. For information on how you can lower your risk of skin cancer, see *Skin Cancer Prevention and Early Detection*.

*Source:* Snowden, R. V. (2010, May 27). Study links tanning bed use to increased risk of melanoma. American Cancer Society. Retrieved April 25, 2011, from http://www.cancer.org/Cancer/news/News/study-links-tanning-bed-use-to-increased-risk-of-melanoma.

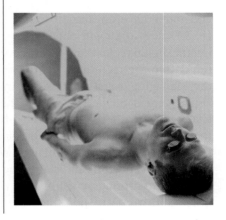

*Healthy People 2020* cancer-reduction objective. For high school students, the baseline was 15.6% who used tanning beds and lights in 2009; the target is a decrease to 14%. For adults, the baseline was 15.2% in 2008; the target is a decrease to 13.7%.[30]

# Cancers with Unknown Causes

**Prostate Cancer** The prostate is a walnut-sized accessory sex organ in men. It lies beneath the bladder, surrounding the urethra, and secretes part of the seminal fluid. (See Chapter 5 for more information on this gland.)

Prostate cancer is the most prevalent cancer in men, and the second most prevalent cause of cancer deaths in men (see Table 133). (Lung cancer is the most prevalent cause of cancer death in men.) The signs and symptoms of prostate cancer mimic those of benign prostatic hypertrophy (BPH) and other noncancerous conditions of the prostate (see the Managing Your Health essay in Chapter 5 titled "Enlargement of the Prostate"). Therefore, experiencing symptoms that include uneven flow of urine while urinating, incomplete emptying of the bladder, reduced urine flow, and urinating more frequently at night does not necessarily mean a man has prostate cancer. However, serious signs and symptoms that are more likely to be related to prostate cancer are pain in the floor of the pelvis, sudden development of impotence, and presence of blood in the urine.

In the United States, African Americans have the highest prostate cancer incidence rate, followed by whites, Hispanics, Native Americans, and Asian/Pacific Islanders, in that order. Advanced age and heredity are strong risk factors for prostate cancer. Along with family history of prostate cancer, having certain genetic mutations, such as *BRCA2*, increase risk. This disease is rare in men younger than 45 years, but its incidence rises as men age. The median age of death from prostate cancer is 80 years.[3]

The American Cancer Society suggests that maintaining a healthy body weight and being physically active may reduce the risk of developing aggressive prostate cancer. Statins—cholesterol-lowering drugs—may reduce the risk of advanced prostate cancer. Long-term low-dose aspirin therapy may reduce prostate cancer risk as well, but taking aspirin for prostate cancer prevention is not recommended by the ACS.[3] Substituting fish for red meat in the diet may lower prostate cancer risk.[11]

For early detection of prostate cancer, the American Cancer Society recommends that all men 50 years and older have an annual prostate-specific antigen (PSA) test, with or without a digital rectal exam. During the digital rectal exam, a physician inserts a gloved finger into the rectum to feel the prostate gland (see the Managing Your Health essay in Chapter 5 titled "Enlargement of the Prostate"). The PSA is a blood test that detects a protein secreted by the prostate. If the protein concentration in the blood is elevated, it indicates that the prostate may be abnormal but not necessarily cancerous and should be checked further. The topic of prostate screening and the use of the PSA test is controversial. The United States Preventive Services Task Force recommends that healthy men not be screened for prostate cancer using the PSA because the test has been shown to not save lives. The American Cancer Society suggests that men make this decision with their physician after being fully informed of the risks and benefits of test results.[31] Chapter 5 describes methods of screening the prostate.

Physicians may treat localized prostate cancer by surgically removing the prostate and some surrounding tissue. However, this treatment can result in impotence, incontinence, and other complications. New surgical techniques with fewer side effects have been developed, leading to a resurgence of prostate surgery as a treatment. Advanced prostate cancer is sometimes treated with drug/hormone therapy or by removal of the testicles to reduce male sex hormone levels, which may influence the progression of this cancer. Chemotherapy, radiation, or a combination of therapies may be used if the cancer has metastasized.[3]

Prostate cancer is, in many cases, a slow-growing cancer. Many prostate cancer patients die *with* prostate cancer rather than *of* it. Because the side effects of prostate cancer treatment can be quite serious, physicians carefully consider "watchful waiting" as the treatment of choice for this cancer.[3]

**Testicular Cancer** The testicles, or testes, are the organs in which sperm develop and are located in the scrotal sac beneath the penis. Cancer of the testicles is a rare and highly curable cancer. Only 1% of cancers in men occur in the testicles.

The signs and symptoms of testicular cancer are a painless, swollen testis and a sensation of heaviness or aching in the testis. Men who perform testicular self-examination might feel a small lump in one testis.

Youth is a risk factor for testicular cancer. This cancer strikes primarily men between the ages of 20 and 54 years. Another risk factor for testicular cancer is the failure of one or both of the testicles to descend into the scrotum by age 1 year. White males are at highest risk, Latino males are at less risk, and African American men are at least risk. Men with a family history of testicular cancer are at increased risk as are men who are infected with HIV or have AIDS. Men who have had testicular cancer in one testicle may develop it in the other.[32]

To detect testicular cancer early, the American Cancer Society recommends that men perform a **testicular self-examination (TSE)** once a month after a warm bath or shower (see the Managing Your Health box titled "Testicular Self-Exam"). The heat relaxes the scrotal skin, making tumors easier to detect. If detected and treated early, testicular cancer is one of the most curable cancers. Surgery is most often used, frequently in conjunction with radiation or chemotherapy.

**Ovarian Cancer** The ovaries are female organs in which eggs mature and are ovulated each month. Ovaries also produce the female sex hormones estrogen and progesterone. Cancer of the ovaries is difficult to detect, especially in its early stages when most women have no symptoms. However, as the cancer progresses and the ovarian tumor enlarges, many women develop symptoms such as frequent urination or bloating and pressure in the abdomen. Thus, advanced ovarian cancer is confused frequently with other urinary and gastrointestinal tract disorders. Additionally, postmenopausal women may experience vaginal bleeding, while premenopausal women may have irregular or heavy menses.

Advancing age is a risk factor for ovarian cancer. Most deaths from this disease occur in women 55 years and older. Other than advanced age, the risk factors for ovarian cancer are similar to those of breast and endometrial cancer: early menarche, late menopause, and not bearing children. The links between

# Managing Your Health

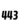

## Testicular Self-Examination

### How the Test Is Performed

Perform this test during or after a shower. This way, the scrotal skin is warm and relaxed. It's best to do the test while standing.

1. Gently feel your scrotal sac to locate a testicle.
2. Hold the testicle with one hand while firmly but gently rolling the fingers of the other hand over the testicle to examine the entire surface.
3. Repeat the procedure with the other testicle.

### Why the Test Is Performed

A testicular self-exam is done to check for testicular cancer. Normal testicles contain blood vessels and other structures that can make the exam confusing. Performing a self-exam monthly allows you to become familiar with your normal anatomy. Then, if you notice any changes from the previous exam, you'll know to contact your doctor.

You should perform a testicular self-exam every month if you have or have had any of the following risk factors:

1. Family history of testicular cancer
2. Previous testicular tumor
3. Undescended testicle
4. Are a teenager or young adult (to about 35 years old)

### Normal Results

Each testicle should feel firm but not rock hard. One testicle may or may not be lower or slightly larger than the other.

Always ask your doctor if you have any doubts or questions.

### What Abnormal Results Mean

If you find a small hard lump (like a pea), have an enlarged testicle, or notice any other concerning differences from your last self-exam, see your doctor as soon as you can.

### Consult your doctor if:

- You can't find one or both testicles—the testicles may not have descended properly in the scrotum.
- There is a soft collection of thin tubes above the testicle—it may be a collection of dilated veins (varicocele).
- There is pain or swelling in the scrotum—it may be an infection or a fluid-filled sac (hydrocele), causing blockage of blood flow to the area.

Sudden, severe (acute) pain in the scrotum or testicle is an emergency. If you experience such pain, seek immediate medical attention.

### Considerations

A lump on the testicle is often the first sign of testicular cancer. Therefore, if you find a lump, see a doctor immediately. Keep in mind that some cases of testicular cancer do not show symptoms until they reach an advanced stage.

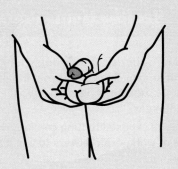

*Source:* MedlinePlus Medical Encyclopedia. (updated September 2009). Testicular self-examination. Retrieved April 21, 2011, from http://www.nlm.nih.gov/medlineplus/ency/article/003909.htm

these risk factors and ovarian cancer, however, are not as well defined as they are in breast and endometrial cancer. Additional risk factors include having had breast cancer, having a family member who had breast or ovarian cancer, and having mutations in the *BRCA1* or *BRCA2* breast cancer genes.[33]

Research results show that the use of oral contraceptives that contain both estrogen and progesterone lower a woman's risk of developing ovarian cancer. Estrogen replacement therapy without progesterone increases a woman's risk of this cancer.[33]

No accurate routine screening test for women at average risk for ovarian cancer is available. However, screening techniques are available for women who have symptoms of or are at high risk for ovarian cancer. Screening techniques include a thorough pelvic examination, transvaginal ultrasound, a blood test for tumor marker CA125, and a CT or MRI scan of the pelvic area. Ovarian cancer is treated with surgery, chemotherapy, and, rarely, radiation.[33]

## Healthy Living Practices

- [ ] To lower your risk of developing lung cancer, do not smoke cigarettes, avoid inhaling airborne asbestos fibers, and avoid exposure to radon gas.
- [ ] If you are exposed to lung carcinogens at your place of work, explore ways to avoid future exposure.
- [ ] To prevent the development of larynx, mouth, and esophagus cancers, avoid smoking and chewing tobacco and excessive drinking of alcoholic beverages.
- [ ] Have a complete oral examination annually for early cancer detection.
- [ ] To lower your risk of developing cancer of the bladder and kidney, avoid smoking cigarettes.
- [ ] To lower your risk of pancreatic cancer, avoid smoking cigarettes and inhaling chemical fumes.
- [ ] To lower your risk of developing stomach cancer, avoid eating salt-cured, nitrate-cured, or smoked foods. Also avoid smoking cigarettes and drinking excessive amounts of alcoholic beverages.
- [ ] To reduce your risk of developing colorectal cancer, follow the American Cancer

Society's screening guidelines and remove precancerous polyps.
- [ ] If you are female, you can reduce your risk of breast cancer by exercising and avoiding alcoholic beverages.
- [ ] To detect breast cancer in its early stages, follow the ACS guidelines for breast clinical examination and mammography. Be aware of any changes in your breasts.
- [ ] If you are female, you can reduce your risk of developing endometrial cancer by losing weight if you are overweight and by controlling diabetes mellitus if you have this disease.
- [ ] Discuss the impact of estrogen replacement therapy on the development of endometrial cancer with your healthcare provider if you are considering or are taking this medication.
- [ ] If you are female and older than 40 years, have annual pelvic examinations for early detection of endometrial cancer.
- [ ] If you are a sexually active woman with multiple partners or with nonmonogamous partners, you can lower your risk of cervical cancer by using male or female condoms to protect yourself against HPV. Young women can be vaccinated against certain types of HPV.
- [ ] All women can lower their risk of cervical cancer by avoiding cigarette smoking.
- [ ] If you have been sexually active and are age 21 years or older, the American Cancer Society recommends that you have annual Pap tests to screen for cervical cancer. See the ACS guidelines for detailed recommendations.
- [ ] To protect against skin cancer, stay out of the sun, wear sunscreen when outdoors, and do not use tanning beds or lights.
- [ ] Detect melanoma early by checking your skin for growths that exhibit these warning signs: asymmetry, irregular border, multiple colors, and large diameter. Be aware that fast-growing melanomas may be red, raised, and itchy with symmetrical borders.
- [ ] If you are male and older than 50, talk to your healthcare provider about annual digital rectal exams and PSA tests for the early detection of prostate cancer.
- [ ] If you are male, perform a testicular self-examination once every month to detect this cancer early.

# Managing Your Health

## Reducing Your Risk for Cancer

### DO'S

- Eat a diet low in red meats, especially high-fat and processed meats.
- Eat a variety of fruits and vegetables daily.
- Follow the American Cancer Society's recommendations for screening tests to detect cancer in its early stages.
- Men should perform monthly testicular self-examinations.
- Know the warning signs of cancer and see your healthcare provider immediately if you detect any of them.
- Sexually active women with multiple partners or with nonmonogamous partners should use male or female condoms during sexual intercourse to protect themselves against infection with human papillomavirus.
- Maintain a healthy weight.
- Women should consult their healthcare providers regarding the use of oral contraceptives and estrogen replacement therapy with respect to cancer prevention and risk.
- Exercise most days of the week.

- When in the sun, wear wide-brimmed hats and sunglasses that block UV radiation.
- Wear sunscreen on sun-exposed skin.

### DON'TS

- Don't smoke cigarettes. If you can't quit, cut down.
- Avoid breathing environmental tobacco smoke.
- Don't chew tobacco products.
- Don't drink excessive amounts of alcoholic beverages.
- Women should avoid drinking alcoholic beverages to reduce the risk of breast cancer.
- Avoid unnecessary exposure to ionizing radiation, such as x-rays and ultraviolet light.
- Don't lie in the sun or in tanning beds.
- Avoid direct sun exposure between 10 A.M. and 4 P.M.
- Avoid exposure to toxic chemicals, such as certain occupational carcinogens.
- Avoid inhaling chemical fumes, such as gasoline fumes.
- Avoid breathing asbestos dust and radon gas.
- Avoid eating salt-cured, nitrate-cured, or smoked foods.

## Reducing Your Risk for Cancer

You cannot change some of your cancer risk factors: heredity, age, ethnicity, lifelong exposure to naturally produced estrogen (in women), and the nondescent of testes (in male children). However, you can avoid many risk factors, thereby reducing your risk of developing one or more cancers. The Managing Your Health box titled "Reducing Your Risk for Cancer" lists modifiable cancer risks and actions you can take to lower your risk.

A summary of the American Cancer Society's recommendations for the early detection of cancer is listed in the Managing Your Health box titled "Screening Guidelines for the Early Detection of Cancer in Average-Risk Asymptomatic People" earlier in this chapter. Finally, the next Managing Your Health box lists cancer's seven warning signs. In ad-

dition to being aware of these signs, you can learn the more detailed early warning signs for the various cancers described in this chapter. If you have concerns about your risk of developing cancer, discuss them with your healthcare provider. Early detection and treatment are critical to winning the war against cancer.

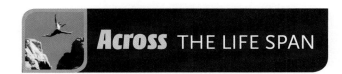

**Across** THE LIFE SPAN

### CANCER

Most cancers arise in people older than 50 years, and the risk continues to rise as people grow older. The only cancers described in this chapter that are prevalent in young adults are malignant melanoma, testicular cancer, cervical cancer, and breast cancer. Additionally, only 1% of cancers occur in children.

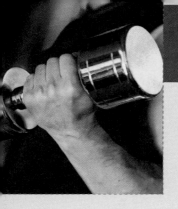

# Managing Your Health

## Cancer's Seven Warning Signs

You can remember the following signs easily by knowing that they are a CAUTION: These signs do not necessarily mean you have cancer but that you should see your healthcare provider to evaluate the sign.

**C**hange in bowel or bladder habits
**A** sore that does not heal
**U**nusual bleeding or discharge
**T**hickening or lump in breast or elsewhere
**I**ndigestion or difficulty in swallowing
**O**bvious change in a wart or mole
**N**agging cough or hoarseness

However, cancer is the most frequent cause of death from disease in American children older than 1 year of age. The most prevalent cancers of children up to 5 years old are listed in *Table 13.8*.

Adult cancers rarely occur in children. These cancers are largely related to the effects of cancer-causing agents acting on cells over a lifetime, while children's cancers seem more often related to genetic factors.

Although pediatric cancers usually grow more rapidly than adult cancers do, they are, in general, more responsive to anticancer drugs than are adult cancers. For this reason chemotherapy is the treatment of choice for most childhood cancers, while surgery and radiation are the primary treatments for adult cancers. Effective cancer chemotherapy has produced a remarkable decline in childhood deaths resulting from cancer over the past 30 years.

### Table 13.8

### The Most Prevalent Cancers of Children up to Age 5 Years

Leukemia (cancer of the blood)

Central nervous system cancers

Lymphomas (cancer of the lymph nodes)

Nervous system tumors (often in adrenal glands)

Wilms' tumor (cancer of the kidney)

Bone cancer

Retinoblastoma (cancer of the eye)

Liver cancer

go.jblearning.com/alters6e

## Summary

Cancer is a variety of diseases that have common characteristics: Their cells exhibit abnormal growth, division, and differentiation and have the potential to spread from where they develop. These cells form masses called malignant tumors that interfere with normal body processes.

Cancer develops in cells that have damaged or mutated genes. Mutations can be inherited or can occur from exposure to low-dose radiation, drugs, toxic chemicals, or certain viruses. Successive genetic changes must take place for a normal cell to change into a cancer cell. Therefore, the probability of developing cancer generally increases with age and with exposure to cancer-causing substances.

This chapter organizes the discussion of cancers according to factors that appear to be most significant in their development. Advanced age is a risk factor for most cancers; heredity is a significant risk factor in some cancers.

Tobacco use causes cancers of the lung, larynx, oral cavity, esophagus, kidney, bladder, pancreas, stomach, blood, and cervix. To lower the risk of developing any of these cancers, avoid smoking and chewing tobacco products. Additionally, avoid drinking excessive amounts of alcoholic beverages to lower the risk of developing larynx, oral, and esophageal cancer. Have a complete oral examination annually for early cancer detection in this area.

Diet accounts for a significant number of cancers and has both a positive and a negative effect on the development of cancer. A primary risk factor in the development of stomach cancer is eating salt-cured, nitrate-cured, or smoked foods. To lower the risk of developing this cancer, avoid eating these foods. To reduce the risk of developing colorectal cancer, avoid having more than one alcoholic drink per day and eat a diet adequate in vegetables and fruits. Refer to the ACS recommendations for screening recommendations for colon cancer in persons over the age of 50.

The cancers related to hormone function are breast cancer and endometrial cancer. These cancers are associated significantly with prolonged exposure to estrogen. Risk factors associated with these cancers are early menarche, late menopause, not bearing children, and delaying pregnancy. Exercising helps reduce breast cancer risk in women. Avoiding alcoholic beverages also reduces the risk. For early cancer detection, women aged 20 to 39 years should have a breast clinical examination every 3 years, and every year at age 40 and after. Women should become aware of the normal condition of their breasts and seek medical attention if they notice any changes. Women aged 40 and older should have mammography every year. For early detection of endometrial cancer, women at menopause should report any unexpected bleeding or spotting to their physician.

Certain viruses are implicated in the development of a variety of cancers. The virally related cancer most prevalent in the United States is cervical cancer. The virus implicated in this disease, human papillomavirus (HPV), is transmitted by infected men to their female partners during sexual intercourse, and vice versa. Sexually active women with multiple partners or with nonmonogamous partners can lower their risk of cervical cancer by using male or female condoms to protect themselves against HPV. Women can also lower their risk by avoiding cigarette smoking. Young women can be vaccinated against certain types of HPV.

The ultraviolet radiation in sunlight is the most important factor that influences the development of cancer of the skin. There are three main types of skin cancer: basal cell carcinoma, squamous cell carcinoma, and malignant melanoma. Of these cancers malignant melanoma results in the most deaths because it is a fast-growing metastatic cancer. Light-skinned, fair-haired whites are a high-risk group for developing skin cancer. To protect against skin cancer, stay out of the sun and wear sunscreen when outdoors. Detect melanoma early by checking your skin for growths exhibiting these warning signs: asymmetry, irregular border, multiple colors, and large diameter. Seek medical attention for any suspicious lesions that do not heal.

Cancers with unknown causes include prostate cancer, testicular cancer, and ovarian cancer. The risk factors for prostate cancer are age and heredity. For early detection of this cancer, men older than 50 should have annual prostate-specific antigen blood tests with or without a digital prostate exam. Men between the ages of 20 and 54 years are at the highest risk for testicular cancer. For early detection of this disease, all males 15 years and older should perform monthly testicular self-examinations. Ovarian cancer is primarily a disease of postmenopausal women.

Childhood cancers, although rare, are the most frequent cause of death from disease in American children older than 1 year. Children develop cancers as a result of hereditary or developmental reasons. Occasionally, environmental agents are the cause. Treatment for childhood cancers is highly effective.

# Applying What You Have Learned

**Critical Thinking**

1. Imagine that you or a female friend had an annual Pap test. The report from the lab stated that cells exhibiting dysplasia were seen in the smear. What does this statement mean? How would these cells look different from normal cells? What would be your or your friend's next course of action? **Application**

2. List three cancer risk factors over which a person has no control. Suppose that at least one of them was a risk factor for you. List this hypothetical (or real) factor and the cancer(s) related to this risk. What might you do regarding cancer prevention if you are aware of this (these) factor(s)? **Application**

3. Your good friend is a heavy drinker, eats lots of spicy food, and experiences heartburn regularly. He takes antacids, but recently they have not helped. He also tells you that he seems to have some difficulty swallowing, but he's not quite sure. He thinks it's "all in his head." What would you advise your friend to do? Might cancer be causing his problems? If so, which type?

Which symptoms led you to this conclusion? **Application**

4. List two dietary factors related to the development of cancer and two dietary factors related to lowering the risk of cancer. Name the cancers to which these dietary factors relate. Now list, as best you can remember, the foods you ate for the past 2 days. What is your intake of the types of foods related to cancer development and prevention? Based on this analysis, should you make changes in your diet to lower your risk of certain cancers? **Evaluation**

5. With respect to the cancers discussed in this chapter, which cancer(s) are you at least risk for developing? Why? Which cancers are you at highest risk for developing? Why? **Synthesis**

6. Referring to your answer to question 5, what can you do to lower your risk of developing the cancers for which you are at high risk? State rationales for each suggestion. Why will these lifestyle changes lower your risk? **Evaluation**

---

**Application**
using information in a new situation.

**Synthesis**
putting together information from different sources.

**Evaluation**
making informed decisions.

**Key**

## *Reflecting on Your Health*

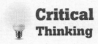

**Critical Thinking**

1. In what ways have your attitudes about cancer changed since reading this chapter?
2. Were you aware of all the ACS recommendations for the early detection of cancer prior to reading this chapter? If you were not, which recommendations were new to you? Will you follow these recommendations? Why or why not? If you were aware of all the ACS recommendations, do you follow those recommendations for your sex and age group? Why or why not?
3. Do you know anyone who has or has had cancer, or have you read stories written by cancer patients about their disease? What did you learn about cancer from them that affected your life?
4. Complete the assessment "What Are Your Cancer Risks?" in the Student Workbook pages at the end of this text. Do your cancer risks match your self-perception of your risks? Did the self-assessment identify cancer risks of which you were unaware? After reading this chapter, develop a list of things you could do to reduce the risks you identified.

## *References*

1. Abt, S. (1999, July 26). Armstrong wins tour and journey. *The New York Times.*
2. BBC News. (2011, February 16). Lance Armstrong confirms retirement from cycling. Retrieved on April 17, 2011, from http://news .bbc.co.uk/sport2/hi/other_sports/cycling/9399280.stm
3. American Cancer Society. (2010). *Cancer facts and figures, 2010.* Atlanta, GA: Author. Retrieved on April 17, 2011, from http:// www.cancer.org/acs/groups/content/@epidemiologysurveilance /documents/document/acspc-026238.pdf
4. Davila, M. L. (2011). Photodynamic therapy. *Gastrointestinal Endoscopy Clinics of North America, 21*(1):67–79.
5. Mroz, P., et al. (2011). Stimulation of anti-tumor immunity by photodynamic therapy. *Expert Review in Clinical Immunology, 7*(1):75–91.
6. National Cancer Institute. (2011, March 1). Targeted cancer therapies. Retrieved on April 19, 2011, from http://www.cancer.gov /cancertopics/factsheet/Therapy/targeted
7. Jain, K. K. (2010). Personalized cancer vaccines. *Expert Opinion on Biological Therapy, 10*(12):1637–1647.
8. American Cancer Society. (2010). *Cancer prevention and early detection facts and figures, 2010.* Atlanta, GA: Author. Retrieved on April 18, 2011, from http://www.cancer.org/acs/groups/content /@epidemiologysurveilance/documents/document/acspc-027876 .pdf
9. U.S. Department of Health and Human Services. (2004). *The health consequences of smoking: A report of the Surgeon General.* Washington, DC: U.S. Government Printing Office. Retrieved on April 18, 2011, from http://www.surgeongeneral.gov/library/smoking consequences/
10. U.S. Department of Health and Human Services. (2010). *How tobacco smoke causes disease: The biology and behavioral basis for smoking-attributable disease.* Washington, DC: U.S. Government Printing Office. Retrieved on April 18, 2011, from http://www .surgeongeneral.gov/library/tobaccosmoke/report/full_report.pdf
11. Khan, N., et al. (2010). Lifestyle as risk factor for cancer: Evidence from human studies. *Cancer Letters, 293*(2):133–143.
12. U.S. Public Health Service. (1964). *Smoking and health: Report of the advisory committee to the Surgeon General of the Public Health Service* (PHS Publication No. 1103). Atlanta, GA: U.S. Department of Health, Education, and Welfare, Public Health Service, CDC. Retrieved on April 18, 2011, from http://profiles.nlm.nih.gov/ps /access/NNBBMQ.pdf
13. Taylor, H. S., & Manson, J. E. (2011). Update in hormone therapy use in menopause. *Journal of Clinical Endocrinology and Metabolism, 96*(2):255–264.
14. Key, T. J. (2011). Fruit and vegetables and cancer risk. *British Journal of Cancer, 104*(1):6–11.
15. U.S. Department of Health and Human Services. (2006). *The health consequences of involuntary exposure to tobacco smoke: A report of the Surgeon General.* Atlanta, GA: U.S. Department of Health and Human Services. Retrieved on April 18, 2011, from http://www .surgeongeneral.gov/library/secondhandsmoke/report/fullreport. pdf
16. Marur, S., et al. (2010). HPV-associated head and neck cancer: A virus-related cancer epidemic. *Lancet Oncology, 11*(8):781–789.
17. Lowrance, W. T., et al. (2010). Obesity is associated with a higher risk of clear-cell renal cell carcinoma than with other histologies. *BJU International, 105*(1):16–20.

18. American Cancer Society. (2011, March 11). Colorectal cancer early detection. Retrieved on April 20, 2011, from http://www.cancer.org/acs/groups/cid/documents/webcontent/003170-pdf.pdf

19. Rothwell, P. M., et al. (2010). Long-term effect of aspirin on colorectal cancer incidence and mortality: 20-year follow-up of five randomized trials. *Lancet, 376*(9754):1741–1750.

20. Chan, A. T., & Giovannucci, E. L (2010). Primary prevention of colorectal cancer. *Gastroenterology, 138*(6):2029–2043.

21. Mayo Clinic staff. (2010, April 15). Stool DNA test. Retrieved on April 20, 2011, from http://www.mayoclinic.com/health/dna-stool-test/MY00623

22. American Cancer Society. (2009). *Breast cancer facts and figures, 2009–2010.* Atlanta, GA: Author. Retrieved on April 20, 2011, from http://www.cancer.org/acs/groups/content/@nho/documents/document/f861009final90809pdf.pdf

23. Li, C. I. (2003). Relationship between long durations and different regimens of hormone therapy and risk of breast cancer. *Journal of the American Medical Association, 289*(24):3254–3263.

24. American Cancer Society. (2007). *Breast cancer facts and figures, 2007–2008.* Atlanta, GA: Author. Retrieved on April 20, 2011, from http://www.cancer.org/acs/groups/content/@nho/documents/document/bcfffinalpdf.pdf

25. Luo, J., et al. (2011). Association of active and passive smoking with risk of breast cancer among postmenopausal women: A prospective cohort study. *British Medical Journal, 342*:d1016.

26. Njeh, C. F., et al. (2010). Accelerated partial breast irradiation (APBI): A review of available techniques. *Radiation Oncology, 5*:90.

27. Srikantia, N., et al. (2009). Endometrioid endometrial adenocarcinoma in a premenopausal woman with multiple organ metastases. *Indian Journal of Medical and Paediatric Oncology, 30*(2):80–83.

28. National Cancer Institute. (2010). Surveillance, Epidemiology and End Results (SEER) stat fact sheets: Cervix uteri. Retrieved on April 21, 2011, from http://www.seer.cancer.gov/statfacts/html/cervix.html

29. Martorell-Calatayud, A., et al. (2011). Defining fast-growing melanomas: Reappraisal of epidemiological, clinical, and histological features. *Melanoma Research, 12*(2):131–138.

30. HealthyPeople.gov. (2011). *Healthy People 2020* topics and objectives: Cancer. Retrieved on April 21, 2011, from http://www.healthypeople.gov/2020/topicsobjectives2020/overview.aspx?topicid=5

31. Shannon Brownlee and Jeanne Lenzer. (2011, October 5). Can cancer ever be ignored? *The New York Times Magazine.* Retrieved on October 11, 2011 from http://www.nytimes.com/2011/10/09/magazine/can-cancer-ever-be-ignored.html?_r=1

32. American Cancer Society. (2011). Testicular cancer. Retrieved on April 21, 2011, from http://www.cancer.org/cancer/testicularcancer/detailedguide/testicular-cancer-risk-factors

33. MedlinePlus. (2010, December). Ovarian cancer. Retrieved on April 21, 2011, from http://www.nlm.nih.gov/medlineplus/ency/article/000889.htm

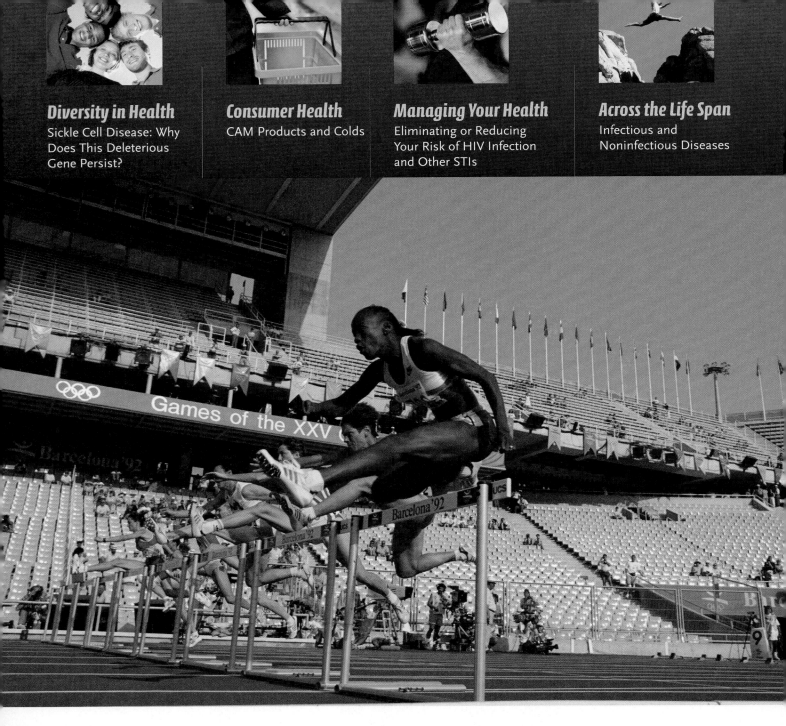

**Diversity in Health**
Sickle Cell Disease: Why Does This Deleterious Gene Persist?

**Consumer Health**
CAM Products and Colds

**Managing Your Health**
Eliminating or Reducing Your Risk of HIV Infection and Other STIs

**Across the Life Span**
Infectious and Noninfectious Diseases

## Chapter Overview

Causes of noninfectious diseases

Symptoms of and treatments for noninfectious diseases

Trends in infectious diseases since 1900

How the chain of infection works

How nonspecific and specific immunity work

How to protect yourself against infectious disease

Symptoms of sexually transmitted infections

Treatments and prevention methods for sexually transmitted infections

## Student Workbook

Self-Assessment: STI Attitude Scale

Changing Health Habits: Reducing Your Risk of Contracting an STI

## Do You Know?

How to protect yourself from sexually transmitted infections?

If over-the-counter cold remedies really work?

Which types of diseases you can catch and which you cannot?

## CHAPTER 14

# Infection, Immunity, and Noninfectious Disease

**J**ackie Joyner-Kersee: Olympian gold, silver, and bronze medalist. The photo shows Kersee leading her competitors in the 100 meter hurdle portion of the women's heptathlon. Some consider Joyner-Kersee the greatest woman athlete ever. At this writing, she is the heptathlon world record holder and the American record holder in the indoor long jump. She has won six Olympic medals, more than any woman in track and field history. Joyner-Kersee officially retired from track and field in 2001.

In late 2004, Joyner-Kersee was honored by USA Track & Field, the national governing body for track and field, long-distance running, and race walking in the United

*"Exercise-induced asthma has not deterred this outstanding athlete from making her indelible mark in the world of sports..."*

States. They cited Joyner-Kersee's breaking of her own women's heptathlon world record at the 1988 Olympic Games as the ninth greatest moment in U.S. track and field history in the last 25 years. In mid-2007, Joyner-Kersee was named one of six "women of power" by the National Urban League. In 2010, she was one of the first inducted into the new St. Louis Sports Hall of Fame, which honors achievements of St. Louis teams and athletes past and present. Clearly, exercise-induced asthma has not deterred this outstanding athlete from making her indelible mark in the world of sports, nor has it deterred other athletes.

Exercise-induced asthma is a condition in which the airways narrow after sustained exertion, making it more difficult than usual for a person to breathe. What triggers this problem is the cooling and reheating of the airways as

**disease** A process that affects the proper functioning of the body and is usually accompanied by characteristic signs and symptoms.

**infectious (in-FEK-shus) disease** A disease caused by bacteria, rickettsias, viruses, fungi, protozoans, or parasitic worms.

**pathogen** (PATH-oh-jen) A disease-causing agent of infection; the first link in the chain of infection.

**noninfectious (NON-in-FEK-shus) disease** Illness caused by genetic abnormalities, by interactions between hereditary and environmental factors, or solely by environmental factors.

**inherited disease** A genetic disease transmitted solely by gene transfer from parents to offspring.

**mutation** (mew-TAY-shun) In reference to human biology, a change in a gene or a chromosome.

**cystic fibrosis** (SIS-tik fie-BROH-sis) (CF) A common, lethal, inherited disease that affects the glands that secrete mucus and sweat, resulting in multiple disorders of the lungs and pancreas.

a person exercises. As exercise begins, a person begins to breathe deeply and rapidly. During this deep and rapid inhalation, more air is moistened and warmed in the respiratory passageways than before exercise began, which draws moisture and heat from the airways. After a person is warmed up, the breathing rate falls, and the airways return to their normal temperature. Health scientists do not know how airway cooling and reheating triggers asthma attacks.

Asthma is one of a variety of noninfectious diseases. **Diseases** are processes that affect the proper functioning of the body and are usually accompanied by characteristic signs and symptoms. **Infectious diseases**, such as colds or the flu, are caused by **pathogens**, which are agents of infection: bacteria, rickettsias, viruses, fungi, protozoans, and parasitic worms. (Infectious diseases are discussed later in this chapter.) **Noninfectious diseases** are caused by abnormalities in the hereditary material (genetic diseases), interactions between heredity and environmental factors (especially those related to lifestyle, such as asthma), or environmental factors alone, as in repetitive-use injuries or lead poisoning (see Chapter 16, "Environmental Health").

## ◻ *Noninfectious Diseases*

## Genetic Diseases

There are two types of genetic diseases: inherited diseases and diseases caused by errors in cell division when gametes (sex cells) are formed.

**Inherited Diseases Inherited diseases** are transmitted solely by gene transfer from parents to offspring. They occur more frequently among close relatives than in the general population and show patterns in their transmission. An inherited disease may strike only males, for example.

Inherited diseases are caused by disorders of *genes*, the physical and functional units of heredity. Genes are segments of *DNA*, a complex chemical compound that codes for the production of proteins. Genes carry information about every aspect of an organism and may carry normal instructions for a particular characteristic in one person and defective instructions in another. A defective gene in the eggs or sperm of an individual can be passed on to a child unless the person dies before reaching reproductive age.

Defective genes arise through mutation. A **mutation** is a change in a gene or a chromosome. A chromosome is a strand of DNA with associated protein; humans have 23 pair of chromosomes. One member of each pair is inherited from the mother and one pair from the father.

A mutation can be inherited from a parent and passed on to children, or it can arise suddenly in a person and be passed on to children. Mutations in eggs and sperm can occur for no apparent reason or from exposure to a variety of environmental sources. One source is ionizing radiation such as x-rays, which is the reason the dentist places a protective lead shield over your pelvic area when taking x-rays of your teeth. Another source of damage to genes is drugs such as lysergic acid diethylamide (lysergide, LSD) or marijuana (*Cannabis sativa*). Chapter 7 describes these drugs and their effects on the body in more detail. Toxic chemicals are a third source of genetic damage. Poisoning, another effect of toxic chemicals, is discussed in Chapter 16. People often come into contact with toxic chemicals in the workplace and do not realize the danger because they feel no ill effects.

Three hereditary diseases that are common in the United States are sickle cell disease, cystic fibrosis, and muscular dystrophy. The Diversity in Health essay "Sickle Cell Disease: Why Does This Deleterious Gene Persist?" discusses this hereditary disease, which is common among African Americans.

**Cystic fibrosis (CF)** is the most common lethal genetic disease in the white population. (It seldom affects African Americans, Asians, or Jews.) Cystic fibrosis affects the glands that secrete mucus and sweat. In CF patients, the sweat glands produce an abnormally salty secretion and the mucous glands produce an exceptionally thick and sticky secretion that builds

# Diversity in Health

## Sickle Cell Disease: Why Does This Deleterious Gene Persist?

Sickle cell disease is one of the most common genetic disorders among African Americans, having arisen in their African ancestors. It has also been observed in people whose ancestors came from the Mediterranean basin, the Indian subcontinent, the Caribbean, and parts of Central and South America (particularly Brazil). The sickle cell gene has persisted in these populations—even though the disease eventually kills its victims—because of a curious interaction between this disease and another disease prevalent in these regions. Today, an estimated 70,000 to 100,000 Americans of African and Hispanic origins have the disease. Medical researchers estimate that 1 out of 10 African Americans and 1 out of 100 Hispanic Americans carry the trait.

Sickle cell disease gets its name from the curved (sickle) shape of the red blood cells of individuals with this disease (**Figure 14.A**). Anemia, or a low number of red blood cells, results from the short life of these abnormal cells. An error in the gene that codes for hemoglobin, the oxygen-carrying molecule in red blood cells, is responsible for the signs and symptoms of sickle cell disease.

These sickle-shaped cells cause pain when they become trapped in the small blood vessels of the body. This condition results in oxygen depletion to the tissues surrounding the blocked vessels, which damages tissues and causes infections. Most sickle cell patients die in their 40s or 50s from conditions such as stroke, infection, kidney failure, or congestive heart failure.

To have sickle cell disease, a person must inherit two defective hemoglobin genes—one from each parent. A person who inherits a single defective gene is a carrier and is said to have *sickle cell trait*. People with sickle cell trait do not have sickle cell disease, but they do have something in common with sufferers of sickle cell disease—resistance to malaria.

Those with the sickle cell gene have a survival advantage in regions of the world in which malaria is prevalent. The map in **Figure 14.B** shows where malaria is widespread; notice from the listing of affected populations in the first paragraph that sickle cell disease is prevalent in these areas as well. Although many of these peoples have since migrated from these areas, this ancestral gene persists in their populations.

How does a defective hemoglobin gene protect against malaria? In sickle cell trait, red blood cells sickle under a variety of conditions, such as when the oxygen tension is low (at high altitudes, for example) and if these cells become acidic. Results of research show that infection of the red blood cells by malaria parasites causes the infected cells to become acidic as a result of the metabolism of the parasite. This change induces the red blood cells to sickle, which interrupts multiplication of the parasite. The spleen, an organ that destroys worn-out red blood cells, traps the sickled cells. Under these conditions, the parasites die and malaria does not develop. For populations who live in regions where malaria is prevalent, the sickle cell gene persists because people who harbor the gene are more likely to live to reproductive age than those who do not have the gene and die from malaria. Therefore, this "deleterious" gene is beneficial to those with sickle cell trait living in malaria-infested areas and is passed from generation to generation. Unfortunately, some offspring inherit sickle cell disease and not simply sickle cell trait.

Healthcare providers alleviate symptoms in those with worsening anemia and sickle cell complications by administering painkillers and blood transfusions. Those receiving transfusions to prevent stroke must continue transfusions indefinitely or the risk of stroke returns. Penicillin is given to children aged 1 to 5 years to ward off infection. The drug hydroxyurea reduces the frequency of pain, hospital admissions, and life-threatening complications by about 50%. Bone marrow stem cell trans-

### Figure 14.A

**Normal and Sickled Red Blood Cells.** The red blood cells to the left have a normal, rounded shape. Those to the right have the curved shape of sickle cell disease, which results in their becoming trapped in the small blood vessels of the body.

*Source:* © Dr. Stanley Flegler/Visuals Unlimited.

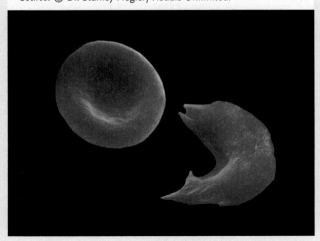

*(Continues)*

## Figure 14.B

**Areas of the World in Which Malaria Is Prevalent.** Malaria is a serious infectious disease in the tropical and subtropical regions of the world. Sickle cell disease is prevalent in these regions as well.

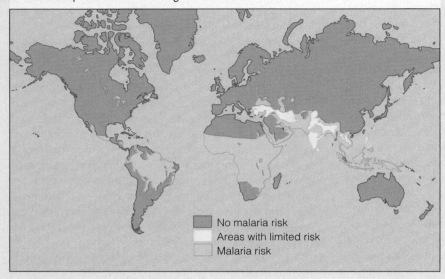

No malaria risk
Areas with limited risk
Malaria risk

counseling, educational initiatives, and community outreach programs and provides patients with federal matching funds for sickle cell disease–related services under Medicaid. In addition, this law has initiated the development of sickle cell treatment centers across the country and has established a National Coordinating and Evaluation Center Sickle Cell Disease and Newborn Screening Program.

Couples can be screened to detect if they are carriers of the trait to help them in their family planning decisions. Researchers are studying new medications and treatments for sickle cell anemia, and eventually, medical experts may discover a way to weed out this life-threatening gene in populations no longer living in malaria-prone areas.

plantation is also used to treat sickle cell disease. Bone marrow stem cells are undifferentiated cells that give rise to all types of blood cells.

The Sickle Cell Treatment Act of 2003 helps expand services for patients with this blood disorder. The federal government provides states with funding for patient

*Sources:* Centers for Disease Control and Prevention. (2010, January 21). Sickle cell disease (SCD). Retrieved on April 26, 2011, from http://www.cdc.gov/NCBDDD/sicklecell/index.html; St. Jude Children's Research Hospital. (2011). Disease information: Hematologic disorders: Sickle cell disease. Retrieved on April 26, 2011, from http://www.stjude.org/stjude/v/index.jsp?vgnextoid=0f3c 061585f70110VgnVCM1000001e0215acRCRD&vgnextchannel=bc4fbfe 82e118010VgnVCM1000000e2015acRCRD.

up and plugs the ducts of glands and other passageways. Although the pancreas (an organ that secretes digestive juices) is often seriously affected, lung disease accounts for most of the illness and nearly all deaths from CF. Multiple disorders of the lungs arise when mucus blocks the airways. Infections result and breathing becomes impaired. According to the Cystic Fibrosis Foundation, in 2009 the median predicted age of survival with CF was in the mid-30s, which means that half of those with CF would be expected to live to that age.[1]

**Duchenne/Becker muscular dystrophy (DBMD)** is the most common type of muscular dystrophy (*dys* means "abnormal"; *trophy* means "growth"). DBMD is a disease in which the muscles gradually weaken and degenerate. The two versions of the disease are similar, but Becker muscular dystrophy has a later onset than Duchenne and a slower progression

of symptoms. Recent estimates by the Centers for Disease Control and Prevention (CDC) reveal that DBMD occurs in 1.3 to 2.6 newborn males in the United States per 10,000, usually striking before the age of 5 years, which is the average age at diagnosis.[2]

Children with DBMD are usually slow to walk and talk. Their thigh and pelvic muscles gradually deteriorate, resulting in unsteadiness in standing, walking, climbing stairs, and getting up from a seated position. As the muscles of the shoulder, trunk, and back weaken, the child's spine begins to curve and the posture becomes swayback. This abnormal body posture interferes with the functioning of internal organs, especially the lungs. Although heart problems sometimes cause sudden death in DBMD patients, these children and young adults usually die in their teens or 20s of respiratory infections or respiratory failure when the diaphragm (a sheetlike muscle that

## Figure 14.1

**Down Syndrome.** (a) This girl has Down syndrome. She exhibits the stocky build, short hands, and flattened facial features characteristic of this genetic condition. (b) Down syndrome is called trisomy 21 because it is caused by the presence of an extra 21st chromosome, as shown in the karyotype, the array of chromosomes in a cell. In addition, individuals with Down syndrome experience delays in physical and intellectual development. Although some individuals with Down syndrome function in the low average range of intellectual capability, the majority function in the mild to moderate range of intellectual disability.

*Source:* Part B Courtesy of Viola Freeman, Associate Professor, Faculty of Health Sciences, Dept. of Pathology and Molecular Medicine, McMaster University.

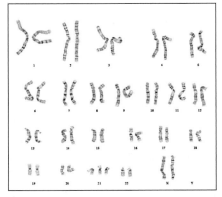

(a)

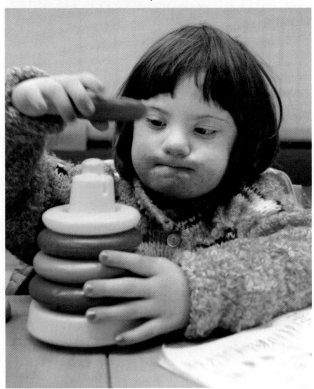

(b)

**Duchenne/Becker muscular dystrophy** (do-SHAYN BECK-er MUSS-ku-lar DIS-tro-fee) (DBMD) An inherited disease in which the muscles gradually weaken and degenerate. It usually strikes boys before the age of 6 years.

**Down syndrome** A genetic disease usually caused by the presence of three (rather than two) number 21 chromosomes; the child is usually mentally retarded, with a short body and a broad, flat face.

forms the floor of the chest cavity and that is essential to breathing) becomes affected. Survival of patients with DBMD is enhanced by the use of noninvasive mechanical ventilation at night along with the use of assisted coughing techniques and medications that protect the heart.[3]

**Diseases Caused by Errors in Sex Cell Division** Gametes, or sex cells, are produced in the ovaries or testes. Sometimes eggs or sperm are made that have too many or too few chromosomes. Other times gametes may be formed in which parts of chromosomes have been lost, gained, or moved to new positions. If conception takes place with a gamete that has a severe defect, the usual result is a spontaneous abortion. However, some genetic defects result in a fertilized egg that is capable of developing into a full-term baby. The child may be born with structural or functional problems, or both.

**Down syndrome**, which affects approximately 1 in 1,000 newborns,[4] is a common genetic disorder caused by improper cell division in gametes. Cell division problems occur more often in eggs than in sperm because men produce new sperm throughout their lives, while women are born with all the potential eggs they will ever have. Therefore, a woman's eggs age as she ages. Each month, a single egg reaches maturity. During this maturation process, a division of the potential egg takes place. The division may result in an error in the number of chromosomes in the mature egg. The majority of Down syndrome children have three number 21 chromosomes instead of the usual pair (**Figure 14.1**). For this reason, Down syndrome is also called *trisomy 21*. As the graph in **Figure 14.2** shows, the risk of bearing a child with Down syndrome or another chromosomal abnormality rises dramatically after the maternal age of 30. This association between the incidence of Down syndrome and increasing age is not observed in fathers.[5] Various screening methods have been developed to detect whether a fetus is affected with trisomy 21 or other chromosomal problems. Prenatal diagnosis is discussed in Chapter 5.

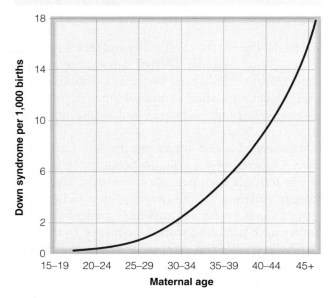

### Figure 14.2

**The Effect of Maternal Age on the Incidence of Down Syndrome.** As maternal age increases, the age of a woman's eggs also increases and genetic abnormalities become more common. The graph shows that the incidence of Down syndrome rises significantly as maternal age increases beyond 30 years.

## Noninfectious Disease and the Interaction of Genetic Factors with the Environment

The genetic diseases just discussed have simple and predictable inheritance patterns. They involve a change in a single gene or an error in sex cell division. Other noninfectious diseases have no simple and predictable inheritance patterns like genetic diseases do, but their development involves interplay between genetic and environmental factors. For example, a person with a family link to type 2 diabetes is more likely to develop this disease if he or she becomes overweight or obese than is a person without the genetic link. Moreover, even in those genetically predisposed, type 2 diabetes can be prevented or managed with weight loss and regular physical activity.

Until recently, scientists were able to look at genetics only in a limited way when studying disease. They did not have the tools to identify genetic factors and the roles they play in diseases with complex genetic links, such as type 2 diabetes, heart disease, and cancer. However, in 1989 an international effort began that would change this narrow view of genetics and health. Research scientists around the world set out to map the entire set of human genes—the human genome—determining its complete DNA sequence. With this endeavor, called the Human Genome Project, a new branch of molecular biology was born: *genomics*. This science focuses on understanding the structure and function of the genome. By 2003, researchers had mapped the entire human genome, revealing the "genetic code" of humans.

Genomics holds promise for helping researchers understand how genetic factors interact with environmental factors, resulting in health or disease. Researchers can now look for genetic variations that increase the risk of certain diseases and may, in turn, be able to develop more effective approaches to prevention and treatment of those diseases. In the future, diagnosis and treatment could be based on an individual's unique genetic makeup.

Asthma, ulcers, diabetes, migraine headaches, cardiovascular disease, and cancer are common noninfectious diseases that have both genetic and environmental causes. Ulcers are sores in the lining of the esophagus, stomach, or duodenum. They are discussed in Chapter 3. Diabetes is a group of diseases in which a person does not metabolize carbohydrates properly. Diabetes is discussed in Chapter 9. Migraine headaches are thought to be an inherited disorder that can be triggered by a variety of environmental factors. Migraines are discussed in Chapter 3. The nation's number one killers—cardiovascular disease and cancer—are discussed in separate chapters (Chapters 12 and 13, respectively) because they affect the nation's health so significantly.

**Asthma**, the most common chronic illness in childhood, is a disease of the airways. The bronchioles of asthmatics narrow in response to certain stimuli much more easily than do the bronchioles of nonasthmatics. (Bronchioles are air passageways, about the diameter of a pencil lead, that lead to the air sacs of the lungs [**Figure 14.3**].) When these airways become narrowed, airflow to and from the lungs is blocked. As a result, asthmatic people have trouble breathing and begin to wheeze, which people refer to as having an asthma attack.

Environmental factors such as air pollution, respiratory infections, tobacco smoke, and allergens such as dust mites often trigger asthma attacks. (Dust mites are microscopic organisms that live in carpets, mattresses, pillows, and curtains.) As mentioned in the opening paragraphs of this chapter, exercise may also stimulate asthma attacks. Breathing warm, moist air is best for the athlete with exercise-induced asthma. For example, swimming in a warm pool will usually

**The Respiratory System.** The bronchioles are the narrow air passageways that branch from the bronchi and lead to the air sacs of the lungs. The bronchioles are covered with muscle tissue that constricts during asthma attacks, narrowing these passageways and making it difficult to breathe.

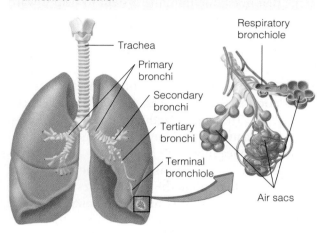

- Trachea
- Primary bronchi
- Secondary bronchi
- Tertiary bronchi
- Terminal bronchiole
- Respiratory bronchiole
- Air sacs

cause fewer problems than snow skiing. Also, warming up before exercise reduces the likelihood of an exercise-induced asthma attack. With other types of asthma, the key to management is discovering what stimulates attacks and avoiding these factors. For example, if a trigger is house dust mites, exposure can be reduced by not using carpeting or draperies, and washing bedding often in hot water. Medication is another important tool for asthma management.

## Noninfectious Conditions with Environmental or Unknown Causes

Many conditions are caused by exposure to various substances in the environment. In general, environmental factors that are the sole cause of disease are toxic chemicals (see Chapter 16). Not only are toxic chemicals present in the home, workplace, and environment, they are also used and abused in ways that seriously affect health. The adverse effects of drug and alcohol abuse are described in Chapters 7 and 8, respectively. The toxic chemicals found in tobacco products are discussed in Chapter 8.

A few noninfectious conditions are caused by the ways in which people use their bodies. Temporomandibular disorder, characterized by pain in the jaw and chewing muscles that often results from grinding or clenching the teeth, is discussed in Chapter 3. **Carpal tunnel syndrome**, a painful condition of the

hands and fingers, results from improper positioning of the wrist while engaging in repetitive activities that use the hands, wrists, and arms. Ten percent of the population experiences occasional symptoms of this syndrome.

Carpal tunnel syndrome is usually the result of repetitive use. Activities such as using power tools frequently, typing for a long time, and playing piano or guitar often result in such injuries because people hold the wrist in a bent position rather than holding it straight. The injury causes inflammation and a buildup of fluid in a tunnel that runs through the bones of the wrist, or carpals. The fluid presses on the nerves and blood vessels in the tunnel. Other conditions such as arthritis, diabetes, and pregnancy may also contribute to pressure in the carpal tunnel. To help avoid injury when typing for a long time, place your computer keyboard at elbow height and keep your wrists unbent as shown in **Figure 14.4**. Use wrist rests and arm rests only when you are resting, not when you are typing.

 **Healthy Living Practices**

- [ ] The risk of chromosomal abnormalities in a woman's eggs increases significantly after her 30th birthday. Therefore, if you and your partner are considering a pregnancy at or beyond this age, consult your healthcare provider for advice regarding options to increase your chances of having a healthy infant.

- [ ] If you have asthma, learn your asthma triggers and avoid them. If you have exercise-induced asthma, consider restricting your activity on cold days or when the pollen count or air pollution levels are high.

- [ ] Abusing drugs, or living and working under toxic conditions, can damage the hereditary material of your cells, particularly the sex cells. Therefore, to protect your health and possibly that of your offspring, avoid exposure to toxic substances.

☐ Carpal tunnel syndrome often results from bending the wrists while engaging in a repetitive activity such as typing, using hand tools, or completing various household chores. To help prevent repetitive-use injury, always keep your wrists unbent while engaging in such activities.

# ☐ Trends in Infectious Disease

In 1900, the three leading causes of death were infectious diseases: pneumonia, tuberculosis, and enteritis (inflammation of the intestine, causing severe diarrhea). Since that time, the United States (and other industrialized countries) has made achievements in public health that have changed this picture dramatically. Early in the twentieth century, U.S. departments of public health were established, whose activities provided for clean drinking water, uncontaminated food, and proper sewage disposal and treatment. These actions have reduced the transmission of pathogens tremendously. *Antibiotics*, which are medications that kill bacteria, and *vaccines*, which are preparations that boost the immune system to help it ward off infection from specific pathogens, combat infection as well. Additionally, new treatments for certain viral illnesses such as influenza have been developed. As a result, after a century, the three leading causes of death in 2007 were no longer infectious diseases, but were noninfectious diseases: heart disease, cancer, and stroke. The only infectious diseases in the "top 15" were pneumonia and influenza, together ranked as the eighth leading cause of death.[6]

Although infectious diseases are not significant contributors to death in the United States at this time, the worldwide picture is much different. Infectious diseases are the leading cause of death in the world. At least 30 new diseases have emerged in the past 30 years, including HIV infection, Ebola viral hemorrhagic fever, and a new strain of hepatitis—hepatitis C. Additionally, many bacterial diseases once easily cured with antibiotics are appearing as incurable diseases, resistant to the variety of antibiotics available at this time. "Old" diseases that once seemed under control, such as diphtheria and tuberculosis, are making a comeback as well.

With international travel commonplace, transmission of infection is a worldwide concern, not just a concern in our own country, state, or city. The resistance of many strains of bacteria to antibiotics and the reemergence of serious diseases once thought conquered make complacency to infection a dangerous attitude. In this time of increasing illness and death from infectious disease in the global community, it is important to understand how infectious diseases are transmitted and how pathogens interact with the body. This knowledge is key to avoiding infection and staying healthy.

## ☐ The Chain of Infection

Infection results from the interaction between a pathogen (also called an agent of infection) and a **host**, the organism that supports the growth of the pathogen. The pathogen is considered the first link in the **chain of infection**. The host is the third and last link. Joining these two links is **transmission**, the

## Figure 14.4

**The Proper Sitting Position for Typing at the Computer.** The screen should be at eye level or slightly lower. The keyboard should be at elbow height, the forearms parallel to the floor, the back supported, the thighs parallel to the floor, and the feet flat on the floor or foot rest.

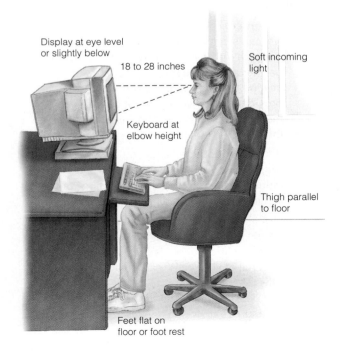

Display at eye level or slightly below

18 to 28 inches

Soft incoming light

Keyboard at elbow height

Thigh parallel to floor

Feet flat on floor or foot rest

route by which the pathogen gets to the host. **Figure 14.5** depicts the chain of infection, the relationship among the factors important in the development of infectious diseases.

## The First Link: Pathogens

The severity of an infectious disease depends on a variety of factors:

- The type of pathogen (such as a bacterium or virus)
- Its virulence (how easily it causes disease)
- Its ability to multiply and spread within the body
- Its ability to combat the defense mechanisms of the body
- The body's reaction to this invader

This chapter first describes pathogens that cause infectious diseases. A later section focuses on the host's defense mechanisms.

**Bacteria and Rickettsias Bacteria** produce infections such as strep throat, bacterial pneumonia, food poisoning, and infected cuts. These organisms are unicellular and microscopic, with a simple cell structure.

When bacteria enter the body, they adhere to the surfaces of host cells and grow and multiply there. Some bacteria penetrate deeply into the tissues (moving between body cells). Many pathogenic bacteria produce one or more chemicals that aid their invasion. A few types of bacteria produce toxins, or poisons, that cause diseases such as certain types of food poisoning.

*Rickettsias* are bacteria-like organisms that live *within* host cells. These organisms cause diseases

such as typhus, which is transmitted by lice, and Rocky Mountain spotted fever, which is transmitted by ticks.

**Viruses Viruses** cause many diseases with which you are familiar: the common cold, influenza (the flu), mumps, measles (**Figure 14.6**), chicken pox, hepatitis, and **acquired immune deficiency syndrome (AIDS)**. Viruses are very different from bacteria and, in fact, are very different from any organism: They do not have a cellular structure. Because the basis of life is the cell, viruses are not considered living organisms. They are simply hereditary material surrounded by a coat of protein.

**host** In reference to disease, an organism that supports the growth of a pathogen; the third, and last, link in the chain of infection.

**chain of infection** The relationship among the factors important in the development of infectious diseases: the pathogen, transmission, and the host.

**transmission** In reference to disease, the means by which a pathogen gets to a host; the second link in the chain of infection.

**bacteria** Unicellular, microscopic organisms with a simple cell structure; some are pathogenic to humans and produce infections such as strep throat, bacterial pneumonia, food poisoning, and infected cuts.

**virus** Hereditary material surrounded by a coat of protein; some viruses are pathogenic to humans and produce infections such as the common cold, influenza, mumps, measles, chicken pox, hepatitis, and AIDS.

**acquired immune deficiency syndrome (AIDS)** A set of certain diseases and conditions that results from infection by the human immunodeficiency virus (HIV).

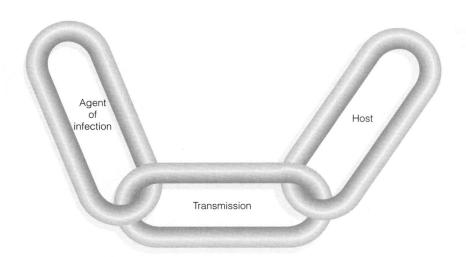

Agent of infection

Transmission

Host

### Figure 14.5

**The Chain of Infection.** Infection is the invasion of the body by disease-causing organisms, or pathogens. Infection results when the pathogen (the first link in the chain) is transmitted (the second link) to a host (the third link). The host is the organism that supports the growth of the pathogen.

Figure 14.6

**Child with the Typical Rash of Measles.** This highly contagious viral disease is characterized by a spreading rash. The rash consists of small, red spots; some of the spots may be raised.

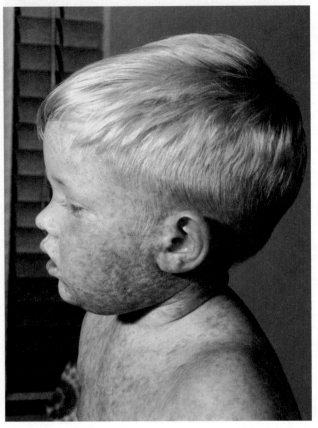

Like bacteria, viruses cause disease by adhering to host cells, but unlike bacteria, viruses enter the cells of the body and use those cells to make more virus particles. The new virus particles break open the infected cell, killing it, and are then ready to infect additional body cells. The death of body cells causes many of the signs and symptoms of viral disease.

Certain types of viruses invade cells but enter a *latent state* during which time infective virus particles are not produced. Although no signs or symptoms of the viral infection are apparent, latency may cause changes in a cell that lead to cancer (see Chapter 13). In many instances, the latent viral hereditary material can become reactivated and replicate once again, causing disease.

Some infections are characterized by a cycling of latent and actively replicating periods, such as the sexually transmitted infection (STI) genital herpes. During the usual course of this disease (discussed later in this chapter), a person suffers active episodes when he or she can transmit this disease to others. The infection then subsides (latency) only to reappear at another time, often triggered by stress or other factors.

**Fungi** You have probably heard of, or may have experienced, yeast infections or athlete's foot (**Figure 14.7**), which is a type of ringworm (a fungal infection of the skin, hair, or nails). These diseases are caused by **fungi**, more commonly known as molds and yeasts. Fungi cannot make their own food and, therefore, grow on a wide range of organisms that they use as food sources, such as rotting logs, spoiling fruit, and the human body. Most human fungal infections, with the exception of yeast infections, are caused by molds.

Medical researchers know less about how fungi cause disease in humans than they know about the other agents of infection. However, fungi appear to invade humans in much the same way as do bacteria. Humans have a high degree of resistance to fungi, which may explain why humans become infected with fungi less often than with bacteria or viruses. Fungi are considered *opportunistic* organisms; that is, they invade the human body when the host has another disease or condition that diminishes its ability to combat fungal infection. People with diabetes or AIDS, for example, are more likely to contract fungal infections than people with no underlying illness.

Figure 14.7

**Athlete's Foot.** Athlete's foot, or tinea pedis, is a fungal infection that usually arises between the toes or on the soles of the feet. This condition often develops when a person wears enclosed footwear without socks or stockings, and the feet become moist for long periods. To help avoid athlete's foot, dry the feet between the toes after bathing or showering and use powder to help keep the feet dry.

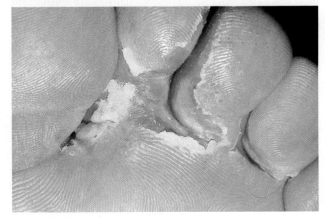

**Other Types of Pathogens** Two additional groups of organisms cause infections in humans: *protozoans* and *worms*. Protozoans cause diseases such as malaria (a tropical disease transmitted by mosquitoes) and trichomonas urogenital infections, or "trich" infections. All protozoans that cause infectious diseases in humans are single-celled organisms, but they differ from one another in the ways they cause disease.

The other group of infectious organisms is the parasitic worms: certain types of roundworms, flatworms (tapeworms), and flukes. Tapeworms are contracted by eating infected pork or beef; these worms live in the intestines, producing digestive disturbances. Adult roundworms also inhabit the intestinal tract and cause digestive disorders; they enter the body in various ways depending on the species of worm. Flukes differ in that they can inhabit the intestine, the liver, the lungs, or the veins depending on the species; they are contracted from water infected with human feces and are not prevalent in the United States.

One other group of organisms important to mention is the *arthropods*. Certain species of this group live on or in the skin of humans, a condition usually referred to as *infestation* rather than infection. Arthropods are organisms such as lice, fleas, mites, and ticks. Some STIs are caused by certain lice and mites (discussed later in this chapter). Ticks only occasionally infest humans but may transmit other pathogens to humans, as can mosquitoes, lice, and flies.

# The Second Link: Transmission

Some infectious diseases are passed from person to person and others are not. Those that are spread from person to person, such as colds, flu, strep throat, and STIs, are **communicable** diseases. Diseases that are not transmitted from person to person, including both infectious and noninfectious diseases, are **noncommunicable**.

**Noncommunicable Infectious Diseases** Noncommunicable infectious diseases can be caused in various ways: by the growth of bacteria that normally inhabit the body, the ingestion of poisons produced by some bacteria, or infection with pathogens from environmental or animal sources.

Many species of bacteria normally reside on and in the human body. However, these beneficial bacteria can cause occasional problems. For example, *Staphylococcus* bacteria normally present on the skin can multiply and cause skin infections, especially in persons with chronic diseases such as diabetes.

**fungi** (FUN-jeye) Cellular organisms that cannot make their own food; some are pathogenic to humans and produce infections such as athlete's foot, ringworm, and yeast infections. *Fungus* is the singular term.

**communicable** (ka-MYOO-ni-kah-bl) Transmissible from person to person.

**noncommunicable** Not transmissible from person to person.

Noncommunicable infections can also be caused by the ingestion of *toxins*, or poisons, produced by some bacteria. Staphylococcal food poisoning (formerly called ptomaine poisoning), for example, is caused by taking in a toxin that certain staphylococcal bacteria produce when they grow on foods. Dairy products and poultry are the foods most commonly contaminated with staphylococcal bacteria from their animal sources or from infected food handlers. The staphylococcal bacteria grow well in high-protein, high-carbohydrate foods. Most often, staphylococcal food poisoning occurs when people eat foods such as potato salad, chicken salad, custard, or cream pies that have not been refrigerated properly after preparation. Picnics are a common time of infection because such foods are left out under warm conditions for long periods of time, which allows the bacteria to grow and produce toxin. Because the bacteria grow on the food and not in the body, this type of noncommunicable infection is more properly called *intoxication* (poisoning) rather than infection. Staphylococcal food poisoning should not be confused with *Salmonella* food infection, in which the bacteria are taken in with food and multiply in the small intestine.

Botulism is another type of food poisoning, caused by a powerful toxin produced by the bacterium *Clostridium botulinum*. This organism most often grows in improperly home-canned, low-acid foods such as green beans and green peppers. Boiling home-canned foods for 10 to 15 minutes inactivates the toxin. (Infants can contract botulism from raw honey [see Chapter 9].)

A third type of noncommunicable infection is caused by pathogens that infect people via environmental or animal sources. Legionnaire's disease, caused by the bacterium *Legionella pneumophila*, is an infectious disease contracted from an environmental source. Under favorable conditions, this pathogen can grow in and be dispersed by any apparatus that provides a water aerosol or mist, such as air conditioners, whirlpool spas, humidifiers, decorative fountains, showerheads, and water faucets. When this water mist is inhaled, these microbes lodge in the lungs and multiply, producing a pneumonia-like disease that includes high fever, cough, chest pain, and diarrhea. This disease is quite serious; 5% to 30% of its victims die, but victims are often those who are older (65 years and older), are smokers, have a compromised immune system, and/or have chronic lung disease. To reduce the growth of this organism and protect against infection, periodically clean and thoroughly disinfect mist-creating items, such as those mentioned previously, and maintain an appropriate concentration of chlorine in home spas.[7]

Lyme disease is an example of a noncommunicable infection contracted from an animal source. Named for the small community of Lyme, Connecticut, where the disease was first recognized in 1975, this bacterial disease is transmitted by ticks that infest animals such as white-footed mice and white-tailed deer. The ticks ingest the bacterial pathogen that causes Lyme disease from infected animals. When a tick harboring this bacterium bites a human, it injects the bacterium into the bloodstream. Usually a painless but large rash (sometimes looking like a bull's-eye) appears at the site of the bite from a few days to 1 month after being bitten (**Figure 14.8**). This rash is generally accompanied by severe headaches, fatigue, chills, and fever. If the disease is not treated with antibiotics at this early stage, it may develop into severe inflammation of the heart muscle or nervous system weeks to months later. Within 2 years, if untreated, arthritic attacks develop (inflammation of the joints) that can become chronic.

In the United States, Lyme disease is found primarily in the Northeast, the mid-Atlantic (Virginia and North Carolina area), and the upper Midwest. It has also been reported in several areas in northwestern California. Deer ticks favor a moist, shaded environment, particularly areas of woods, brush, or tall grass. If you are walking, gardening, or engaging in other activities in these types of areas and in which deer and mice live (and therefore deer ticks [**Figure 14.9**]), wear long pants and a long-sleeved shirt. Tuck your pant legs into your socks or boots. Spray insect repellent containing at least 30% DEET on your clothing and exposed skin. (Do not spray it on your face.

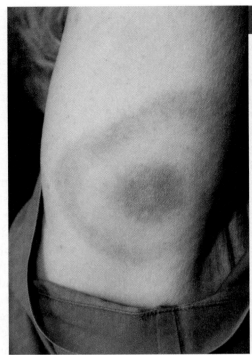

### Figure 14.8

**The "Classic" Rash That Develops at the Site of a Tick Bite in Lyme Disease.** Not everyone who contracts Lyme disease will develop this type of rash.

### Figure 14.9

**Deer Tick.** Deer ticks transmit the bacterium that causes Lyme disease from infected animals to humans.

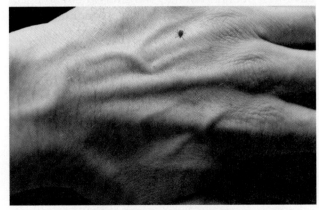

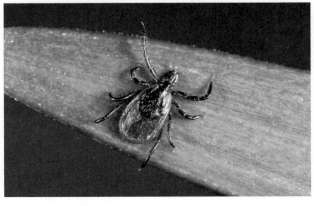

Spray it on your hands and pat that on your face. Use products with no more than 10% DEET on children.) Check yourself carefully for ticks, removing any you find with tweezers.

A Lyme disease vaccine was introduced in 1999, but the manufacturer withdrew the vaccine from the market in 2002, citing poor sales. Moreover, the public was concerned about possible serious side effects of the vaccine even though preliminary evidence showed the vaccine was safe. As of mid-2011, there was no vaccine available to prevent Lyme disease in humans.[8]

**Communicable Infectious Diseases** Communicable diseases are transmitted from person to person by direct or indirect contact, by means of a common vehicle, through the air, and by means of vectors such as mosquitoes.

Some infectious diseases, such as STIs, are passed from person to person by close physical (direct) contact. In the case of STIs, of course, the close contact is usually vaginal intercourse, anal intercourse, genital contact without intercourse, or oral sex. Other diseases such as colds and the flu are often transmitted by direct contact also, such as shaking hands. Therefore, it is important to wash your hands well and frequently to help avoid transmitting or contracting such communicable diseases. These diseases can also be transmitted indirectly by means of an object, such as a shared drinking glass, or through close contact with droplets sneezed or coughed by a person. Strep throat and measles are spread in this way.

Frequently, a source contaminated with pathogens from humans may transmit an infectious disease to many people. Examples of common sources of infection are a blood supply contaminated with human immunodeficiency virus, food contaminated with the hepatitis virus by an infected food handler, and water contaminated by the feces of a person infected with typhoid fever. A variety of infectious diseases are transmitted via food or water.

Some communicable diseases can be transmitted from infected persons to noninfected persons through the air on microscopic water droplets or on dust particles. Certain disease-causing organisms of the respiratory tract, such as the bacterium that causes tuberculosis, can be transmitted in this way, propelled into the air when an infected person coughs or sneezes. When not in isolation, persons with communicable tuberculosis should wear surgical or other types of masks to help prevent transmission of their disease.

Other communicable diseases are spread indirectly by means of vectors. A *vector* is an organism (other than a human) that transmits a pathogen from one person to another. Usually a part of the life cycle of the pathogen takes place in or on the vector. For example, the malaria organism is a protozoan that carries out part of its life cycle in humans and another part in the gut of *Anopheles* mosquitoes. When a mosquito bites an infected person, it ingests blood that contains the protozoan. After the organism undergoes sexual reproduction in the mosquito, its progeny can infect new hosts when the mosquito bites them.

## The Third Link: The Host

Why do you remain healthy sometimes, yet get sick at other times? How did you avoid getting the cold that everyone else seems to have? Why didn't your spouse come down with the flu like the rest of the family? So far we've seen that some of the answers to these questions have to do with the pathogen and certain of its characteristics, such as its virulence. Transmission may also mean the difference between infection and health. Persons exposed frequently to pathogens are likely to become infected more often than those exposed less frequently. The other answers to these questions have to do with your body's resistance to the invading microbe.

As described in Chapter 3, stress can be one factor that reduces your resistance to infection. High-intensity or exhaustive exercise, such as running more than 60 miles per week or for 3 or more hours per session, also suppresses the immune system. Moderate exercise, however, such as running fewer than 20 miles per week or walking for 45 minutes per day for 5 days per week, stimulates the immune system. Exercising when you are sick lowers the body's defenses.

Race and age affect an individual's resistance or susceptibility to certain diseases. Africans or people with African ancestry, for example, have a higher resistance to tropical diseases such as malaria and yellow fever than do non-Africans. Asians are more resistant to the sexually transmitted infection syphilis than are non-Asians. Children are more likely to contract certain "childhood" infectious diseases such as measles and chicken pox, while older adults are more susceptible to pneumonia and influenza. And, as mentioned earlier, people with other diseases, such as AIDS, diabetes, and cancer, have weakened defense mechanisms.

Your body has two main types of defenses against infectious agents: mechanisms of nonspecific resistance, which are a variety of defenses that combat any foreign invader, and the immune system, which is a specific defense system that combats the particular invading pathogen. The following sections describe these two major defense mechanisms.

## Healthy Living Practices

- Refrigerate cold starchy and protein-rich foods and cold foods made with dairy products or poultry immediately after preparation. At picnics, keep these foods chilled until it is time to eat.
- Boil all low-acid home-canned foods before eating or avoid eating home-canned foods.
- Periodically clean and thoroughly disinfect mist-creating items such as humidifiers and maintain an appropriate concentration of chlorine in home spas.
- Avoid close contact with people who have communicable diseases.
- Wash your hands well and frequently to help avoid contracting communicable diseases, such as colds and the flu.
- Do not share drinking glasses and eating utensils with others.
- Do not share hypodermic needles with others because they may be contaminated with pathogens such as the hepatitis B virus or the AIDS virus.
- Use a condom when engaging in sex unless you are in a long-term, mutually monogamous relationship with an uninfected partner. Infectious bodily secretions can be passed from one partner to another during sexual activity.
- Use insect repellents formulated to repel ticks and flying insects that may be carriers of disease-producing organisms.
- Do not drink the water when traveling in developing countries. Also avoid raw fruits, vegetables, and salads because they may have been washed with contaminated water.
- Avoid the following hazardous foods when traveling in developing countries: uncooked or poorly cooked beef, pork, fish, and seafood and unpasteurized milk and other local dairy products.
- Avoid stress; high levels of stress reduce your resistance to infection.
- Avoid high-intensity or exhaustive exercise because it reduces your resistance to infection.
- Engage in moderate exercise to boost the immune system.

## Immunity

**Immunity** is protection from disease, particularly infectious disease. You have two types of immunity: nonspecific and specific. **Nonspecific immunity** comprises a variety of defense mechanisms that combat any type of damage to the body, including the invasion of infectious agents. **Specific immunity** is carried out by the immune system. The **immune system** recognizes and combats pathogens and other foreign cells (such as cancer cells or tissue transplants) with cells and proteins that are specific for particular invaders. The immune system is discussed later in this chapter.

### Nonspecific Immunity

Pathogens can enter the body at sites called **portals of entry** (**Figure 14.10**). The mucous membranes lining the respiratory, digestive, urinary, and reproductive systems are all portals of entry. Whether resulting from a cut, insect bite, burn, or injection, broken skin is a portal of entry. The placenta may be a portal of entry for a fetus, which may become infected with pathogens (mostly viruses) from an infected mother. Unbroken skin is a portal of entry only for some fungi and the larvae of certain parasitic worms.

**The Skin and Mucous Membranes** The skin provides a *mechanical barrier* to pathogens. The hardened cells at the surface of the skin provide a waterproof barrier that most infective agents cannot penetrate. In addition, acidic skin oils and sweat help make the skin an inhospitable environment for most organisms.

Body openings, such as the eyes, and tubes that open to the outside, such as the digestive and respiratory tracts, are lined with tissue called *mucous membranes*. Most mucous membranes have a thin layer of cells that produces a sticky, viscous secretion called mucus. Mucus keeps the membrane moist and traps foreign particles and organisms.

Another defense mechanism that works with the mucous membranes is *cilia*. These short, hairlike structures project from the surfaces of the cells lining the upper respiratory tract. As they beat in wavelike fashion, they move mucus that contains trapped foreign material such as dust and bacteria up toward the

## Figure 14.10

**Portals of Entry of the Human Body.** Portals of entry are areas of the body where pathogens can intrude: the skin and mucous membranes lining the respiratory, digestive, urinary, and reproductive systems; the placenta; broken skin; and unbroken skin (only for some fungi and the larvae of certain parasitic worms).

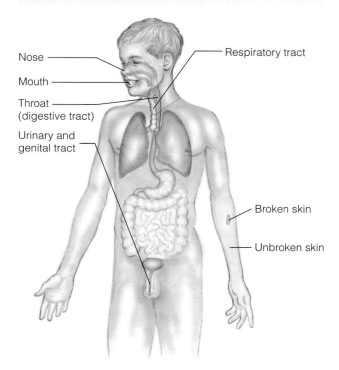

Nose

Mouth

Throat
(digestive tract)

Urinary and
genital tract

Respiratory tract

Broken skin

Unbroken skin

**immunity** (im-MYOU-nih-tea) Resistance to disease.

**nonspecific immunity** A variety of defense mechanisms that combat any type of damage to the body, including the invasion of infectious agents.

**specific immunity** Defense mechanism carried out by the immune system.

**immune system** A collection of cells and organs of the body that recognizes and combats pathogens and other foreign substances with cells and proteins that are specific for particular invaders. The immune system has two branches: antibody-mediated immunity and cell-mediated immunity.

**portal of entry** Site on or in the body where pathogens enter.

**leukocytes** (LEWK-oh-sites) White blood cells; active in both specific and nonspecific defenses of the body.

**phagocytosis** (FAG-oh-sigh-TOE-sis) The process of white blood cells ingesting foreign cells and debris, such as the dirt or dead cells in a cut.

**lymph** (limf) Tissue fluid.

help protect the body against infection and are part of the immune system.

**The Lymphatic System** The lymphatic system, another key player in nonspecific immunity, is composed of vessels and nodes through which tissue fluid, or **lymph**, flows. Pictured in **Figure 14.12**, the

back of the mouth where it can be swallowed, keeping it away from lower respiratory structures, especially the lungs.

Other tissues have a *chemical defense* mechanism. The lacrimal glands (located above the upper, outer corners of the eyes) produce tears that wash away foreign material on the eyes and also contain a chemical called *lysozyme* that kills certain bacteria. Lysozyme is also found in saliva. Another structure that provides a nonspecific chemical defense is the stomach. Stomach acid kills most of the microorganisms ingested with food.

**White Blood Cells and Phagocytosis** Another nonspecific line of defense is the action of certain white blood cells, or **leukocytes**, that ingest foreign cells and debris, such as the dirt or dead cells in a cut. This process is **phagocytosis** (literally, *phago*, "eating," and *cyto*, "cell") and is shown in **Figure 14.11**. Two types of leukocytes—the neutrophils and the macrophages—are important phagocytes in the human body. Other white blood cells called *lymphocytes*

## Figure 14.11

**White Blood Cell Ingesting Bacteria.** This is a highly magnified, colorized photo of a white blood cell called a macrophage (yellow/orange). Macrophages are the scavengers of the body and protect it by "eating" bacteria and other foreign material. The bacteria (green) it is ingesting cause tuberculosis in humans.

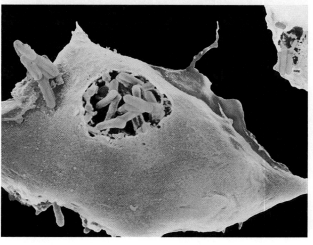

## Figure 14.12

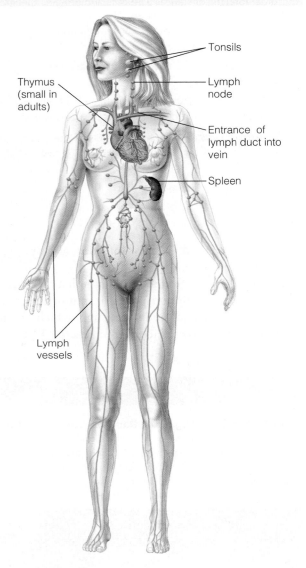

**The Lymphatic System.** The lymphatic system is made up of blind-ended vessels, nodes, and a few organs. Tissue fluid, derived from the blood, flows through the lymphatic vessels and is cleansed of debris and microorganisms by white blood cells that reside in the nodes. The fluid eventually returns to the blood.

Tonsils

Thymus (small in adults)

Lymph node

Entrance of lymph duct into vein

Spleen

Lymph vessels

taining lymphocytes and macrophages. The nodes cleanse tissue fluid by trapping microorganisms and other foreign substances in their weblike structures; macrophages in the nodes phagocytize this material.

The tonsils are large groups of lymph nodes located at the back of the oral cavity; they rid the nose and mouth area of bacteria and other debris. The spleen, located in the upper left corner of the abdominal cavity (see Figure 14.12), not only performs the function of a lymph node but also destroys worn-out red blood cells and stores red blood cells to provide an emergency supply in the case of severe loss. The thymus, located just above the heart at the midline of the chest, is the place where the lymphocytes destined to be T cells mature during fetal life and early childhood (see the section titled "Specific Immunity" later in this chapter). (These T cells then reside in the lymphatic tissue and produce new T cells when the thymus is no longer active.)

**Inflammation** Can you remember the last time you got a splinter or a cut? If so, you can probably remember (quite well!) your body's response. The inflammatory response is a series of events that takes place when the body is harmed by occurrences such as bacterial or viral invasion (infection), cuts, chemical damage, and burns. This response can be *local*, as in the case of getting a splinter in your finger, or *systemic* (affecting the whole body), as in the case of contracting a cold. Inflammation involves a variety of defense mechanisms that isolate and destroy the pathogens or other injurious agents and then remove the foreign materials and damaged cells so that the body can repair itself.

The presence of infectious agents or damage to the body triggers the inflammatory response. As a result, many chemicals are released. Some of these chemicals, such as histamine, cause an increase of blood flow to the affected area, which brings phagocytes and other white blood cells to ingest microorganisms and debris—pieces of a splinter, for example. In addition, other chemicals stimulate phagocytes to move to the affected area, where they leave the blood and enter the damaged tissues. Yet other chemicals allow the surrounding blood vessel walls to leak, permitting phagocytes, certain blood-clotting factors, and other chemicals that enhance the inflammatory response to enter the tissues. The blood-clotting factors wall off the infected area, which prevents the spread of the infection. **Figure 14.13** illustrates the inflammatory process.

The signs and symptoms of local inflammation are redness, heat, swelling, pain, and a loss of func-

lymphatic system also consists of lymphocytes and three lymphatic organs: the tonsils, the spleen, and the thymus (which is only active until puberty). The lymphatic system removes microorganisms and other foreign substances from the tissue fluid, the fluid surrounding the cells that is derived from the blood.

Lymph nodes are located at many points along the lymphatic vessels. Lymphatic vessels enter and exit each lymph node, which is a mesh of tissue con-

**The Inflammatory Process.** (a) A splinter damages the skin, thrusting bacteria deep into the wound. Injured cells release chemicals such as histamine that cause the blood vessels to widen, bringing more blood to the area. (b) White blood cells squeeze through vessel walls and migrate to the bacteria, where they phagocytize them. Blood clots and connective tissue wall off the area.

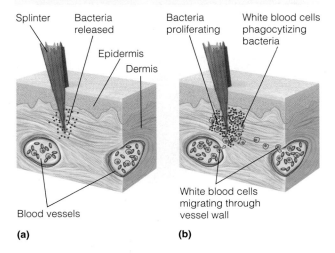

(a)  (b)

**interferons** (IN-ter-FEAR-onz) Proteins produced by the body during a viral infection that protect uninfected cells from viral invasion.

**antigens** (AN-tih-jenz) Proteins that are foreign or recognized as "nonself" by the body.

tion. The redness, heat, and swelling are results of increased blood flow to the affected area, including movement of fluids into surrounding tissues. Pain results as nerves are stimulated by the swelling and the chemicals released during inflammation. The pain, tissue damage, and swelling may contribute to a temporary loss of function of the affected body part.

Systemic inflammation occurs when you have a widespread infection such as a cold, the flu, strep throat, or pneumonia. Systemic inflammation has the same signs as local inflammation, but additional processes occur that result in more significant signs. The red bone marrow, located in the ends of certain bones, produces and releases large numbers of white blood cells. In addition, invading microorganisms and white blood cells release chemicals that affect the body's temperature-regulating system in the brain, resulting in a fever.

A *fever* is a rise in the internal body temperature from the human average of about 98.6°F. A fever lower than 104°F helps the body fight infection by enhancing phagocytosis and inhibiting the growth of certain microorganisms. However, a prolonged fever of 104°F, or a fever higher than 104°F, is dangerous because it can destroy proteins in the body. Other symptoms of systemic inflammation are fatigue, aches, and weakness.

The inflammatory process continues until the pathogens are killed or inactivated, or other injurious agents are walled off from the rest of the body and no longer pose a threat. Phagocytes ingest cellular debris and other organic material as the tissues recover from the infection.

**Natural Killer Cells** Natural killer cells are specialized white blood cells that attack cancer cells and body cells invaded by viruses. Natural killer cells secrete a chemical that pokes holes in the membranes of these two types of cells, destroying them. The response of natural killer cells to viral infections or developing cancer cells is quick, providing the body with protection until the immune system takes over (see the section titled "Specific Immunity" that follows).

**Interferons** Released from virally infected cells, **interferons** are proteins that protect uninfected cells from viral invasion. Interferons stimulate these cells to produce a protein that breaks down the hereditary material of the virus. When the damaged viruses enter cells, they are unable to replicate and the viral infection is eventually halted. Interferons enhance the activity of the phagocytes as well as the action of other, more specific immune system responses. In this role, interferons enhance the body's ability to fight invasions from most disease-causing agents, not just viruses.

## Specific Immunity

Specific immunity is a function of the immune system. The immune system is made up of cells residing in tissues scattered throughout the body. These cells can react to specific pathogens and foreign molecules.

The immune system has two branches: *antibody-mediated immunity* and *cell-mediated immunity*, which are discussed shortly. Each branch works slightly differently to attack foreign invaders and stop an infection. The immune system also has a memory: cells that react quickly to subsequent attacks by an invader.

**Antigens: The Triggers of Specific Immunity**
**Antigens** are usually foreign, or "nonself," proteins. Sometimes, entire infectious agents act as antigens. In other instances, parts of pathogens or the poisons they may secrete act as antigens. Noninfectious

agents such as plant pollens, blood transfusions, or tissue transplants are antigenic, although the response to these antigens may differ from person to person. Unfortunately, the body sometimes perceives its own cells as foreign, attacking them and causing localized and systemic reactions, as in the case of **autoimmune diseases** such as *rheumatoid arthritis* (see Chapter 3). In this disease, the reactions include inflammation and deformity of the joints. The following sections describe how the immune system reacts to antigens that enter the body.

**Antibody-Mediated Immunity** The antibody-mediated portion of the immune system reacts to *extracellular* antigens, that is, antigens that reside outside of body cells, such as most bacteria and any toxins they produce. **Antibodies** are proteins that interact in a lock-and-key fashion with antigens. When they bind with an antigen, antibodies interfere with the normal functioning of the antigen. Antigen–antibody binding also stimulates the inflammatory response and promotes phagocytosis of the antigen.

The workhorses of antibody-mediated immunity (the cells that produce antibodies) are specialized white blood cells called *B lymphocytes*, or **B cells**. Each B cell has receptors on its membrane that bind to a specific antigen. When a foreign antigen enters the body, B cells bind to it. After stimulation by lymphocytes called helper T cells, the B cells reproduce in large numbers and become plasma cells, which produce antibodies. **Figure 14.14** illustrates the antibody-mediated immune response.

Some of the stimulated B cells do not differentiate into plasma cells. These cells circulate as *memory B cells*, which respond more rapidly and forcefully whenever the antigen is encountered in the future. Memory cells confer immunity (resistance) to a disease. Many infections stimulate lifelong immunity (measles and chicken pox, for example); others, such as diphtheria, confer immunity for only a few years. Unfortunately, not all infectious agents stimulate the formation of memory cells, so no immunity is produced as a result of their infection. Examples of such infections are strep throat and gonorrhea (an STI).

**Cell-Mediated Immunity** The cell-mediated portion of the immune system reacts to *intracellular* antigens; that is, antigens that reside inside our body cells, such as viruses, fungi, a few types of bacteria, and parasites. It also acts against foreign tissues such as organ transplants and controls the growth of tumor cells.

Lymphocytes called **T cells** function in cell-mediated immunity. T cells reside in lymphoid tissues and in the bloodstream with the B cells. The body con-

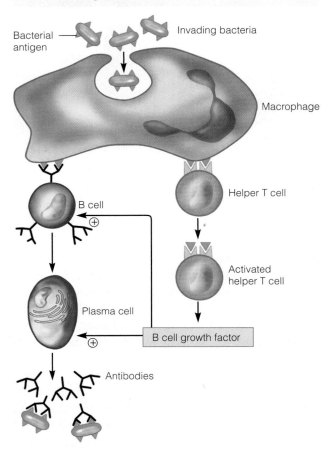

### Figure 14.14

**The Antibody-Mediated Immune Response.** White blood cells called macrophages ingest invading microbes and display their antigenic parts. Helper T cells and B cells specific to the antigens attach to them, which activates both types of cells. The helper T cells produce a chemical that stimulates the growth of the B cells. These B cells, now called plasma cells, secrete proteins called antibodies. Antibodies attach to and promote the death of the invading microbes.

Bacterial antigen

Invading bacteria

Macrophage

B cell

Helper T cell

Activated helper T cell

Plasma cell

B cell growth factor

Antibodies

tains thousands of different T cells. Upon binding to antigens, T cells reproduce and differentiate into four types: cytotoxic T cells, helper T cells, suppressor T cells, and memory T cells.

*Cytotoxic T cells* destroy invading intracellular pathogens (primarily viruses) by secreting chemicals that break apart infected host cells. By destroying host cells, the cytotoxic T cells take away what a virus or any other intracellular infective agent needs to reproduce or replicate. Cytotoxic T cells destroy nonself tissue transplants or tumorous growths in much the same way (**Figure 14.15**).

*Helper T cells* and *suppressor T cells* regulate the activities of both branches of the immune system.

Figure 14.15

**The Cell-Mediated Immune Response.** Cytotoxic T cells are key to the cell-mediated immune response. Here, whole T cells, not just antibodies, attach to cells infected with viruses, to cancer cells, or to tissue transplants. The T cell then secretes chemicals that destroy the host cell before the virus can enter the nucleus and begin to replicate.

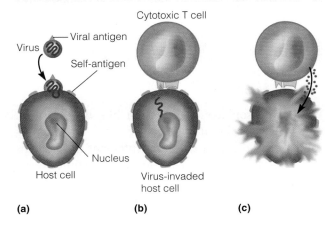

Cytotoxic T cell

Viral antigen

Virus

Self-antigen

Nucleus

Host cell

Virus-invaded host cell

(a)                (b)                (c)

autoimmune diseases Diseases in which the body perceives its own cells as foreign, attacking them and causing localized and systemic (whole-body) reactions.

antibodies Proteins that interact in a lock-and-key fashion with antigens, interfering with the normal functioning of the antigen.

B cells Specialized white blood cells (lymphocytes) that function in antibody-mediated immunity and produce antibodies.

T cells specialized white blood cells (lymphocytes) that function in cell-mediated immunity; there are four types of T cells.

acquired immunity Specific resistance to infection that is not inherited but develops during a person's lifetime.

Helper T cells secrete various chemicals that enhance the activity of cytotoxic T cells and suppressor T cells and attract phagocytes to the area. Some helper T cells secrete chemicals that enhance the development and reproduction of B cells.

When the infection has subsided, suppressor T cells shut down the immune system. Although these cells inhibit the activity of various immune system cells, they increase in number more slowly than do other T cells. Therefore, suppressor T cells shut down the immune response only after it has successfully done its job.

A group of stimulated T cells circulates as *memory T cells*. Like memory B cells, memory T cells respond rapidly and forcefully during subsequent encounters with antigens, resulting in immunity to a disease.

## Interactions Between Nonspecific and Specific Immunity

The mechanisms of nonspecific and specific defense work together to prevent infection or combat infection when it occurs. For example, the intact skin, mucous membranes, and chemicals in body fluids are effective barriers against viral invasion. However, if viruses gain entry to the body, macrophages phagocytize them before they can enter body cells. Activated helper T cells secrete chemicals that stimulate the B cells to become antibody-producing cells.

If some of the virus particles enter body cells despite these defenses, the infected cells produce interferons, which protect uninfected cells. Natural killer cells poke holes in the infected cells, killing them, thus destroying the virus's host. After binding to infected cells, cytotoxic T cells reproduce, developing large populations specific for this viral infection. As armies of cytotoxic T cells break apart infected cells, the freed viruses are phagocytized by macrophages and inactivated by antibodies. Usually this complex process stops the viral infection. The memory B cells and T cells continue to circulate and recognize this same virus quickly if it reenters the body. Most likely, the virus will never again cause infection because it will have been stopped before it could gain a foothold in the cells.

## Protection Against Infectious Diseases

A variety of factors determine whether a person develops an infectious disease. In general, to prevent infectious disease, you must break the chain of infection. This chapter offers many tips on breaking the chain of infection and preventing disease. However, one of the best ways to protect yourself against infection is to increase your resistance.

Specific immunity is either inborn or acquired. *Inborn immunity* is inherited, such as immunity to infectious diseases that attack other organisms (your cat or dog, for example) but not humans. **Acquired immunity** is not inherited; it develops during a per-

**vaccine** A preparation of a killed or weakened pathogen or its antigenic parts to be administered to a person to induce immunity and thereby prevent infectious disease.

**antibiotics** (AN-tie-by-OT-iks) A group of chemicals that kill bacteria or inhibit their growth.

## Healthy Living Practices

☐ Protect yourself against infection by having the appropriate vaccinations before traveling.

☐ Protect children from infection by having them immunized according to the most recent childhood immunization schedule.

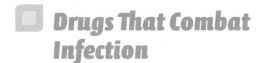

## Drugs That Combat Infection

son's lifetime. Acquired immunity develops in a variety of ways: either actively or passively, and by natural or artificial means.

*Active acquired immunity* is an immune system response developed as a result of contact with a pathogen, which includes development of memory B cells or T cells. Contact with the pathogen can occur naturally, during day-to-day life. It can also occur artificially, by a **vaccine** prepared from a killed or weakened pathogen or its antigenic parts. Depending on how the vaccine is prepared, it may have long- or short-term effects. That is why people need booster vaccinations every few years against some infectious diseases.

Children develop active acquired immunity to many serious childhood diseases by being vaccinated according to a schedule recommended by the American Academy of Pediatrics and the American Academy of Family Physicians. The CDC, at www.cdc.gov/vaccines, lists the current childhood and adolescent immunization schedule. In addition, immunization of adults and children prior to travel to foreign countries leads to active acquired immunity to diseases not generally found in the United States. If you are traveling outside the United States, consult your physician 4 to 6 weeks prior to your trip for the required and recommended immunizations. The CDC provides health-related travel information at www.cdc.gov/travel.

*Passive acquired immunity* is conferred when a person is given antibodies. Passive immunity can be acquired naturally when antibodies from a mother cross the placenta and enter the bloodstream of a developing fetus. After birth, a breast-fed infant passively acquires antibodies from its mother's milk. These antibodies help a newborn resist disease for the first month of life until its own immune system becomes functional. Passive immunity can also be acquired artificially, when a person receives an injection of antibodies after exposure to a serious infection (such as hepatitis A or rabies) or a lethal poison (such as certain snake venoms).

Once a person has an infection like the common cold, what can he or she do to combat it? Most often, getting rest and drinking sufficient fluids helps the body as it mounts its defense. Sometimes over-the-counter cold medications, such as decongestants, antihistamines, and cough medicines can help relieve symptoms. Many products are also available that are considered part of complementary and alternative medicine. See the Consumer Health feature "CAM Products and Colds" for more information. For other infections, individuals can obtain specific recommendations from a physician. These medical practitioners often prescribe medicines to inhibit the growth of or inactivate the infectious agent.

**Antibiotics** are a group of chemicals that kill bacteria or inhibit their growth. Antibiotics work by attacking parts of bacterial cells or bacterial processes that differ from human cells. When taking an antibiotic, it is important to finish the medication your physician prescribed, even though your symptoms may be gone prior to that time. All the bacteria may not have been killed, and the infection could return.

Antibiotics do nothing to combat viral infections and may kill some of the body's normal bacterial inhabitants. These bacteria control the growth of troublesome microorganisms; when they are gone, it is easier for unwanted disease-causing bacteria to multiply and cause a secondary bacterial infection. Therefore, *taking antibiotics when they are unnecessary can be harmful.* Furthermore, the unnecessary use of antibiotics provides additional opportunities for antibiotic-resistant strains of bacteria to develop.

Various topical antibiotics (those applied to the skin, such as bacitracin) are available without prescription to treat or prevent minor skin infections. Over-the-counter topical antifungal drugs are also

# Consumer Health

## CAM Products and Colds

Adults have an average of two to four colds per year, and children have more—about six to eight. Each year Americans experience many colds, making the market for cold/cough/flu remedies huge and manufacturers anxious to tap into it. The last time you had a cold or the flu, you likely roamed the aisles of your local pharmacy trying to find a product to shorten the duration of your illness and lessen its symptoms.

Pharmacy shelves are stocked with the usual over-the-counter kinds of decongestants, cough suppressants, and antihistamines. However, you might have noticed other products packaged as cold or flu treatments and labeled "homeopathic medicine" or "dietary supplement." These are two types of *alternative* cold products. Complementary and alternative medicine (CAM) is a diverse group of healthcare systems, treatments, and products that differ from conventional (scientific or evidence-based) medicine. Chapter 1 describes CAM in more detail and provides a classification of CAM systems and treatments. Can the alternative cold treatments available on pharmacy shelves help support your immune system, quiet your cough, shorten the duration of your cold or flu infection, relieve your sinus pain and pressure, or dry up your nasal congestion as they claim?

### Homeopathic Products

Within the CAM classification framework, homeopathic (ho-me-oh-PAH-thick) "medicine," or *homeopathy* (ho-me-AH-pah-thee), is a type of alternative medical system. Developed in Germany more than 200 years ago, homeopathy operates on the principle of "similar" or "like cures like." Proponents believe that a disease or condition can be cured by using small amounts of a substance that in much larger amounts causes those same symptoms in healthy people. For example, homeopaths use substances from onions to stop the watery eyes and runny nose of a cold—the same substances that cause tears when an onion is cut during food preparation.

To prepare homeopathic products, the "principle of dilutions" is used, which states that the lowest dosage possible has the greatest effect. Therefore substances are diluted with water in a stepwise fashion, with a special and specific type of shaking occurring after each dilution. Scientific and mathematical analyses have determined that no molecules of the original substance are present in most preparations after the dilution process. However, homeopaths believe that the "essence" of the original substance remains because the water used in the dilutions has a "memory" of it and can therefore stimulate the body to heal itself. These basic principles, beliefs, and methods of homeopathy oppose the basic principles, understandings, and methods of science and evidence-based medicine.

A variety of products labeled "homeopathic medicine" can be found on drugstore shelves claiming "to reduce the duration and severity of flu-like symptoms," "to shorten the duration of the common cold," or "for sinus pain, nasal congestion, sinus pressure, and headache pain." The "active ingredients" listed on the package are the substances used at the beginning of the dilution process and can be a single item, a few, or a long list. These substances come from plants, animals, or minerals.

Are these products safe, and are they effective? The National Center for Complementary and Alternative Medicine (NCCAM) of the National Institutes of Health (NIH) states that "there is little evidence to support homeopathy as an effective treatment for any specific condition." Edzard Ernst, physician and director of the Complementary Medicine Peninsula Medical School at the Universities of Exeter in the United Kingdom, agrees with this NCCAM assessment and notes, "Today, about 200 clinical trials of homeopathy are available. Collectively these data fail to provide good evidence that the clinical effects of homeopathic remedies are different from those of placebos." Placebos are sugar pills or sham therapies that often make patients feel better solely because of their belief that they are being given a helpful treatment.

Although the NCCAM notes that the side effects and risks of homeopathic products have not been well researched, it adds that most homeopathic products contain little to no active ingredients. Therefore, the NCCAM concludes that these products are likely safe but ineffective.

### Dietary Supplements and Supplement Drops

Alongside homeopathic products in the cough/cold section of your local pharmacy, you will also find products labeled as "dietary supplements," or "supplement drops" for "immune support," to help combat or prevent colds or flu, or to calm your cough. Within the CAM classification framework, these products are considered biologically based treatments. They generally contain a variety of vitamins and minerals along with various herbal extracts. Garlic, echinacea, vitamin C, and zinc are among the dietary supplements often included in over-the-counter cold and flu remedies. The following sections describe the results of scientific research that has been conducted on these substances to determine their effectiveness to prevent and treat colds.

*(Continues)*

### Garlic (Allium sativum)

Garlic is touted to have many and varied health benefits, including clearing acne, reducing high blood cholesterol, preventing cancer, and repelling mosquitoes. It is also said to have antimicrobial, antiviral, and anti-inflammatory properties, which work to relieve colds. Garlic contains various substances, such as sulfur-containing compounds, that could result in positive health effects when ingested.

Laboratory studies show that garlic appears to have some antiviral and antimicrobial properties. Few studies have been conducted on the effects of garlic on human health, however. Weak evidence shows that garlic may prevent occurrences of colds, but much more evidence is needed.

### Echinacea

Extracts of the flowering plant *Echinacea* (eh-kih-NAY-sha) are used to make over-the-counter products claiming to reduce the severity and duration of colds and flu and prevent these upper respiratory infections when taken regularly. Results of studies with mice show that various compounds from echinacea appear to stimulate white blood cells, act against viruses, and help reduce inflammation, which lends credence to these claims. However, it is difficult to study the effects of echinacea products in humans because over-the-counter echinacea products differ greatly. Products are formulated from different species and parts of the plant, by using differing extraction processes, and by combining echinacea with other substances.

There is some evidence that echinacea preparations made of the above-ground parts of *Echinacea purpurea* (**Figure 14.C**) might shorten the duration or decrease the severity of symptoms of a cold when taken as soon as symptoms appear. There is no evidence to support its prolonged use for cold prevention, and its long-term safety has not been established. Side effects are reported infrequently. Well-designed studies are needed to confirm the effects of echinacea in humans and to characterize its active ingredients and mechanism of action.

### Vitamin C

Vitamin C is essential for good health, and most balanced diets provide a sufficient quantity. Eating a citrus fruit or drinking its juice along with having a serving of another vitamin-C-containing vegetable or fruit, such as broccoli, butternut squash, pineapple, or strawberries, is adequate to achieve the recommended dietary allowance. As mentioned in Chapter 9, the tolerable upper limit to avoid side effects or toxicity is 2,000 milligrams (mg) per day. Although it is a water-soluble vitamin, which means that it dissolves in bodily fluids and the excess is flushed out in the urine, vitamin C can cause a variety of side effects, including diarrhea, heartburn, cramps, headache, and kidney stones if too much is ingested.

Among the many jobs it performs in the body, vitamin C enhances various functions of the immune system. Therefore, it has been used for the treatment of a variety of ills, including treating and preventing colds. Although taking vitamin C does not appear to prevent colds, regular vitamin C ingestion (200 mg/day, for example) might reduce the duration, and possibly the severity, of cold symptoms.

### Zinc

Zinc is a mineral that is an essential part of the diet. It plays a variety of roles in metabolism and is involved in proper immune function. Zinc is stored in bone and skeletal muscle, but infection can cause a drop in normal blood levels of the mineral. (Common food sources of zinc are listed in Table 9.10.)

Zinc is sold in various forms including lozenges, tablets, capsules, and nasal sprays for the treatment of colds. Scientists hypothesize that zinc may compete for cold virus receptors in the lining of the nose, and this is the reasoning behind zinc nasal sprays. Put simply, if the cold virus receptors in the nose are saturated with zinc, the viruses cannot gain entry into the body.

According to results of recent studies, zinc-containing nasal sprays appear to shorten the duration of cold symptoms and lessen symptoms. However, a loss of smell—possibly a permanent loss—has been reported and appears to be a major roadblock to the study and use of zinc nasal sprays.

Along with competing for cold virus receptors in the lining of the nose, zinc also appears to inhibit the repli-

## Figure 14.C

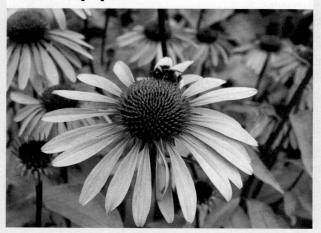

***Echinacea purpurea.***

cation of the cold virus, which makes it an excellent candidate as a cold treatment when taken orally. A review of decades of scientific studies on the use of zinc as a treatment for colds concludes that zinc reduced the duration and severity of cold symptoms when taken within 24 hours of the onset of symptoms. Supplementation of the diet with zinc over a 5-month period also reduced the incidence of colds. Zinc lozenges, however, can produce undesirable side effects, such as stomach disturbances and diarrhea. Scientists are unable to make recommendations concerning which formulation of zinc might be used, and how much might be taken and for how long for the possible prevention and treatment of colds.

Complementary and alternative products for the prevention and treatment of colds can differ dramatically from one another. In addition, the scientific evidence supporting their usefulness is often weak or absent. When evidence supporting the usefulness of a therapy becomes strong, it usually becomes accepted by the scientifically based (conventional) medical community and is no longer considered "alternative." Being an informed consumer will help you make the best choices for your health. Always check with your physician before taking any new medications or other treatments, including CAM products; they can react with medications you are already taking or have adverse effects of which you are unaware.

*Sources:* Barrett, B., et al. and the CRD. (2011). *Echinacea* for upper respiratory infection (structured abstract). *Cochrane Library Database of Abstracts of Reviews of Effects,* no. 2; D'Cruze, H., et al. (2009). Is intranasal zinc effective and safe for the common cold? A systematic review and meta-analysis. *Journal of Primary Health Care, 1*(2):134–139; Ernst, E. (2011). Pharmacists and homeopathic remedies. *American Journal of Health-System Pharmacy,* 68:478; Heimer, K. A., et al. (2009). Examining the evidence for the use of vitamin C in the prophylaxis and treatment of the common cold. *Journal of the American Academy of Nurse Practitioners,* 21:295–300; Hemilä, H., et al. (2010). Vitamin C for preventing and treating the common cold (Review). Cochrane Database of Systematic Reviews, *Cochrane Library,* no. 3; Linde, K., et al. (2009). *Echinacea* for preventing and treating the common cold (Review). Cochrane Database of Systematic Reviews, *Cochrane Library,* no. 4; Lissiman E., et al. (2009). Garlic for the common cold (Review). Cochrane Database of Systematic Reviews, *Cochrane Library,* no. 4; National Center for Complementary and Alternative Medicine. (2010, August). Homeopathy: An Introduction. National Institutes of Health. Retrieved on April 29, 2011, from http://nccam.nih.gov/health/homeopathy/; Singh, M., & Das, R. R. (2011). Zinc for the common cold (Review). Cochrane Database of Systematic Reviews, *Cochrane Library,* no. 3.

available to treat fungal infections of the skin, such as athlete's foot and ringworm, and vaginal yeast infections. Antifungal drugs that must be taken orally for more serious fungal infections require a prescription.

Progress in the production of effective antiviral drugs has been slow because viruses reside inside the body's cells. Therefore, a drug must inactivate the virus without harming its host. A few antiviral drugs treat infections caused by the herpesvirus (such as genital herpes, cold sores, and chicken pox) and others treat diseases associated with AIDS. Antiviral medications have been developed to control influenza (flu) infection.

Specific medications have also been developed to treat protozoal diseases such as malaria, amebic dysentery, and trichomoniasis. Likewise, prescription medicines are available to treat infestations of worms such as tapeworms and pinworms.

## Healthy Living Practices

☐ If you contract a localized infection such as an infected sore or wound, consult your physician for specific recommendations on treating it.

☐ If you contract a systemic infection such as a cold or the flu, rest and drink sufficient fluids to help your body mount its defense.

☐ If you are prescribed a medication to combat an infection, follow all instructions and take the prescribed amount.

# Sexually Transmitted Infections

**Sexually transmitted infections (STIs),** which are also called sexually transmitted diseases (STDs), are spread from person to person by the intimate contact that occurs during sexual activity, primarily vaginal intercourse and anal intercourse. In general, the pathogens that cause STIs are passed from the sores, secretions, or tissues of an infected individual's reproductive system to the mucous membranes or broken skin of the reproductive system and surrounding tissue of another. (As you read the rest of this chapter, please refer to Figure 5.1, which shows the male reproductive organs, and Figure 5.3, which shows the female reproductive organs.) Infectious organisms can also be transferred from the mouth to the genitals and vice versa during oral sex.

Contracting a sexually transmitted infection is more likely when other STIs are present. For example, infection with the herpes simplex virus (HSV) or with syphilis has been shown to increase the risk of human immunodeficiency virus (HIV) transmission by as much as 10- to 100-fold for a single act of intercourse. Both HSV and syphilis cause sores on the genitals, which apparently facilitate the transfer of the human immunodeficiency virus.

Most pathogens that cause STIs cannot survive long (or at all) outside the human body. Therefore, most STIs cannot be contracted by genital contact with contaminated toilet seats or bed linens. Most STIs are passed directly from one person to another.

Some sexually transmitted infections are caused by yeasts, protozoans, mites (organisms closely related to spiders), and lice (organisms closely related to fleas). Most STIs are caused by bacteria and viruses.

Before you read more of this chapter, complete the "STI Attitude Scale" self-assessment in the Student Workbook pages at the end of this text. A high score on this assessment indicates a predisposition toward high-risk STI behavior. A low score indicates a predisposition toward low-risk STI behavior. This chapter can help you develop low-risk behaviors.

### Healthy Living Practices

☐ To protect yourself and others against the transmission of sexually transmitted infections, use latex condoms during sexual intercourse.

## Sexually Transmitted Infections Caused by Viruses

Sexually transmitted infections caused by viruses are extremely serious because they cannot be cured. Certain medications ease the discomfort of viral STI symptoms, but virus particles remain in the tissues and can cause recurrent symptoms. Also, the virus can be passed continually from chronically infected individuals to others during sexual activity.

In addition to causing STIs, three sexually transmitted viruses have been implicated in the development of particular cancers: HIV, human papillomavirus (HPV), and **hepatitis B virus (HBV)**. Therefore, contracting any one of these viruses not only results in an incurable infectious disease but also increases the risk of developing particular types of cancers. HPV is discussed later in this chapter. HBV causes a serious inflammation of the liver and can result in liver cancer. Although hepatitis is caused by a variety of hepatitis viruses (such as A, B, C, and D), hepatitis B virus is the one most commonly transmitted by sexual contact. Although hepatitis B is a serious and long-term disease, people can recover from it.

Human immunodeficiency virus is the most serious viral sexually transmitted pathogen. HIV infection not only raises the risk of developing the cancer Kaposi's sarcoma, also the virus attacks the immune system, disabling the body's defenses. Eventually, the immune system of an HIV-infected individual becomes so weakened that he or she succumbs to an array of illnesses (the syndrome known as AIDS) that lead to death.

## Human Immunodeficiency Virus

As of January 1995, AIDS became the leading cause of death among Americans aged 25 to 44 years. By 1996 death rates from AIDS began to decline, by 1997 AIDS had dropped to the fifth leading cause of death in this age group, and by 2001 it was the sixth leading cause of death (**Figure 14.16**). In the United States, about three-fourths of new HIV infections each year occur in men.[9]

Since AIDS was first recognized in the early 1980s, the number of known deaths in all age groups in the United States increased annually through 1995.

**Figure 14.16**

**Leading Causes of Death Among Persons 25–44 Years of Age: United States, 1997–2007.** Although AIDS was the leading cause of death in this age group in 1995, the graph shows that by 1997 AIDS had dropped to the fifth leading cause of death. By 2001, AIDS was the sixth leading cause of death in this age group and remained so through 2007.

*Source:* Data from Centers for Disease Control and Prevention, National Center for Health Statistics. (2011, February). *Health, United States, 2011 with special feature on death and dying.* Retrieved on on May 4, 2011, from http://www.cdc.gov/nchs/data/hus/hus10.pdf

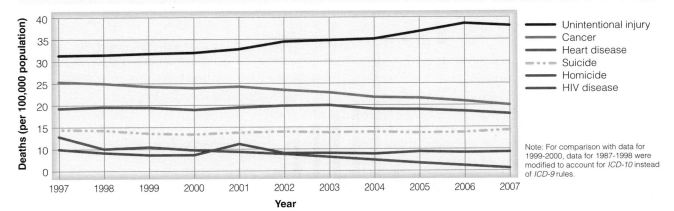

Then, with the introduction of antiretroviral therapy, deaths declined in 1996 through 1998. Antiretroviral therapy uses combinations of medications to slow the replication (copying) of the AIDS virus and reduce its levels in the bloodstream. Deaths have leveled off since the decline (**Figure 14.17**).

The annual number of new AIDS cases increased steadily from 1984 until its dramatic increase in 1993. Much of the 1993 increase is to the result of a change in the definition of AIDS, which broadened the list of conditions reportable as AIDS and included measures of immune system function. Beginning in 1994, the annual number of new AIDS cases declined steadily through 2001. This decrease reflects, in part, the waning effect of the 1993 definition change. A slight decline occurred beginning in 2006 and extending through 2009.

Globally, HIV infection is a widespread epidemic disease. Approximately 33.3 million people were living with HIV in 2009. In that same year, approximately 2.6 million people became newly infected, and about 1.8 million died from HIV/AIDS.[10] The majority of new HIV infections occur in sub-Saharan Africa, a poor, developing part of the continent. Although death rates from AIDS have not fallen as dramatically in developing regions of the world as they have in industrialized countries, they are falling somewhat because of antiretroviral therapy, which has finally become more available and affordable.

Overall, United Nations Programme on HIV/AIDS (UNAIDS) reports that the global AIDS epidemic has stabilized and the annual number of new HIV infections has been declining worldwide.

**The Progression of the Disease: HIV Infection and AIDS** Although medical researchers realized in 1981 that AIDS was a new disease, its cause (infection with human immunodeficiency virus) was not discovered until 1983. AIDS is a *syndrome*, a set of signs and symptoms occurring together. Being infected with HIV does not mean that a person has AIDS; infection leads to AIDS. Current data suggest that all infected individuals will develop AIDS eventually because HIV infection results in a continuous, prolonged, and ongoing disease process that still cannot be cured.

Approximately 1 to 3 weeks after becoming infected with HIV, most people experience a brief flulike illness that lasts for 1 to 2 weeks. During this stage of infection, people usually do not know that they are infected with HIV and think that they have a particularly bad case of the flu. When this initial illness subsides, the HIV-infected person seems to be healthy but is in the *asymptomatic phase* of HIV disease, which usually lasts about 8 to 10 years. (*Asymptomatic* means that no disease symptoms are apparent.) This time varies widely among individuals; it can be as short as a few months or longer than 10 years. During this time, many HIV-infected individuals do

Sexually Transmitted Infections Caused by Viruses  **477**

**Figure 14.17**

**Reported Cases and Known Deaths from AIDS, United States, 1984–2008/9.** The extreme rise in reported cases in 1993 is the result of a change in the definition of AIDS, which broadened the list of conditions reportable as AIDS and included measures of immune system function.
*Source:* Data from National Center for Health Statistics, National Vital Statistics System. U.S. Department of Health and Human Services, Centers for Disease Control and Prevention.

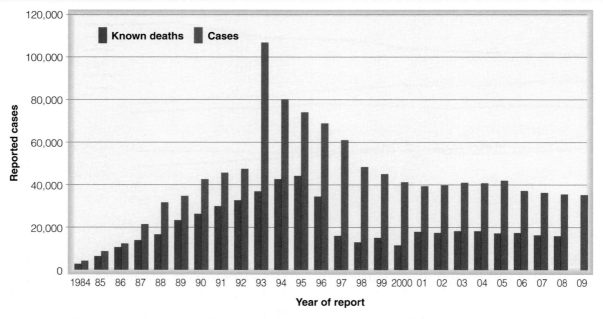

*Note:* Includes Guam, Puerto Rico, the U.S. Pacific Islands, and the U.S. Virgin Islands.

not realize that they are infected and may pass the virus on to others.

Although people with asymptomatic HIV infection may feel well, the virus is actively killing helper T cells in their bodies. Gradually, the number of helper T cells declines.

Although various laboratory tests can detect abnormalities in infected asymptomatic patients, these persons remain relatively symptom-free until they enter the *symptomatic phase* of HIV disease. The symptomatic phase usually begins when mature helper T cells (also called CD4 cells) have declined to about 500 cells (or fewer) per cubic millimeter of blood (500 cells/mm³). The normal level is 800 to 1,200 helper T cells/mm³. When the T cell count drops to 500/mm³, the body begins to have trouble warding off infections that a normal, healthy body resists. These infections are called *opportunistic infections* because they are caused by organisms that normally cannot produce infections except in people with lowered resistance.

During this phase of disease, the HIV-infected individual experiences a tremendous array of signs and symptoms. Some of these are nonspecific; that is, they are not in response to any opportunistic infection. These nonspecific signs and symptoms include fever, night sweats, headache, and fatigue. Chronic diarrhea usually occurs as opportunistic organisms infect the digestive system. Also, the HIV-infected individual often contracts minor oral infections such as thrush, caused by the yeast *Candida albicans* (KAN-de-dah AL-bih-kanz) (**Figure 14.18**). These symptoms and infections of the symptomatic phase are not usually life threatening, but the infected individual has trouble maintaining the normal pace of his or her lifestyle.

As the helper T cell count declines further to about 200/mm³, the rate of contracting serious opportunistic diseases increases. Common infections at this stage include *Pneumocystis carinii* pneumonia (a fungal infection of the lungs), *Cryptococcus* meningitis (a fungal infection of the coverings that surround the

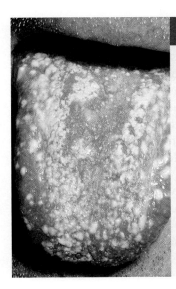

**Figure 14.18**

**Thrush, or Oral Candidiasis.** This oral infection is caused by the yeast *Candida albicans* and is a common infection of the symptomatic stage of HIV infection. It can also occur in persons taking broad-spectrum drugs or medications that suppress the immune system. Infants can acquire the disease during birth from mothers with vaginal candidiasis.

**Figure 14.19**

**Kaposi's Sarcoma.** Named after an Austrian dermatologist, this cancer is a serious, opportunistic disease of the HIV-infected person. It begins in the skin and metastasizes to the lymph nodes and body organs.

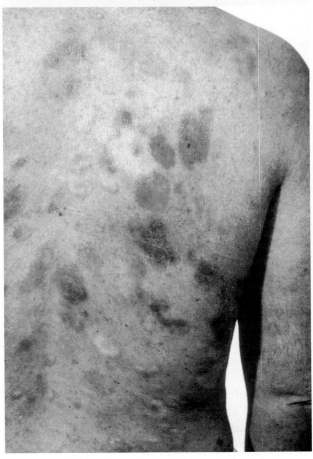

brain), toxoplasmosis (a protozoal infection of the brain, heart, and/or lungs), Kaposi's sarcoma (a type of cancer; **Figure 14.19**), and cytomegalovirus retinitis (a viral infection of the retina). A condition called *wasting syndrome* can also occur at this stage, which includes a marked loss of weight and a decrease in physical stamina, appetite, and mental activity. A person with HIV infection is usually diagnosed as having AIDS when the helper T cell count falls below 200/mm³ and one of these conditions (or another condition typical of this stage) is present.

On average, if treated with antiretroviral therapy, people live about 22 years from their initial HIV diagnosis[11] and about 5 years with AIDS.[12] Again, the amount of time varies tremendously from individual to individual. But as the T cell count falls below 50/mm³, the risk of death increases dramatically.

**How HIV Is Transmitted** Human immunodeficiency virus is transmitted in three ways: sexual contact with an infected person; exposure to infected blood or blood products; and placental transfer during fetal development, during labor and delivery, and during breastfeeding. These transmission routes are related in that, with the exception of breastfeeding, they all require the blood of the uninfected person to come into direct contact (or close contact, as in the case of placental transfer) with the blood, semen, or vaginal secretions of an infected person.

In 2008, approximately 47% of all HIV/AIDS cases diagnosed were men who had sex with men. One-fifth (19%) of cases were both men and women exposed through heterosexual sex.[13] Sexual behaviors that carry risk of HIV infection are unprotected anal

intercourse between men and unprotected anal or vaginal intercourse between a man and a woman. However, any sexual behavior that results in the contact of infected blood, semen, or vaginal secretions with the blood of an uninfected individual is risky because it may result in HIV transmission. Because minor abrasions or tears in the skin and mucous membranes of the genitals often occur during sex without partners being aware of it, such contact may take place much more readily than might be thought. Another primary route of HIV transmission is the sharing of contaminated needles and syringes among injecting drug abusers. (Chapter 7 describes drug abuse in detail.)

Some children and adults with AIDS acquired the disease by receiving contaminated blood during blood transfusions. These incidents occurred before blood banks instituted HIV antibody testing. However, staff at U.S. blood banks use new, sterile needles and syringes with each person who donates blood so that donating blood never has been a risk and is not a risk now.

Most children with AIDS contracted it during the birth process from their infected mothers. The fetus is thought to become infected during labor contractions, after the rupture of the membranes, or while in the birth canal. Elective cesarean section is one way to prevent mother-to-child transfer of the virus during the birth process and does not always present higher risk than vaginal delivery for the mother.[14] An HIV-infected pregnant woman can also take the drug zidovudine (AZT) to decrease the chance of HIV being transmitted to her fetus.

Transmission of HIV also occurs via breastmilk. Therefore, women with HIV who live in industrialized countries such as the United States, where infant formula is available and safe, should not breastfeed their children.

**How HIV Is Not Transmitted** There is no need to worry about contracting HIV disease if you work, go to school, and come into casual contact with a person who is infected with HIV. People in certain professions, such as health professionals and police officers, are at some risk of HIV infection because they may come into contact with HIV-infected blood. The results of numerous studies show that HIV is not transmitted by sharing such things as telephones or drinking fountains. Likewise, living with an HIV-infected person and sharing personal items such as combs, towels, eating utensils, and dishes do not transmit the virus.

Although HIV has been detected in saliva, it does not appear to be transmitted by kissing, except in the remote chance of transfer during open-mouth, deep kissing with an infected person who has bleeding gums or other spots in the mouth.[15] HIV transmission can take place through oral sex, but the level of risk is lower than with vaginal or anal intercourse.[16] Transmission of the virus by mosquitoes or other insects does not occur.[17]

**Protecting Yourself Against HIV Infection** The primary means of protecting yourself against becoming infected with HIV is not to engage in any behavior that puts your blood in contact with the blood, semen, or vaginal secretions of an infected person. Abstaining from sex with infected individuals eliminates that particular risk of HIV infection. Engaging in sex in a mutually monogamous relationship in

which neither partner is infected also eliminates that risk. HIV testing before engaging in sex can assure both of you that there is no risk of contracting the disease. Of course, both of you must *remain* monogamous throughout your relationship.

Unfortunately, you may not know if a potential sexual partner is infected; also, the partner may be unaware of his or her own infection. Therefore, to reduce your risk of HIV infection, reduce your number of sexual partners. *Table 14.1* lists the characteristics of high-risk partners. Avoid casual sexual encounters (having sex with people you do not know well) so that you have time to evaluate whether potential partners have any of these characteristics.

Always use a latex condom or a polyurethane vaginal pouch (female condom) during each act of sexual intercourse. Both types of condoms provide a barrier between you and the body fluids of another. Never use a male condom and a female condom at the same time. The two materials may tear as they rub against one another and the condoms may not stay in place. Also, do not use contraceptives that contain the spermicide nonoxynol-9. Some contraceptives containing this chemical might increase the risk of transmission of HIV and other STIs.[18] (See Chapter 5 for more detailed information on the use of condoms.) Using a cut-open condom or a dental dam (a rectangular sheet of latex used in dentistry) as a physical barrier

### Table 14.1

### People at High Risk for HIV Infection (United States)

Injecting drug users

People who have had sex with injecting drug users

Homosexual or bisexual men

Women who have had sex with bisexual men

People who received blood transfusions between 1978 and 1985

People with hemophilia

People who have another STI, particularly syphilis or herpes

Women from countries where heterosexual transmission is common (Latin America, the Caribbean, and Africa)

# Managing Your Health

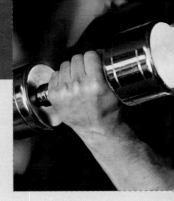

## Eliminating or Reducing Your Risk of HIV Infection and Other STIs

### How to Eliminate Your Risk of Becoming Infected with HIV or Other STIs

Abstain from sex. If that is not an option:

- Do not have sex with HIV-infected individuals or those infected with any STI.
- Engage in sex only in a monogamous relationship in which it is certain that neither partner is infected.
- Abstain from using drugs.

Note: People in certain professions, such as healthcare workers and police officers, have additional risks of infection because of the nature of their work. Such risks are not eliminated by these practices. These people can become infected with hepatitis B virus or HIV if their blood mixes with the blood or bodily secretions of an infected person.

### How to Reduce Your Risk of Becoming Infected with HIV or Other STIs

- Reduce your number of sexual partners.
- Avoid having sex with high-risk partners.
- Avoid having sex with people you do not know well.
- Avoid having sex while under the influence of drugs, including alcohol.
- Use a new latex condom during each act of anal or vaginal intercourse.
- Never share needles or syringes.
- Do not use contraceptives containing the spermicide nonoxynol-9.
- Use a cut-open condom or a dental dam during oral sex.

---

between the mouth and the genitals or anus during oral sex can reduce the likelihood of HIV or other STI transmission.[16]

Another risk factor for HIV infection is drug abuse of both injecting and noninjecting drugs. Eliminate this risk by abstaining from using drugs. Injecting drug abusers are primarily at risk because HIV-contaminated needles transmit the virus to anyone who shares the contaminated needles. Noninjecting drug abusers are also at an increased risk of contracting HIV because drug abusers engage in risky sexual behaviors while under the influence of drugs.

If you use drugs, you can reduce your risk of HIV infection by never sharing needles or syringes. If you do share needles and syringes, cleaning this equipment with bleach and then rinsing it with water will reduce your risk of infection. Do not have sex while under the influence of drugs.

In summary, medical researchers have discovered the ways in which HIV is transmitted and the ways in which it is not. This information was used to develop the lists shown in the Managing Your Health box "Eliminating or Reducing Your Risk of HIV Infection and Other STIs." One list summarizes the behaviors that virtually eliminate your risk of HIV infection and the other summarizes the behaviors that reduce your risk.

**Treatment of HIV Infection** There is no cure for HIV infection and AIDS. Thus far, attempts to develop an effective vaccine to protect against HIV infection have been unsuccessful. Because of the variability of the virus, developing an effective HIV vaccine is extremely difficult. It is unlikely that a vaccine will be available before 2020.[19]

Researchers are continually working on ways to treat HIV infection by boosting the immune system, inactivating the virus, or protecting immune system cells from infection. All approved anti-HIV drugs interfere with viral replication. However, the virus becomes immune to the drugs quite quickly as it mutates. Therefore, combinations of drugs appear to work best to retard HIV.

AIDS researchers consider a life-long drug regimen referred to as ART (antiretroviral therapy; also called HAART [highly active antiretroviral therapy]) as the best treatment for HIV/AIDS. ART combines three or more HIV drugs that suppress HIV replication. Researchers have found that the concentration of HIV in the bloodstream of some patients declines to undetectable levels with ART treatment. When HIV is suppressed, the concentration of mature helper T cells (CD4 cells) rises. HIV-infected patients who respond in this way to ART treatment may have their CD4 cell concentrations return to normal levels with long-term ART treatment. Although ART is extending the lives of AIDS patients, it has serious side effects with long-term use, including cardiovascular problems and bone demineralization.

ART may be used to prevent HIV; it appears to reduce susceptibility to infection in HIV-uninfected individuals. A vaginal gel incorporating the antiretroviral drug tenofovir has also shown promising results in reducing the rate of HIV transmission. The gel is still under study and not yet approved for use in the United States.[20]

Another promising area of research in the treatment of HIV/AIDS is *gene therapy*. In this approach, the HIV-infected cells of an AIDS patient are replaced with cells engineered to resist virus replication. Progress has been slow, but the results of clinical trials suggest that this approach may be useful.[21]

## Genital Herpes

**Genital herpes** (herpes simplex virus-2; HSV-2) is another STI that many people fear contracting because it is painful and incurable. When asked, "Do you worry about contracting an STI?" one health student responded: "I am really worried about getting herpes. Once you have it, you can't get rid of it. That's scary!"

The herpes "scare" began in the United States in the 1970s, and the number of initial visits to doctors' offices for concerns about HSV-2 has increased since then as **Figure 14.20** shows. Because HSV-2 is not a disease that must be reported to the CDC, epidemiologists (medical researchers who study such topics as the spread of disease) use data such as visits to doctors' offices and the results of blood tests to estimate its prevalence. (Reportable STIs are gonorrhea, syphilis, chlamydia, and chanchroid, a disease that is rare in most parts of the United States and is not discussed in this chapter.) CDC data show that the prevalence of HSV-2 based on the number of the persons aged 14–49 years who tested positive for the virus has decreased in the past two decades or so, from 21% in years 1988–1994 to 16.2% in years 2005–2008. The CDC notes, however, that "most persons with HSV-2 have not received a diagnosis," and that the increase in the number of doctor visits "may indicate increased recognition of infection."[22]

Like all STIs, HSV-2 is contracted through vaginal and anal intercourse with an infected individual. In addition, HSV-1 (which causes cold sores/fever blisters in the mouth) can infect the genital and anal areas during oral sex, and HSV-2 can infect the mouth. Either virus gains a foothold in the body by first infecting the skin cells in the immediate area of contact and spreading to surrounding cells. During an incubation period (the time between exposure to the pathogen and the onset of symptoms) that lasts about a week, the virus begins to replicate and destroy skin cells. The patient may experience irritation at these sites of infection prior to the eruption of skin lesions. The first lesions appear as groups of tiny, raised, solid bumps that turn clear or yellowish and become filled with fluid. These blisters eventually break open, oozing fluid containing viruses, and then develop into painful sores. The sores turn gray, crust over, and heal usually in 5 to 10 days. With this initial infection, the patient often experiences a headache, fever, weakness, and muscle pain.

HSV-2 usually infects the labia, vagina, and cervix in women and the penis in males, but it can also infect

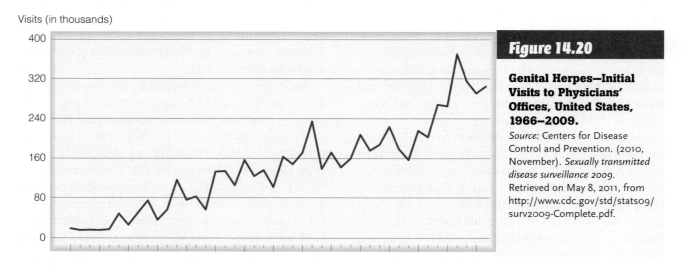

Visits (in thousands)

**Figure 14.20**

**Genital Herpes—Initial Visits to Physicians' Offices, United States, 1966–2009.**
*Source:* Centers for Disease Control and Prevention. (2010, November). *Sexually transmitted disease surveillance 2009.* Retrieved on May 8, 2011, from http://www.cdc.gov/std/stats09/surv2009-Complete.pdf.

tissues in the genital/anal area that are not protected by a condom. Therefore, the use of latex condoms can only *reduce* the risk of herpes transmission; it does not eliminate the risk for neighboring tissues. The tenofovir vaginal gel being tested to reduce HIV transmission has been shown to reduce transmission of HSV as well.[20] Follow the practices outlined in the section "Protecting Yourself Against STIs" (later in this chapter).

Transmission of HSV occurs when the infected tissues of a person who is shedding virus come in contact with the mucous membranes or with small cracks in the skin in the genital, anal, or oral areas of another. A person sheds virus when the virus is present in the skin cells, usually just prior to the appearance of sores and when they first appear. Often, a person shedding virus is unaware of this danger; he or she may have no symptoms of disease at the time. The sexual partners of a person shedding virus may not see sores or other indications that their partner is infected.

When the sores heal, the herpes infection is not cured—the virus is establishing itself in the nervous system for life. The virus particles enter the nerve endings in the area of infection and move up these nerves until they are close to the base of the spinal cord. There, the virus particles lie dormant. During the dormant phase, the infected person shows no signs or symptoms of herpes and is not shedding the virus.

From time to time, the virus becomes reactivated. Researchers are unsure about the exact mechanisms of reactivation, but infected individuals appear to have triggers that initiate a recurrence of infection. Common triggers are stress, lack of sleep, and menstruation. During a recurrence, the virus descends along the nerves close to the areas of original infection. No symptoms may be present, but the person sheds virus and can infect others during this time. Often, skin lesions appear, but these sores are not usually as painful nor do they last as long as during the initial infection. Most individuals experience five to eight recurrences per year. However, treatment with the drug acyclovir reduces the recurrence rate dramatically. Some persons have no recurrences for as long as 2 years. There is no vaccine to protect against HSV-2, and a recent trial failed of a vaccine that held promise.[23]

Herpesvirus can also infect newborns as they pass through the cervical opening and vagina of a mother with an active infection. Infected newborns may die or suffer damage to their nervous systems. In cases of active maternal infection, cesarean section (deliv-

ering the baby surgically, by cutting through the abdominal wall and the uterus) is often recommended.

## Genital Warts

**Genital warts** (*Condylomata acuminata*) are not painful, unlike the sores of herpes infection, but some of the viruses that cause this STI are associated with the development of cervical cancer. This association with cancer and the possible transmission of this disease to the respiratory tract of infants during birth are the gravest concerns of this disease.

Warts are noncancerous skin tumors, masses of cells that result from uncontrolled cell growth. All warts are called *papillomas* and are caused by the *human papillomavirus* (PAP-ih-LOW-mah-vigh-rus) (HPV). However, there are more than 60 types of papillomaviruses (named HPV-1, HPV-2, and so on); each affects only certain areas of the body.

About 40 types of HPV can infect the genital tract, but visible genital warts are usually caused by HPV-6 and HPV-11. These viruses cause warts particularly in the cervical, vaginal, and vulvar areas in women and various parts of the penis in men. They can also infect the urethra and anal areas in both sexes (**Figure 14.21**). The HPV types that infect the genital area but do not result in the growth of warts cause tissue changes that a physician usually can see by using special techniques. Some of these viruses, particularly HPV-16 and HPV-18, are associated with cancer of the cervix and less often with cancer of the vulva and penis. The American Cancer Society recommends that women have regular Papanicolaou tests (Pap smears) to detect atypical, precancerous, or cancerous cells within the cervix (see Chapter 13, the American Cancer Society "Managing Your Health" for specific recommendations) and that men consider having any abnormal tissue growth in the genital area microscopically examined for the presence of cancer. In addition, the HPV DNA test, which is used along with the Pap test, can determine whether a woman is infected with one of the 13 high-risk types of HPV.

Healthcare professionals are not required to report cases of genital warts to the CDC, so data are collected on initial visits to physicians' offices to receive

Figure 14.21

*Condylomata acuminata* **(Genital Warts).** These warts are growing around the anus of a man, nearly obscuring that opening.

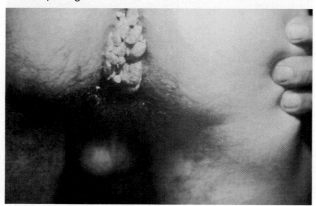

medical care for this STI, as shown in **Figure 14.22**. The number of initial visits for warts fell from 1987 to 1997 but has been rising since then. In 2009, the number of initial visits to physicians' offices for genital warts was slightly above that for herpes.

To avoid infection with this cancer-causing virus, follow the precautions in "Protecting Yourself Against STIs." Remember, however, that HPV, like genital herpes, can infect genital and anal tissue that is not protected by a condom. Additionally, because skin-to-skin contact can transmit HPV, infection can occur even if anal or vaginal intercourse does not take place. Transmission is also possible during oral sex, so a person with genital HPV could infect the lips, tongue, or palate of an uninfected sexual part-

ner. Adults as well as infants can develop warts on the larynx, or voice box, if the virus is breathed in. Furthermore, infants may acquire such infections from an infected mother during the birth process.

Although genital warts may go away on their own, the virus particles may remain in the tissue and can reactivate and infect others. These warts may also persist, grow larger, and spread. The removal of genital warts involves applying medications to the skin that break down the wart tissue, freezing them with liquid nitrogen, cauterizing (burning) them, or treating them with carbon dioxide lasers. Treatment for hard-to-remove warts involves the injection of the antiviral agent alpha-interferon directly into the tumorous growths. If you contract genital warts, you may want to discuss the benefits and drawbacks of various treatments with your physician. Many treatments are far more painful than the warts, interferon treatments can be costly, and medical researchers are unsure whether treatment to remove warts reduces the risk of transmission.

In June 2006, the U.S. Food and Drug Administration (FDA) approved a new vaccine (Gardasil) that protects against four major types of HPV: HPV-16 and HPV-18 that cause about 70% of cervical cancers and HPV-6 and HPV-11 that cause about 90% of genital warts. The vaccine is recommended for adolescent girls who have not yet had sex because they have not yet been exposed to HPV. Once infection with a type of HPV occurs, the vaccine cannot protect against it. A girl's or young woman's physician is the best person to determine whether she should be vaccinated. In 2009, the FDA expanded the approval of Gardasil for use in boys and young men to prevent genital warts and approved a second HPV vaccine

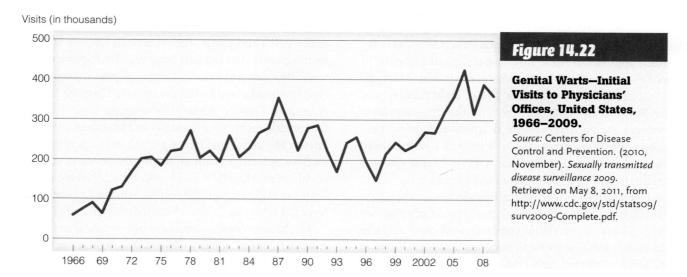

Visits (in thousands)

Figure 14.22

**Genital Warts—Initial Visits to Physicians' Offices, United States, 1966–2009.**

*Source:* Centers for Disease Control and Prevention. (2010, November). *Sexually transmitted disease surveillance 2009.* Retrieved on May 8, 2011, from http://www.cdc.gov/std/stats09/surv2009-Complete.pdf.

The following article was written to inform the general public about additional approved uses of the cervical cancer vaccine Gardasil. Explain why you think this article is a reliable or an unreliable source of information. Use the model for analyzing health information to guide your thinking; the main points of the model are noted here. The model is fully explained in Chapter 1.

1. Which statements are verifiable facts, and which are unverified statements or value claims?
2. What are the credentials of the source making these health-related claims? Does the source have the appropriate background and education in the topic area? What can you do to check the credentials of this source?
3. What might be the motives and biases of the source making the claims?
4. What is the main point of the article? Which information is relevant to the issue, main point, product, or service? Which information is irrelevant?
5. Is the source reliable? What evidence supports your conclusion that the source is reliable or unreliable? Does the source of information present the pros and cons of the topic or the benefits and risks of the product?
6. Does the source of information attack the credibility of conventional scientists or medical authorities?

Based on your analysis, do you think that this article is a reliable source of health-related information? Summarize your reasons for coming to this conclusion.

## Gardasil Approved to Prevent Anal Cancer

**FDA Press Office**

The U.S. Food and Drug Administration today approved the vaccine Gardasil for the prevention of anal cancer and associated precancerous lesions due to human papillomavirus (HPV) types 6, 11, 16, and 18 in people ages 9 through 26 years.

Gardasil is already approved for the same age population for the prevention of cervical, vulvar, and vaginal cancer and the associated precancerous lesions caused by HPV types 6, 11, 16, and 18 in females. It is also approved for the prevention of genital warts caused by types 6 and 11 in both males and females.

"Treatment for anal cancer is challenging; the use of Gardasil as a method of prevention is important as it may result in fewer diagnoses and the subsequent surgery, radiation or chemotherapy that individuals need to endure," said Karen Midthun, M.D., director of the FDA's Center for Biologics Evaluation and Research.

Although anal cancer is uncommon in the general population, the incidence is increasing. HPV is associated with approximately 90 percent of anal cancer. The American Cancer Society estimates that about 5,300 people are diagnosed with anal cancer each year in the United States, with more women diagnosed than men.

Gardasil's ability to prevent anal cancer and the associated precancerous lesions [anal intraepithelial neoplasia (AIN) grades 1, 2, and 3] caused by anal HPV-16/18 infection was studied in a randomized, controlled trial of men who self-identified as having sex with men (MSM). This population was studied because it has the highest incidence of anal cancer. At the end of the study period, Gardasil was shown to be 78 percent effective in the prevention of HPV 16– and 18–related AIN. Because anal cancer is the same disease in both males and females, the effectiveness data was used to support the indication in females as well.

Gardasil will not prevent the development of anal precancerous lesions associated with HPV infections already present at the time of vaccination. For all of the indications for use approved by the FDA, Gardasil's full potential for benefit is obtained by those who are vaccinated prior to becoming infected with the HPV strains contained in the vaccine.

Individuals recommended for anal cancer screening by their health care provider should not discontinue screening after receiving Gardasil.

As of May 31, 2010, more than 65 million doses of Gardasil had been distributed worldwide, since its approval in 2006 according to the manufacturer, Merck and Co. Inc, of Whitehouse Station, N.J. The most commonly reported adverse events include fainting, pain at the injection site, headache, nausea, and fever. Fainting is common after injections and vaccinations, especially in adolescents. Falls after fainting may sometimes cause serious injuries, such as head injuries. This can be prevented by keeping the vaccinated person seated for up to 15 minutes after vaccination. This observation period is also recommended to watch for severe allergic reactions, which can occur after any immunization.

*Source:* Food and Drug Administration. (2010, December 22). FDA news release. Retrieved on October 13, 2011, from http://www.fda.gov/NewsEvents/Newsroom/PressAnnouncements/ucm237941.htm.

(Cervarix), which acts against HPV-16 and HPV-18 only.[24] See the Analyzing Health-Related Information feature on the previous page for more information on another approved use of Gardasil.

### Healthy Living Practices

☐ To virtually eliminate your risk of contracting HIV infection, do not have sex with infected persons or share needles and syringes.

☐ To reduce your risk of contracting HIV, use a new latex condom with each act of sexual intercourse.

☐ Adolescent girls and young women, and boys and young men, should consult with their physician to determine whether they should receive an HPV vaccine.

## Sexually Transmitted Infections Caused by Bacteria

In contrast to viral STIs, bacterial STIs can be cured with treatment. Nevertheless, bacterial infections can be quite serious. If not treated, or not treated promptly and properly, bacterial STIs can damage the reproductive system, possibly resulting in infertility. Some diseases such as syphilis can cause even more devastating health effects. Therefore, it is crucial to seek medical attention immediately if you suspect that you are infected and to refrain from sex to avoid transmitting the disease to others.

## Syphilis

For centuries, **syphilis**, a serious STI caused by the bacterium *Treponema pallidum* (TREP-oh-NEE-mah PAL-ih-dum), has been a dreaded disease. Historically, the infection rate of syphilis reached a peak in the United States at the end of World War II. Physicians were soon able to demonstrate the effectiveness of the antibiotic penicillin against the syphilis bacterium. Although syphilis is not as prevalent as it once was, its incidence increased in the late 1980s, declined dramatically through 2000, and increased overall from 2001 to 2009, as **Figure 14.23** shows. The increases between 2001 and 2009 were primarily among men who have sex with men. Female infection rates dropped from 2001 to 2003 and then remained relatively steady through 2009. The male-to-female rate ratio (see Figure 14.23) was about 6 to 1 in 2009. Syphilis remains an important problem in the South and in some urban areas in other regions of the country.[22]

An individual can contract syphilis by having sex with a person who has sores caused by *T. pallidum*. These bacteria enter the body through a break in the skin of an uninfected person. Some syphilis bacteria remain in the skin at the site of entry, where a dime-sized sore called a chancre forms. Some of these bacteria move to the lymph nodes.

The incubation period for syphilis is about 3 weeks. The first sign of the disease is a chancre, which is characteristic of the first stage of syphilis, *primary syphilis*. Most often this sore appears in the genital or anal areas, but it can occur on the lips, tongue, breast,

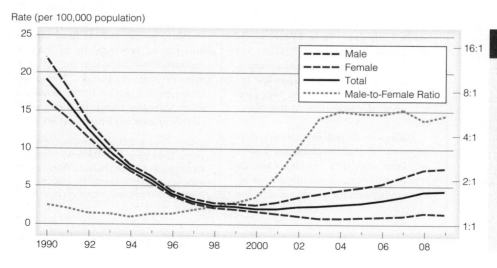

Rate (per 100,000 population)

### Figure 14.23

**Primary and Secondary Syphilis—Rates by Sex and Male-to-Female Rate Ratios, United States, 1990–2009.**

*Source:* Centers for Disease Control and Prevention. (2010, November). *Sexually transmitted disease surveillance 2009.* Retrieved on May 8, 2011, from http://www.cdc.gov/std/stats09/surv2009-Complete.pdf.

or fingers. The chancre first appears as a dull, red, flat spot, but becomes raised and then ulcerates. **Figure 14.24** is a photograph of a chancre on the penis. Although it looks as though it would be extremely painful, a chancre does not hurt. If untreated, a chancre usually heals in 3 to 6 weeks. During that time, however, *T. pallidum* is multiplying in the body; the disease is not gone.

After the chancre heals, the signs and symptoms of *secondary syphilis* appear. These symptoms are throughout the body because the bloodstream has distributed the bacteria to most of the tissues. Common symptoms of secondary syphilis are sore throat, weakness, headache, weight loss, fever, and muscle pain. In some patients, wartlike growths develop in moist areas of the body such as the genital region and under the arms. Most persons develop a rash that covers the body—even the soles of the feet. Although the appearance of this rash varies from person to person, it is often scaly.

When the symptoms of secondary syphilis subside, the infected person is said to be in *latent syphilis*. He or she has no outward signs of disease but is still infected. This stage may last a lifetime, or the infected individual may enter *tertiary syphilis*. During the tertiary stage of infection, tissue-destroying lesions called *gummas* develop. Gummas not only affect the skin but can destroy any type of tissue in the body—even bones. This stage of syphilis is, therefore, often disfiguring. If the tissues of the heart, major blood

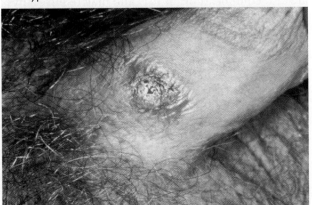

### Figure 14.24

**A Syphilitic Chancre of the Penis.** These painless sores can occur on the genital or anal areas, lips, tongue, breast, or fingers. They are characteristic of the first stage of syphilis.

**syphilis** (SIF-ih-lis) An STI that can progress from skin sores to more generalized symptoms (e.g., weight loss and muscle pain) to life-threatening, tissue-destroying skin abnormalities.

**gonorrhea** (GON-ah-REE-ah) An STI characterized by infection of the urethra in men and the cervix in women, usually resulting in a thick discharge from the penis or vagina.

vessels, or brain are destroyed, paralysis and death can result.

Since the introduction of antibiotics, few people with syphilis in the United States reach this stage of the disease. Most people are given antibiotics for various infectious diseases over a period of years; even if they are not treated specifically for syphilis, the administration of penicillin for any reason will kill *T. pallidum*. Nevertheless, approximately 40–50 people each year die in the United States as a result of untreated tertiary syphilis.

Unfortunately, the syphilis bacterium can cross the placenta during pregnancy, infecting the fetus. Infants infected with *T. pallidum* are born with a wide variety of serious conditions, such as bone deformities, low birth weight, lung damage, brain damage, deafness, and blindness. In addition, the infant can be infected during birth or after birth by coming into contact with the mother's lesions.

## Gonorrhea

The incidence of gonorrhea declined dramatically between 1975 and 1996, remained relatively stable through 2006, and declined through 2009 (**Figure 14.25**). In 2009, the age group with the highest prevalence of gonorrhea infection was young men and women aged 15 to 29 years.[22] This fact is worrisome to health officials because gonorrhea can cause irreversible damage to the reproductive tract.

**Gonorrhea** is caused by tiny, spherical bacteria called *Neisseria gonorrhoeae* (neye-SEE-ree-ah GON-ah-REE-ah) that enter the body via the mucous membranes. The bacteria infect primarily the urethra in men and the cervix in women. Therefore, condoms are an excellent measure to prevent gonorrhea because they protect these areas well.

The incubation period of gonorrhea is from 2 to 8 days. In men, infection with gonorrhea bacteria usually causes urethritis, an inflammation of the urethra, the tube through which urine exits the body. Urethritis is also commonly known as a urinary tract

Rate (per 100,000 population)

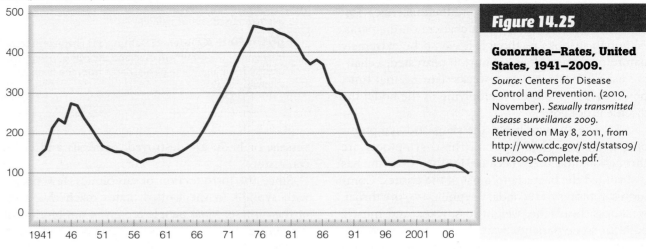

**Figure 14.25**

**Gonorrhea—Rates, United States, 1941–2009.**

*Source:* Centers for Disease Control and Prevention. (2010, November). *Sexually transmitted disease surveillance 2009.* Retrieved on May 8, 2011, from http://www.cdc.gov/std/stats09/surv2009-Complete.pdf.

infection (UTI). A UTI caused by the gonorrhea bacterium results in a pus-containing discharge from the urethra (**Figure 14.26**). (Pus is a thick fluid made up of tissue fluid, white blood cells, dead microorganisms, and dead body cells.) The infected male then experiences painful urination and an urgency to urinate. Most men seek attention quickly because of these symptoms, but if untreated, within several weeks to several months their body's natural defenses will suppress the infection. Until an infection is suppressed, however, a man can spread it to his sexual partners.

Gonorrhea infection in females may cause urethritis, but it more commonly causes inflammation of the cervix and uterus, resulting in a pus-containing vaginal discharge, uterine bleeding, and abnormally long and heavy menstrual periods.

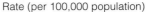

**Figure 14.26**

**Pus-Containing Discharge from the Penis as a Result of Gonorrhea.**

The bacteria can infect the prostate, epididymis, and seminal vesicles in males. Although infection of these male reproductive structures is rare, it does occur and can result in sterility. Women are more prone to widespread infection of the reproductive tract than are men. Infection of the uterine (fallopian) tubes or other female reproductive organs is called *pelvic inflammatory disease (PID).*

Gonorrhea is the most common cause of PID, a serious, painful condition. Its symptoms are lower abdominal pain, pain during sexual intercourse, abnormal menstrual periods, bleeding between periods, and sometimes fever. Often, the uterine tubes become constricted from infection, resulting in sterility or in ectopic pregnancy. An *ectopic pregnancy* occurs when a fertilized egg implants outside of the uterus, most often in a uterine tube (see Figure 5.7). Ectopic pregnancies are extremely serious situations. Abscesses (collections of pus) on the pelvic organs are also complications of PID and may require a hysterectomy, an operation to remove some or all of a woman's reproductive organs.

Another complication of gonorrhea is that the eyes of newborns can become infected with *N. gonorrhoeae* during birth if the mother is infected. If untreated, blindness may occur. For this reason, the eyes of all newborns in the United States are treated with antibiotic ointment or silver nitrate immediately after birth.

Gonorrhea can be treated with a variety of antibiotics. In recent years, many antibiotic-resistant strains of bacteria have emerged, sometimes making treatment difficult. However, laboratory testing of the particular strain can determine the most effective antibiotic to administer. Although gonorrhea is curable, reinfections are possible.

## Chlamydial Infections

*Chlamydia trachomatis* (klah-MID-dee-ah trah-ko-MA-tiss) causes **chlamydial infections**, which are similar to gonorrhea. The bacteria that cause both STIs infect mucous membranes in the genital area, primarily infecting the urethra in males and the urethra and cervix in females. The symptoms of both infections are similar, and both organisms can travel throughout the reproductive tract to spread infection. Both can cause PID in women. One difference is that the incubation period for gonorrhea is from 2 to 8 days, and that of chlamydial infections is from 2 to 3 weeks.

Chlamydia is the most frequently reported STI in the United States and its rate is increasing, as **Figure 14.27** shows. One reason for its prevalence is that infection with the organism causes only mild symptoms or no symptoms in most people. Therefore, many infected people transmit the disease unknowingly to their sexual partners. This disease is important to diagnose, however, because women with silent chlamydial infections are at a high risk for developing more serious illness such as PID, and they can transmit the infection to their children during birth. Men rarely develop serious disease from *C. trachomatis* infection, but men with undiagnosed infection continue to transmit the organism to women.

The symptoms of chlamydial infection in men are painful urination and a whitish or clear discharge from the urethra. The amount of discharge and the level of pain are usually much milder than with gonorrheal infections, so men tend to wait longer to seek treatment than with gonorrheal infections. Occasionally, *C. trachomatis* travels to other parts of the male reproductive tract and causes epididymitis, an inflammation of the epididymides, tubules located on the back of the testes in which sperm mature. This bacterium also infects the rectum in people who engage in anal sex.

Some women develop urethritis when they are infected with *C. trachomatis*. Most often, the main site of female infection is the cervix, and a vaginal discharge may occur.

One of the most serious consequences of infection with chlamydia is pelvic inflammatory disease. No matter which organism causes it, PID has similar symptoms and can result in sterility or ectopic pregnancy, even though chlamydia causes less painful infection than other organisms such as *N. gonorrhoeae*.

Babies born to mothers with chlamydial infections not only can develop serious eye infections but their lungs can become infected also. Chlamydial pneumonia in a newborn can cause long-term damage to the lungs, which affects lung function throughout childhood.

*Chlamydia trachomatis* infections are treated with various antibiotics. The CDC suggests using latex condoms to reduce the risk of contracting chlamydial infections and following suggestions such as those in the section entitled "Protecting Yourself Against STIs."

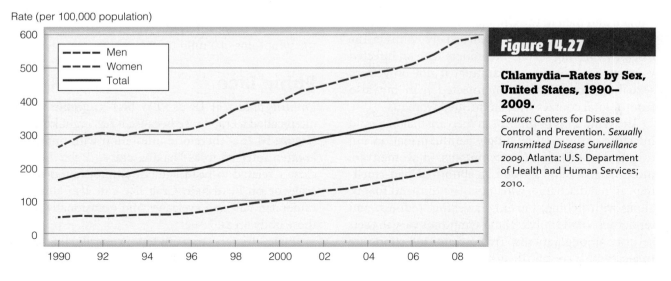

**Figure 14.27**

**Chlamydia—Rates by Sex, United States, 1990–2009.**

*Source:* Centers for Disease Control and Prevention. *Sexually Transmitted Disease Surveillance 2009.* Atlanta: U.S. Department of Health and Human Services; 2010.

## Other Sexually Transmitted Infections

Organisms other than bacteria and viruses also cause sexually transmitted infections. The itch mite (a close relative of spiders) and the pubic louse (a close relative of fleas) cause sexually transmitted *infestations*, conditions in which these organisms live on the skin in the genital area. The yeast *Candida albicans* causes an infection of the genital tract, primarily in women, that can be acquired sexually or in nonsexual ways. *Trichomonas vaginalis*, a protozoan (a single-celled organism much more complex than a bacterium), causes an infection of the lower genital tract of both men and women.

### Trichomonas Vaginalis Infections

As the name of this organism implies, **T. Vaginalis infections** (trichomoniasis) are more of a problem for women than for men. Women are 20 times more likely to contract trichomoniasis than are men. The reason for higher infection rates in women is that *T. vaginalis* lives on the surface tissues of the reproductive tract, such as the walls of the vagina, and uses glucose (a sugar) as a principal nutrient. This nutrient is more abundant in the reproductive tract of women than men. However, *Trichomonas* does not grow well in acidic conditions, which is the normal environment of the vagina (and of the male urethra). If the acid environment of the vagina changes, such as when a woman has another genital infection, is taking antibiotics, or when she is pregnant, the organism will grow easily if she becomes infected.

According to the CDC, an estimated 7.4 million women and men in the United States are infected annually with *Trichomonas*. Men usually contract the disease by having sexual intercourse with an infected woman, but women can contract it not only from sexual intercourse with an infected man but also from genital contact with an infected woman.

The symptoms of this STI in men are that of a mild infection of the urethra: mildly painful urination and urgency to urinate. The symptoms in women are more extensive and serious: an abnormal, bad-smelling vaginal discharge, which may be thin and foamy, along with itching, burning, swelling, redness, and tenderness of the vulva. These symptoms vary in their severity among patients. *Trichomonas* infections are treated with a specific drug that kills the organism.

## Yeast Infections

**Yeast infections** (candidiasis) are common among women and are acquired in a variety of ways, including sexual intercourse. *Candida albicans* is the organism most commonly responsible for yeast infections. (These infections are *not* caused by the yeasts used to make certain baked products or beer.) These organisms are thought to be always present in the genital-anal area (as are a variety of bacteria) because they are present in fecal material. The bacteria that normally inhabit the vagina in high numbers keep yeast and other bacteria from growing because they produce acids and outcompete other organisms for nutrients and space. However, under certain conditions, yeast may grow in the vagina.

Yeast may begin to grow and produce a vaginal infection during antibiotic use or pregnancy. Women who have poorly controlled diabetes or other STIs are also prone to yeast infections. Yeast grow best under warm and moist conditions, so clothing that is tight and poorly ventilated in the crotch may also contribute to the development of yeast infections. All these factors change the vaginal environment, allowing the yeast to grow.

The most common symptom of yeast infections in women is itching in the genital area. Other symptoms are soreness, burning, irritation, swelling, and a vaginal discharge that is white and looks somewhat like cottage cheese. Although numerous over-the-counter preparations are available to treat yeast infections, women should report symptoms to their healthcare providers before self-treatment.

Women infected with *Candida* can pass the infection to their male partners during sexual intercourse. Typically, the penis becomes infected; parts of this organ, the scrotum, and the groin may become irritated and swollen and may develop a rash, white patches, or both. Infected men may also experience the symptoms of a mild urethritis.

## Pubic Lice

*Phthirus pubis* (THIR-us PEW-bis) is a **pubic louse**, often called a crab louse because it has crablike claws (**Figure 14.28**). Therefore, infestation with pubic lice is often referred to as "having crabs." Pubic lice are closely related to head lice but are not found in the scalp or on head hair. Crab lice can also attach to underarm hair and eyelashes and occasionally infest these body areas.

Pubic lice are transmitted primarily by sexual contact and are rarely spread via contaminated toi-

## Figure 14.28

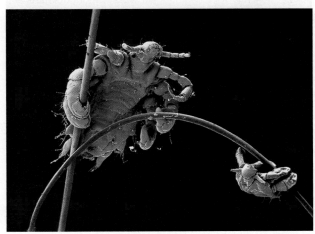

**The Pubic Louse.** This color-enhanced scanning electron microscope image shows two pubic lice, one adult and one juvenile, magnified about 40 times. They are hanging from pubic hair by their massive, crablike claws.

let seats and bed linens, although these routes of infestation are possible. They move from the pubic hairs of an infected individual to a partner when the genital areas touch. The lice then anchor themselves by grasping pubic hairs. For nourishment, pubic lice pierce the host's skin with their mouthparts and suck the blood of their host. When a person contracts pubic lice, he or she may notice tiny droplets of blood on the underwear before the symptoms of itching, swelling, redness, and irritation begin.

Pubic lice also reproduce in the pubic area. Female lice lay their eggs and then glue them to pubic hairs, where they eventually hatch and mature. Unless the infestation is treated, the lice will continue to reproduce and infest their host.

Both nonprescription and prescription medications are available to treat infestations of pubic lice, but a healthcare provider should be consulted to confirm the diagnosis. Bed linens and clothing should be washed in hot water and dried to kill any eggs or lice. Sexual partners must also be treated at the same time, as with all STIs, so that reinfestation (or reinfection) does not occur.

## Scabies

**Scabies** (*Sarcoptes scabiei*) (sar-COP-tees SKAY-bee-ee) produce infestations of the pubic area similar to those of the pubic louse. These spider-like organisms

---

**T. vaginalis infection** An STI caused by a protozoan, resulting in infection of the urethra in men and of the urethra and walls of the vagina in women.

**yeast infection** A condition in which the fungus *Candida albicans* grows in the vagina or on the penis; also known as candidiasis or moniliasis.

**pubic louse** A close relative of fleas that causes sexually transmitted infestation; also called crabs.

**scabies** (SKAY-beez) An infestation of the pubic area in which a spider-like organism burrows into the skin and lays eggs there.

(often called *itch mites*) burrow into the skin and lay eggs there. Therefore, one sign of infestation with scabies is thin, red lines or bumps in the skin, which result from burrowing and egg laying. In addition to the pubic region, these organisms infest other areas of the body (**Figure 14.29**).

Itch mites are transmitted by prolonged, close, personal contact, including sexual intercourse. However, if one member of a family becomes infested, the infestation can spread to other family members via infected bed linens, towels, or other household items. Outbreaks also occur in institutional settings such as hospitals and nursing homes. Scabies is treated with prescription medications that are applied to the skin and sometimes with accompanying oral medications.

## Protecting Yourself Against STIs

The first step in protecting yourself against sexually transmitted infections is to realize that STIs can strike anyone who is sexually active. Regardless of your age, gender, ethnicity, or socioeconomic status, if you are sexually active, you can contract an STI.

The Managing Your Health box in this chapter lists behaviors that will help protect you from infection with HIV and other STIs. Of course, you may choose to abstain from sexual activity and drug use, which virtually eliminates your risk of contracting a sexually transmitted infection. If you choose not to abstain from sex, having sex with noninfected individuals also eliminates your risk. How do you know if your partner is infected?

The best way to know if you are having sex with an uninfected partner is to be in a long-term, monogamous relationship in which you and your partner

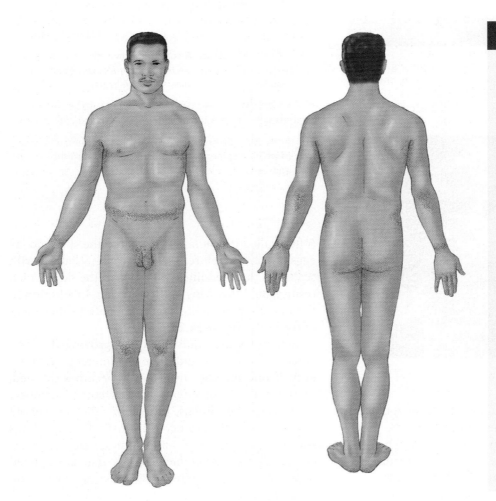

**Figure 14.29**

**The Distribution of Scabies Skin Lesions.** The red dotted areas show where infestation usually occurs. The areas without dots are rarely affected.

have been tested for STIs. A monogamous relationship is one in which a person has only one mate or partner at any one time. Unfortunately, monogamy is not foolproof. You must be absolutely certain that your partner is not having sex with anyone else. Consider the comment by a health student when asked, "Do you know someone who has a sexually transmitted infection? What was their reaction when they found out?":

*A married friend of mine went to the doctor right away after she suspected she had a sexually transmitted infection. The doctor said she had herpes. She was so upset with her husband; she later divorced him.*

Apparently, this "monogamous" relationship was one-sided. It obviously did not eliminate this woman's risk of contracting an STI. Also, don't equate *serial monogamy* with elimination of risk. Having sex with only one person for a short period and then having sex only with a new partner, and so on, does not

eliminate your risk of contracting a sexually transmitted infection.

Because it is difficult to eliminate your risk of contracting an STI (or to be certain that you have no risk), it is prudent to adhere to behaviors that reduce your chances of becoming infected.

Limiting your number of sexual partners statistically reduces your chances of contracting any STI. With regard to the partners you have, you will lower your risk if you delay having sex with people until you know them well enough to assess their risk as sexual partners. Although you may question your partner about his or her previous sexual experiences, history of STIs, and drug use habits, be aware that people often conceal this information. Avoid having sex with individuals who consistently have sex with multiple partners. Also avoid having sex with individuals who are in the high-risk categories listed in Table 14.1. If you choose to have sex with a person in one or more of these categories, avoid penetrating activities: anal, vaginal, and oral sex. Also, do not use contraceptives that contain nonoxynol-9, which might increase the risk of transmission of STIs.

If you use drugs, you are putting yourself in jeopardy of contracting an STI. To avoid contracting STIs, never share needles and syringes if you are an injecting drug user, and never have sex while under the influence of drugs or alcohol. While under the influence, you are more likely to engage in sexually risky and dangerous behaviors.

The most effective strategy to prevent HIV and other STIs is to refrain from anal and vaginal intercourse as well as oral sex with infected partners. The second most effective strategy is to use latex condoms during sexual activity. According to the CDC, condom use substantially reduces the risk for contracting the following STIs: gonorrhea, HSV infection, syphilis, HIV infection, hepatitis B, and chlamydial infection. By reducing the risk of gonorrheal and chlamydial infections in women, condoms also reduce their risk of contracting pelvic inflammatory disease.

Although the use of synthetic condoms will reduce your risk of becoming infected, they do not provide a guarantee against transmission because they may tear or slip (although with proper use, this is unlikely) and they do not cover the entire genital area. Condoms made of natural membranes such as sheep intestine are not effective barriers. HIV and other sexually transmitted viruses can penetrate this type of condom, so use latex ones. When using latex condoms, however, do not use oil-based lubricants such as petroleum jelly, mineral oil, vegetable oils, massage oils, and body lotions, which can weaken the latex. Apply only water-based lubricants such as K-Y Jelly.

Another practice to avoid is storing condoms in hot cars or wallets for extended periods of time; keep them in a cool, dry place and out of direct sunlight. Do not use them after the expiration date, or if the packaging on the condom shows signs of damage or deterioration, such as brittleness, stickiness, or discoloration.

It is important to use condoms consistently (a new one for each act of intercourse) and properly for them to be effective in reducing your risk against STIs. As you use a condom, handle it carefully, being sure not to damage it with your fingernails, teeth, or other sharp objects. Figure 5.18 and the accompanying text show and describe the correct procedure for putting on a male condom.

Female polyurethane condoms are also available. Laboratory tests show that viruses such as HIV cannot pass through the polyurethane; studies with actual use show the female condom to be effective in preventing transmission of STIs. In 2009, the FDA approved the "second-generation" female condom (FC2).[25]

The female condom is a plastic sheath that covers the cervix much like a diaphragm, lines the vagina, and covers the labia. The same precautions and care regarding the use of male condoms should be followed when using female condoms. Figure 5.19 and the accompanying text show and describe the correct procedure for using a female condom. Female condoms can also be used as protection during anal intercourse.

Condoms can be slit open and used flat to cover the genital areas during oral sex to help prevent STI transmission. Dental dams (flat pieces of latex) are useful for this purpose as well.

## Healthy Living Practices

☐ If you are sexually active, you are at risk for contracting sexually transmitted infections. You can virtually eliminate your risk by abstaining from sex or by engaging in sex only within a mutually monogamous relationship in which you and your partner are free of disease.

☐ You can reduce your risk by limiting your number of sexual partners, never sharing needles and syringes during drug use, and not engaging in sex while under the influence of alcohol or drugs.

☐ Another way to reduce your STI risk is by using synthetic condoms for each act of anal or vaginal intercourse. In addition, you can use a flat piece of latex to cover the genital areas during oral sex. If you choose not to use condoms, you can reduce STI risk by having both yourself and your partner screened for STIs before engaging in sex.

## Across THE LIFE SPAN

### INFECTIOUS AND NONINFECTIOUS DISEASES

Noninfectious diseases and conditions that are present at birth are termed *birth defects*. According to the

CDC, 1 in 33 babies in the United States are born with a birth defect, and more than 5,500 of these children die.[26]

Some birth defects are caused by environmental influences such as fetal exposure to teratogens—drugs, alcohol, viruses, or other substances that directly damage the tissues of the embryo (during weeks 3 to 8 of pregnancy) or fetus (during week 9 of pregnancy through birth). Table 5.1 lists some teratogens known to cause birth defects. Chapter 7 describes problems that can occur during prenatal development when a pregnant woman takes drugs. Chapter 8 discusses fetal alcohol spectrum disorders. Dietary deficiencies during pregnancy can also cause birth defects.

*Metabolic diseases* are also types of birth defects. An infant born with a metabolic disease lacks an enzyme necessary for normal metabolism. Such problems are genetic and result in an infant's cells being unable to make a necessary body compound. Sometimes abnormal substances are made that build up in the blood and urine; these substances can damage tissues in the body such as the liver, brain, and kidney.

Most metabolic diseases are rare; two of the more well-known are Tay-Sachs disease and phenylketonuria. In Tay-Sachs disease, which occurs predominantly among Ashkenazi Jews (the descendants of Jews who settled in eastern and central Europe), certain fatlike molecules accumulate in the brain and other tissues, retarding development and causing death by the age of 3 to 4 years. In phenylketonuria (PKU), cells are unable to convert the amino acid phenylalanine to other needed compounds. Phenylalanine and related chemicals build up in the blood and damage tissues, causing intellectual disability. Because the ill effects of this disease can be avoided by restricting the amount of phenylalanine in the diet, most newborn infants are tested for this disorder.

Although many genetic diseases claim the lives of infants and children, genetic disorders persist in those children who survive to become adolescents or young adults. Down syndrome, cystic fibrosis, and Duchenne muscular dystrophy are all noninfectious diseases, discussed earlier in this chapter, that affect children. The hope for curing these and other genetic diseases is *gene therapy*, in which corrected copies of defective genes are inserted into the hereditary material of infected individuals. A preventive measure is genetic counseling, in which prospective parents seek advice regarding the probability that they will have a child with particular genetic disorders. Couples can use this information to make family planning deci-

sions (see the Managing Your Health essay "Genetic Counseling and Prenatal Diagnosis" in Chapter 5).

Most genetic diseases strike early in life. However, one disease, Huntington's chorea (also called Huntington's disease), does not become evident until approximately age 40 years. By this time, victims may have already passed on the genes for this disease to their children. In Huntington's chorea, the patient makes involuntary, purposeless, rapid motions such as flexing and extending the fingers or raising and lowering the shoulders. (*Chorea* refers to involuntary muscle twitching.) The mental faculties of the person also deteriorate. Fifteen years or so after the onset of the disease, the patient dies. Although there is no cure or effective treatment for this disease, certain medications can relieve or lessen some of the symptoms. Genetic testing is available so that young adults who have affected parents can learn whether they carry the lethal gene. The gene is dominant, which means that if you inherit one gene from either parent, you will develop this disease. This information allows people at risk for this disease to make informed reproductive choices.

Other than heart disease, cancer, and stroke, which are discussed in Chapters 12 and 13, one of the most well-known noninfectious diseases of older adults is Alzheimer's disease. This disease has a strong genetic link and is discussed in Chapter 15.

Infectious diseases also have a variety of effects across the life span. As life begins, infection can do harm. Viral infections can be dangerous to a pregnant woman because many viruses can cross the placenta, the organ through which the fetus absorbs nutrients and excretes wastes. Certain viruses, such as the German measles virus, can cause birth defects, including deafness, heart defects, and intellectual disability. Other viruses, such as the human immunodeficiency virus (HIV), can infect the fetus, resulting in an infected newborn. Most bacteria cannot cross the placenta, but if bacteria infect the birth canal at the time of delivery, the baby can become infected as it passes through, as in the case of gonorrhea (discussed earlier).

In the past, certain bacterial diseases (e.g., diphtheria and whooping cough) and viral diseases (e.g., measles, mumps, and German measles) were common childhood infectious diseases in the United States. However, vaccines for these diseases have been developed, and most children are immunized routinely in the United States according to a schedule. Occasionally, serious outbreaks of these diseases occur in people who are not immunized. These childhood diseases are still prevalent in developing countries.

Other than contracting common infections such as colds and the flu, sexually active adolescents, teens, and young adults are at highest risk for contracting STIs because they frequently have unprotected intercourse. The one nonsexually transmitted infectious disease prevalent in adolescents and young adults is infectious mononucleosis. "Mono" primarily strikes young adults ranging in age from 15 to 25 years (although some suggest this age range extends from 10 to 35).

Infectious mononucleosis has been nicknamed the "kissing disease" because it is spread via infectious saliva. However, it is also contracted by inhaling infectious droplets sneezed or coughed into the air by an infected person or by drinking from an infected person's glass. This disease is usually not serious, but the Epstein-Barr (EB) virus (a herpesvirus), which causes mononucleosis, has been associated with the subsequent development of two forms of cancers: Burkitt lymphoma in certain African populations and nasopharyngeal (nose and throat) carcinoma in Asian populations. Furthermore, infection with EB virus can cause a prolonged period of exhaustion, lasting up to 2 to 3 months. Rest is the primary treatment.

The most common symptoms of infectious mononucleosis are a sore throat; low-grade, long-term fever; swollen lymph nodes and spleen (which may result in pain in the upper left side of the abdomen);

fatigue; and weakness. However, the symptoms can vary and may include a rash, headache, or nausea. Previously, mono was difficult to diagnose in some cases, but healthcare practitioners can now test for mono in their offices.

Infections are a major cause of illness and death among older adults; respiratory infections are the sixth leading cause of death in persons 85 years and older, and the seventh leading cause of death for those aged 75–84 years. Bacterial pneumonia and influenza, for example, together have well more than 100 times the fatality rate for persons 75–84 years than for those between the ages of 25 and 34 years and nearly 600 times the fatality rate for persons 85 years and older.[6]

Older adults are more susceptible to infections and have a more difficult time recovering from them than do younger persons for a variety of reasons. The cell-mediated component of the immune system functions less well as people age. Also, the respiratory tract changes during the aging process, resulting in decreased elasticity of the lungs and a diminished cough reflex, making elderly people more susceptible to respiratory infections. Other organ systems may also experience structural and degenerative changes that predispose elderly persons to infection. Many elderly people have chronic diseases too, which lower their organs' functional reserves and contribute to their decreased resistance to infection. However, older adults are in a low-risk category for contracting STIs because they usually have fewer sexual partners than younger people do.

# CHAPTER REVIEW

## Summary

Noninfectious diseases are processes that affect the proper functioning of the body, are usually accompanied by characteristic signs and symptoms, and are not caused by pathogens, but rather, abnormalities in the hereditary material, factors in the environment, or an interaction of the two cause noninfectious diseases.

Genetic factors are the sole cause of some noninfectious diseases; such genetic diseases are inherited or are caused by mistakes during cell division when gametes are formed. Inherited diseases are caused by disorders of the hereditary material, or genes. Two inherited diseases that are prevalent in the United States are cystic fibrosis and Duchenne/Becker muscular dystrophy. Down syndrome is a genetic disease caused by errors during gamete formation.

Some diseases are caused by an interaction of genetic and environmental factors. Genetic factors can predispose a person to a disease. Diseases having both genetic and environmental causes include asthma, ulcers, diabetes mellitus, and migraine headaches.

Some noninfectious conditions have environmental or unknown causes. Many of these conditions are discussed in Chapter 16, "Environmental Health." A few noninfectious conditions are caused by improperly performing certain activities. Carpal tunnel syndrome, for example, is a painful condition of the hands and fingers that results from improper positioning of the wrist while engaging in repetitive activities that use the hands, wrists, and arms.

Birth defects are noninfectious conditions present at birth that affect either the body's structures or how it functions. Anatomic defects can be caused by genetic or environmental factors or a combination of both. Metabolic defects are genetic and affect a person throughout life. Alzheimer's disease, which is discussed in Chapter 15, is a prominent noninfectious disease of older adults.

Infectious diseases affect the proper functioning of the body, are usually accompanied by characteristic signs and symptoms, and are caused by disease-producing (pathogenic) bacteria, viruses, fungi, protozoans, or worms. Some infectious diseases are communicable; that is, they are spread from person to person either directly or by means of an intermediary organism called a vector. Other infectious diseases are noncommunicable; they are caused by organisms such as bacteria that normally (and usually harmlessly) reside on a person's body, by the ingestion of toxins produced by pathogens, or by pathogens from environmental or animal sources.

The severity of a disease's symptoms depends on a variety of factors: the type of organism; its virulence; the manner in which it enters, multiplies, and spreads in or on the body; the chemicals it produces, if any; its ability to combat the defense mechanisms of the body; and the body's reaction to the invading microbe.

Two primary causes of infectious diseases are bacteria and viruses. Bacteria, microscopic organisms that have a simple cell structure, cause disease by first adhering to the surfaces of cells. Some penetrate more deeply into tissues, and many bacteria produce chemicals that break down the connections between cells, aiding their invasion. Viruses are noncellular, nonliving, protein-coated pieces of hereditary material. They cause infection by adhering to cells also, but then enter cells and use them to make more viruses, killing the cells in the process.

The human body has two main types of immunity, or defense against disease: nonspecific and specific immunity. Nonspecific immunity combats any foreign invader. Mechanisms of nonspecific immunity include the skin and mucous membranes, white blood cells and their phagocytic properties, the lymphatic system, the inflammatory response, natural killer cells, and interferons.

Specific immunity combats each specific invading pathogen and is carried out by the immune system. The immune system has two branches: antibody-mediated immunity and cell-mediated immunity. Antibody-mediated immunity reacts to antigens (foreign proteins) that reside outside of the body cells, such as most bacteria and the toxic products they produce.

Cell-mediated immunity reacts to antigens that reside inside body cells, such as viruses, fungi, a few types of bacteria, and parasites. It also acts against foreign (nonself) tissues such as transplanted organs and controls the growth of tumor cells.

Immunity is either inborn or acquired. Inborn immunity is inherited, such as immunity to infectious diseases that attack other organisms but not humans. Acquired immunity develops during a person's lifetime. Immunity is acquired either actively or passively and by natural or artificial means.

Many drugs have been developed to combat infection. Antibiotics kill or inhibit the growth of bacteria and are in wide use. Antiviral drugs are limited in availability and scope. Specific medications have been developed to treat protozoal diseases and infections caused by worms.

Sexually transmitted infections (STIs) are infectious diseases spread from one person to another during sexual activity, primarily sexual intercourse. Most pathogens that cause STIs can survive for only a short time outside of the body; therefore, transmission of these diseases from objects, such as toilet seats, is either impossible or rare, depending on the STI. Sexually transmitted infections are caused primarily by viruses and bacteria, but some infections and infestations are caused by yeast, protozoans, mites, and lice. The transmission of STIs is often facilitated in persons infected with other STIs.

Sexually transmitted infections caused by viruses are incurable, although the body may clear itself of some human papillomavirus (HPV) infections. In addition to causing STIs, three sexually transmitted viruses have been implicated in the development of particular cancers: human immunodeficiency virus (HIV), HPV, and hepatitis B virus (HBV).

The most serious viral STI is HIV infection because it not only raises the risk of developing a particular type of cancer, but also the virus attacks the immune system, disabling the body's defenses. Eventually, the immune system of an HIV-infected individual becomes so weakened that he or she succumbs to an array of illnesses that lead to death. This stage in HIV infection is called acquired immunodeficiency syndrome (AIDS). The best ways to protect yourself against contracting this deadly disease or any STI are to refrain from having sex with infected individuals, reduce your number of sexual partners, avoid sex with high-risk partners, and use a latex condom with each act of sexual intercourse.

Sexually transmitted infections caused by bacteria are curable with antibiotics. Three prevalent bacterial STIs are syphilis, gonorrhea, and chlamydial infections.

One protozoan, *Trichomonas vaginalis*, causes a sexually transmitted infection primarily in women. The yeast *Candida albicans* may cause troublesome, itchy infections in women that can be transmitted sexually. The crab louse, *Phthirus pubis*, and itch mite, *Sarcoptes scabiei*, both can cause sexually transmitted infestations of the genital area.

Adolescents and young adults are in the highest-risk age category for contracting sexually transmitted infections. Infants are at risk of infection from infected mothers. Middle-aged and older people are less likely to contract sexually transmitted infections because they are less likely to have multiple sex partners. However, anyone who practices high-risk behaviors or who has sex with an infected person can contract a sexually transmitted infection.

## Applying What You Have Learned

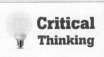

**Critical Thinking**

1. Based on the information in this chapter, describe two ways in which you can lower your or your unborn children's risk of contracting noninfectious diseases. **Analysis**

2. The human immunodeficiency virus (HIV) attacks helper T cells. Why is this attack so devastating to the body's ability to resist disease? **Application**

3. Think about the last infectious disease you contracted. Outline what you think might have been the chain of infection for this disease. Could you have done anything to break the chain of infection and avoid becoming infected? **Analysis**

4. Analyze your behaviors regarding your risk for contracting STIs. What can you do to lower your risk of contracting a sexually transmitted infection? **Analysis**

5. A man develops a sore on his genitals but is too busy to go to his healthcare provider. The sore heals, so he decides that he "got better" on his own. State two reasons why his reasoning is faulty and dangerous. With which STI(s) might this man be infected? Support your answer with evidence. **Synthesis**

6. State a behavior or behaviors that you could adopt or change to help you become more resistant to infection in general. How would this behavioral change increase your resistance to infection? **Evaluation**

**Key**

**Application**
using information in a new situation.

**Analysis**
breaking down information into component parts.

**Synthesis**
putting together information from different sources.

**Evaluation**
making informed decisions.

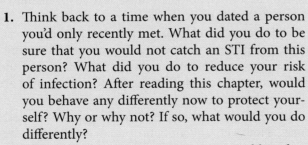

# *Reflecting on Your Health*

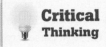
**Critical Thinking**

1. Think back to a time when you dated a person you'd only recently met. What did you do to be sure that you would not catch an STI from this person? What did you do to reduce your risk of infection? After reading this chapter, would you behave any differently now to protect yourself? Why or why not? If so, what would you do differently?

2. When you have a common communicable infectious disease like a cold or the flu, do you do anything to protect others, such as members of your family, from catching your illness? If so, what? Would you do anything differently after reading this chapter? If so, what?

3. Have you ever traveled outside the United States? If so, to what countries did you travel? Think back to your trip(s) and describe what you did before departing to protect yourself from infection. What did you do to protect yourself while you were there? Has reading this chapter alerted you to additional steps you should take to protect yourself from infection? If so, what? If you have never traveled outside of the country, pick a country to which you would like to travel and explain what steps you would take before you left to protect yourself from infection. What steps would you take while you were there?

4. Do any hereditary diseases run in your family? If you are not sure, ask your family members, including parents, grandparents, uncles, aunts, and cousins, if possible. What steps can you take to protect your future children from a hereditary disease? Include specifics about diseases that run in your family, if any.

5. Many strains of bacteria are becoming resistant to the antibiotics used to treat them. One reason for this is that people pressure their healthcare providers for antibiotics when they do not have bacterial illnesses. Also, some people stop taking antibiotics before their physician says they should. Both these situations provide an opportunity for resistant strains of bacteria to develop and replicate. Do you practice either of these behaviors? If so, why? What have you learned in this chapter that may cause you to change those behaviors?

# References

1. Cystic Fibrosis Foundation. (2011, January 31). About cystic fibrosis: Frequently asked questions. Retrieved on April 26, 2011, from http://www.cff.org/AboutCF/Faqs/

2. Centers for Disease Control and Prevention. (2009, October 16). Prevalence of Duchenne/Becker muscular dystrophy among males aged 5–24 years—four states, 2007. *Morbidity and Mortality Weekly Report, 58*(40):1119–1122.

3. Ishikawa, Y., et al. (2011). Duchenne muscular dystrophy: Survival by cardio-respiratory interventions. *Neuromuscular Disorders, 21*(1):47–51.

4. University of California San Francisco Medical Center. (2011, January 20). Down syndrome. Retrieved on April 27, 2011, from http://www.ucsfhealth.org/education/down_syndrome/

5. Allen, E. G., et al. (2009). Maternal age and risk for trisomy 21 assessed by the origin of chromosome nondisjunction: A report from the Atlanta and National Down Syndrome Projects. *Human Genetics, 125*:41–52.

6. Xu, J., et al. (2010, May 20). Deaths: Final data for 2007. *National Vital Statistics Reports, 58*(19):1–136. Retrieved on April 27, 2011, from http://www.cdc.gov/nchs/data/nvsr/nvsr58/nvsr58_19.pdf

7. Mayo Clinic staff. (2010, December 10). Legionnaires' disease: Risk factors. Retrieved on April 27, 2011, from http://www.mayoclinic.com/health/legionnaires-disease/DS00853/DSECTION=risk-factors

8. Schuijt, T. J., et al. (2011). Lyme borreliosis vaccination: The facts, the challenge, the future. *Trends in Parasitology, 27*(1):40–47.

9. Centers for Disease Control and Prevention. (2011, April 22). HIV surveillance—epidemiology of HIV infection (through 2009). Retrieved on May 4, 2011, from http://www.cdc.gov/hiv/topics/surveillance/resources/slides/general/index.htm

10. United Nations Programme on HIV/AIDS (UNAIDS). (2010). *UN-AIDS report on the global AIDS epidemic.* Retrieved on May 4, 2011, from http://www.unaids.org/globalreport/documents/20101123_Global Report_full_en.pdf

11. Harrison, K. M., et al. (2010). Life expectancy after HIV diagnosis is based on national HIV surveillance data from 25 states, United States. *Journal of Acquired Immune Deficiency Syndrome, 53*(1):124–130.

12. Schneider, M. F., et al. (2005). Patterns of the hazard of death after AIDS through the evolution of antiretroviral therapy: 1984–2004. *AIDS, 19*(17):2009–2018.

13. Centers for Disease Control and Prevention. (2010, June). Diagnoses of HIV infection and AIDS in the United States and dependent areas, 2008.

14. *HIV Surveillance Report, 20.* Retrieved on May 4, 2011, from http://www.cdc.gov/hiv/surveillance/resources/reports/2008report/index.htm

15. Chama, C. M., & Morrupa, J. Y. (2008). The safety of elective caesarean section for the prevention of mother-to-child transmission of HIV-1. *Journal of Obstetrics and Gynaecology, 2*:194–197.

16. Centers for Disease Control and Prevention. (2010, August 11). Basic information about HIV and AIDS. Retrieved on May 4, 2011, from http://www.cdc.gov/hiv/topics/basic/

17. Centers for Disease Control and Prevention. (2009, June). Oral sex and HIV risk. Retrieved on May 4, 2011, from http://www.cdc.gov/hiv/resources/factsheets/pdf/oralsex.pdf

18. Crans, W. J. (2010, June 1). Why mosquitoes cannot transmit AIDS. Rutgers Center for Vector Biology. Retrieved on May 4, 2011, from http://www.rci.rutgers.edu/~insects/aids.htm

19. Moscicki, A.-B. (2008). Vaginal microbicides: Where are we and where are we going? *Journal of Infection and Chemotherapy, 14*:337–341.

20. Willyard, C. (2010, July 15). Tiny steps toward an HIV vaccine. *Nature, 466*(7304):S8.

21. Centers for Disease Control and Prevention. (2010, December 17). Sexually transmitted diseases treatment guidelines, 2010. *Morbidity and Mortality Weekly Report, 59*(RR-12):1–110. Retrieved on May 8, 2011, from http://www.cdc.gov/std/treatment/2010/STD-Treatment-2010-RR5912.pdf

22. Tsygankov, A. Y. (2009). Current developments in anti-HIV/AIDS gene therapy. *Current Opinion in Investigational Drugs, 10*(2):137–149.

23. Centers for Disease Control and Prevention. (2010, November). *Sexually transmitted disease surveillance 2009.* Retrieved on May 8, 2011, from http://www.cdc.gov/std/stats09/surv2009-Complete.pdf

24. Cohen, J. (2010). Immunology. Painful failure of promising genital herpes vaccine. *Science, 330*(6002):304.

25. American Cancer Society. (2010). *Cancer prevention and early detection facts and figures, 2010.* Atlanta, GA. Rtrieved on April 18, 2011, from http://www.cancer.org/acs/groups/content/@epidemiologysurveilance/documents/document/acspc-027876.pdf

26. Witte, S. S., et al. (2010). Can Medicaid reimbursement help give female condoms a second chance in the United States? *American Journal of Public Health, 100*(10):1835–1840.

27. Centers for Disease Control and Prevention. (2011, March 29). National Center for Birth Defects and Developmental Disabilities: About us. Retrieved on May 9, 2011, from http://www.cdc.gov/ncbddd/AboutUs/index.html

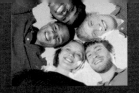

## Diversity in Health
Hunting for
Supercentenarians

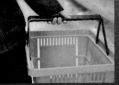

## Consumer Health
Choosing a Long-Term
Care Facility

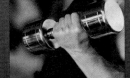

## Managing Your Health
After the Death of a Loved
One

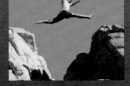

## Across the Life Span
Dying and Death

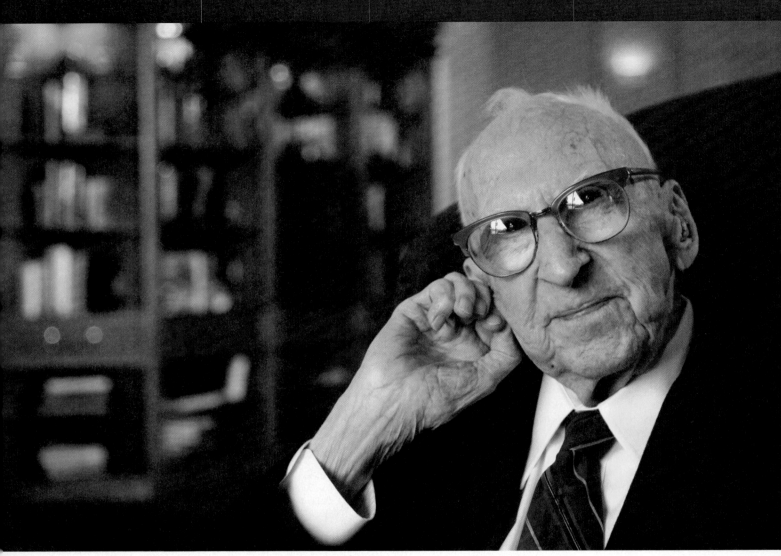

## Chapter Overview

The status of aging Americans

Why we age

The effects of aging on health and well-being

The spiritual and emotional aspects of dying

The options for terminal care

The definition of death

How to prepare for death

## Student Workbook

Self-Assessment: Preparing for Aging and Death

Changing Health Habits: Can Changing a Health Habit
Extend Your Life?

## Do You Know?

Who was the oldest person to ever live?

What happens to your body as you age?

How to increase your chances of living a long and healthy
life?

## CHAPTER 15

# Aging, Dying, and Death

On April 15, 2011, Walter Breuning died in Montana. You might be thinking, "So what?" When Walter died of natural causes, he was *114* years of age—the oldest man in the world. Walter's recipe for living more than 100 years included the following recommendations:

- Accept change. "Every change is good."
- Take care of your mind and body.
- Eat two meals a day.
- Work as long as possible.
- Help others.
- Accept death. "You're born to die."[1,2]

> "Take care of your mind and body."

*Centenarians* are people who are older than 100 years of age; people who are at least 110 are *super*centenarians. Why are centenarians able to live such long lives? Lifestyle, environmental, and social factors are known to influence *longevity*, but genetic differences play a major role in determining whether a person lives to be at least 100 years of age.[3]

**gerontologists** Scientists who study aging.

**aging** The sum of all changes that occur in an organism during its life.

**life span** The maximum number of years that members of a species can expect to live when conditions are optimal.

**senescence** (seh-NES-ens) The stage of life that begins at age 65 years and ends with death.

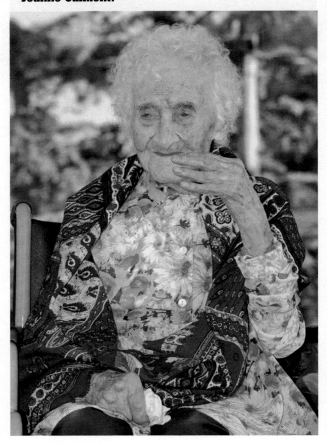

**Figure 15.1**

Jeanne Calment.

In December 2010, nearly 72,000 Americans were 100 or more years of age.[4] Today in the United States, more people are living to be 100 years old than in past decades. According to the U.S. Census Bureau, more than 600,000 Americans will be centenarians by 2050.[5]

**Gerontologists**, scientists who study aging, note that individuals who have the genetic potential to live longer than average often eliminate this advantage by adopting unhealthy lifestyles, such as using tobacco and being physically inactive.[6] Therefore, an important key to enjoying a long and healthy life is taking actions now to improve your health and well-being.

For humans, growing old is a natural and universal process. The prospect of aging and dying, however, has troubled people for centuries. Instead of dreading this time of life, many older adult Americans are busy pursuing a variety of enjoyable and rewarding activities. Healthy people do not let the aging process interfere with their active lifestyles.

The Across the Life Span sections of each chapter of this textbook highlight specific health concerns of older adults. This chapter provides more detailed information concerning the aging process, including ways to enjoy good health and a positive sense of well-being while growing old. Additionally, this chapter examines dying and death as well as ways of coping with loss and grief. To determine if you are prepared for aging and death, answer the questions in the assessment activity for this chapter in the Student Workbook section of this text.

## Aging

We can define **aging** as the sum of all changes that occur in an organism during its life. The **life span** is the maximum number of years that members of a species can live when conditions are optimal. The life span of an adult mayfly is a few days; the life span of a human is 122 years. In 1997, Jeanne Calment of Marseilles, France, died at the age of 122. According to official records, Ms. Calment lived longer than any other person (**Figure 15.1**). However, very few people live longer than 105 years. Contrary to popular belief, there are no regions of the world where populations usually live more than 100 years (see the Diversity in Health feature "Hunting for Supercentenarians" that follows).

Medical experts customarily divide the human life span into stages or periods (see Chapter 1, Table 1-7). Most people reach physical maturity or adulthood by the time they are 25 years old, but *adulthood* usually refers to the period spanning 21 through 65 years of age. Older adulthood, or **senescence**, is the stage of life that begins at 65 years of age and ends with death. In this chapter, the terms *older adulthood, old, aging, older adult*, and *elderly* are interchangeable with *senescence*. The ages that define these life stages are arbitrary; there are no obvious physical signs that indicate the precise ages when one passes from young adulthood into middle age or from middle age into senescence.

# Diversity in Health

## Hunting for Supercentenarians

Despite the high standard of living and excellent quality of medical care in the United States, few Americans live to be 100 years old. According to verifiable records, no one in the United States has lived longer than 120 years. Yet in certain isolated parts of the world, hundreds of people claim to be more than 120 years old (supercentenarians). Do people who live in these places actually live longer than Americans or the rest of the world's population?

In the first half of the twentieth century, reports emerged concerning the extreme longevity of people living in the Hunza area of northern Pakistan, in the village of Vilcabamba in Ecuador, and in the Caucasus region in the eastern European country of Georgia. Scientists visited these regions to question the very old people and determine factors that were associated with their extreme longevity. After interviewing the oldest people in these regions, some experts concluded that living in an isolated and unpolluted rural environment, eating a simple nutritious diet, avoiding the use of alcohol and tobacco, and maintaining an active daily schedule were the keys to superlongevity.

By the 1970s, however, the real story began to unfold concerning the existence of the so-called supercentenarians. As some investigators returned to locate and interview the same old people that they had met previously, their elderly subjects gave ages that did not match. For example, if 5 years had lapsed since the first interview, instead of being 5 years older, the old person reported being 7 or 10 years older. It did not take researchers long to realize that these elderly people typically inflated their ages. How could so many people have been fooled into believing that supercentenarians existed?

It is difficult to verify the ages of very old individuals who live in rural, undeveloped places. During the 1800s, birth records that could document the ages of very elderly persons were not kept, or they were destroyed. In some cases, investigators initially believed the authenticity of an extremely old individual's birth record, but later rejected it after determining that the person shared the name of a long-dead ancestor who was the rightful owner of the document. Even if individuals who claim to be extremely old have their birth records, the documents' value is questionable because birth dates can be altered.

Why would elderly people add years to their actual ages? In many isolated and impoverished places, conditions are not ideal for enjoying a lengthy life. Aged members of these populations know that the longer they live, the more fame, respect, and status they can expect to receive from younger members of the population. Government officials often do little to refute citizens' astounding superlongevity claims because the notoriety attracts a steady stream of curious international visitors whose money supports the local economy.

Scientists who study individuals who claim to be supercentenarians think that their subjects are old, but not that old. They may be older than 80 years of age, but few are older than age 90. Thus, no convincing evidence exists that supports the amazing longevity claims of supercentenarians. Many people, however, persistently believe stories that there are concentrations of extremely old people living in certain regions of the world.

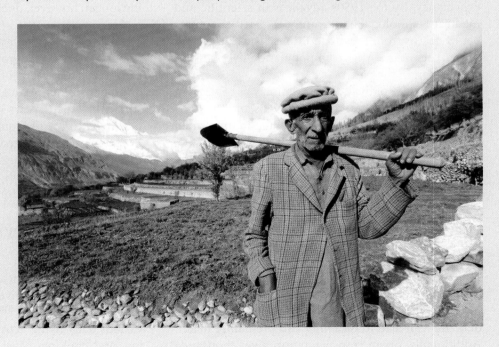

# Life Expectancy

**Life expectancy** is the average number of years that an individual who was born in a particular year can expect to live. In the United States, life expectancies vary according to age, sex, and socioeconomic status. Overall, American females outlive American males by about 5 years.[7] As a result, the older adult population consists of about one-third more women than men. The reasons for these differences are unclear, but hormonal, genetic, and socioeconomic factors are thought to influence life expectancy.

As mentioned in Chapter 1, life expectancies increased dramatically during the twentieth century, especially for people who live in developed countries. In the United States, for example, individuals born in 1900 could expect to live 47 years; individuals born in 2009 can expect to live 78 years.[7] An increase in life expectancy generally occurs when fewer people die during the earlier stages of life rather than in the later ones.

In the first part of the twentieth century, people lived past 65 years of age, but so many younger individuals died from serious injuries, infections, and in childbirth that these statistics lowered overall life expectancy. By the 1950s advances in scientific and medical technology significantly reduced the number of deaths from these conditions. Today, a greater proportion of the American population lives beyond age 65 than in the past.

In 2009, 13% of the U.S. population was 65 years of age and older.[4] Between the mid-1940s and the mid-1960s, the birthrate was unusually high in the United States. As a result, experts estimate that almost 20% of the U.S. population will be 65 years and older by the year 2030.[5] **Figure 15.2** shows estimates of the number of Americans who are or will be 65 or more years of age in 2020, 2030, and 2040.

Scientists are learning more about the causes of aging and are seeking ways to extend life expectancy. Their efforts have led to the development and testing of new therapies for today's major killers: cancer and cardiovascular disease. Advances in genetic engineering offer ways to prevent and treat inherited disorders that can lead to disability and premature death. Additionally, organ transplantation gives thousands of dying individuals the opportunity to survive by replacing their failing organs with healthy ones. Liv-

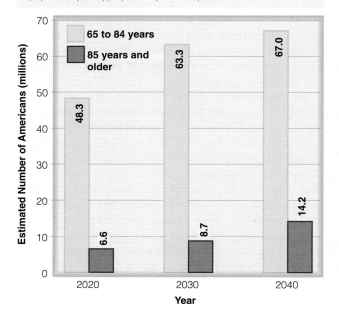

## Figure 15.2

**Estimates of the U.S. Population 65 Years of Age and Older in 2020, 2030, and 2040.** The number of older adults in the United States is expected to increase significantly in the next 30 years.
*Source:* U.S. Census Bureau. (n.d.). *U.S. population projections.* Retrieved on on May 29, 2011, from http://www.census.gov/population/www/projections/summarytables.html

ing longer, however, does not necessarily mean living better.

Preserving the quality of life becomes increasingly important as people grow older. By the time Americans reach 65 years of age, chronic illnesses and disabilities often reduce their quality of life. A measurement called "years of healthy life" estimates the negative impact that quality of life can have on life expectancy. A broad goal of *Healthy People 2000* was to increase years of healthy life from 64 years to at least 65 years.[8] Presently, Americans can still expect to live in good health for about 67 years.[9]

# The Characteristics of Aged Americans

The majority of Americans older than 65 years of age own their homes or live with family members, and they can handle their financial matters and manage various daily living activities such as bathing, dressing, and cooking. Most older adults suffer from at least one chronic health problem, particularly hypertension, heart disease, arthritis, cancer, and diabetes.[10]

## Figure 15.3

**Independent Living.** Adding certain features to homes, such as "grab bars" in and next to the shower stall and supportive arms around the toilet, can help older adults with physical disabilities live independently.

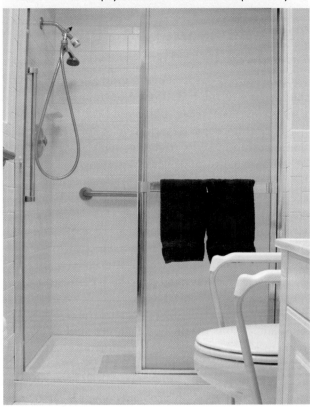

Many older adults with mild physical disabilities live independently by making some adaptations to their homes. For example, installing elevated toilets, grab bars, and shower seats makes it easier for people with physical conditions such as arthritis to take care of their personal hygiene (**Figure 15.3**).

In July 2009, 5.6 million Americans were 85 years or older.[4] This population is increasing so rapidly, experts think about 21 million people will be in this age group by 2050. People who are 85 years old and older, the "oldest of the old," are more likely to be severely disabled and unable to live independently than the "young old" who are 65 to 74 years. In 2009, about 4% of Americans 65 years and older lived in institutional settings, such as extended-care or long-term care facilities ("nursing homes").[10] However, more than 14% of people 85 years or older lived in these places.

A significant number of older adults are independent and financially secure, often because they planned for their retirement needs when they were young. Today, fewer older Americans live in poverty than in the late 1960s, thanks largely to federal programs such as Social Security, Medicaid, and Medicare. Nevertheless, many older Americans must live on lower incomes than when they were younger. In 2009, about 9% of older adults had incomes that were less than the federal government's poverty level.[10] Older adults who are members of minority groups, particularly African Americans and Latinos, are more likely to have lower retirement incomes and live in poverty than are elderly white people.

Although some of their expenses are less because they are no longer working, healthcare costs of retirees are generally higher than those of younger individuals. Almost all older American adults have **Medicare**. Medicare is a federal health insurance program that provides benefits for people 65 years of age and older. The program, however, does not pay for every medical expense. Thus, elderly people must often buy additional health insurance. The cost of health care is not a major barrier to health care for most older adults. Nevertheless, people with low incomes and less education often have difficulty paying for medical expenses not covered by insurance. Without adequate insurance, serious chronic health conditions can drain the financial resources of older adults and their families. Many older adults continue working beyond the usual retirement age to help pay for health insurance and other expenses.

## Why Do We Age?

People age at different rates. A person's *chronological age*, as measured in years, may not match his or her *physiologic age*, as measured in functional ability. For example, some 50-year-old people experience the physical changes of aging earlier than average; they look, act, and feel older than others who are the same age. Inheritance accounts for some of this variation because a person's genes determine when certain physiologic events occur.

*Genes* are hereditary material located on *chromosomes* within a cell's nucleus. Genes provide chemical instructions for the production of vital proteins that are needed for cellular activities. For example, most body cells can divide to form new cells. A cell's genes control the number of times it can divide. After di-

**macular degeneration** A leading cause of vision loss for people age 60 years and older.

**cataracts** A chronic condition in which the lens of the eye becomes cloudy and opaque, impairing vision.

viding its maximum number of times, the cell dies. Most tissues produce a surplus of cells, so they can afford the death of some cells. As people age, however, the rate of new cell production in tissues normally slows and the number of living cells declines as existing cells die.

*Telomeres* are structures that form the tips of chromosomes. Telomeres play a major role in the aging process by serving as biological clocks that control the number of times cell division can occur. Each time a normal cell divides, its telomeres shorten. When telomeres reach a certain length, they cannot become shorter and chemical processes that initiate cellular death occur. Theoretically, people who inherit instructions to produce chromosomes with longer telomeres have the genetic potential to live longer than those who inherit instructions to produce shorter telomeres. More research, however, is needed to determine the role of telomere length in the human aging process.

External factors such as environment and lifestyle also influence the aging process. For example, exposure to certain environmental conditions can damage genes. Damaged genes make mistakes in copying and transferring information concerning protein production. Young cells can correct many of these errors, but aging cells are less efficient at correcting such mistakes. When the parts of cells that manufacture proteins receive faulty instructions from the genes, they are unable to produce these compounds. Without an adequate supply of proteins, the affected cells eventually die.

An organ fails if it does not contain enough functioning cells. The systems of the body are interrelated, so when the organs of one system fail, the organs of the other systems soon lose their functional capacities. For example, when a heart that has been weakened by disease cannot pump blood efficiently, the lungs and kidneys are not able to function properly. As a result, other organs fail to perform their jobs, and death occurs.

Radiation, pollution, and some drugs and viruses may damage genes, thereby accelerating the rate of aging and shortening life expectancy. By limiting contact or exposure to these agents, you may be able to lengthen your life expectancy. Furthermore, adopting a lifestyle that includes regular exercise and that avoids

smoking can reduce your risk of heart disease, stroke, and cancer. Eating more fruits and vegetables may lower your risk of cancer also. The "Changing Health Habits" feature of this and the other chapters can help you identify and change unhealthy practices (see the Student Workbook section at the end of the book).

# The Effects of Aging on Physical Health

People begin to experience a gradual and irreversible decline in the functioning of their bodies when they are about 30 years old. Even healthy people experience this progressive decline as they grow older. Some common signs of aging, such as menopause, delayed sexual responsiveness, graying and thinning hair, loss of height, and *presbyopia*, the inability to see close objects clearly, reflect normal changes associated with growing old. *Table 15.1* describes some significant physical changes that are associated with normal senescence. As you can see, growing old affects every system of the body.

Aging is an individual process. There is no timetable that specifies at what age people can expect a particular physical change to occur. The rate at which these alterations occur, however, accelerates after 65 years of age. As a result of these normal changes, the aging body is less able to adapt to stress, repair itself, and resist or fight infection. Infections and accidents that were minor health problems when a person was young can become disabling or deadly experiences when a person is old.

Compared to young adults, elderly people are more likely to develop nutritional deficiencies, especially of vitamins D and $B_{12}$, because aging bodies are less able to absorb or use certain nutrients. The serious health problems that often affect older adults, such as heart disease and hypertension, are associated with lifestyle and are preventable to some extent. Previous chapters discuss cardiovascular disease, hypertension, osteoporosis, and cancer in depth.

Although certain chronic conditions such as arthritis commonly affect elderly people, they are not normal aspects of aging. These ailments may not be life threatening, but they frequently reduce the quality of life.

**Age-Related Macular Degeneration** In the United States, **macular degeneration** is a leading cause of vision loss for people age 60 and older.[11] The macula is a small region in the eye that enables you to see objects in your central line of vision clearly. As many people age, the light-sensitive cells in the

## Table 15.1

### Biological Effects of Normal Aging

| System | Normal Changes |
|--------|----------------|
| Cardiovascular | Heart function remains normal, but the heart muscle thickens; arterial walls thicken; pulse rate declines |
| Skeletal | Bone loss occurs, which can be abnormal if excessive (osteoporosis) |
| Nervous | Brain weight decreases, especially in the cerebral cortex; neurotransmitter levels decline, nervous message transmission and muscular responses slow; short-term memory becomes less efficient; visual and hearing ability decreases; the ability to taste bitter and salty foods declines; sleep disturbances, such as taking longer to fall asleep and frequent awakening during the night, often occur |
| Immune | Immune response against pathogens or developing cancer cells declines |
| Endocrine | Many hormone levels decline, including insulin (regulates carbohydrate metabolism), aldosterone (regulates sodium metabolism), and thyroid, estrogen, and growth hormones |
| Digestive | Tooth loss becomes more likely as gums recede; levels of stomach acid drop; intestinal absorption of calcium is less efficient; constipation can occur, often the result of medications or poor diet |
| Muscular | Muscle mass declines, resulting in less strength; stamina reduction occurs |
| Reproductive | Menopause occurs in women, resulting in thinning of vaginal lining, less vaginal lubrication, and shrinkage of reproductive organs; breast tissue shrinks; prostate gland enlarges in men; sexual responsiveness slows so that it takes longer for erections to occur; orgasms are shorter and less intense |
| Urinary | Kidneys become less efficient at filtering wastes from the blood |
| Skin (integument) | Skin becomes drier and less elastic, resulting in wrinkles; scalp hair growth slows, and its loss increases; hair growth in the nose and ears increases; fingernails often become yellow, develop ridges, and split |

macula gradually die, resulting in distorted, blurry, or lost central vision. People with macular degeneration have difficulty reading, driving, and viewing television or a computer monitor. To test your vision for macular degeneration, visit www.amd.org/living-with-amd/resources-and-tools/31-amsler-grid.html.

In about 10% of cases, tiny blood vessels form under the macula and leak fluid and bleed, causing severe vision loss ("wet" or advanced macular degeneration). Medication and laser surgery can stop the bleeding in early stages of wet macular degeneration, but these treatments cannot restore lost vision. There is no effective treatment for the "dry" form of macular degeneration, and this condition can lead to the "wet" form.

Preventing macular degeneration is important. Aging people who smoke and have a family history of macular degeneration have a high risk of developing the condition. Other risk factors include age, obesity, and female sex. Eating a diet that contains plenty of dark green leafy vegetables, such as spinach, collards,

and mustard greens, may protect against macular degeneration. For people who have been diagnosed with the disease, zinc and antioxidant supplements may slow the deterioration of the macula. However, these dietary substances can be toxic and should not be taken without consulting a physician.

**Cataracts** Although the reasons for their occurrence are unclear, **cataracts** are common in people older than 50 years of age. A cataract forms when the normally transparent lens of the eye becomes cloudy and opaque with aging. Clouded lenses scatter light

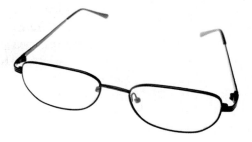

as it enters the eyes, making it difficult to see images clearly. Symptoms of cataracts include blurry and double vision, sensitivity to bright light, and seeing halos around objects. Without surgery to remove damaged lenses, cataracts can lead to blindness. In many cases, surgeons can replace natural lenses with artificial ones; in others, they remove the damaged lenses and prescribe eyeglasses or contact lenses.

Some medical experts think that exposure to ultraviolet light can cause cataracts. You may be able to reduce your risk of cataracts by wearing sunglasses to shield your eyes, when you are outdoors.

**Glaucoma** Glaucoma is another ailment that frequently affects the vision of aged people. In this condition, an abnormal amount of fluid accumulates in the eyeball. Over time, the high fluid pressure causes vision loss by permanently damaging the optic nerve, the nerve that transmits visual information to the brain. Eye pain, headache, and loss of peripheral vision are symptoms of glaucoma. Risk factors for developing glaucoma include family history, African ancestry, diabetes, and cardiovascular disease. In most cases, placing medicinal drops into the eyes can control the condition. In severe cases of glaucoma, surgery is necessary to reduce the fluid pressure within the eyeball.

Glaucoma may not produce noticeable symptoms; therefore, early detection is the best way to control the effects of the disorder. A simple, painless screening test is available that can identify the disease before serious damage to the optic nerve occurs. Thus, you can prevent the irreversible effects of glaucoma by having a physician or optometrist perform periodic screenings.

**Arthritis** Arthritis is a broad group of chronic joint diseases characterized by inflammation, pain, swelling, and loss of mobility ("stiffness") of affected joints. Rheumatoid arthritis, osteoarthritis, "lupus," fibromyalgia, and gout are forms of arthritis. Rheumatoid arthritis and lupus can affect multiple organs and cause a wide variety of symptoms (**Figure 15.4**).

According to the Centers for Disease Control and Prevention, an estimated 50 million adult Americans suffer from doctor-diagnosed arthritis.[12] Regardless of age, arthritis is the leading cause of disability among Americans.[12] In *osteoarthritis*, the cartilage that protects the ends of bones and keeps them from rubbing together at joints wears away and breaks down. As a result, tiny bits of cartilage or bone float in the fluid that fills the joint and the joint becomes misshapen (**Figure 15.5**). People often confuse osteoarthritis with osteoporosis, a different condition that affects older adults. Information about osteoporosis is in Chapter 9.

Older adults are more likely to develop osteoarthritis than young persons are.[12] Joints simply wear out as a person ages. Other contributing factors include heredity, overuse, injury, and obesity. Overuse and injury of joints can occur when performing sports or jobs that place excessive stress on joints. Obese older adults have a high risk of developing osteoarthritis because carrying around extra weight stresses joints, especially the knees.

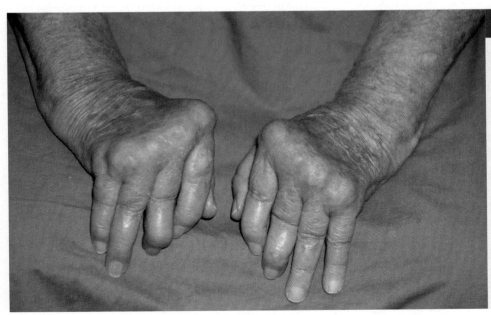

### Figure 15.4

**Effects of Arthritis on the Hands.** Arthritis damages joint tissue, resulting in deformities and the loss of flexibility.

**Effects of Osteoarthritis on Joints.** (a) In a healthy joint, such as the knee joint, the ends of bones are encased in smooth cartilage. The bone ends are protected by a joint capsule line with a synovial membrane that produces synovial fluid. The capsule and fluid protect the cartilage, muscles, and connective tissues. (b) This illustration shows a knee joint severely affected by osteoarthritis. Note that the cartilage has worn away. Spurs grow out from the edge of the bone, and synovial fluid within the joint increases. As a result, the joint is difficult to move and it is sore.

*Source:* National Institute of Arthritis and Musculoskeletal and Skin Diseases. (revised May 2006). OsteoArthritis. Retrieved on July 20, 2007, from http://www.niams.nih.gov/hi/topics/Arthritis/oahandout.pdf.

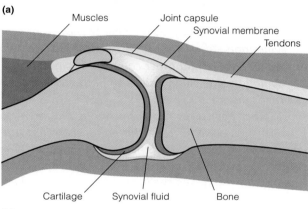

(a)

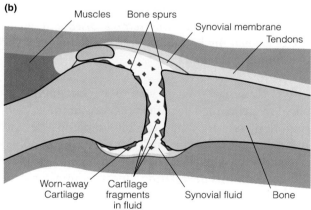

(b)

**urinary incontinence** The inability to control the flow of urine from the bladder.

**Alzheimer's disease (AD)** An incurable, progressive, degenerative disease that affects the functioning of the brain.

Although arthritis is a chronic disease, symptoms tend to come and go. Treatment for osteoarthritis includes medications to relieve inflammation and pain, and exercises to strengthen muscles and improve or maintain joint mobility. Losing weight reduces stress on weight-bearing joints in obese people. In some cases, surgery is necessary to replace damaged joints with artificial implants.

**Urinary Incontinence Urinary incontinence**, the inability to control the flow of urine from the bladder, is an embarrassing and costly problem for millions of Americans. As people age, the muscles that control bladder emptying weaken, making it easier for urine to leak out when people move, sneeze, cough, or lift heavy things. Additionally, many older adults experience involuntary contractions of their bladders that cause some urine to be eliminated unexpectedly. Medications, infections, strokes, tumors, history of childbirth in women, and enlargement of the prostate gland in men can contribute to urinary incontinence.

The fear of leaking urine accidentally while in public often makes many incontinent people avoid social situations. If family members cannot manage an incontinent elderly relative at home, they often find it necessary to place him or her in an extended-care facility.

Many older adults restrict their fluid intake to reduce their urine production. This practice can lead to dehydration. The majority of individuals who experience urinary incontinence can benefit from treatment, such as behavioral techniques that enable them to be more aware of the bladder's state of fullness. By learning to empty the bladder more frequently, a person may be able to avoid the leakage. People can learn and practice a series of exercises that strengthen the pelvic muscles that control urination. These exercises, called *Kegel* exercises, involve imitating the same muscular movements that individuals make when they voluntarily stop urinating. Incontinent people can also wear absorbent pads and undergarments designed to prevent incidents of urine leakage. Medication and surgery may alleviate incontinence. Embarrassment or concerns about surgery, however, keep many incontinent people from discussing this common problem with personal physicians.

**Alzheimer's Disease** You cannot find your keys; you forget an appointment; you sometimes call your child by your cat's name. Do you ever have the feeling that you are losing your mind? It may be reassuring to know that everyone has these and other similar annoying experiences from time to time, but many middle-aged Americans worry that instances of forgetfulness are early symptoms of **Alzheimer's disease (AD)**. According to the Alzheimer's Association, the most common early sign of the disease is difficulty recalling newly learned information.[13]

AD is an incurable, progressive, degenerative disease that affects the functioning of the brain. People with AD have abnormal amounts of a protein that forms clumps between cells in the brain. These clumps interfere with brain cells' ability to communicate with each other. Furthermore, tangled bundles of useless protein fibers form within the brain cells, disrupting cell function. As an increasing number of brain cells die, the signs and symptoms of AD become more apparent.

Experts with the Alzheimer's Association estimate that 5.4 million Americans, mostly elderly persons, had AD in 2011.[14] As the baby boom generation ages, 10 million more people will be added to this number. By the year 2050, three times as many Americans will suffer from this dreaded disease.

AD is the most common form of **dementia**, a brain disorder that seriously affects normal *cognitive* (thinking) abilities, such as recalling information and solving problems. Strokes and Parkinson's disease also are major causes of dementia. Common features of AD include memory loss, mental confusion, and loss of control over behavior and body functions. Although AD is incurable, a few medications can be prescribed to slow the decline in cognitive functioning, control certain inappropriate behaviors of patients, and improve patients' moods.

Age and family history are major risk factors for AD. Although the disease is common among older adults, it is not a normal feature of growing old. What are the signs of AD? Is it preventable?

In the early stages of Alzheimer's, affected people may notice lapses in their memories and cognitive abilities. For example, they may have unusual difficulty remembering events that happened recently, learning new information, and using information to make reasonable conclusions. These symptoms typically begin between 40 and 60 years of age. Over time, people with the disease become increasingly forgetful, confused, disoriented, restless, and moody. Communicating becomes difficult as their speech deteriorates; depression is common. These changes are distressing to patients with AD, their family members, and their associates. One woman recalls her affected mother-in-law's gradual loss of cognitive functioning:

*The first time I had a feeling that my elderly mother-in-law might have a serious problem with her memory occurred in April when she got lost while driving to our house. We live close to her and she had made the short trip dozens of times. When I told my husband that this was unusual behavior for her and could be a sign of a memory problem, he disagreed and said it was "easy" to make a wrong turn on the way to our house. A few months later, I was driving Mother to a store when she insisted that I should be making a right turn instead of a left one at a familiar intersection in our town. When I told her she was wrong, she became angry and argued with me about the directions to the store. When I finally reached the store, she recognized the place but didn't apologize for her behavior. At Christmas, Mother was very quiet and seemed to be in a fog. My husband and his sister finally recognized that she was "not herself," and they took her to the doctor's for an evaluation. After a series of medical tests to rule out minor strokes and other causes of brain damage, her condition was diagnosed as mild-to-moderate Alzheimer's disease.*

*Mother now takes two medications that seem to help her memory a little. At this point, she is not supposed to drive and she needs help with housework. She still cooks, but I'm concerned she'll forget that she's making something and she'll start a fire in her kitchen. My husband and his sister are thinking about selling Mother's house and placing her in a special group home for people with this terrible disease. I dread the day when my husband greets his mother and she doesn't recognize him.*

As AD progresses, its victims neglect their personal hygiene; their facial expressions become "flat" (emotionless); and they exhibit inappropriate and unpredictable behaviors such as undressing in public and attacking caregivers. In the terminal stages, individuals with this devastating illness require constant care. They are bedridden and unable to talk and eat. Nothing can be done to stop the relentless progression of the disease. After diagnosis, the average person can expect to survive about 8 years. Some people with AD live only 4 years after diagnosis, whereas others are able to live for 20 years with the disease.[14] Death often results from pneumonia and starvation as the degenerating brain is unable to control vital functions such as breathing, swallowing, and digestion. In 2009, about 79,000 Americans died of AD, making it the sixth leading cause of death.[7]

Physicians often diagnose AD when patients cannot answer questions like those listed in **Table 15.2**.

## Table 15.2

### Simple Memory Test for Identifying Dementia

**Ask the person:**

1. His or her age
2. His or her date of birth
3. The time to the nearest hour
4. His or her address
5. The current year
6. Where he or she is
7. The names of two people who are pictured in family photos
8. The years of World War II
9. The name of the current president of the United States
10. To count backwards from 100 to 1
11. His or her phone number

*Source:* Adapted from Wattis, J. (1996). What an old age psychiatrist does. *British Medical Journal, 313*:101–104.

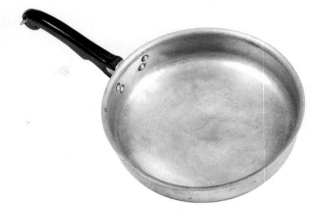

Using aluminum cookware does not increase the risk of Alzheimer's disease.

Until recently, the only way to confirm the diagnosis was by examining the patient's brain after death. Brain imaging techniques such as magnetic resonance imaging (MRI) scans can now detect shrinkage in areas of the cerebral cortex, the thinking part of the brain. Such brain shrinkage is a sign of AD.

The factors that cause AD are unclear. At least two forms of the disorder are inherited. Although genetic testing is available to determine whether relatives of patients with AD have the genes associated with the condition, many people who test positive do not develop the disease. Other forms of AD may be the result of slow-acting brain viruses, brain injury, or exposure to pollutants. At one time, scientists thought that aluminum poisoning caused the disease because higher than normal amounts of this metal are found in the brains of patients who died of AD. Many people are concerned about the safety of using aluminum cookware and the natural presence of this element in drinking water. However, most experts think that the unusual concentration of aluminum in the brains of persons with AD is a result, not a cause, of the disorder. Nevertheless, scientists are investigating whether environmental factors, such as exposure to other minerals, may contribute to AD.

Can Alzheimer's disease be prevented? Lifestyle factors appear to play a role in reducing the risk of AD. Keeping physically active, being involved in a variety of intellectually stimulating activities, and maintaining an extensive social network are associated with a lower risk of AD.[15] Making certain dietary changes may also help. Results of one study indicated that people who eat high amounts of salad dressing, fruit, nuts, fish, tomatoes, cruciferous vegetables (broccoli and cabbage, for example), dark green and leafy vegetables, and low amounts of high-fat milk products, red meat, and butter have lower risk of AD than people who did not eat this dietary pattern.[16] More research is needed to determine whether a particular dietary pattern protects against AD.

Elevated blood cholesterol levels, particularly LDL cholesterol, are associated with increased risk of AD.[17] Results of recent studies, however, do not support taking cholesterol-lowering medications, such as certain *statins*, to reduce the risk of AD.[17,18] Nevertheless, more research is needed to confirm these findings.

Inflammation and the effects of excess oxidation in the body, especially in the brain, may increase the risk of AD.[19] Thus, herbal preparations and substances in foods that have anti-inflammatory and antioxidant activity may protect against AD. *Curcumin*, a chemical with anti-inflammatory and antioxidant activity, may help prevent the disease.[20,21] The spice and food coloring agent turmeric contains curcumin. *EGb 761*, an extract made from leaves of the ginkgo biloba tree, has antioxidant activity. Promoters of dietary supplements that contain ginkgo claim their products can treat memory loss, confusion, depression, and other conditions associated with Alzheimer's disease.[22]

The following article is an abbreviated version of "Alzheimer's: Few Clues on the Mysteries of Memory" that appeared in *FDA Consumer* magazine. Read the article and evaluate it using the model for analyzing health-related information. The main points of the model are noted on the following page; the model is fully explained in Chapter 1.

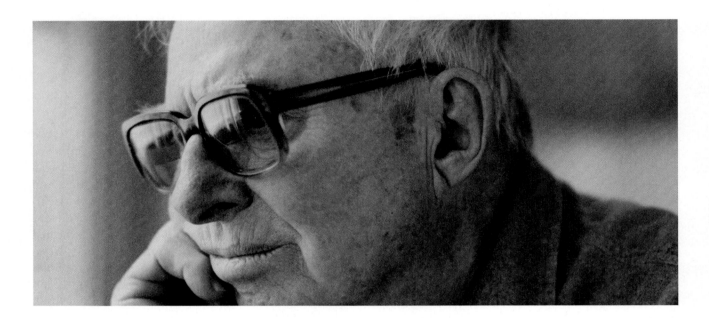

## Alzheimer's

### Few Clues on the Mysteries of Memory

by Audrey T. Hingley

It happened some years ago but the memory is still firmly implanted in my mind. One sunny afternoon I heard the sound of a car pulling into our driveway, peered out of my living room window, and saw one of my father's friends, Sam (not his real name), then in his early 80s. Sam got out of his car and walked just a few steps. I watched as he stood for a few moments, gazing at our house with an expressionless face. Then he silently returned to his car, got in, and drove away, without ever knocking on our door or communicating with us in any way.

I thought the incident puzzling, but it wasn't until months later that I learned the reason for it. Sam had Alzheimer's, a progressive disease in which nerve cells in the brain degenerate and brain substance shrinks.

A widower living alone, Sam clearly was in a dangerous position. Once he was followed home by a police officer, who told his grown children he had found Sam stopped by the side of the road, not able to remember how to get home by himself.

Sam's story is being played out in the lives of up to 4 million Americans who suffer from Alzheimer's disease. The disease plays no favorites, attacking rich and poor, famous and ordinary. Among its most famous sufferers: former President Ronald Reagan.

With an average lifetime cost of care per patient of $174,000, it is the third most expensive disease in America, fol-

lowing only heart disease and cancer. But perhaps even more staggering than the monetary costs are the emotional and psychological costs borne by both patients and their families.

"People are very frightened of the possibilities because they know it represents a loss of one's self," says Steven T. DeKosky, M.D., director of the Alzheimer's Disease Research Center at the University of Pittsburgh and a practicing neurologist. "It's a very frightening prospect to see a loved one who looks the same but doesn't talk or act the same."

### "I Have Lost Myself"

Alzheimer's disease, a progressive, degenerative disease attacking the brain and resulting in impaired thinking, behavior and memory, was first described by Alois Alzheimer, M.D., in 1906. German researchers recently found an important set of notes from Alzheimer's journal of the world's first documented case of the disease. The patient exhibited many of the symptoms seen in Alzheimer's patients today. But perhaps most poignant of all is the patient's own description of the disease: "I have lost myself."

In Alzheimer's, nerve cells in the part of the brain responsible for memory and other thought processes degenerate for still-unknown reasons. Some of the most severely affected cells normally use acetylcholine, a brain chemical, to communicate. Tacrine (brand name Cognex, also called THA), the first drug approved by the Food and Drug Administration specifically to treat Alzheimer's disease, works by slowing the breakdown of acetylcholine. This results in relieving some memory impairment.

Tacrine does not cure Alzheimer's or slow the disease's progression. It has only been studied in those with mild to moderate Alzheimer's disease who were otherwise in generally good health. Because tacrine can increase the blood levels of a liver enzyme that can indicate liver damage, regular monitoring is necessary. Other side effects include nausea, vomiting, diarrhea, abdominal pain, skin rash, and indigestion.

Aricept (generic name donepezil hydrochloride, also called E2020), approved by the FDA in 1996, is by far the most used drug for Alzheimer's treatment. Like tacrine, Aricept inhibits the breakdown of acetylcholine but does not cause the kind of increase in liver enzymes that tacrine does. It can also cause diarrhea, vomiting, nausea, fatigue, insomnia, and

anorexia, but in most cases, such side effects are mild and decline with continued use of the drug. Again, the drug helps only those patients with mild to moderate symptoms of Alzheimer's and does not stop or slow the disease's progression.

## Forgetfulness or Alzheimer's?

While most people understand at least some of the horrifying aspects of Alzheimer's disease, DeKosky says a big challenge is educating people regarding the widely held assumption that people are supposed to have memory impairment as they age.

"There's this huge prejudice where we think people should have severe mental impairment as they get older," he says. Memory loss, disorientation, and confusion are not part of the normal aging process, he explains. They are symptoms of dementia, and the most common form of dementia is Alzheimer's.

"You need to look at the functional consequences of what someone cannot remember," DeKosky says. "If mom forgets where she put her car in the parking lot at the mall, that's not abnormal. But if she walks home from the mall because she forgot she took her car, that's not normal. Memory is the first and worst change, but you will also see social withdrawal and less willingness to interact with others."

## The Need for Answers

Although no cure for Alzheimer's is available now, planning and medical/social

management can help ease the burden on both patient and family members. Physical exercise, good nutrition, and social activities are important. A calm, structured environment may also help the person to continue functioning.

At some point, however, people with Alzheimer's require 24-hour care. The financing of such care, including diagnosis costs, treatment, and paid care, is estimated to be $100 billion annually, according to the Alzheimer's Association. The federal government covers $4.4 billion and the states another $4.1 billion, with much of the remaining costs borne by patients and their families.

"It's a national imperative to find effective means to diagnose, treat and prevent this disease," says David Banks, R.Ph., a public health specialist in the FDA's Office of Special Health Issues. "When you look at it demographically, the nearly 80 million baby boomers living in the United States . . . now have an average life expectancy of approximately 78 years. One in five Americans could be age 65 or older by 2030, and tens of millions of baby boomers will live into their 80s. The Alzheimer's Association projects that as many as 14 million Americans could have Alzheimer's disease in 2050. When viewed in the context of accelerating Social Security and Medicare costs . . . , the future monetary costs of Alzheimer's disease may be unsustainable. The human costs could be even greater."

*Note:* Audrey T. Hingley is a freelance writer in Mechanicsville, Virginia.

1. Which statements are verifiable facts, and which are unverified statements or value claims?
2. What are the credentials of the person who wrote the article? Does this person have the appropriate background and education in the topic area? What can you do to check the person's credentials?
3. What might be the motives and biases of the person who wrote the article?
4. What is the main point of the article? Which information is relevant to the issue, main point? Which information is irrelevant?

5. Is the source reliable? What evidence supports your conclusion that the source is reliable or unreliable? Does the source of information present the pros and cons of the topic?
6. Does the source of information attack the credibility of conventional scientists or medical authorities?

Based on your analysis, do you think that this article is a reliable source of health-related information? Explain why you think it is or is not. Summarize your reasons for coming to this conclusion.

Although a review of several scientific studies indicated EGb 761 can improve cognitive functioning, the extract's beneficial effects were slight.[23] Results of the Ginkgo Evaluation Memory Study indicate ginkgo had no effect on memory loss or AD.[24]

Vitamins E and C have antioxidant effects. According to results of certain studies, populations that consume vitamin E–rich diets have lower risk of Alzheimer's disease.[25] No such benefit, however, was observed in groups of people taking high amounts of vitamin E, multivitamin, or other vitamin supplements.[24] Researchers continue to investigate the association between dietary sources of antioxidants, such as fruits, vegetables, and vegetable oils, and the risk of Alzheimer's disease. At present, there is no conclusive scientific evidence that supports the effectiveness of any specific dietary supplement in preventing the disease.[24]

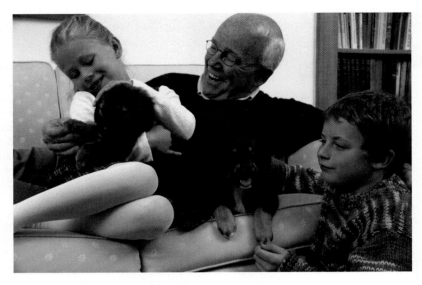
Older adults often enjoy caring for their grandchildren.

Patients with Alzheimer's often live at home until they reach the terminal stage and require the care provided in a skilled nursing care facility. Living with an affected loved one can be emotionally stressful and physically demanding. While caring for a patient with this disease, family members must try to maintain their own health and well-being. To provide assistance, many communities have special "adult day care" centers where persons with AD can spend a few hours during the day before returning to their homes. Not every community offers this service, so if you need help caring for someone with AD, check with your local mental health association or Alzheimer's Association for information about adult day care centers in your area. The following Analyzing Health-Related Information feature involves evaluating excerpts of an article about AD.

## The Effects of Aging on Psychological Health

As they approach the end of middle age, most employed people face retirement, and many aging parents have grown children with families who have moved away. If older adults equate retirement from jobs and separation from their families with being old and useless, they may experience serious psychological distress. Additionally, the dramatic reduction of financial resources that often accompanies retirement can mean a serious loss of economic stability.

Many older adults began planning for their future financial security while they were young. Therefore, not every older adult dreads the prospect of retiring from job and family responsibilities. Many people approach retirement with a positive outlook and look forward to this time of life. Retired individuals often find pleasure from traveling, volunteering in their communities, caring for their grandchildren, and exploring new interests. Other retirement-age adults choose to continue working, especially if they enjoy what they do and their work is intellectually stimulating and personally fulfilling. Older adults often have a wealth of knowledge and experience that they can share with younger members of society.

Older adults, especially those older than 85 years of age, frequently experience deteriorating health, difficult social circumstances, and poor economic conditions. Deaths of spouses and friends, separations from family, and reductions in financial resources create emotional stress. As a result, elderly persons often suffer depression.

Regardless of one's age, depression is associated with an increased risk of suicide. In the United States, older adults are twice as likely to commit suicide when compared to people who are 10–24 years of age.[26] Divorced or widowed elderly persons are more likely to kill themselves than married older adults are.[27] Additionally, poor health is a risk factor for suicide. Older adults suffering from chronic conditions, particularly mental illness, heart failure, obstructive lung disease, and pain, are more likely to commit suicide than older adults who did not have these conditions.[28]

Like younger people, depressed or isolated aged individuals can benefit from participation in social and physical activities. In addition, antidepressant medications or psychotherapy may be necessary to help them regain and maintain their emotional balance.

## The Effects of Aging on Social Health

Although a large segment of the U.S. population is older than 65 years, our society is highly youth-oriented. Not surprisingly, middle-age Americans often worry that aging will mean losing their jobs to younger people, being forced into early retirement, becoming widowed, and suffering from debilitating illnesses. Growing old in America can have serious social impacts on older adults; they may be ignored, neglected, and abused by younger members of the population.

Some people in our society have negative attitudes toward older adults. For example, they stereotype elderly people as poor, sick, useless, and dependent. Additionally, some young adults believe that older adults demand too much from the rest of society. **Ageism** is a bias against older adults. Ageism creates conflict between the generations because the old do not trust the young and vice versa. To combat ageism, people need to recognize that growing old does not always mean having poor health, living in an institution, depending on public support, and being useless.

Older adults represent a valuable social asset that is not well used. Aging parents and grandparents often have experience and wisdom that they can share with younger family members. Additionally, many retirees have a variety of talents and special organizational skills that enable them to serve as consultants, managers, or advisors in business, governmental, or educational settings. Both young and old benefit when each accepts, values, and trusts the other.

## Successful Aging

Many people would like to believe that it is possible to prevent aging or delay the process. Restricting caloric intakes without creating nutritional deficiencies may slow the rate of aging.[29] The modern search for a "fountain of youth" has resulted in the promotion of pills, potions, diets, or treatments that are touted as having "anti-aging" or "life-extending" capabilities. Contrary to the claims of advertisers, none of these substances or regimens prevents or slows aging.[30]

Instead of searching for magic formulas to extend your life, you can take various actions while you are young to increase your chances of aging successfully. Although there is no generally agreed upon definition for "successful aging," people who age successfully have good physical functioning.[29] Other characteristics of such healthy older adults include having positive attitudes toward themselves and the future and being connected socially with others.

To increase your chances of aging successfully, evaluate your health status and lifestyle, identify specific unhealthy or risky behaviors, and then work at changing those behaviors. Although modifying all unhealthy behaviors is commendable, certain practices are associated more closely with lengthening one's life span than others are.

Physically active people live longer than people who are sedentary.[31] Engaging in regular exercise throughout your life will help you control your body weight as well as improve your circulation, strengthen your heart, and maintain your muscle and bone mass. People older than 65 years of age who perform regular exercise improve their physical strength and flexibility, features that can enhance their quality of life.[31] Exercise may improve some cognitive abilities of aging adults, such as memory, and delay the onset of Alzheimer's disease.[32] More research, however, is needed to further support these findings. **Table 15.3** lists some basic recommendations for enhancing your health and quality of life as you age, such as managing stress, maintaining relationships, and developing a positive attitude. The other chapters of this textbook provide more detailed information about these recommendations. It is worth remembering the words of Eubie Blake, a jazz musician who died in 1983 at the age of 100, "If I had known that I was going to live this long, I would have taken better care of myself."

### Healthy Living Practices

☐ Planning for your future financial needs while you are still young can help you enjoy your retirement years.

☐ To age successfully, evaluate your present health and lifestyle, identify risky behaviors, and then consider changing those behaviors.

**Table 15.3**

## Tips for Successful Aging

**Taking the following actions now, while you are still young, may help you enjoy a healthier, longer life:**

- Maintain a healthy weight and eat a nutritious, low-fat diet that includes plenty of whole grains, fruits, and vegetables.
- Be physically active; exercise daily.
- Do not smoke, drink too much alcohol, or abuse other drugs.
- Manage stress; take time to relax daily.
- Have regular physical examinations.
- Adopt safer sex practices.
- Do not drive while under the influence of alcohol or other drugs; always wear a seat belt in vehicles.
- Protect your skin and eyes from sunlight.
- Obtain enough sleep.
- Be concerned about your safety at home, work, or play.
- Maintain social networks with your family and friends.
- Be flexible; expect changes.
- Develop a positive attitude; have a sense of humor.
- Find opportunities to learn new skills or information.
- Get involved with living while accepting your mortality.

*Sources:* Adapted from Kerschner, H., & Pegues, J. A. (1998). Productive aging: A quality of life agenda. *Journal of the American Dietetic Association, 98:*1445–1448; and Turner, L. W., Sizer, F. S., Whitney, E. N., & Wilks, B. B. (1992). *Life choices: Health concepts and strategies.* Minneapolis, MN: West Publishing.

## Dying

Many Americans, including health professionals, fear dying and death, especially the possibility that dying will be premature and painful. Fearing death makes it difficult to be around someone who is dying. One reason many Americans fear dying and death is that few have had contact with dying persons or dead bodies. Usually an ambulance rushes the critically injured or terminally ill person to a hospital, where he or she is connected to a variety of life-support machines and placed in an intensive care unit (**Figure 15.6**). Most hospitals permit family members to visit the seriously ill patient for only a few minutes each hour. In other instances, elderly or incurably ill pa-

**Figure 15.6**

**Intensive Care.** Treatment of a critically injured or terminally ill person may include being connected to a variety of life-support machines in a hospital's intensive care unit.

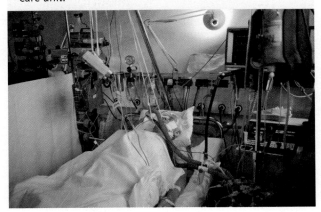

tients die in long-term care facilities with few or no family members present. In the United States, dying often becomes a mechanized, isolated, and depersonalized process.

Dying was very different a hundred years ago. In that era, nearly everyone died at home, surrounded by family and friends. Shortly after death, the body was cooled, and it often remained in the home for the funeral ceremony. It was even customary for people to have photographs taken of their deceased loved ones to remember them (**Figure 15.7**). These practices helped survivors accept dying and death as a part of life.

## The Spiritual Aspects of Dying

Some people who have been revived after being unresponsive describe "near-death" experiences and relate them as spiritually uplifting events. They report that they were aware of what was happening before they recovered consciousness. They often recall feeling temporarily disengaged from their bodies and having unusual but peaceful sensations. Accounts of near-death experiences often include some features of the person's spiritual or religious beliefs. People who have been in these situations are often profoundly affected by their experiences, but scientists have no ways of verifying their stories.

People who believe in an afterlife may have less fear of dying and death. Many people believe that a soul exists, which leaves the body after death and goes to heaven or hell. Others believe in reincarnation, com-

**Figure 15.7**

**Remembrance Photo, Circa 1896.** A hundred years ago, nearly everyone died at home, surrounded by their families and friends. It was customary for people to have photographs taken of their deceased loved ones to remember them. This African-American mother is posing with her dead infant.

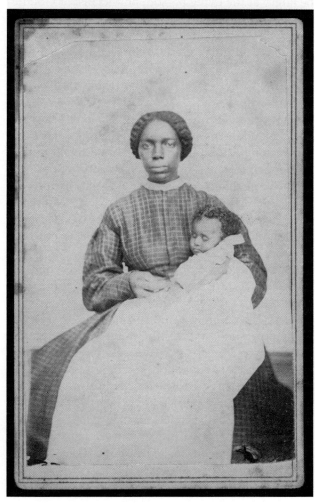

ing back to life as another person or organism after death. Some individuals are not concerned with what happens to them after death. In many instances, cultural and religious backgrounds provide the foundation for a person's feelings about life after death.

## The Emotional Aspects of Dying

Although coping with the death of a beloved person is one of life's most difficult experiences, knowing that your own death is near is especially difficult. In the late 1960s, Elisabeth Kübler-Ross, a psychiatrist at the University of Chicago Billings Hospital, pio-

neered efforts to understand the psychological processes of dying and death.[33] After interviewing more than 200 terminally ill patients, she formulated a five-stage model to describe the emotional responses that people often experience as they face their deaths (**Table 15.4**).

The first stage of this coping process is denial. People in denial may act shocked after receiving news of their terminal condition. Frequently, they do not believe their physician's prognosis. While in denial, dying individuals may ignore their troublesome symptoms or seek more optimistic outlooks from other physicians. Some dying patients completely lose faith in the value of conventional medical care; some maintain hope of "beating this thing" by using untested alternative treatments.

As the dying begin to accept their situation, they may enter the second stage, anger. In this stage, dying people are provoked easily; they may lash out at loved ones, medical staff, and anything or anybody. They often demand to know "Why me? Why not someone else?" It is important for people who care for or visit dying individuals to expect this reaction and not take such anger personally.

## Table 15.4

### Kübler-Ross's Stages of Emotional Responses to Dying

| Stage | Typical Responses |
|---|---|
| Denial | Feels emotionally numb, avoids thinking about his or her condition, ignores the reality of his or her condition |
| Anger | Lashes out at healthcare providers and loved ones |
| Bargaining | Makes deals with healthcare providers, loved ones, or God to live long enough to do special things or experience certain events |
| Depression | Mourns his or her impending death, withdraws socially |
| Acceptance | Realizes that his or her condition is terminal, gives away cherished items, makes funeral plans |

*Source:* Data from Kübler-Ross, E. (1969). *On death and dying.* New York: Macmillan.

**hospice** Health care specifically designed to give emotional support and pain relief to terminally ill people in the final stage of life.

The third emotional stage of dying is bargaining. Incurably ill individuals may make deals with medical staff or God, promising to exchange exceptionally good behavior for a few more years of life or a painless death. In the fourth stage, depression, dying people become increasingly aware that their condition will not improve. Terminally ill individuals mourn for themselves after realizing that they will not live long enough to enjoy experiences such as watching their children mature or playing with their grandchildren.

The final emotional stage of dying is acceptance. Although terminally ill people continue to hope for cures, they accept the possibility that nothing can be done to save them. Friends, family members, and caregivers can help maintain the self-esteem and dignity of the dying by visiting and touching them, as well as by listening to their concerns.

Critics of Kübler-Ross's research charge that she focused on people who were dying prematurely of chronic illnesses and had time to experience each stage. Therefore, her findings may have been different if she had studied people who were dying of acute illnesses or very sick elderly persons. Some people, particularly the elderly, may not experience all five stages of dying. Additionally, aged people who are terminally ill may accept their impending deaths more readily than people who face the prospect of dying while they are still young. The Kübler-Ross model, however, is useful for understanding the complex emotions of dying people.

Dying people are usually under extreme emotional distress. They often feel helpless and hopeless, and they have difficulty relaxing. Treatments such as surgery, chemotherapy, or radiation add to their discomfort. Some terminally ill people fight the prospect of dying; others accept what is happening to them and choose to make the most out of the time they have remaining. In modern societies, death can be the final stage of personal fulfillment if dying people have opportunities to satisfy their social and emotional needs. Thus, some terminally ill people choose to spend more time with their friends and families; others travel far from home.

As the end of life nears, terminally ill people may become more detached from others and the environment. They tend to sleep more often and may lapse in and out of consciousness. When awake or conscious, dying persons may not want to talk as much as they did before reaching this stage. According to Kübler-Ross, dying individuals are almost without feelings; most die without fear.

When you know that a beloved person is dying, you may experience a variety of intense emotions. You may be afraid of enduring the emotional pain of watching a close friend or relative die. You may be angry at the dying person, physicians, or God because you feel they are responsible for the impending death, or they are unable or unwilling to prevent it. You may feel guilty about your feelings toward the dying individual. Recognizing that someone is terminally ill forces us to face the reality that we will someday die.

Family and friends of a dying person typically feel helpless and intensely sad. As a result, they may avoid the person because such feelings are difficult to hide and uncomfortable to bear. This reaction does little to boost the dying person's dignity and sense of well-being. Being avoided makes the dying person feel isolated and rejected at a time when he or she usually has a high need for the compassionate support and comfort of others.

Physicians and family members have become increasingly aware that positive thinking, including hopefulness, can improve the well-being of the dying. Meeting the emotional and spiritual needs of terminally ill persons can help them live better while dying. Many physicians actively seek the participation of their seriously ill patients and their families in decisions concerning treatment. Medical practitioners can enhance the dignity and self-worth of dying patients by discussing the serious nature of their conditions with them, listening carefully to their concerns, and allowing them to make decisions regarding their medical care.

## Terminal Care: The Options

The majority of Americans die in hospitals or extended-care facilities such as nursing homes. The goal of hospital-based health care is to provide technologically sophisticated medical care that enables sick people to become well. Because hospital care is costly, elderly patients who are too ill or frail to return home often move into nursing homes. These extended-care facilities offer less comprehensive medical care than hospitals, but they are designed and equipped to manage the long-term care of people recovering from surgery or illness. Not every condition is curable; many chronically ill patients die while residing in these care centers.

# Consumer Health

## Choosing a Long-Term Care Facility

The most important feature to consider when choosing a residential facility is the quality of medical care that it provides. Before making this decision for a loved one, visit a few facilities, observe the condition of the buildings, its rooms, and residents, and answer the following questions:

1. Is the facility licensed by the state?
2. Is the facility clean, well maintained, and free of objectionable odors?
3. Are staff members friendly, helpful, and respectful to visitors and residents?
4. Are the rooms clean, comfortably furnished, well lit, and cheerful?
5. Do the residents appear to be appropriately dressed, clean, and well groomed? Do they appear to be alert?
6. Are there enough staff members to take care of the number of residents?
7. Are there handrails along the hallways and grab bars in the bathrooms?
8. Does the facility have rehabilitation and exercise areas, a quiet place with reading material, and a chapel?
9. Does the facility have an activities director and scheduled social events that are appropriate for elderly people?
10. Are the dining room and kitchen clean?
11. Are menus nutritious? Do menus indicate that a variety of foods is offered? Can you sample a meal? How are the special dietary needs of patients handled?
12. If you have an opportunity, ask some residents and staff (privately) what they like and dislike about the facility.
13. What are the monthly fees? Can you afford this facility? Does the facility accept Medicaid?
14. Contact your state's Division of Aging to obtain information about the facility's inspection reports.

Before making a final decision, visit the facility at least one additional unscheduled time to make another set of observations.

*Source:* Adapted from Goldsmith, S. B. (1990). *Choosing a nursing home.* New York: Prentice Hall.

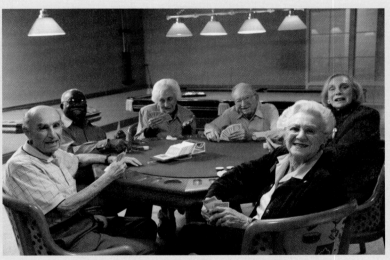

Older adults enjoying a social activity at a long-term care facility.

Choosing to place an aged parent or relative into a nursing home is often an emotionally difficult decision. Family members may have to select an available facility quickly and without researching their options. The Consumer Health feature "Choosing a Long-Term Care Facility" lists some important questions to answer when selecting a residential facility that provides long-term and/or skilled nursing care.

When patients have only a few months to live, their personal physicians may refer them to hospice. **Hospice** is health care specifically designed to give emotional support and pain relief to terminally ill people in the final stage of life (palliative care). This care may be provided in the patient's home or in a hospice center. The primary goal of hospice care is not to save dying patients with aggressive treatments but to relieve their discomfort. Hospice physicians often prescribe powerful medications to keep terminally ill patients as free from pain as possible. Freedom from extreme pain permits the dying person to manage his or her activities more effectively and die with dignity.

Hospice staff receive specialized training to work closely with and to provide emotional and spiritual support to dying patients and their families. Staff encourage patients and their relatives to participate in decision making regarding care. Most terminally ill people and their families can obtain hospice services in their homes from a team of medical professionals. Family members are taught simple medical procedures such as care of surgical wounds or maintenance of feeding tubes. Hospice nurses make home visits to check patients' conditions and are available to answer questions concerning their care. Dying at home allows patients to remain in a comfortable and familiar environment where they can participate in holiday and other family-oriented events.

Some dying patients receive hospice care in clinical settings that have rooms designed to look more like patients' homes than hospitals. The staff encourage patients to decorate their rooms with favorite possessions to foster a homelike environment. Visiting family and friends provide additional social, emotional, and spiritual support and often participate in caring for their ill loved ones. Regardless of whether the terminally ill person dies at home or in a hospice center, hospice staff provide grief counseling services for survivors.

Many nursing homes and hospitals offer hospice services that are covered by health insurance plans. To find such resources in your community, contact local hospitals or check the Yellow Pages under Hospice. Social workers in these facilities can provide information about local support groups for the terminally ill and their families. The National Hospice and Palliative Care Organization can also provide information about hospice programs in your area; this group's toll-free phone number is 1-800-658-8898.

## Death

Many people have a difficult time thinking about and discussing death. For example, they may avoid using the term *died*, preferring to use euphemisms such as *passed away*. Whether people believe in an afterlife or not, most are reluctant to handle matters concerning their own dying and death, such as preparing a will or signing an organ donor card.

### What Is Death?

**Death**, the cessation of life, occurs when the heart or lungs stop functioning. When this happens, no oxygen is available for metabolism, and brain cells begin to die. Within 4 to 5 minutes, the dying person loses consciousness. As remaining body cells die, other signs of death become obvious.

When a person dies, the muscles that control voluntary and involuntary movements no longer function. As a result, the body eliminates the contents of the bladder and rectum, and reflexes are absent. *Reflexes* are neuromuscular responses that do not require thinking, such as eye blinking. Gradually, skeletal muscles become rigid, and body temperature cools until it matches that of the environment. Unless the body is chilled or treated with embalming chemicals, it decomposes rapidly. Decomposition occurs because the immune system no longer prevents bacteria and other microorganisms from breaking down the organic material of the body.

The physician who attended the dying patient is usually responsible for certifying that the patient has died. Then, the medical staff informs family members. In most cases, they deliver the body to a funeral home or medical school, according to the deceased person's wishes. If there are any questions or suspicions about the cause of death, the family, physicians, or coroner can request an **autopsy**. During an autopsy, a specially trained physician conducts various medical examinations and tests that usually determine the cause of death.

In 1968, a team of experts at the Harvard Medical School defined death according to four irreversible physical criteria:

- The absence of electrical activity in the brain
- No spontaneous muscular movements, including breathing
- No reflexes
- No responses to the environment

These criteria define what is commonly referred to as *brain death*. The majority of state laws recognize these criteria as the basis for defining death. A legal definition of death is important for criminal cases that involve murder. Defining death is necessary for physicians who need to establish that patients are dead before removing tissues or organs for transplantation.

Since the 1980s, advances in medical technology have made it necessary for medical experts to reconsider the traditional definition of death. By using *cardiopulmonary resuscitation* (CPR), *respirators* (devices that assist breathing), and feeding machines, physicians can often save the lives of certain seriously ill persons and, in some instances, may sustain patients who have virtually no chance of recovering.

**Cerebral Death** The cerebral cortex of the brain controls thoughts, interprets sensory information, and integrates voluntary muscular activities. An individual who experiences severe damage to his or her cerebral cortex is **comatose**, that is, unresponsive to the environment and in a *coma*. If the damage is irreversible, it is unlikely that the person will regain consciousness. In some comatose patients, the areas of the brain that control and regulate vital activities, including digestion and breathing, continue to function. Although their conditions do not meet the standard criteria for brain death, such individuals have experienced *cerebral death*. With specialized care, a person with a nonfunctioning cerebral cortex can exist in an irreversible coma, a **persistent vegetative state**, for years.

The level of care required to maintain patients in persistent vegetative states is stressful for their families, as well as expensive. Under what circumstances can physicians remove life-sustaining care from a patient in an irreversible coma? The U.S. Supreme Court decision in the Quinlan case provides an answer.

In 1975, Karen Ann Quinlan, a 21-year-old New Jersey woman, was hospitalized in an unconscious state after allegedly consuming a combination of alcohol and tranquilizers. After realizing that she would not recover, Ms. Quinlan's parents requested that the medical staff and hospital administrators allow their daughter to die by disconnecting her respirator. However, the administrators and attending physicians denied the parents' request, noting that the young woman was not dead according to established criteria.

After lower state courts supported the hospital's position, the Quinlans took their daughter's case to the New Jersey Supreme Court. In 1976, this court ruled that because Karen had previously told her mother and some friends that she would not want to live in a persistent vegetative state, her parents had the right to ask physicians to remove her respirator. After being removed gradually from the ventilation device, Karen was able to breathe without the machine's assistance, but she continued to be fed through tubes. The Quinlans moved their comatose daughter to a nursing home, where she died 10 years later.

Since the Quinlan case, several states have passed laws that establish steps for withholding or removing life-sustaining care in similar cases involving the terminally ill. A later section of this chapter describes how you can inform other people in advance about your wishes concerning such medical care.

> **comatose** The condition in which a person is unresponsive to the environment and in a coma.
>
> **persistent vegetative state** The condition in which a person has a nonfunctioning cerebral cortex and is in an irreversible coma.

# Euthanasia and the Right to Die

Euthanasia is the practice of allowing permanently comatose or incurably ill persons to die. In cases of active euthanasia, physicians hasten the deaths of dying people by giving them large doses of pain-relieving medications that can completely suppress breathing. Passive euthanasia involves cases in which terminally ill people die because physicians do not provide life-sustaining treatments, or they withdraw such care.

Since the Quinlan case, the courts have decided several right-to-die cases, particularly those involving people who were seriously ill but not dying. Some chronically ill individuals decide that life is not worth living, or that they are tired of living in pain. To hasten death, these people may refuse life-prolonging medical treatment, demand that it be withdrawn, or remove it themselves. In recent years, the courts often have made or upheld decisions that give such seriously ill people the right to die. After physicians discontinued their life support, many of these patients died naturally within a couple of weeks.

In some instances, the seriously ill person is too physically or mentally incapacitated to actively end his or her life. Concerned relatives, friends, or caregivers risk criminal prosecution by helping people commit suicide. Although most physicians strive to preserve life, some assist in the suicides of dying patients by prescribing overdoses of certain drugs. In the 1990s, retired physician Jack Kevorkian focused national attention on the controversial practice of physician-assisted suicide by helping more than 125 people end their lives. In 1999, a judge sentenced Kevorkian to prison for injecting a deadly dose of drugs into a man who was suffering from an incurable deadly disease. Kevorkian spent about 8 years in prison before being paroled. In 2011, Kevorkian died after a brief illness.

Oregon, Montana, and Washington are the only states that allow physicians to prescribe drugs to terminally ill patients so that they can end their lives. Oregon and Washington maintain records concerning the number of deaths attributed to physician-assisted suicide each year. Between 1998 and 2010, 525 Oregonian patients chose to end their lives by taking a prescribed dose of deadly medications.[34]

In 1990, 26-year-old Terri Schiavo's heart failed and the young woman's body entered a persistent vegetative state after a significant number of her brain cells died from the lack of nutrients and oxygen (**Figure 15.8**). For several years, Terri's parents fought legal battles with her husband over their desire to keep her alive in a long-term care facility by providing nourishment through tube feedings. Terri's husband contended that her life-supporting care should be withdrawn, because before her heart attack, she had indicated to him that she would not want to be kept alive in such a manner if she were incapacitated. By spring of 2005, the parents' legal options were exhausted after courts ruled consistently in Terri's husband's favor. When the comatose woman's feeding tube was removed, the tragic case made headline news in the United States and around the world, rekindling debate over euthanasia. Terri died almost 2 weeks after her feeding tube was withdrawn.

## Preparing for Death

Young adults may see the need to plan for a comfortable retirement, but planning for a good death seems too morbid to consider. A dying person has a good death if he or she maintains a high degree of dignity and experiences little physical and emotional pain during the dying process. Additionally, a good death causes minimal amounts of emotional trauma for the person's survivors.

Not everyone has time to prepare for a good death; death can be premature and unexpected, such as in cases of homicides or fatal accidents. Healthy people, however, can make various legal, financial, emotional, and spiritual preparations for their deaths. Such planning can reduce their survivors' confusion and anxiety.

**Advance Directives** The Patient Self-Determination Act gives people the right to prepare advance directives that indicate their wishes concerning treatment if they become incapacitated. The act also allows physicians and administrators of certain medical facilities to withhold or remove life-support care from comatose patients who have no hope of regaining consciousness and who would not want to be kept alive in such conditions.

A living will or a durable power of attorney document can specify your wishes concerning your medical care in the event that you become permanently incapacitated. **Figure 15.9** shows a sample living will. Not every state honors such documents. For example, your state may exclude the right to have artificial feeding and hydration (water) tubes removed, regardless of your wishes.

Although some states do not sanction living wills, they allow other advance directives such as a durable power of attorney. In this document, you identify a mentally competent individual to serve as a healthcare surrogate or proxy. A healthcare proxy will make decisions concerning your care if you become unable to do so. Additionally, you may indicate which life-

### Figure 15.8

**Terri Schiavo.** These photographs show Terri before and after a heart attack deprived her brain of oxygen and resulted in a persistent vegetative state.

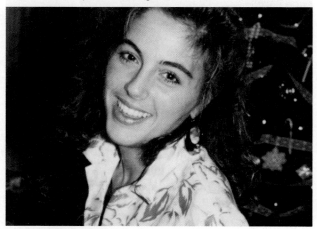

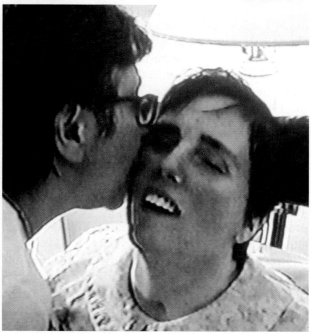

**Figure 15.9**

**A Living Will.** While still able, a person can sign a living will to specify wishes concerning medical care in the event that he or she becomes permanently incapacitated. This advance directive is for the District of Columbia.

*Source:* © 2005 National Hospice and Palliative Care Organization. Revised 2011. All rights reserved. Reproduction and distribution by an organization or organized group without the written permission of the National Hospice and Palliative Care Organization is expressly forbidden.

**DISTRICT OF COLUMBIA DECLARATION – PAGE 1 OF 2**

INSTRUCTIONS

PRINT THE DATE

PRINT YOUR NAME

Declaration made this _____ day of _____.
(date)                    (month, year)

I,

_____,
(name)

being of sound mind, willfully and voluntarily make known my desires that my dying shall not be artificially prolonged under the circumstances set forth below, do declare:

If at any time I should have an incurable injury, disease or illness certified to be a terminal condition by two physicians who have personally examined me, one of whom shall be my attending physician, and the physicians have determined that my death will occur whether or not life-sustaining procedures are utilized and where the application of life-sustaining procedures would serve only to artificially prolong the dying process, I direct that such procedures be withheld or withdrawn, and that I be permitted to die naturally with only the administration of medication or the performance of any medical procedure deemed necessary to provide me with comfort care or to alleviate pain.

ADD OTHER INSTRUCTIONS, IF ANY, REGARDING YOUR ADVANCE CARE PLANS

THESE INSTRUCTIONS CAN FURTHER ADDRESS YOUR HEALTH CARE PLANS, SUCH AS YOUR WISHES REGARDING HOSPICE TREATMENT, BUT CAN ALSO ADDRESS OTHER ADVANCE PLANNING ISSUES, SUCH AS YOUR BURIAL WISHES

ATTACH ADDITIONAL PAGES IF NEEDED

Other directions:

_____
_____
_____
_____
_____
_____
_____
_____
_____
_____
_____

© 2005 National Hospice and Palliative Care Organization 2011 Revised.

**DISTRICT OF COLUMBIA DECLARATION — PAGE 2 OF 2**

In the absence of my ability to give directions regarding the use of such life-sustaining procedures, it is my intention that this declaration shall be honored by my family and physician(s) as the final expression of my legal right to refuse medical or surgical treatment and accept the consequences from such refusal.

SIGN AND DATE THE DOCUMENT AND PRINT YOUR ADDRESS

I understand the full importance of this declaration and I am emotionally and mentally competent to make this declaration.

Signed _____ Date_____

Address _____

WITNESSING PROCEDURE

TWO WITNESSES MUST SIGN AND DATE HERE

I believe the declarant to be of sound mind. I did not sign the declarant's signature above for or at the direction of the declarant. I am at least eighteen years of age and am not related to the declarant by blood, marriage, or domestic partnership, entitled to any portion of the estate of the declarant according to the laws of intestate succession of the District of Columbia or under any will of the declarant or codicil thereto, or directly financially responsible for declarant's medical care. I am not the declarant's attending physician, an employee of the attending physician, or an employee of the health facility in which the declarant is a patient.

Witness _____ Date_____

Witness _____ Date_____

© 2005 National Hospice and Palliative Care Organization 2011 Revised.

prolonging medical actions are acceptable or necessary under certain circumstances. The results of surveys indicate that most Americans would want limited care if they became incapacitated. Few Americans, however, have prepared living wills or other advance directives.

Before preparing an advance directive, it is a good idea to discuss your wishes with family and address their concerns. Your physician can probably answer questions that you or your family may have about life-support care. Family members or the person who agrees to serve as your healthcare surrogate and your personal physician will need copies of these documents. It is a good idea to store your copy along with your other important documents in a safety deposit box.

**Estate Management** In addition to an advance directive, it is important to have a will, a legal document that specifies how you want your property to be distributed after your death. To prepare a formal will, it is a good idea to consult an attorney, preferably one who specializes in estate administration. For the will to be valid, you must be of "sound mind" (aware of your actions) when you write and sign your will, and the document must be signed and witnessed by at least two people.

Most Americans die without having a will. When this happens, probate courts follow state laws concerning the division and distribution of the deceased person's estate. An estate includes the individual's sources of money, such as checking and savings accounts, life insurance policies, and retirement plans. In addition, possessions that can be sold, such as jewelry, real estate, furniture, and collectibles, are part of one's estate. A carefully constructed will can ensure that these assets go to whomever you want, and not to whom the courts choose. Furthermore, a will can eliminate much unhappiness, stress, and confusion among your survivors. If family members feel that provisions stated in your will unfairly distribute the estate, they can contest it in court.

In addition to making a will, it is a good idea to appoint an executor to manage your estate after your death. The executor uses income from the estate to pay your debts and funeral costs. If you have young children, it is important to identify and ask a person who will act as their legal guardian in case they become orphans. Most people choose a guardian who is a close relative or friend to whom they can entrust the care of their children.

In addition to having a will and an executor, you can protect your survivors' assets by having enough health and life insurance to cover your final medical and funeral expenses. The best time to buy life and health insurance is while you are young and healthy.

**Organ Donation** In dying, people can make a priceless contribution to the living by donating their tissues or organs. Soon after death, a donor's kidneys, liver, skin, heart, and corneas can be removed and transplanted into people whose organs or tissues are failing. Many seriously ill patients who would have died without receiving donated organs are able to live nearly normal lives after having the procedures.

As of May 31, 2011, more than 111,400 people in the United States were on waiting lists to receive organ transplants.[35] Patients are more likely to need kidneys and/or livers than other organs. Unfortunately, the demand for organs is greater than the supply. In 2010, more than 7,100 Americans died while waiting for matching organs to become available for transplantation.[36] Although people may express an interest in having their organs donated when they die, they often do not make their wishes known to others nor do they document them formally. For example, potential donors may fail to inform family members of their decision or sign organ donor cards. In most states, family members can override the deceased person's wishes concerning organ donation.

People can help those who need healthy tissues and organs by completing and signing uniform donor cards like the one shown in **Figure 15.10**. This card should be kept in a person's wallet. Additionally, people can fill in and sign the organ donor declaration on the back of their driver's license. Additionally, individuals who would like to become organ donors when they die should inform their relatives of their wishes. Although there are no guarantees that

## Figure 15.10

**A Uniform Donor Card.** By completing and signing a donor card like this one, people can help others who need healthy tissues and organs.
*Source:* Reprinted with permission from the National Kidney Foundation.

**NATIONAL KIDNEY FOUNDATION**
*Please keep this card in a safe place and inform your family of your wishes to be a donor.*

This is to inform you that, should the occasion ever arise, I would like to be an organ and tissue donor. Please see that my wishes are carried out by informing the attending medical personnel that I have indicated my wishes to become a donor. Thank you.

*Signature* _____ *Date* _____

For further information contact:
**NATIONAL KIDNEY FOUNDATION**
(800) 622-9010 • www.kidney.org

- - - - - - - - - - - - - - - - - - - - - - - - - - - - - - -

**ORGAN AND TISSUE DONOR CARD**

*Of* _____
(print or type name of donor)

In the hope that I may help others, I hereby make this anatomical gift, if medically acceptable, to take effect upon my death. The words and marks below indicate my wishes.

I give: ☐ any needed organs or tissues
☐ only the following organs or tissues

_____
(specify the organ[s], tissue[s])

for the purposes of transplantation, therapy, medical research or education;
☐ my body for anatomical study if needed.

Limitations or special wishes, if any: _____

- - - - - - - - - - - - - - - - - - - - - - - - - - - - - - -

Signed by the donor and the following two witnesses in the presence of each other:

_____        _____
*Signature of Donor*        *Date of Birth of Donor*

_____        _____
*Date Signed*        *City and State*

_____        _____
*Witness*        *Witness*

This is a legal document under the Anatomical Gift Act or similar laws.

☐ Yes, I have discussed my wishes with my family. For further information consult your physician or

 **National Kidney Foundation**
30 East 33rd Street, New York, NY 10016

surgeons will be able to transplant a person's tissues after death, it may be reassuring for some people to know that, even after death, they might be able to help others.

## Some Final Thoughts on Death

Funeral and memorial services can help friends and family members deal with the loss of a loved one. You can ease some of the emotional and financial burdens of your survivors by planning your funeral arrangements. A funeral can be very costly, and it is often a difficult emotional task for families to make such arrangements when a loved one dies.

Many mortuaries offer prearranged funerals that enable you to specify the kind of funeral you want and the most affordable services. For example, you could choose to have a simple memorial service, your body *cremated* (burned), and your ashes placed in a container and given to your survivors. You can contact mortuaries in your area for more information about making funeral and burial prearrangements.

In addition to making funeral and burial arrangements, you can prepare spiritually for your death.

One spiritual arrangement you can make in preparation for death is to write your own obituary or death notice. Many obituaries include a brief biography. If you prepare these documents, you can give copies of them to your survivors and let them know where to send them. Newspapers, college alumni associations, and professional organizations usually print death notices.

After a beloved person dies, survivors often experience confusion and distress because they cannot locate the deceased person's will and other important documents. To reduce the likelihood that this situation will occur after your death, share copies of these personal papers with your spouse, adult children, the executor, and the individual who has the power of attorney. A safety deposit box is a safe place to store such documents. To help your survivors find these important papers, you can keep a small card in your wallet that lists their location.

### Healthy Living Practices

- ☐ If you would like to be an organ donor when you die, complete a uniform donor card or sign the declaration on the back of your driver's license. Inform your relatives of this decision.
- ☐ Preparing a will can help your survivors manage your estate.
- ☐ To convey your wishes concerning treatment in case you become severely disabled and cannot communicate, consider preparing an advance directive.

**grief** An emotional state that usually occurs after the loss of something or someone special.

**mourning** The culturally defined way in which survivors resolve the grief surrounding a death.

## Grief

**Grief** is the emotional state that nearly everyone experiences when they lose something special or someone with whom they enjoyed a close relationship. Losing someone you love is one of the most significant emotional events that can occur during your life. Some of life's losses are predictable, such as the death of beloved grandparents, parents, and spouses. Unexpected or premature losses, such as the death of a child or the sudden death of a spouse, can be emotionally devastating to the surviving parents, spouse, and other family members.

Regardless of the circumstances surrounding a death, resolving the grief that follows the loss of a loved one (*bereavement*) involves regaining emotional balance and stability. **Mourning**, the culturally defined way in which survivors observe bereavement, can be a difficult and lengthy process.

The emotional and physical reactions to the death of a beloved person vary; some people have a more difficult time coping with the loss than others do. People's emotional reactions are usually more severe after unexpected deaths than after anticipated deaths. Typically, the initial responses of survivors are psychological shock, disbelief, and denial. They next enter the acute mourning stage, which is characterized by crying, withdrawal, and other symptoms of depression. In many societies, people in mourning are expected to display their grief, for example, by crying and by wearing somber clothing. After mourning, survivors are often able to accept the death of their loved one, recognize that they have grieved, and regain a sense of emotional balance.

The most intense period of grieving normally lasts about 4 to 6 weeks after the death. It is not uncommon for people to continue mourning for a year or longer after the loss. Some people experience psychological and physical problems if they are unable to resolve their feelings of grief.

Much of the research that examines the impact of grieving on health involves people whose spouses have recently died. Most widowed people experience some signs and symptoms of depression, such

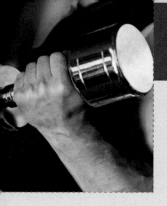

# Managing Your Health

## After the Death of a Loved One

The "Managing Grief" sections of this box provide some suggestions that may help you cope with the death of a beloved individual. The "Managing Legal, Social, and Financial Concerns" sections provide some actions that you can take to manage various concerns that often arise after the death of a spouse or other beloved person.

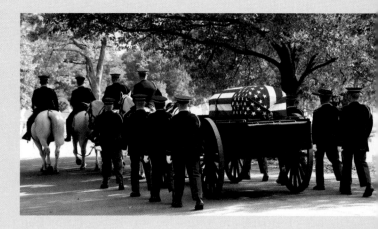

### Immediate Actions and Concerns

*Managing Grief*

- Resolve to survive the first few days of the sorrowful event.
- Accept the support and company of clergy, friends, and family.
- Permit yourself to vent your feelings, for example, to cry or to feel anger.

*Managing Legal, Social, and Financial Concerns*

- Notify your attorney; obtain the deceased person's will and make several photocopies of it.
- Order several copies of the death certificate; the funeral director may do this for you.

### Within the First 4 Weeks

*Managing Grief*

- Acknowledge those who sent food or flowers or who made memorial donations. Consider responding to those who visited or sent cards. This is an emotionally difficult task, but the process may be beneficial in itself.
- Anticipate feelings of grief: the tears, anger, guilt, and blame. Delayed or prolonged absence of grief may lead to negative physical and psychological consequences.
- If troubled by sleeplessness, nightmares, agitation, headaches, and even skin rashes, consult your physician for help to alleviate these conditions.
- Note changes in your appetite.

*Managing Legal, Social, and Financial Concerns*

- Notify relevant government agencies and other organizations of the death, such as the Social Security Administration, Veterans Administration, and insurance companies.
- Submit insurance claims and apply for refunds and benefits where applicable. Keep records of all response letters from agencies and organizations.
- Notify the deceased person's banks, credit card accounts, custodians of mutual funds and annuities, and accountant of the death.

### Within 6 Months

*Managing Grief*

- Join a grief support group. For information concerning support groups in your area, contact social workers at a local hospital or hospice or your local United Way.
- Adapt to lifestyle changes. You may need to learn how to do unfamiliar chores such as maintaining the house, tracking investments, cooking meals, or paying bills.
- Continue previous activities such as participating in hobbies or clubs if they are satisfying.
- Participate in healthful physical activities such as walking, swimming, or golfing. Join a health spa or similar organization.

*Managing Legal, Social, and Financial Concerns*

- Share meals with friends and accept the invitations of others to dine out with them.
- Update your will: change beneficiaries, trustees, or executors if necessary.
- Consult your accountant; your tax situation may have changed.

### Long-Term

*Managing Grief*

- Establish your own identity to function independently. Your degree of dependence and attachment to the deceased may determine the time needed for adjustment.
- Establish new relationships; continue existing relationships.
- Consider participating in activities or organizations that help others.

*Managing Legal, Social, and Financial Concerns*

- Plan for the future. Do not rush into making major changes or decisions.

as sadness, withdrawal, and sleep disorders. With the support of family and friends, however, grieving individuals can often regain their emotional balance within a few months. Survivors may become saddened again over the loss of a spouse, especially on anniversaries, on holidays, and during family reunions. An estimated 10% to 20% of widowed people suffer severe depression that lasts a year or more after their spouses die. The Managing Your Health feature "After the Death of a Loved One" contains some suggestions that can help people endure the first year after the death of a spouse or other beloved individual.

In addition to affecting emotional health, bereavement often influences the physical health of survivors. Most grieving people are emotionally distressed, and such stress often has a negative impact on their immune systems. Individuals who have weakened immune systems are at risk of developing frequent infections and chronic health problems such as cardiovascular disease. Additionally, grieving people may not take good care of themselves; for example, they may not eat nutritious foods or exercise, and some may abuse drugs, including alcohol.

People who undergo an abnormal grieving process may have had a poor relationship with the deceased person. According to Kübler-Ross, grief includes some degree of anger that is directed toward the dead individual. Survivors may hide their anger; others may express it by lashing out at someone else or by grieving for an unusually long period. **Table 15.5** lists the signs of abnormal grieving. People with these signs may need professional counseling.

## Healthy Living Practices

☐ Consider seeking professional counseling if your grief is severe or does not subside over time after the death of a loved one.

## Across THE LIFE SPAN

### DYING AND DEATH

In the United States, parents often find it difficult to discuss death with their children until someone or something, such as a pet, is dying or has died. Young children have difficulty grasping the concepts of dying and death (**Figure 15.11**). For example, if a 4-year-old child attends a funeral and views a loved one's body, the youngster may think this person is asleep.

Children as young as 2 years old miss a familiar person who has died, especially if the deceased was a parent. Preschool-aged children, however, do not express grief as older children or adults do. At this age, children typically grieve differently from how adults grieve; they may act unconcerned about the death and become intensely involved in play activities or misbehave.

School-age children are able to understand that dead things do not come back to life, and they respond to the loss much like adults: crying, withdrawing, or being angry. Older children often associate death with being old, particularly if they have experienced the death of a grandparent. Thus, they may have a great deal of difficulty coping when a peer dies.

Adults need to be honest and straightforward when discussing terminal illness and death with children. They should consider the child's ability to understand

---

### Table 15.5

### Grieving Danger Signs

**Professional counseling to handle grief may be necessary if the grieving person:**

- Doubts that his or her grieving is normal
- Experiences frequent outbursts of anger
- Finds little or no pleasure in life and has persistent suicidal thoughts
- Is preoccupied with thinking about the deceased loved one, or has hostile or guilty feelings that persist for more than a couple of years
- Experiences significant weight loss, weight gain, or persistent insomnia
- Begins engaging in risky behaviors such as abusing drugs or practicing unsafe sex
- Loses interest in taking care of personal hygiene for more than two weeks

*Source:* Adapted from Kouri, M. K. (1991). *Keys to dealing with the loss of a loved one.* Hauppauge, NY: Barrons Educational Series.

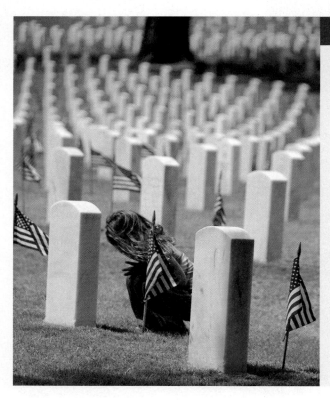

## Figure 15.11

**Children's Responses to End-of-Life Concepts.** Young children have difficulty grasping the concepts of dying and death. When faced with the loss of a loved one, preschool children typically grieve differently from how adults grieve.

the meaning of death. Frequently, children begin to understand and accept death when caring people share what is happening with them. Adults need to allow grieving children to express their concerns and feelings about dying and death. Professional counseling may be necessary if the child's responses are excessive, if the young person becomes preoccupied with death, or if the child becomes depressed.

## Healthy Living Practices

☐ If your child becomes preoccupied with death or depressed after someone or something has died, professional counseling can help him or her deal with the loss.

# Summary

Aging is the sum of all changes that occur in an organism over its life span. The human life span is divided into stages. The final stage, senescence, generally refers to the stage of life that begins at 65 years of age.

The overall life expectancy of Americans has increased since 1900. In the United States, a person born in 2009 can expect to live for about 78 years. Life expectancies, however, vary according to age, sex, and socioeconomic status. For example, American females outlive American males by about 5 years.

As of 2009, 13% of the U.S. population was 65 years of age and older. By the year 2030, nearly 20% of Americans will be in this age group. This segment of the American population is increasing at a rapid rate.

Aged people must often live on incomes that are lower than when they were younger. In the United States, older adult members of certain minority groups are more likely to have lower retirement incomes and live in poverty than are white aged persons. With appropriate financial planning, Americans who have adequate incomes when they are young may be able to maintain adequate incomes during their retirement years.

A gradual and irreversible decline in the functioning of the human body begins to occur around 30 years of age. However, people age at different rates. Genetic, environmental, and lifestyle factors influence the rate of aging.

Some of the physical changes associated with the aging process, such as gray hair, presbyopia, and menopause, are normal and inevitable. Other age-related physical changes such as heart disease, cancer, and osteoporosis are not normal and are signs of disease processes. People who modify their lifestyles while they are young may be able to prevent or delay such conditions.

According to Kübler-Ross, the typical emotional responses to dying include denial, anger, bargaining, depression, and acceptance. However, death can be the final stage of personal fulfillment if dying people have opportunities to satisfy their social and emotional needs. Family, friends, and medical care providers can help terminally ill individuals live better while dying by taking steps to enhance their dignity and self-worth.

Death occurs when the heart or lungs cease functioning and cells in the brain do not receive oxygen. The criteria for brain death include no brain waves, no spontaneous muscular movements, no reflexes, and no responses to the environment. A brain-dead person can exist in a persistent coma for years as long as the heart is functioning, nutritional needs are met, and the supply of oxygen to the heart is maintained by the use of a respirator. Euthanasia is the practice of allowing a permanently comatose or an incurably ill person to die.

The Patient Self-Determination Act gives people the right to prepare advance directives, documents that indicate a person's wishes concerning life-support measures if the individual becomes incapable of making such decisions.

Nearly everyone experiences grief with the loss of something special or someone with whom he or she enjoyed a close relationship. Although it is normal to grieve after such a loss, grief can have negative effects on health. To resolve grief, a person accepts the death of a loved one, recognizes that he or she has grieved for this person, and regains a sense of emotional balance. An individual who grieves for a prolonged period may require professional counseling.

Preschool children do not understand the concept of death, yet they still experience distress over the missing loved one. At this age, children may mourn by acting disinterested about the death or by misbehaving. Older children often grieve like adults by crying, withdrawing, and being angry. Grieving youngsters need to express their concerns and feelings about death. Like adults, children may need professional counseling if their emotional responses to death are severe or prolonged.

# Applying What You Have Learned

**Critical Thinking**

1. Develop a will that reflects your wishes concerning the distribution of your assets after death. **Application**
2. Analyze how your present lifestyle may affect your life span. **Analysis**
3. Propose a special program that would prevent ageism by promoting understanding and cooperation between young and old members of your community. **Synthesis**
4. Choose a position concerning the issue of euthanasia. How would you defend your position? **Evaluation**

**Key**

| **Application** | **Analysis** | **Synthesis** | **Evaluation** |
|---|---|---|---|
| using information in a new situation. | breaking down information into component parts. | putting together information from different sources. | making informed decisions. |

# Reflecting on Your Health

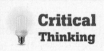
**Critical Thinking**

1. How do you feel about growing old? Are you undergoing the age-related changes that Table 15.1 describes? Which age-related changes trouble you the most? Are you making any lifestyle changes that will increase your chances of living a long and healthy life? If you answered yes to the previous question, what changes are you making, and how do you think they will affect your longevity?
2. If you suffered severe brain damage in an accident, would you want to be maintained in a persistent vegetative state? Why or why not? If so, for how long would you want to be kept alive? Why?
3. Do you intend to donate your organs if you die in an accident? Why or why not? Have you signed an organ donor card or the back of your driver's license, enabling survivors to donate your organs when you die? If you have not signed an organ donor card on the back of your license, explain why.
4. Have you ever known someone who knew he or she was dying? If so, describe any stages of Kübler-Ross's emotional responses to dying that you observed in that person.
5. If someone you loved has died, how did the grieving process affect your psychological, social, and spiritual health? What did you do to overcome the grief?

# References

1. Volz, M. (2011). World's oldest man dies in Montana at 114. *Associated Press*. Retrieved on May 29, 2011, from http://www.foxnews.com/us/2011/04/14/worlds-oldest-man-dies-age-114/
2. Colton, A. (2011, April). Survival skills: World's oldest man. *Men's Journal*, p. 126.
3. Flachsbart, F., et al. (2009). Association with FOXO3A variation with human longevity confirmed in German centenarians. *Proceedings of the National Academy of Sciences, 106*(8):2700–2705.
4. U.S. Census Bureau. (2011, March). Older Americans Month: May 2011. Retrieved on May 29, 2011, from http://www.census.gov/

newsroom/releases/archives/facts_for_features_special_editions/cb11-ff08.html

5. U.S. Census Bureau. (n.d.). *U.S. population projections.* Retrieved on May 29, 2011, from http://www.census.gov/population/www/projections/summarytables.html

6. Kahana, E., et al. (2002). Long-term impact of preventive proactivity on quality of life of the old-old. *Psychosomatic Medicine, 64*(3):382–394.

7. Kochanek, K. D., et al. (2011). Deaths: Preliminary data for 2009. *National Vital Statistics Reports, 59*(4):1–68. Retrieved on May 29, 2011, from http://www.cdc.gov/nchs/data/nvsr/nvsr59/nvsr59_04.pdf

8. U.S. Department of Health and Human Services. (1991). *Healthy People 2000: National health promotion and disease prevention objectives.* Washington, DC: U.S. Government Printing Office.

9. Centers for Disease Control and Prevention. (2010, December). Life expectancy free of chronic condition-induced activity limitations among white and black Americans, 2000–2006. *Vital and Health Statistics, 3*(34). Retrieved on May 29, 2011, from http://www.cdc.gov/nchs/data/series/sr_03/sr03_034.pdf

10. Department of Health and Human Services, Administration on Aging. (2011, February). A profile of older Americans: 2010. Retrieved on May 29, 2011, from http://www.aoa.gov/aoaroot/aging_statistics/Profile/2010/docs/2010profile.pdf

11. U.S. National Library of Medicine, National Eye Institute. (2011, May). Facts about age-related macular degeneration. Retrieved on May 29, 2011, from http://www.nei.nih.gov/health/maculardegen/armd_facts.asp

12. Centers for Disease Control and Prevention, Chronic Disease Prevention and Health Promotion. (2011, February). Arthritis: Meeting the challenge. *At a Glance* Retrieved on May 29, 2011, from http://www.cdc.gov/chronicdisease/resources/publications/aag/pdf/2011/Arthritis-AAG-2011-508.pdf

13. Alzheimer's Association. (2011, May 18). What is Alzheimer's? Retrieved on May 29, 2011, from http://www.alz.org/alzheimers_disease_what_is_alzheimers.asp#basics

14. Alzheimer's Association. (2011). 2011 Alzheimer's disease facts and figures. *Alzheimer's and Dementia, 7*(2):208–244. Retrieved on May 29, 2011, from http://www.alzheimersanddementia.com/article/PIIS1552526011000367/fulltext

15. National Institute on Aging. (2011, January). Looking for the causes of AD. Retrieved on May 30, 2011, from http://www.nia.nih.gov/Alzheimers/Publications/Unraveling/Part3/causes.htm

16. Gu, Y., et al. (2010). Food combination and Alzheimer's disease risk: A protective diet. *Archives of Neurology, 67*(6):699–706.

17. McGuinness, B., & Passmore, P. (2010). Can statins prevent or help treat Alzheimer's disease? *Journal of Alzheimer's Disease, 20*(3):925–933.

18. Ligthart, S. A., et al. (2010). Treatment of cardiovascular risk factors to prevent cognitive decline and dementia: A systematic review. *Vascular Health and Risk Management, 6*:775–785.

19. Lau, F. C., et al. (2007). Nutritional intervention in brain aging: Reducing the effects of inflammation and oxidative stress. *Subcellular Biochemistry, 42*:299–318.

20. Frank, B., & Gupta, S. (2005). A review of antioxidants and Alzheimer's disease. *Annals of Clinical Psychiatry, 17*(4):269–286.

21. Cole, G. M., et al. (2007). Neuroprotective effects of curcumin. *Advances in Experimental Medicine and Biology, 595*:197–212.

22. Evans, J. G., et al. (2004). Evidence-based pharmacotherapy of Alzheimer's disease. *International Journal of Neuropsychopharmacology, 7*(3):351–369.

23. Burns, A., et al. (2006). Clinical practice with anti-dementia drugs: A consensus statement from British Association for Psychopharmacology. *Journal of Psychopharmacology, 20*(6):732–755.

24. Dwyer, J., & Donoghue, M. D. (2010). Is risk of Alzheimer disease a reason to use dietary supplements? *American Journal of Clinical Nutrition, 91*(5):1155–1156.

25. Morris, M. C., et al. (2005). Relation of the tocopherol forms to incident Alzheimer disease and to cognitive change. *American Journal of Clinical Nutrition, 81*(2):508–514.

26. Centers for Disease Control and Prevention. (2009, September). National suicide statistics at a glance: Trends in suicide rates among both sexes, by age group, United States, 1991–2006. Retrieved on May 30, 2011, from http://www.cdc.gov/violenceprevention/suicide/statistics/trends02.html

27. Podgorski, C. A., et al. (2010). Suicide prevention for older adults in residential communities: Implications for policy and practice. *PLoS Medicine, 7*(5):e10000254.

28. Juurlink, D. N., et al. (2004). Medical illness and the risk of suicide in the elderly. *Archives of Internal Medicine, 164*(11):1179–1184.

29. Jeste, D. V., et al. (2010). Successful cognitive and emotional aging. *World Psychiatry, 9*(2):78–84.

30. Perls, T. T. (2010). Antiaging medicine: What should we tell our patients? *Aging Health, 6*(2):149–154.

31. Warburton, D. E., et al. (2006). Health benefits of physical activity: The evidence. *Canadian Medical Association Journal, 174*(6):801–809.

32. Larson, E. B., et al. (2006). Exercise is associated with reduced risk for incident dementia among persons 65 years of age and older. *Annals of Internal Medicine, 144*(2):73–81.

33. Kübler-Ross, E. (1969). *On death and dying.* New York: Macmillan.

34. Oregon Department of Human Services. (2011). *Death with Dignity Act annual reports.* 2010 Summary. Retrieved on May 28, 2011, from http://public.health.oregon.gov/ProviderPartnerResources/EvaluationResearch/DeathwithDignityAct/Documents/year13.pdf

35. United Network for Organ Sharing. (2011, May 31). Data: Waiting list candidates. Retrieved on May 31, 2011, from http://www.unos.org

36. U.S. Department of Health and Human Services, Health Resources and Services Administration, Organ Procurement and Transplant Network. (2011). Death removals by region by year. Retrieved on May 31, 2011, from http://optn.transplant.hrsa.gov/latestData/viewDataReports.asp

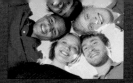
### Diversity in Health
Hunger, the Environment, and the World's Population

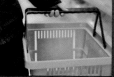
### Consumer Health
Carbon Monoxide Detectors: Are They Reliable?

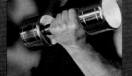
### Managing Your Health
Tips to Prevent Poisonings | Avoiding ELF Radiation | Reducing Pesticide Levels in the Food You Eat

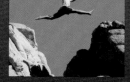
### Across the Life Span
Environmental Health

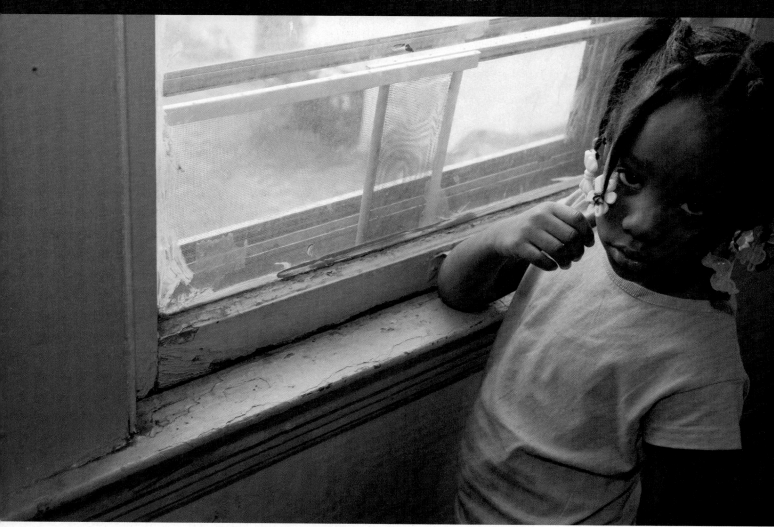

## Chapter Overview

Which types of poisoning are prevalent in the United States?

How to avoid poisoning in the home

Which toxic chemicals are prevalent in the workplace?

What factors contribute to indoor air pollution?

How water supplies become contaminated

Why air pollution is a threat to health

How noise pollution affects hearing

## Student Workbook

Self-Assessments: Poison Lookout Checklist | Checklist for the Prevention of Carbon Monoxide Poisoning

Changing Health Habits: Can You Reduce Environmental Threats to Your Health?

## Do You Know?

If you work or go to school in a "sick" building?

If you are in danger of pesticide poisoning?

If your house or apartment is painted with lead-based products?

# CHAPTER 16

# Environmental Health

zarcon, greta, litargirio, and pay-loo-ah ... if you have Hispanic or Asian ancestry, the names of one or more of these traditional ethnic remedies may be familiar to you. Greta and azarcon are Mexican remedies for empacho, a colicky digestive disorder. Pay-loo-ah is a Southeast Asian tonic for rash or fever. All three are fine powders and may be given as a tea, or a pinch may be added to a baby's bottle. They also can be mixed with milk or sugar and administered by teaspoon. Litargirio is used as an antiperspirant/deodorant and as a folk remedy for burns and fungal infections of the feet. Family members who rely on folk medicine give these remedies regularly to children.

*"[One way] in which U.S. children are poisoned by lead... by eating lead-based paint chips..."*

Many folk remedies contain substances that are useful in medical practice. In fact, pharmaceutical companies often start looking for new drugs by chemically analyzing the herbs and other plants used in many traditional folk remedies that have been part of a culture for generations. However, some remedies, like those mentioned above, can cause harm. Azarcon, greta, litargirio, and pay-loo-ah all contain high levels of lead. Even seemingly harmless over-the-counter herbal dietary supplements have been found to be associated with high lead levels in women. Some Ayurvedic "medications" contain lead as well.[1-4] Ayurveda (AH-yer-VAY-da) is a type of traditional or folk medicine practiced in India and other South Asian countries.

**environmental health** The effects of environmental factors on humans and the effects of humans on their environments.

**ozone holes** Depleted areas of the ozone ($O_3$) layer in the upper atmosphere.

**municipal solid waste** Nonhazardous refuse generally collected from homes and offices.

**toxic chemicals** Poisonous substances present in the home, workplace, or outdoor environments that affect human health.

**toxicity** (tok-SIH-si-tea) Poisonous quality.

Lead is only one of the many substances in our environment that can cause serious illness. The major ways in which U.S. children are poisoned by lead are by eating lead-based paint chips and by inhaling lead particles in contaminated dust or soil.[5] In adults in the United States, about 95% of lead poisoning occurs from occupational exposure, such as the mining and smelting of lead ore, the manufacture of batteries, and construction work involving lead-based products.[6] Nonetheless, folk remedies containing lead, and lead-based paints and other products in the home, pose a serious health risk for both children and adults.

The study of the effects of environmental factors on humans and the effects of humans on their environments is called **environmental health**. People often affect the environment in ways that later influence their health. For example, people emitted chlorofluorocarbons (CFCs) into the atmosphere when they used certain spray can propellants prior to their being banned in 1979. CFCs contribute to the depletion of the ozone layer in the upper atmosphere. These depleted areas are commonly referred to as **ozone holes**. The upper atmospheric ozone layer protects people from some of the sun's harmful ultraviolet (UV) radiation, which can cause skin cancer. (Chapter 13 discusses the relationship between UV radiation and skin cancer.) Many automobile air conditioners still contain chemicals harmful to the ozone layer. In another example, people in industrialized countries such as the United States produce millions of tons of **municipal solid waste** per year—all of those items that trash collectors pick up from homes and offices each week. This waste is usually placed in landfills. Along with running out of space for this trash, a problem with landfills is that chemicals may seep into the ground from these massive waste sites and pollute water supplies. We discuss water pollution from various sources later in this chapter.

Many **toxic chemicals** present in the home, workplace, or outdoor environments affect human health. They may be in the form of dusts, fumes, particles, or liquids and are found in a wide variety of substances, such as household products, plants, products manufactured or used in the workplace, and prescription and illegal drugs. (The adverse effects of drug abuse are described in Chapter 7, and of alcohol abuse in Chapter 8. The hazardous substances in tobacco products are also discussed in Chapter 8.) Additionally, toxic chemicals are present in the air we breathe and the water we drink.

Toxic chemicals result in poisoning, or **toxicity**, which damages body tissues and affects bodily functioning in various ways. Toxins may affect chemical reactions of the body. They may also hinder the normal functioning of body cells. Additionally, toxins may cause cells in the body to release chemicals that may have an adverse effect on certain body structures. The consequences of these effects are a variety of conditions such as dermatitis (inflammation of the skin), asthma, lung disease, and immune system disorders.

## Environmental Health in and Around the Home

### Poisoning

The Toxic Exposure Surveillance System (TESS) is composed of participating poison centers that report on human poisoning incidents. Begun in 1983, TESS grew from 16 participating centers to a high of 73 centers in 1991; in 2009, TESS was made up of 60 centers. TESS data are compiled by the American Association of Poison Control Centers (AAPCC). Because the number of centers composing TESS has changed from year to year, the data from 1983 to the present cannot be used to determine a trend in human poisoning incidents. TESS reported that there were nearly 2.5 million human poisonings in 2009.[7]

Most human poisonings in 2009—about 91%—occurred in the home. About 1.5% occurred in workplaces, 1.3% in schools, and less than 1% each in healthcare facilities and restaurants. Approximately 82% of poisonings were unintentional, which included medication errors, bites and stings, food poisonings, and occupational mishaps. Fourteen percent were intentional and included suicides and drug abuse. The remaining 4% or so were to the result of causes such as malicious intent and adverse reactions to drugs or food.[7]

## Table 16.1

### Substances Most Frequently Involved in Pediatric (≤ 5 years) Exposures (Top 25)*

| Substance Category | Number | %⁺ |
|---|---|---|
| Cosmetics/personal care products | 174,073 | 12.97 |
| Analgesics | 130,213 | 9.70 |
| Cleaning substances (household) | 125,394 | 9.34 |
| Foreign bodies/toys/miscellaneous | 93,574 | 6.97 |
| Topical preparations | 91,127 | 6.79 |
| Vitamins | 53,717 | 4.00 |
| Antihistamines | 48,046 | 3.58 |
| Cold and cough preparations | 45,033 | 3.36 |
| Pesticides | 41,882 | 3.12 |
| Plants | 39,771 | 2.96 |
| Gastrointestinal preparations | 38,615 | 2.88 |
| Antimicrobials | 37,009 | 2.76 |
| Arts/crafts/office supplies | 27,241 | 2.03 |
| Alcohols | 27,087 | 2.02 |
| Hormones and hormone antagonists | 26,729 | 1.99 |
| Cardiovascular drugs | 26,566 | 1.98 |
| Electrolytes and minerals | 24,389 | 1.82 |
| Deodorizers | 22,851 | 1.70 |
| Dietary supplements/herbals/homeopathic | 20,897 | 1.56 |
| Sedative/hypnotics/antipsychotics | 16,258 | 1.21 |
| Other/unknown nondrug substances | 15,290 | 1.14 |
| Hydrocarbons | 14,798 | 1.10 |
| Asthma therapies | 14,671 | 1.09 |
| Antidepressants | 14,310 | 1.07 |
| Information calls | 12,726 | 0.95 |

*Includes all children with actual or estimated ages ≤5 years old. Results do not include "Unknown Child" or "Unknown Age."

⁺Percentages are based on the total number of substances reported in pediatric exposures (1,341,999).

*Source:* Bronstein, A. C., et al. (2010, December). 2009 annual report of the American Association of Poison Control Centers' National Poison Data System (NPDS): 27th annual report. *Clinical Toxicology, 48*:979–1178.

Only about 0.06% of all human poisoning incidents in 2009 were fatal. Ninety-one percent of poisoning fatalities occurred in adults aged 20 years and older.[7] Nonfatal poisonings are most often caused by the ingestion of household products and over-the-counter or prescription drugs. In 2009, they occurred in children younger than the age of 6 years approximately 68% of the time.[6] **Table 16.1** lists the substances most frequently involved in the poisoning of children younger than 6 years. **Table 16.2** lists

## Table 16.2

### Frequently Ingested Products by Children (≤ 5 years) That Are Usually Nontoxic

| | |
|---|---|
| Antacids | Hand dishwashing detergents |
| Antibiotics | Hydrogen peroxide (3%) |
| Baby oil | Lotions |
| Ballpoint pen ink | Noncoloring shampoos |
| Bath oil | Paint (latex) |
| Bubble bath | Pencil graphite |
| Calamine lotion | Perfume |
| Candles | Petroleum jelly |
| Chalk | Play-Doh |
| Clay (modeling) | Poinsettia (*Euphorbia pulcherrima*) |
| Conditioners | Shaving cream |
| Cosmetics | Silica or charcoal dehumidifying packets |
| Crayons | Soaps |
| Deodorants | Toothpaste |
| Deodorizers | Topical steroids (e.g., hydrocortisone cream) |
| Diaper rash products | Vitamins |
| Etch-A-Sketch | Water colors |
| Fabric softener | Water-based paints |
| Furniture polish | White glue |

Note: Some of these products, although considered nontoxic, may present a choking hazard.

*Sources:* Muller, A. A. (2005). Common nontoxic pediatric ingestions. *Journal of Emergency Nursing, 31*(5):494–496; Mofenson, H. C., et al. (1984). Ingestions considered nontoxic. *Clinics in Laboratory Medicine, 4*(3):587–602

## Figure 16.1

**The Path of Toxic Substances Through the Body.** The body absorbs toxic substances via the digestive system if they are ingested or via the respiratory system if they are inhaled. Some toxic substances can be absorbed through the skin. Once in the body, toxic substances reach the blood and lymph, which brings them to all the cells. Body cells (principally the liver) metabolize toxins; the products of metabolism are stored or excreted.

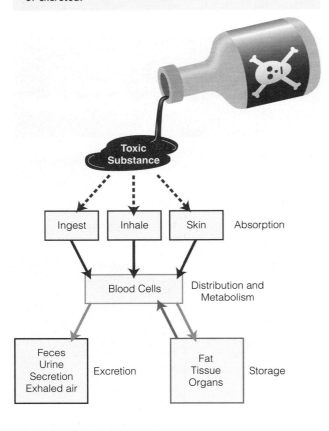

substances that are usually not toxic. See the self-assessment "Poison Lookout Checklist" in the Student Workbook pages at the end of this text to determine whether your home is free of substances that can lead to poisoning.

Unless a child or adult is observed ingesting a toxic substance, it may be difficult to determine whether he or she is poisoned. Poisoning does not always start the moment exposure occurs. Also, symptoms vary depending on the substance and how it entered the body, which can occur by ingestion, inhalation, or skin contact (**Figure 16.1**).

Suspect poisoning in a person who becomes suddenly ill with symptoms that affect many systems of the body, appears drowsy and indifferent, or exhibits bizarre behavior. Also, consider poisoning as a possibility in children or young adults with chest pain; they may have ingested poison or an overdose of drugs. If poisoning may have occurred, call the local poison control center immediately. If the suspected poisoning victim is experiencing severe symptoms such as unconsciousness, seizures, intense chest pain, or repeated vomiting, he or she should be rushed to the emergency room of the closest hospital. Follow the tips in the following Managing Your Health box titled "Tips to Prevent Poisonings" to lessen the chances of being accidentally poisoned.

**Toxic Plants** Toxic (poisonous) plants can be the source of poisoning emergencies, especially in children. A wide variety of plants have parts that are poisonous and parts that are not. For example, tomatoes are not poisonous, but the stems and leaves of tomato plants are. Some common plant parts that are poisonous include holly berries, morning glory seeds, narcissus and daffodil bulbs, rhubarb leaves, and sweet pea seeds. The entire hemlock, jimson weed, dieffenbachia, philodendron, and mountain laurel plants are poisonous. Some plants are so poisonous that drinking the water from a vase in which their cut flowers were kept can result in poisoning.

Although many plants are not poisonous—including the poinsettia, which for years has been inaccurately reported to be toxic—house plants and cut flowers should be kept out of reach of children younger than 5 years old, and all children should be instructed that eating house and yard plants can make them sick. Many plants, such as the poinsettia, may be highly irritating when ingested, even if they are not poisonous. If a child ingests a plant, call the local poison control center and describe the plant, where it was growing, and what part of the plant the child ate. If possible, take a leaf from the plant for identification when seeking emergency medical treatment. Only plant experts should rely on their knowledge of whether the plant is poisonous.

In addition to plants, approximately 1% to 2% of mushroom species are poisonous. (Mushrooms are not plants, but fungi.) One type of mushroom is so poisonous that eating one-third of its cap can be lethal.

Symptoms of mushroom poisoning may occur immediately after ingestion and may include increased salivation, tearing, increased urination, diarrhea, difficulty breathing, and an abnormal heartbeat. Other mushroom species have toxins that produce symptoms 12 to 24 hours after ingestion that include headache, jaundice (a yellowish cast to the skin),

# Managing Your Health

## Tips to Prevent Poisonings

*Keep Young Children Safe*

- Keep all drugs in medicine cabinets or other child-proof cabinets that young children cannot reach.
- Never call medicine "candy" when giving medicine to children.
- Be aware of any legal or illegal drugs that guests may bring into your home. Do not let guests leave drugs where children can find them, for example, in a pillbox, purse, backpack, or coat pocket.
- When you take medicines yourself, do not put your next dose on the counter or table where children can reach them.
- Never leave children alone with household products or drugs. If you have to do something else while using chemical products or taking medicine, such as answer the phone, take any young children with you.
- Do not leave household products out after using them. Return the products to a childproof cabinet as soon as you are done with them.
- Identify poisonous plants in your house and yard and place them out of reach of children or remove them.

*Drugs and Medicines*

- Follow directions on the label when you give or take medicines. Read all warning labels. Some medicines cannot be taken safely when you take other medicines or drink alcohol.

- Turn on a light when you give or take medicines at night so that you know you have the correct amount of the right medicine.
- Keep medicines in their original bottles or containers.
- Never share or sell your prescription drugs.
- Keep opioid pain medications, such as methadone, hydrocodone, and oxycodone, in a safe place that can be reached only by people who take or give them.

*Household Chemicals*

- Always read the label before using a product that may be poisonous.
- Keep chemical products in their original bottles or containers. Do not use food containers to store chemical products.
- Never mix household products together. For example, mixing bleach and ammonia can result in toxic gases.
- Wear protective clothing (gloves, long sleeves, long pants, socks, shoes) if you spray pesticides or other chemicals.
- Turn on the fan and open windows when using chemical products such as household cleaners.

*Source:* Adapted from Department of Health and Human Services, Centers for Disease Control and Prevention. (2011, March). Tips to prevent poisonings. Retrieved on October 17, 2011, from http://www.cdc.gov/homeandrecreationalsafety/poisoning/preventiontips.htm.

---

confusion, convulsions, and possible coma. Because poisonous mushrooms can be lethal or cause severe poisoning, do not eat any mushrooms that you find growing wild. Only a person trained in mushroom identification should attempt to distinguish between mushrooms that are safe to eat and those that are not.

**Ingestion of Household Cleaning Aids, Medications, and Vitamins** Children younger than the age of 5 years are most in danger of being poisoned from household cleaning aids and from over-the-counter and prescription drugs and vitamins. The Federal Hazardous Substances Act, passed into law by the Consumer Product Safety Commission in 1966, has been helpful in lowering the incidence of poisoning in children by controlling the concentration of toxic chemicals in household products. The Poison Pre-

vention Packaging Act of 1972 established standards for the packaging of potentially harmful household products and medications by requiring child-resistant caps and packaging on products that present a serious danger to children. The intent of this packaging is to make it difficult for children to open toxic substances so that adults will discover their attempts before they are successful. The use of blister packs in which pills are individually encased is another approach to lessen a child's ability to remove pills from packaging.

Although warning stickers such as Mr. Yuk (**Figure 16.2**) are available for placing on hazardous substances, the results of research suggest that their use does not lower the incidence of poisoning in children.[8] Additionally, children and adults do not view the facial expression of disgust, which Mr. Yuk portrays,

**Figure 16.2**

**Poison Prevention Symbols.** The skull and crossbones used to be the traditional warning symbol of poison, but the symbol was and is used to denote fun things like pirates and adventure. Therefore, Mr. Yuk (left) was developed as a warning label in the early 1970s. Using these labels on toxic substances are unrelieable deterrents, however. Lock all toxic substances in cabinets, away from children.

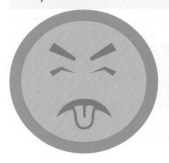

as precautionary; a facial expression of fear might be more appropriate as a deterrent.[9] Because child-resistant packaging can be opened by children (although with difficulty) and because warning stickers do not appear to discourage children from investigating package contents, all dangerous household substances, including medications and cleaning aids, should be locked in cabinets. Special child-proof locks are available that enable an adult to open a cabinet easily but bar the child from doing so. Placing items on high shelves is not a good substitute and is not safe; children easily stack items and climb on them to reach these substances.

Never suggest to a child that any medication or vitamin pill is candy because the child will seek out the pills at another time. Additionally, never take medication or vitamins in front of a young child who may think that it is candy or food and try to do the same.

Children rarely become poisoned by vitamins and mineral supplements in the amounts they accidentally consume (see Table 16.2), but adults become poisoned by intentional overdose. Megadosing with vitamins (taking much greater amounts than that recommended per day) has become a popular practice but may cause health problems. Vitamin overdosing in adults most often occurs with vitamins A and D, two fat-soluble vitamins that are readily stored in the body. Daily overdoses of most fat-soluble vitamins build up, resulting in chronic intoxication. Daily doses of 3 to 10 times the recommended amount of vitamin A over a few months to a few years produce

toxic symptoms. Accutane, a form of vitamin A taken to treat skin conditions, can cause vitamin A toxicity when taken by mouth. Daily doses of 10 times the recommended amount of vitamin D over 6 months to a year produce toxic symptoms as well. Minerals that most commonly cause poisoning are iron, selenium, and zinc. Chapter 9 discusses vitamins and minerals and their roles in the body in more detail. Table 9.8 lists vitamin toxicity symptoms and Table 9.10 lists mineral toxicity symptoms.

**Lead Poisoning** **Lead poisoning** is still a health problem in children in the United States even though many sources of lead poisoning have been eliminated in this country: leaded gasoline, leaded solder in food and soft drink cans, and leaded paint. (Solder is a metal that is heated and then used, when soft, to join other metals. It hardens on cooling and makes the joint solid.)

Even though many sources of lead have been removed from the environment, leaded dangers still exist. Ceramicware that is poorly made can have very high levels of leaching lead (that is, lead that dissolves out of the dishes and passes into food). Car batteries contain lead and should be brought to collection centers for proper disposal or recycling. Some pipes that bring water to homes contain lead-based solder. Additionally, the soil surrounding roads and highways often contains lead from years-past auto emissions.

Houses and apartments built before 1978 were often painted with lead-based paint. Although layers of nonleaded paint may cover leaded paint, the top coats of paint can chip. The exposed leaded paint creates leaded dust that may be inhaled, or the leaded paint may chip and children may eat it. Leaded paint on the exterior of homes and apartments often contaminates the surrounding soil in which children may play.

Decorating techniques that use old, salvaged building components, such as old doors, and old decorative items, such as distressed-looking old furniture, old dishes, and old toys, can be a lead health hazard.[10] Additionally many cases of lead poisoning occur when older homes are remodeled without attention to the containment of leaded dust and paint chips. When doing such work, use a high-efficiency particulate air filter–equipped vacuum cleaner, properly fitted respirators, wet sanding equipment, and protective clothing (**Figure 16.3**). Seal off work areas with heavy-duty polyethylene plastic sheeting, and keep all nonworkers away from the area.

Lead poisoning is serious because it affects the central nervous system and can cause coma, convul-

## Figure 16.3

**Lead Paint Removal.** These experts are removing lead paint from an old home in Providence, Rhode Island. They are using a specialized vacuum cleaner and are wearing protective clothing and respirators.

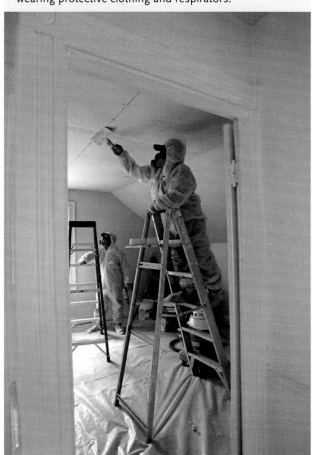

**lead poisoning** A toxic condition that affects the central nervous system, caused by the ingestion or inhalation of the metallic element lead.

**carbon monoxide poisoning** A toxic condition that affects red blood cells' ability to carry oxygen, caused by the inhalation of the gas carbon monoxide.

sions, and even death. Today, deaths resulting from lead poisoning are rare in the United States. Nonetheless, many children are severely affected by this toxin. Whereas adults absorb about 11% of lead reaching the digestive tract, children absorb from 30% to 75%. When lead is inhaled, up to 50% is absorbed.[11]

Low levels of lead in the blood (10 micrograms per deciliter [mg/dl]) are associated with decreased intelligence, learning disabilities, impaired development of the nervous system, and delayed or stunted growth. Behavioral disorders also have been linked to lead poisoning. At slightly higher levels of lead poisoning, the body does not metabolize certain vitamins properly or manufacture red blood cells correctly.

A child with high blood levels of lead (70 mg/dl) will show some of the following symptoms: decreased appetite, vomiting, abdominal pain, consti-

pation, drowsiness, and indifference. Children who have even higher blood levels will exhibit some of the signs and symptoms of degenerative brain disease: coma, seizures, bizarre behavior, impaired muscular coordination, and vomiting. Either situation is a medical emergency and the child should be hospitalized. Tests should be performed to determine the child's lead blood level, and medications will be administered to reduce that level. However, the most important therapy is removing sources of lead from the child's environment. Call the National Lead Information Center at 1-800-424-LEAD for more information on how to avoid lead poisoning or visit its website at www.epa.gov/lead/.

**Carbon Monoxide Poisoning** Carbon monoxide (CO) is a colorless, odorless, tasteless gas that can kill. In fact, unintentional CO poisoning from nonautomotive sources causes about 170 deaths in the United States per year.[12] Carbon monoxide is produced by the incomplete combustion of carbon-containing fuels such as oil, coal, wood, natural gas, charcoal, and gasoline. Fires are a major source of **carbon monoxide poisoning**; persons caught in a fire often die from inhaling carbon monoxide and other toxic gases rather than from the fire. Firefighters also are at risk for carbon monoxide poisoning. Other primary sources of carbon monoxide poisoning are automobile exhaust, malfunctioning furnaces, charcoal fires, gasoline-powered tools, wood stoves, fireplaces, unvented kerosene and gas space heaters, gas cooking stoves and ovens, and tobacco smoking. See the self-assessment "Checklist for the Prevention of Carbon Monoxide Poisoning" in the Student Workbook pages at the end of this text to determine whether your home, auto, cabin, or camper is as safe as it can be.

The proper maintenance and use of tools and appliances that burn fuel cuts down on the amount of CO they produce; these levels are usually not hazardous. Improper maintenance and incorrect use often result in dangerous levels of CO. To protect against these dangers, be certain that home heating stoves or furnaces are vented properly and are inspected regularly for carbon monoxide leakage. Use charcoal grills and gas-powered tools only in well-ventilated areas. (Don't use your charcoal grill in your garage or

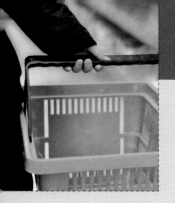

# Consumer Health

## Carbon Monoxide Detectors: Are They Reliable?

Carbon monoxide (CO) detectors should be thought of only as a backup to proper use and maintenance of fuel-burning appliances. The technology of these detectors is still developing, and a variety of types is available for home use. However, none is considered to be as reliable as home smoke detectors.

The U.S. Environmental Protection Agency reports that CO detectors have been laboratory tested with varying results. Some performed well, others failed to alarm at high CO levels, and still others alarmed at low levels that do not pose an immediate health risk. Because CO is invisible and odorless, it is hard to tell if an alarm is false or a real emergency.

When purchasing a CO detector, research the features of various models and brands and use this knowledge, not the price, as your basis for selection. Carefully follow the manufacturer's instructions for its placement, use, and maintenance. CO detectors have an average life span of approximately 2 years, after which they should be replaced. If your CO detector goes off:

- Make certain it is the CO detector alarm and not the smoke detector alarm.
- Seek medical help for anyone experiencing CO poisoning symptoms.
- Ventilate the home with fresh air and turn off all potential sources of CO.
- Have a qualified technician inspect all fuel-burning appliances and chimneys to make sure they are operating correctly and that there is nothing blocking fumes from being vented.

*Source:* Adapted from U.S. Environmental Protection Agency, Indoor Environments Division, Office of Air and Radiation. (2010, September 30). Protect your family and yourself from carbon monoxide poisoning (EPA-402-F-96-005). Retrieved on May 11, 2011, from http://www.epa.gov/iaq/pubs/coftsht.html.

---

in a tent while camping.) Additionally, do not leave a car running in an attached garage where fumes can leak into the house. Run the car engine outdoors only. Carbon monoxide can also leak into a car if the exhaust system is faulty.

Carbon monoxide sensors are available for home use. These products are designed to sound an alarm when indoor air contains dangerously high levels of this toxin. Research results show that the use of carbon monoxide detectors could reduce by half the number of unintentional deaths by CO poisoning in the home. (See the Consumer Health box "Carbon Monoxide Detectors: Are They Reliable?")

Carbon monoxide kills because it binds to the oxygen-carrying molecule hemoglobin in the bloodstream. When CO is bound to hemoglobin, oxygen cannot bind and the person dies of suffocation. Before carbon monoxide poisoning kills, however, it produces signs and symptoms that become more severe as blood levels of this gas increase. At first, a person may have a slight headache that worsens as blood levels rise. (This level of poisoning can even occur if you jog near rush-hour traffic.) Fatigue sets in and the poison victim may become dizzy. As the poisoning continues, nausea, vomiting, a cherry-red skin color, and blurry vision result. Eventually the person collapses, may have convulsions, and dies.

Carbon monoxide poisoning is an emergency; immediately get the victim to fresh air and seek medical help. Healthcare practitioners treat CO poisoning victims with oxygen and test them for other medical problems that may have occurred at the time of the poisoning (such as a blow to the head in a fall). In some circumstances, the poisoning victim is placed in a hyperbaric (pressure) chamber and administered oxygen.

## Inhalation of Asbestos Fibers

Asbestos is a fiber-like mineral that resists damage by fire and other natural processes. Because of these qualities, asbestos has been used in the manufacture of products exposed to fire, such as stoves, furnaces, and appliances; insulation in walls and ceilings; insulation surrounding pipes; patching compounds and textured paints (as a binding compound and texturizer); roofing and siding materials; and vinyl flooring (as a strengthener).

Asbestos-containing products came into use beginning in the 1920s, but by the early 1970s scientists discovered that long-term inhalation of microscopic asbestos fibers can result in asbestosis as well as cancer of the lungs and stomach. During **asbestosis**, scar tissue forms in the lungs as a response to irritation by asbestos fibers. The patient experiences shortness of breath, which progresses to a fatal lack of oxygen or heart failure. Because of the danger that asbestos exposure poses to humans, the U.S. Environmental Protection Agency (EPA) banned the use of various asbestos-containing products during the 1970s and 1980s. In 1989, the EPA announced a ban on all asbestos products by 1996.

Aside from the danger to those who mine asbestos, those in primary danger of asbestos exposure are people who live in homes built between 1920 and 1978. Various asbestos products were developed at different times during those years and were used in home construction. Asbestos was also widely used in schools built between 1950 and 1973. Intact asbestos products do not pose a hazard. Danger exists when asbestos fibers are released from the products of which they were a part and become airborne. Asbestos fibers are released from products that are deteriorating; banged, rubbed, or handled frequently; or disturbed during home remodeling. Asbestos fibers are also released when asbestos-containing flooring is sanded or seriously damaged.

To protect against the inhalation of asbestos fibers, avoid disturbing this material. Do not vacuum particles that may be asbestos-laden; vacuuming them releases microscopic asbestos fibers that are inhaled. If possible, contact the contractor who built the home to determine whether asbestos was used. If this is not possible, contact a certified professional trained in asbestos removal and repair to determine whether the home contains asbestos. Sometimes materials must be sent to a laboratory to assess their content. If so, use a laboratory accredited to perform asbestos analysis. If removal, repair, or sealing of the material is necessary, hire only trained, certified personnel who can do this job safely and properly.

## Electromagnetic Radiation

Are computer screens, television sets, electric blankets, microwave ovens, cell phones, or electric appliances health hazards? Are people putting their health at risk if they live near high-power electric lines or electrical distribution substations? A variety of studies has been conducted regarding the effects on the body of extremely low frequency (ELF) radiation, which is emitted by some of these sources. ELF radiation has been associated with negative effects such as risk of cancer, DNA damage, and changes in human brain electrical activity. So far, however, most

**asbestosis** (AS-bes-TOE-sis) A condition in which scar tissue forms in the lungs as a response to irritation by asbestos.

scientists see no major negative effects and no reason to recommend extreme caution.[13,14] However, taking reasonable preventive measures against undue exposure may be prudent.

Extremely low frequency radiation is a type of *electromagnetic radiation*—electric and magnetic fields of energy that travel at the speed of light through the atmosphere. Sunlight, for example, is electromagnetic energy. Other forms of electromagnetic radiation include x-rays, ultraviolet light, infrared light, and radio waves.

The electric fields of extremely low frequency radiation are not as potentially problematic as are their magnetic fields. Although the strength of both the electric and magnetic fields decreases dramatically and quickly as a person moves away from the source, magnetic fields penetrate the walls of buildings that electric fields cannot.

Cathode ray tube (CRT) televisions and computer monitors produce radiation that spans the electromagnetic spectrum from x-rays to radio waves. However, they were manufactured with protective shielding to prevent most of the radiation from escaping. The small amount that does escape results in electric and magnetic fields in the atmosphere surrounding the user, but the level of radiation where the user sits is well below occupational and exposure limits recommended by governmental and industrial safety standards. CRT televisions and computer monitors are no longer manufactured. Liquid-crystal displays (LCDs) and plasma screens do not emit ELF radiation.

Cell phones and microwave ovens emit a form of electromagnetic radiation called nonionizing radiofrequency (RF) energy. RF energy is not able to break bonds in DNA—the hereditary material—so it cannot cause cancer in that way. However, at high enough levels, RF energy can heat living tissue; this is the principle used in microwave cooking. A person using a microwave often stands away from the oven, and results of studies show that radiation exposure from microwaves during regular use is unlikely to be harmful.

The heat generated by cell phones is small in comparison to that generated by microwave ovens. A cell phone's main source of RF energy is its antenna, which is part of the body of the phone. The closer

The following abstract is from an online environmental health journal, written to inform the general public about research and current thinking on cell phone use and cancer. Explain why you think this abstract is a reliable or an unreliable source of information. Use the model for analyzing health information to guide your thinking; the main points of the model are noted at the end of this abstract. The model is fully explained in Chapter 1.

# Mobile Phones, Brain Tumors, and the Interphone Study: Where Are We Now?

**Anthony J. Swerdlow[1], Maria Feychting[2], Adele C. Green[3,4], Leeka Kheifets[5], and David A. Savitz[6,7], International Commission for Non-Ionizing Radiation Protection Standing Committee on Epidemiology**

[1]Section of Epidemiology, Institute of Cancer Research, Sutton, United Kingdom
[2]Karolinska Institutet, Institute of Environmental Medicine, Stockholm, Sweden
[3]Cancer and Population Studies Unit, Queensland Institute of Medical Research, Brisbane, Australia
[4]School of Translational Medicine, University of Manchester, Manchester, United Kingdom
[5]Department of Epidemiology, University of California at Los Angeles, Los Angeles, California, USA
[6]Department of Community Health
[7]Department of Obstetrics and Gynecology, Brown University, Providence, Rhode Island, USA

## Abstract

### Background

In the past 15 years, mobile telephone use has evolved from an uncommon activity to one with > 4.6 billion subscriptions worldwide. However, there is public concern about the possibility that mobile phones might cause cancer, especially brain tumors.

### Objectives

We reviewed the evidence on whether mobile phone use raises the risk of the main types of brain tumor—glioma and meningioma—with a particular focus on the recent publication of the largest epidemiologic study yet: the 13-country Interphone Study.

the phone (and therefore the antenna) is to the user's head, the higher the user's exposure to the phone's RF energy. Cell phones (and lower-energy cordless home phones) with antennas mounted away from the user are considered safe.

In recent years, many studies and reviews have been conducted regarding cell phone use and an increased risk of cancer or other adverse health effects.

The American Cancer Society has summarized research results with this statement:

*Most studies published so far have not found a link between cell phone use and the development of tumors. However, these studies have had some important limitations that make them unlikely to end the controversy about whether cell phone use affects cancer risk.*[15]

*Discussion*

Methodological deficits limit the conclusions that can be drawn from the Interphone study, but its results, along with those from other epidemiologic, biological, and animal studies and brain tumor incidence trends, suggest that within about 10–15 years after first use of mobile phones there is unlikely to be a material increase in the risk of brain tumors in adults.

Data for childhood tumors and for periods beyond 15 years are currently lacking.

*Conclusions*

Although there remains some uncertainty, the trend in the accumulating evidence is increasingly against the hypothesis that mobile phone use can cause brain tumors in adults.

1. Which statements are verifiable facts, and which are unverified statements or value claims?
2. What are the credentials of the researchers/journal abstract making these health-related claims? Do the researchers/journal abstract have the appropriate background and education in the topic area? What can you do to check the credentials of this source?
3. What might be the motives and biases of the researchers/journal abstract making the claims?
4. What is the main point of the abstract? Which information is relevant to the issue, main point, product, or service? Which information is irrelevant?
5. Are the researchers/journal abstract reliable? What evidence supports your conclusion that the source is reliable or unreliable? Do the researchers/journal abstract present the pros and cons of the topic or the benefits and risks of the product?
6. Do the researchers/journal abstract attack the credibility of conventional scientists or medical authorities?

Based on your analysis, do you think that this abstract is a reliable source of health-related information? Summarize your reasons for coming to this conclusion.

Source: Swerdlow AJ, Feychting M, Green AC, Kheifets L, Savitz DA. International Commission for Non-Ionizing Radiation Protection Standing Committee on Epidemiology 2011. Mobile Phones, Brain Tumors, and the Interphone Study: Where Are We Now? *Environmental Health Perspectives* 119:1534-1538. http://dx.doi.org/10.1289/ehp.1103693

The World Health Organization's International Agency for Research on Cancer (IARC) in a May 31, 2011, press release revealed that it had "classified radiofrequency electromagnetic fields as possibly carcinogenic [cancer-causing] to humans … based on an increased risk for glioma, a malignant type of brain cancer, associated with wireless phone use." The many sources of data that the IARC reviewed suggest a 40% increase in risk for glioma in heavy cell phone users, defined as an average of 30 minutes per day for 10 years. The IARC concludes that further research was needed to clarify links between cancer risk and cell phone use.[16]

To decrease your risk of these adverse health effects, put distance between yourself and your cell phone; RF exposure decreases rapidly with increas-

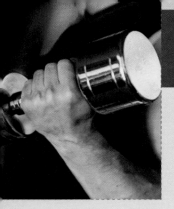

## Avoiding ELF Radiation

- Do not sleep or sit for a long time near electric devices, particularly those with motors.
- Sit a minimum of 18 inches (at arm's length) from your CRT computer screen.
- Turn off your CRT computer monitor when it is not being used.
- Sit several feet away from the back or sides of a CRT computer monitor or television. Follow this rule even if the TV or monitor is in another room; magnetic fields travel through walls.
- Adults and especially children should sit several feet away from a CRT television screen.
- Turn on your waterbed heater or electric blanket before going to bed. Unplug them when you get into bed.
- Use a mobile phone in the car with an antenna located outside the vehicle, or use a cell phone with a headset.

---

ing distance from the source. Thus, use a headset or earpieces and carry the phone away from your body, or use a cell phone connected to a remote antenna. Household cordless phones operate at lower power levels and do not appear to have these adverse health effects. The Analyzing Health-Related Information activity in this chapter contains an article that discusses the results of research on the cancer–cell phone link.

Regarding exposure to ELF radiation of all types, medical researchers have adopted the position of "prudent avoidance" until research data indicate that another course of action should be taken. The Managing Your Health box titled "Avoiding ELF Radiation" gives some tips.

### Healthy Living Practices

- ☐ Teach children not to ingest house or yard plants because they may be poisonous. In homes with young children, substitute safe plants for poisonous ones.
- ☐ Teach children not to ingest house or yard plants because they may be poisonous. In homes with young children, substitute safe plants for poisonous ones.
- ☐ Eat only mushrooms that you are certain are nonpoisonous.
- ☐ In homes with small children, store all dangerous household substances, including medications and cleaning aids, in locked cabinets.

- ☐ Never suggest to a child that medications or vitamin pills are candy.
- ☐ Do not take large doses of fat-soluble vitamins except under the direction of a physician.
- ☐ If you live in a house or apartment built before 1978, be certain that children do not ingest peeling paint. Consult a professional to test for lead, and, if lead is present, to minimize its release into the home.
- ☐ To avoid carbon monoxide poisoning, maintain and use fuel-burning tools and appliances properly, be certain that heating stoves and furnaces are correctly vented, and warm up the car outside rather than in the garage.
- ☐ Seek medical assistance immediately for anyone who exhibits symptoms of carbon monoxide poisoning.
- ☐ Do not disturb asbestos that is deteriorating.
- ☐ Seek professional help for asbestos cleanup.
- ☐ Avoid exposure to ELF radiation.

## Irradiation of Food

Many types of organisms contaminate the food supply. *E. coli* (a common intestinal bacterium) can be found in such foods as hamburger and unpasteurized apple juice. A particularly deadly strain of *E. coli* (O157:H7) has caused illness and death. *Salmonella* bacteria are common contaminants of poultry. Certain insects and their larvae contaminate wheat and wheat flour. A wide range of organisms cause not only foodborne illness but the spoilage of food.

One method of killing organisms in food is irradiation; that is, treating food with radiation. Radiation is the emission of energy by the unstable nuclei of certain atoms in the form of rays or waves. Food is irradiated in its packaging by either exposing it to gamma (g) rays (a form of electromagnetic radiation similar to x-rays) or to high-energy electron beams produced by electron accelerators. Radiation is harmful to living tissue, so it kills living organisms in the food as the energy passes through it, much like microwaves pass through food in a microwave oven. And just as a dentist's x-ray does not make your teeth radioactive, irradiation does not make food radioactive.

Food irradiation is a process that was patented in the United States in 1921 but was not approved for use on the first food products (wheat, wheat flour, and white potatoes) by the Food and Drug Administration (FDA) until the early 1960s. Since then, whether to irradiate food in the United States has been a contentious issue. Approximately 50 years after its approval, irradiation remains in limited use, although the FDA has since approved the use of irradiation on fresh produce, herbs, spices, pork, poultry, and red meat.

Numerous national and international organizations (such as the American Medical Association and the World Health Organization) as well as many university-based research institutes endorse the irradiation of food. Irradiation has been shown to be the only way to rid ground beef of *E. coli* O157:H7 before cooking. (Cooking ground beef thoroughly also kills this pathogen.) Irradiation also kills other bacteria, as well as insects and fungi that can make people sick or spoil food. Additionally, irradiating food inhibits the sprouting of vegetables and delays the ripening of fruits. Using this process makes the food supply safer, provides a better quality of food, and extends the "shelf life" of food.

# Environmental Health in the Workplace

Exposures to some toxins can occur both at home and at work, depending on one's occupation. Accidental carbon monoxide poisoning, for example, is certainly a hazard for automobile mechanics if car exhaust is not properly vented, but carbon monoxide poisoning more frequently occurs in the home. Pesticides are another group of toxic substances that

**pesticides** Chemicals that kill plant and animal pests and that can cause poisoning when ingested.

persons may accidentally ingest at home if these chemicals are placed in unlabeled containers. However, pesticide poisoning more frequently occurs on the job in people who manufacture or apply pesticides. Poisoning by exposure to certain solvents, metals, plastics, and adhesives generally occurs only during their manufacture.

## Pesticide Poisoning

**Pesticides** are chemicals that kill plant and animal pests; they are used on farms and in homes and businesses to control insects, rodents, and weeds. People rarely become poisoned from spraying pesticides in their homes or yards; however, they should be cautious, spray downwind, and protect their skin and eyes. Occasionally, people accidentally drink or eat pesticides (or other toxic chemicals) stored in unmarked food containers in storage areas. For this reason, pesticides always should be kept in clearly marked containers. A person who has ingested pesticides should receive immediate medical attention.

People also ingest pesticides in the food they eat. These pesticides are not simply what is sprayed on fruits and vegetables but are found in fish, seafood, and meat. Animals often ingest foods sprayed with pesticides. Marine and freshwater organisms also eat food contaminated with pesticides when rain washes chemicals from the land into the water. Animals store certain pesticides they eat (and other toxic chemicals such as heavy metals) in their tissues, especially in fat.

Although many harmful pesticides, such as DDT, have been banned in the United States, these toxic chemicals, as well as pesticides being manufactured today, persist in the food chain. In addition, certain harmful pesticides such as DDT are still used in other countries on crops that are imported to the United States. However, pesticide levels in humans from eating supermarket produce are not considered toxic. The FDA, EPA, and Food Safety and Inspection Service of the U.S. Department of Agriculture together ensure that the levels of pesticides in food are not hazardous to the health of consumers. Data collected by the FDA over a 7-year period show that pesticide residues on infant foods and adult foods that infants and children eat are almost always *well below* the highest levels legally allowed by the EPA (and that

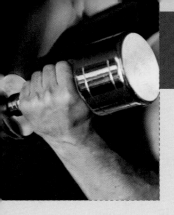

# Managing Your Health

## Reducing Pesticide Levels in the Food You Eat

- Scrub all fruits and vegetables with water for at least 20 seconds.

- Remove and discard the outer leaves of leafy vegetables.
- Trim the fat from red meats.
- Remove the skin and underlying fat from fish and poultry.
- Discard pan drippings and broths from animal products.

includes testing foods such as bananas without washing and peeling them). See the Managing Your Health feature for tips on reducing the level of pesticides in your food.

Most often, pesticide poisoning occurs in workers who manufacture or apply pesticides (**Figure 16.4**). Such workers inhale or have their skin exposed to toxic chemicals over a period of time if their skin and respiratory passageways are not properly protected. The signs and symptoms of poisoning in such cases may be vague and nonspecific at first: headache, intermittent dizziness, and general discomfort. As the poisoning worsens, the symptoms progress to include insomnia, nausea, increased sweating, involuntary eye movements, double or blurred vision, ringing in the ears, and involuntary body movements. If exposure continues, the poisoning victim may have convulsions. Treatment of chronic pesticide poisoning requires careful medical evaluation and is individualized for each patient.

The relationship of high-level exposure to pesticides and cancer has been studied by many researchers. Determining whether a causal link exists between pesticide exposure and cancer is difficult in that occupational exposure may include a variety of pesticides and cancer can have many causes. Cancers that have been associated with heavy pesticide exposure include non-Hodgkin's lymphoma (cancer of the lymphoid tissue), leukemia (cancer of the blood), multiple myeloma (cancer of antibody-producing cells of the bone marrow), as well as cancers of the following organs: brain, breast, prostate, colon, rectum, lung, and skin. Continued research is needed to clarify these associations.[17,18]

## Exposure to and Inhalation of Other Toxic Chemicals

A *solvent* is a liquid in which another substance is dissolved. Solvents are varied and perform a broad range of tasks in business and industry, such as removing unwanted substances (e.g., dry-cleaning solvents remove stains from clothing) or adding coatings such as paints and sealers to surfaces. (In the latter case, the coating is dissolved in the solvent, which then evaporates upon drying.)

Exposure to most solvents slows nerve transmission in the brain and spinal cord, resulting in slowed movements and thought processes. Continued solvent exposure can lead to unconsciousness. Some solvents are irritants that can cause fluid to collect in the lungs or cause the skin to redden. Chronic exposure to solvents can also cause cracking or scaling of the skin.

Metals (such as aluminum, tin, copper, and iron) are elements that are usually shiny, are good conductors of heat and electricity, and can be melted, fused, hammered into thin sheets, or drawn into wires. Metals are extracted from ores by various processes.

### Figure 16.4

**Protection Against Pesticides.** This worker is using proper protection for his skin and respiratory passageways.

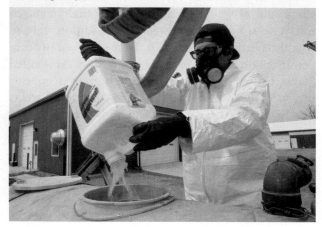

During these processes, ores are crushed, melted, and poured, which results in the production of metal dusts and vapors (**Figure 16.5**). Processing metal ores sometimes uses toxic and caustic chemicals such as sulfuric acid or cyanide, and often produces other toxic gases such as carbon monoxide and sulfur dioxide (discussed later in this chapter). Various industries use metals in the manufacture of products such as bearings, solder, batteries, cutting tools, plumbing, cookware, and roofing materials.

Exposure to heavy metals results in a variety of signs and symptoms depending on the metal and how it enters the body. Inhaling metal dusts or fumes, for example, can cause a variety of lung disorders such as lung scarring, fluid in the lungs, and emphysema (a lung disease in which the air sacs break apart and breathing is difficult). Inhaling fumes of heavy metals can also irritate the eyes and mouth, damage the kidneys, and damage the brain and spinal cord, especially with exposure to lead, mercury, or manganese. Skin contact with fumes can cause burns, rashes, reddening, swelling, and itching. Exposure to many heavy metals also causes cancer.

Adhesives are used to join substances during assembly operations. In order to join parts, other processes may also be used, such as etching, roughening, or solvent cleaning. Each of these processes may introduce its own specific hazards.

In most cases, the U.S. Occupational Safety and Health Administration (OSHA) of the U.S. Department of Labor regulates procedures in industries to protect the health of workers. However, many small companies, such as auto repair shops, are not regulated by OSHA.

### Healthy Living Practices

- Always keep pesticides and other chemicals away from children and stored in sealed, marked containers.
- When working with pesticides, wear clothing that protects your skin, eyes, nose, and mouth.
- If you work with toxic chemicals, take measures to protect yourself from damage to skin and eyes, assess the danger from toxic fumes that may be created as a result of your work, and contact OSHA for more information.

## Indoor Air Pollution

As people became concerned about the excessive use of energy in the 1970s and started creating "tighter" buildings to conserve energy in heating and cooling, they also became concerned about the quality of indoor air. Numerous studies have been conducted during the past two decades to address this concern and determine the cause of "sick building syndrome."

**Sick building syndrome** refers to a variety of symptoms reported by occupants of large buildings. These symptoms are attributed to the physical environments of the buildings. Buildings are identified as problems when a large proportion (sometimes as many as 30%) of their occupants complain about the same vague health-related problems, such as headaches; unusual fatigue; eye, nose, and throat irritation; and shortness of breath.

The results of studies of sick buildings show the predominant problem to be inadequate ventilation. Another cause of health problems is chemical contamination from a variety of sources such as building materials, carpets, paints, adhesives, and furniture. In

### Figure 16.5

**Processing Steel.** This factory worker in east China is working at the furnace of a steel plant. He is wearing an asbestos suit for protection as he takes a sample of the molten ore with a long tool. In the process, he is exposed to metal vapor.

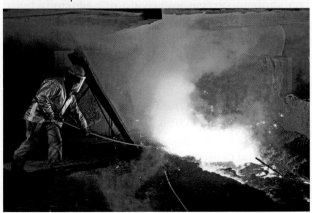

addition, if the building moisture level is too high, it can promote the growth of mold and cause symptoms in those allergic to mold.[19] Other sources of contamination of indoor air include asbestos and combustion-generated pollutants (discussed earlier in this chapter), radon, and formaldehyde. Authors of a study in England, however, conclude that poor psychosocial conditions in a workplace may far outweigh poor physical conditions of a building in causing symptoms of sick building syndrome.[20]

**Formaldehyde** is a chemical used in the manufacture of many building materials and furnishings, which then release formaldehyde into the air. Specific products that are most frequently responsible for high levels of formaldehyde in indoor air are pressed wood products such as fiberboard, particleboard, and hardwood plywood paneling and urea-formaldehyde foam, which is usually used to insulate walls.

Formaldehyde irritates the eyes, nose, and sinuses; people who inhale formaldehyde may have difficulty breathing, experience chest pain, and begin to wheeze. Some people experience headaches, fatigue, nausea, and have difficulty sleeping, while others exhibit gastrointestinal disturbances such as vomiting and diarrhea. Formaldehyde's role in the development of asthma and cancer is controversial.

If formaldehyde contamination occurs in a home or public building (as noted by occupants' symptoms), the source must be determined and removed, or other measures must be taken to reduce the level of this gas in the indoor air. This process may be difficult and expensive. Removing urea-formaldehyde foam insulation from walls is costly and damages the walls. (However, urea-formaldehyde foam insulation installed 5 to 10 years ago is unlikely to still release formaldehyde.) Paneling may need to be removed or furniture discarded. Alternatives are to install an air ventilation system designed to remove toxic substances such as formaldehyde from the air, bring large amounts of fresh air into the building, or seal the surfaces of the formaldehyde-containing products.

**Radon gas** may also contaminate indoor air. Radon is present in the rocks and soils in many areas in the United States. People who live in these regions may be exposed to radon gas if it leaks through cracks in basement walls and collects in their homes. Chapter 13 contains a discussion of this colorless and odorless gas and its relationship to lung cancer.

Homes that were built or remodeled between 2001 and 2008 may have been constructed with defective imported drywall (often called Chinese drywall) that emits various sulfur-containing compounds. Along with causing corrosion in the homes' plumbing and electrical systems, the drywall emissions have been linked to negative health effects in some sensitive individuals.[21]

## Environmental Health in the Outdoors

### Water Pollution

People get the water they drink from underground reservoirs called aquifers and from above-ground sources: lakes, rivers, and man-made reservoirs. Both sources of water can become contaminated with toxic chemicals. Surface water, however, can also become contaminated with pathogens, plant fertilizers, sediments (soil), radioactivity, and heat.

In developed countries, waterborne pathogens are infrequently a cause of disease because sewage plants treat wastewater so that it will not contaminate water supplies. Additionally, public drinking water is chlorinated to kill pathogens. However, infection can occur when water purification and supply systems break down. Waterborne infectious disease is a widespread problem in developing countries, which have no water purification systems.

Plant fertilizers, sediments, and heat, which often contaminate surface waters, do not generally harm humans. The radioactivity emitted by nuclear power plants that enters the water supply is thought to be so low as to be harmless to humans. However, chemical contaminants such as toxic chemical compounds (including pesticides), heavy metals (such as mercury and lead), and acids (from acid precipitation; see the section titled "Air Pollution" later in this chapter) can cause noninfectious diseases and poisoning.

Chemical contaminants pollute both groundwater (aquifers) and surface water. Such pollutants enter surface water when industries spill waste chemicals into waterways, mining wastes flow into rivers, pesticides wash into rivers and lakes during a rain, and salt used to de-ice roads washes into rivers and streams during spring rains.

Heavy metals can also contaminate surface water. Metals enter the water when they are dumped into rivers and streams from industrial sources. However, the Clean Water Act of 1972 and the Federal Water Pollution Control Act of 1972 and their amendments have all been instrumental in prohibiting industry from discharging such toxic chemicals into surface water. Metals also get into drinking water on its way to homes by leaching from lead solder in water pipes. (Leaching is the removal of the dissolvable parts of a substance as water moves through or over it.) The Safe Drinking Water Act and its 1986 amendments authorize the EPA to monitor the safety of drinking water and requires the use of lead-free solder in plumbing pipes.

Groundwater becomes polluted from deteriorating underground petroleum storage tanks at gasoline stations, chemicals from road salting, or agricultural chemicals that leach into the ground. However, **hazardous waste** (toxic chemical waste) is the primary source of groundwater pollution as toxic chemicals leach into aquifers.

In 1980, Congress passed a toxic waste cleanup bill and allocated funds to clean up hazardous substances. Known as the Superfund, it provides money to find the parties guilty of dumping toxic waste at specific sites and forces them to pay cleanup costs. If the government cannot find the guilty parties, it pays to have the sites cleaned up. Since 1980, the Superfund program has fostered the cleanup of hundreds of hazardous waste sites nationwide. Sites are continually being deleted and added to the National Priorities List (NPL), which is the list of hazardous waste sites eligible for cleanup under Superfund.

To ensure the safety of drinking water, purification methods in the United States often involve chlorination to kill unwanted pathogens. In fact, 75% of the nation's drinking water is treated with chlorine. In 1974, however, scientists realized that this chemical interacts with other chemicals in drinking water to form new compounds such as chloroform. Since this discovery, scientists have been studying whether these compounds are associated with the incidence of cancer. At normal levels of consumption, compounds formed from chlorine in drinking water are not likely to produce cancer, miscarriages, or birth defects.

Becoming aware of the potential for water pollution is only the first step in protecting against the short-term and long-term health effects of drinking contaminated water. Tap water can be tested to be

**hazardous waste** Toxic chemical refuse.

**acid precipitation** Rain, snow, or fog combined with sulfur dioxide from fossil fuel emissions.

sure that it does not contain toxic or other unwanted chemicals. If it does, it can be treated using various methods such as carbon filtration. Carbon filters remove many carbon-containing compounds and chlorine from the water, improving its taste, odor, and color. The filters are not useful for all water-treatment needs. Some persons choose to use only bottled water for cooking and drinking. However, bottled water is not necessarily better than tap water. To judge its purity, have your bottled water tested for the presence of toxic chemicals, or write to the International Bottled Water Association (IBWA), 1700 Diagonal Road, Suite 650, Alexandria, VA 22314 for information regarding a specific bottler. Their information hotline is 1-800-WATER-11.

## Air Pollution

Air pollution is also a threat to health. The primary substances in the air that harm humans are sulfur dioxide ($SO_2$), nitrogen dioxide ($NO_2$), carbon monoxide ($CO$), ozone ($O_3$), and particulates. These substances are formed when fossil fuels are burned. Fossil fuels are carbon-containing substances formed over time and under pressure from once-living organisms (both plants and animals). Gasoline, coal, natural gas, and oil are all fossil fuels.

The two main contributors to air pollution are automobiles and coal-fired power plants. The use of small gasoline-powered machines such as leaf blowers, chainsaws, weed cutters, and snow blowers also contributes to air pollution.

Coal-fired power plants generate particulates and sulfur dioxide as their primary pollutants. People who live downwind of such power plants experience the greatest impact from these pollutants. Sulfur dioxide combines with water in the atmosphere to produce sulfuric acid, the major component of **acid precipitation**. Acid precipitation (rain, snow, and fog) damages both living and nonliving things and acidifies surface water. When it falls in cities, it can harm vegetation as well as damage stone statues and buildings, as shown in **Figure 16.6**. Acid water in reservoirs leaches metals from pipes carrying the water into the drinking water supplies. The regions of the United States affected most heavily by acid precipitation are the Great Lakes area and New England. Southern Canada also experiences the effects of American power plant emissions.

Sulfur oxides and particulates also combine with atmospheric moisture to form a grayish haze called **smog** (smoke plus fog). Smog can harm the lungs. Cities with sulfur oxide smog (called *gray-air cities*) are usually located in cold, moist climates and rely on coal and oil for electricity and home heating. The smog in gray-air cities, such as New York City and Paris, France, is worst during cold, wet winters (**Figure 16.7a**).

Of the sulfur oxides and particulates in smog, particulates do the most damage to the lungs. *Particulates* are small particles that are dispersed in the air. Al-

## Figure 16.7

**Two Forms of Smog Created in Two Ways.** (a) New York City exhibits the gray haze of a gray-air city. Its smog is formed from the by-products of coal and oil combustion mixing with moisture in the air. (b) Los Angeles exhibits the brown haze of a brown-air city. Its smog is formed from the by-products of vehicle emissions that react with sunlight.

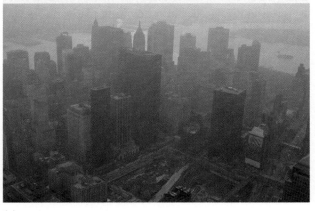

(a)

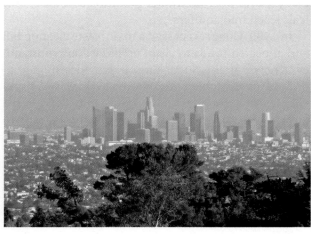

(b)

## Figure 16.6

**The Effects of Acid Rain.** This stone statue is located on the side of a church in England. The pitting of the stone is due to the effects of acid rain.

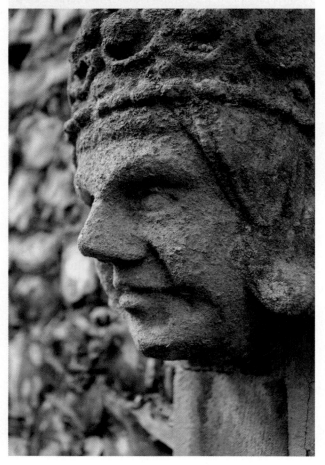

though nasal hairs and mucus in the nose and throat trap large particles, particulates reach the lungs and accumulate over time. Eventually, this material irritates the lungs and blocks their microscopic air sacs, making breathing more difficult. Particulates in the air passageways and lungs can also be a factor in the development of respiratory diseases such as bronchitis, emphysema, and asthma. They also make existing respiratory illness worse.

Sulfur dioxide in the air irritates the mucous lining of the eyes and lungs. Like particulates, sulfur dioxide worsens respiratory illness. Together, particulates and sulfur dioxide have a greater effect on respiratory problems than if only one of these pollutants were present. At highest risk are older adults and people with chronic lung and/or heart disease.

Cities located in the warm, dry climates of the southwestern United States are plagued by smog too, but the smog of these *brown-air cities* is created primarily by the emissions of automobiles. Photochemical smog comprises carbon monoxide (discussed earlier in this chapter), nitrogen dioxide, and ozone. Nitrogen dioxide is formed when nitrogen gas in the air chemically combines with oxygen during the combustion of fuel. This compound irritates the eyes, lungs, and other mucous membranes. It also reacts with hydrocarbons (the hydrogen and carbon in fuel) in the presence of sunlight to produce a secondary pollutant—ozone. In the upper atmosphere, ozone protects us from the sun's damaging ultraviolet rays. But when it is in the air we breathe, ozone is irritating to the lungs. The smog in brown-air cities, such as Los Angeles and Phoenix, is worst during the summer months (**Figure 16.7b**).

The **Air Quality Index (AQI)** is a means by which the public is informed of air quality. Levels of five major air pollutants ($CO$, $NO_2$, $O_3$, $SO_2$, and particulates) are monitored and used to determine AQI values (**Figure 16.8**). The descriptor for air quality (good, moderate, unhealthful, and so forth) is determined by the highest concentration of each pollutant in the air. When the air is unhealthful or worse, the AQI cautionary statements should be heeded; many elderly persons and those with chronic lung or heart conditions can die during times of unhealthful and

hazardous air quality. Since strict amendments to the Clean Air Act were passed in 1970 and even tougher standards were set with the passage of amendments in 1990, the quality of the air in the United States has improved greatly, but many cities and areas of the country still have high levels of pollution.

## Noise Pollution

Noise pollution can have a negative effect on health, but it is unlike any of the environmental dusts, fumes, vapors, gases, and liquids discussed previously. Noise is composed of sound waves. If sound waves were visible, they would look much like ripples on water—areas of compressed air molecules followed by areas in which the molecules are more spread out. These waves in the air are the result of the vibration of an object disturbing the air around it.

The human ear detects these sound vibrations in the air as they hit the eardrum, causing it to vibrate. The vibrating eardrum moves the tiny bones of the middle ear, which, in turn, cause the fluid of the inner ear to move across delicate hairs. The hairs of the inner ear are connected to nerves that send messages to the brain. These messages are interpreted as sound. The fragile hairs, however, can be permanently injured by sound waves that are too loud.

How loud are everyday sounds? **Table 16.3** lists some everyday sounds and their loudness. Sound intensity, or loudness, is expressed in decibels (dB). The faintest sound a human can hear is considered zero (0) dB. As the intensity of sound increases on the decibel scale, each 10-dB increase means a 10-fold increase in the intensity of the sound. Therefore, a 50-dB sound is 10 times louder than a 40-dB sound.

Sounds that are considered quiet or soft are 50 dB or less. The National Institute on Deafness and Other Communication Disorders (NIDCD) states that sounds of less than 75 dB are unlikely to cause hearing loss. When sounds get as loud as 80 dB, they begin to be annoying and can be harmful over time. At 85 dB, hearing is at risk of permanent damage. Pain sets in at 120 dB.

The EPA estimates that 40% of the U.S. population is exposed to enough noise to cause permanent hearing loss. The average person can damage his or her hearing if he or she

- Uses a power lawn mower (90 dB) for 8 hours
- Is at a loud party (90 dB) for 6 to 8 hours

### Figure 16.8

**The Air Quality Index (AQI).**

*Source:* United States Environmental Protection Agency. (2010, September 3). Air Quality Index: A guide to air quality and your health. Retrieved on May 12, 2011, from http://www.airnow.gov/index.cfm?action=aqibasics.aqi

| Air Quality Index (AQI) Values | Levels of Health Concern | Colors |
|---|---|---|
| When the AQI is in this range: | ...air quality conditions are: | ...as symbolized by this color: |
| 0 to 50 | Good | Green |
| 51 to 100 | Moderate | Yellow |
| 101 to 150 | Unhealthy for Sensitive Groups | Orange |
| 151 to 200 | Unhealthy | Red |
| 201 to 300 | Very Unhealthy | Purple |
| 301 to 500 | Hazardous | Maroon |

## Table 16.3

### Loudness of Some Everyday Sounds

| Sounds | dB |
| --- | --- |
| Rustling leaves | 10 |
| Normal conversation | 50 |
| Suburban neighborhood noise | 52 |
| Vacuum cleaner | 70 |
| City noise; busy traffic | 80 |
| Inside a passenger jet (takeoff) | 78–83 |
| Heavy trucks at 50 feet | 76–88 |
| Home shop tools | 65–110 |
| Subway noise | 80–114 |
| Nearby jet airplane | 150 |
| Shooting a gun | 150–170 |

- Uses a chain saw (100 dB) for 2 hours
- Uses a gasoline-powered leaf blower (110 dB) for 30 minutes
- Is at a dance club or rock concert (115 dB) for 15 minutes

Although you may not be at one party for 8 hours, damage to hearing from loud sounds is cumulative. That is, the effects add up. These effects can be devastating; the National Institutes of Health have determined that permanent hearing loss will result from years of exposure, 8 hours per day, to 85-dB and louder sounds. Permanent deafness may result from such continual exposure and can also result from a single exposure, such as being close to an explosion of 140 dB.

How do people know if they are losing their hearing? First, a person may lose the ability to hear high-frequency sounds. He or she may be unable to hear occasional words in conversation or have difficulty hearing on the telephone. Additionally, people with partial hearing loss often experience ringing or roaring in their ears, called tinnitus. Tinnitus makes hearing even more difficult. Hearing aids may be helpful to the person with partial hearing loss but cannot totally compensate for the problem.

Total or partial hearing loss is only one of the effects of listening to sounds that are too loud. Parts of the body other than the ear react to noise. Researchers have shown that exposure to 70-dB noise results in an increase in the heart rate and a rise in blood pressure; muscles tighten and breathing patterns change. Exposure to noise also increases the rate at which stress-related hormones are secreted into the bloodstream. Even moderate daytime noise levels have been shown to increase anxiety and hostile behavior in some persons. Environmental noise exposure has also been linked to impaired learning ability and performance in school.

Paying attention to the noise in your environment will help save your hearing. For example, many health clubs blast loud music as an aerobics instructor yells commands. Often, these sounds top 110 dB. Request that the volume be turned down. If you wear ear protection, use only materials and items manufactured to reduce sound; placing cotton or tissue in your ears does not do an adequate job of protecting your ears.

If you attend loud concerts, check your hearing when you leave. Set your car or home radio to a level at which you can barely hear the words. Then, as soon after the concert as possible, turn on the radio. Can you hear the words? If not, you have sustained short-term hearing loss from the loudness of the music. Frequently listening to such loud music could result in a permanent hearing problem.

### Healthy Living Practices

☐ To avoid hearing loss and the other effects of noise pollution, avoid situations in which the sound is over 80 dB. Pay attention to noise levels and complain if they are too high.

## Across THE LIFE SPAN

### ENVIRONMENTAL HEALTH

Environmental health hazards are a risk for all segments of the population. However, young children are most at risk for unintentional poisoning by ingestion of toxic substances because they lack understanding that these materials are harmful and they put most things in their mouths; this is a normal

# Diversity in Health

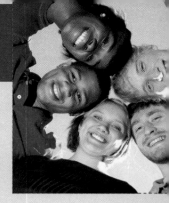

## Hunger, the Environment, and the World's Population

Nearly one of six people in the world suffers from acute or chronic hunger. Hunger is more than appetite, the psychological desire for food, or feeling hungry after not eating for a few hours. Acute hunger, or starvation, is a condition in which a person has not eaten for a prolonged period and will eventually die from lack of food. *Chronic hunger* refers to a long-term condition in which food intake is inadequate. People who experience chronic hunger are undernourished (see Chapter 9) and do not have the nutrients they need for proper growth, development, and body function.

Although many of the factors that lead to hunger are political, social, and economic, environmental conditions play a role in the many perceived causes of world hunger. Overpopulation, environmental limits to food production, and land use problems are factors that scientists debate with regard to their roles in hunger. In fact, many scientists assert that there is no global hunger problem. Instead, they assert, regional hunger problems exist, each with diverse causes.

The world population reached 7 billion people in October 2011. The *2010 Revision of World Population Prospects* issued by the United Nations (UN) in May of 2011 projects that the world population will reach 9.3 billion by 2050 and 10.1 billion by 2100. By the turn of the century, projects the UN, only high-fertility countries such as those in Africa will have populations on the increase. The populations of medium-fertility countries, such as India and the United States, will peak in about 2060 and then very slowly start to decline. Populations in low-fertility countries, such as most countries in Europe, will peak in 2030 and decline more quickly than the populations of medium-fertility countries.

Various experts predict that the world population will level off, reaching its carrying capacity between 12.4 billion and 14 billion people. The carrying capacity is the maximum number of individuals that can be supported by the available resources. However, scientists disagree as to whether the global food output can support that many individuals. Many scientists calculate that even with the use of the best agricultural technologies, the carrying capacity of the Earth will be limited to 7.5 billion people.

Scientists disagree as to whether the increase in food production during the 1980s kept up with the need for food worldwide. They also disagree as to whether technological advances in various areas of agriculture, such as changes in machinery, seed varieties, fertilizers, pesticides, and management practices, as well as the genetic engineering of plants to resist certain crop pests, will allow the world's farmers to produce greater and greater crop yields. Many scientists assert that to increase sufficiently the amount of food produced around the world, farmers must increase the amount of land they cultivate. However, using marginal land (land not well suited for cultivation) may increase the danger of erosion, landslides, and floods. Marginal land is also likely to produce lower crop yields than land already in cultivation. Additionally, the limited availability of water in many regions may constrain agricultural expansion.

Many parts of the Earth cannot support the population that now exists on their lands. A country is overpopulated when its natural resources cannot sustain its people. An example of such overpopulation is Africa, the continent with the fastest population growth in the world. According to the UN's *Revision of World Population Prospects*, in 2010 62% of the African population was younger than age 25 years. Therefore, the size of this population will increase in the next decade and beyond because a large proportion of the population is and will be in its reproductive years. Much of the land in Africa has a low natural carrying capacity. Additionally, its climate is highly changeable and therefore unreliable for growing crops.

The problem of world or regional hunger is serious. Environmental issues such as overpopulation, methods of food production, and approaches to land use interact with political, cultural, social, and economic issues to create situations that can affect the health of many peoples throughout the world.

---

exploratory behavior for small children. Additionally, carbon monoxide and lead are particularly injurious to fetuses and young children because their brains and nervous systems are still developing. Also extremely susceptible to carbon monoxide poisoning or air pollutants are older adults and persons with chronic lung or heart disease, whose lung function may be impaired.

## Summary

In general, environmental factors that are the sole cause of disease are toxic chemicals. Such substances damage body tissues and affect bodily functioning; they are present in the home, workplace, and environment. Toxic chemicals are found in a wide variety of substances, such as household products, plants, products used in the workplace, and prescription and illegal drugs.

Toxic (poisonous) plants can be the source of poisoning emergencies, especially in children. Although many plants are not poisonous, house plants and cut flowers should be kept out of reach of children younger than 5 years old. In addition to plants, approximately 1% to 2% of mushroom species are poisonous.

Children younger than the age of 5 years are those most in danger of being poisoned from household cleaning aids and from over-the-counter and prescription drugs and vitamins. Special packaging that makes it difficult for young children to open hazardous products has lowered the incidence of poisoning in this age group. Nevertheless, such substances should be locked in cabinets in homes in which young children reside or visit often.

Lead poisoning is still a health problem in children in the United States even though many sources of lead poisoning have been eliminated in this country. Lead poisoning is serious because it affects the central nervous system and can cause coma, convulsions, and death. Children can exhibit a wide range of symptoms of lead poisoning, depending on the level of lead in the blood. It is extremely important to remove sources of lead, such as lead-based paint, from a child's environment.

Carbon monoxide poisoning can occur when levels of this gas build up in an enclosed environment. Major sources of carbon monoxide poisoning are fires, automobile exhaust, malfunctioning furnaces, charcoal fires, gasoline-powered tools, woodstoves, fireplaces, unvented kerosene and gas space heaters, gas cooking stoves and ovens, and tobacco smoke. To avoid this hazard, properly maintain and use tools and appliances that burn fuel, avoid running the car in the garage, vent home heating stoves and furnaces properly, and use charcoal grills and gas-powered tools only in well-ventilated areas.

Extremely low frequency (ELF) radiation is emitted by computer screens, microwave ovens, cell phones, television sets, electric blankets, electric appliances, high-power electric lines, and electrical distribution substations. ELF radiation has been associated with negative effects such as risk of cancer, DNA damage, and changes in human brain electrical activity. Nonetheless, scientists have seen no major negative effects in most situations and with most products and see no reason to recommend extreme caution. Medical researchers suggest, however, that people avoid being unnecessarily close to products and power lines that emit ELF radiation. Additional caution is needed with cell phones. It is recommended that cell phones be used with a headset or earpieces, or that a cell phone be connected to a remote antenna.

Many types of environmental hazards exist in the workplace. Common workplace hazards include exposure to pesticides while manufacturing or applying them and exposure to toxins in the industrial manufacture and use of certain solvents, metals, plastics, and adhesives. People who work with toxic chemicals should protect themselves from damage to their skin and eyes and should assess the danger from toxic fumes that may be created as a result of their work.

Indoor air may be contaminated with pollutants such as formaldehyde, asbestos, and combustion-generated products. Some buildings have poor ventilation systems, which appear to be a primary cause of vague health-related symptoms in building occupants.

The air we breathe and the water we drink are also contaminated with toxins to a greater or lesser degree in various parts of the United States. Contaminated drinking water can result in both short-term and long-term health effects. The air is contaminated with emissions from coal-fired power plants and vehicles. When the air is unhealthful, older adults and those with respiratory illness are most at risk for further damage to their health.

Noise pollution can have a negative effect on health. Sounds of less than 75 dB are unlikely to cause hearing loss. To avoid hearing loss and other negative health effects of noise pollution, avoid situations in which the sound is over 80 dB or wear specially designed ear protection in such situations.

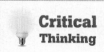

## Applying What You Have Learned

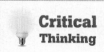
**Critical Thinking**

1. Your 4-year-old cousin is coming to visit for the summer. What steps would you take to make your house or apartment safe for your cousin? **Application**
2. List and then analyze your interactions with the environment in the last 24 hours. Develop a list of environmental threats to your health from these interactions. **Analysis**
3. You have just moved to a part of the country that is new to you. Develop a plan to assess whether you are being exposed to hazardous chemicals and toxins and to evaluate which health hazards might be present, if any. **Synthesis**

4. Develop a fictitious set of at least three outcomes based on question 3. What will be your course of action to diminish or eliminate these threats to your health? **Evaluation**
5. Gather the chemicals that you use in your home, such as cleaning products. Many such products have warnings on their labels about physical hazards, storage, and disposal. Read the labels of the products you have gathered and list the types of warnings you see. State what you learned about safeguarding not only your health but also the health of the environment when using these chemicals. **Synthesis**

## Reflecting on Your Health

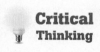
**Critical Thinking**

1. Do you take steps to protect your hearing? If so, what do you do? Do you think about possible hearing loss when you are in noisy environments? Describe three situations in which you regularly are exposed to harmful noise levels and discuss what you can do to avoid hearing loss in these situations.

2. Go through your house or apartment and identify environmental health risks. What can you do to reduce these risks to health?
3. Do you ever put yourself or others at risk for carbon monoxide poisoning? If so, describe your risky behaviors and what you can do to eliminate the risk. If not, identify behaviors in others that

| **Application** | **Analysis** | **Synthesis** | **Evaluation** | |
|---|---|---|---|---|
| using information in a new situation. | breaking down information into component parts. | putting together information from different sources. | making informed decisions. | **Key** |

you have observed that put people at risk for carbon monoxide poisoning. How might you help others avoid such risks?

4. Find out about environmental risks in your area. For example, is your tap water chlorinated to levels that are worrisome? Do you live in a region of the country in which water comes to your home in lead pipes? What might you do in either of these situations to reduce or eliminate your health risks from water? Investigate air pollution in your area.

How can you protect your respiratory health in the region in which you live? Describe any environmental health risks that affect your community and suggest what you might do to reduce health risks to yourself and your family.

5. Do you ever discard toxic waste improperly, such as putting old batteries (especially car batteries), solvents, or paints in the trash? If so, describe the proper disposal methods for these substances in your city or town.

# References

1. Gupta, N., et al. (2011). Lead poisoning associated with Ayurvedic drug presenting as intestinal obstruction: A case report. *Clinica Chimica Acta, 412*(1–2):213–214.

2. Saper, R. B., et al. (2008). Lead, mercury, and arsenic in US- and Indian-manufactured Ayurvedic medicines sold via the Internet. *Journal of the American Medical Association, 8*:915–923.

3. Centers for Disease Control and Prevention. (2005). Lead poisoning associated with use of litargirio—Rhode Island, 2003. *Morbidity and Mortality Weekly Report, 54*(9):227–229.

4. Buettner, C., et al. (2009). Herbal supplement use and blood lead levels of United States adults. *Journal of General Internal Medicine, 24*(11):1175–1182.

5. Gaitens, J. M., et al. (2009). Exposure of U.S. children to residential dust lead, 1999–2004: I. Housing and demographic factors. *Environmental Health Perspectives, 117*:461–467.

6. Centers for Disease Control and Prevention. (2009). Adult blood lead epidemiology and surveillance—United States, 2005–2007. *Morbidity and Mortality Weekly Report, 58*(14):365–369.

7. Bronstein, A. C., et al. (2010, December). 2009 annual report of the American Association of Poison Control Centers' National Poison Data System (NPDS). *Clinical Toxicology, 48*:979–1178. Retrieved on May 10, 2010, from http://www.aapcc.org/dnn/Portals/0/correctedannualreport.pdf

8. Vernberg, K., Culver-Dickinson, P., & Spyker, D. A. (1984). The deterrent effect of poison-warning stickers. *American Journal of Diseases of Children, 138*:1018–1020.

9. Pooley, A. J., & Fiddick, L. (2010). Social referencing "Mr. Yuk": The use of emotion in a poison prevention program. *Journal of Pediatric Psychology, 35*(4):327–339.

10. Sharmer, L., et al. (2010, December). A potential new health risk from lead used in consumer products purchased in the United States. *Journal of Environmental Health, 73*(5):8–12.

11. Farley, D. (1998). Dangers of lead still linger. *FDA Consumer, 32*(1):16–21.

12. U.S. Consumer Product Safety Commission. (2008). Carbon monoxide questions and answers. Retrieved on May 11, 2011, from http://www.cpsc.gov/cpscpub/pubs/466.html

13. Kheifets, L., et al. (2010). A pooled analysis of extremely low-frequency magnetic fields and childhood brain tumors. *American Journal of Epidemiology, 172*(7):752–761.

14. Kheifets, L., et al. (2010). Extremely low frequency electric fields and cancer: Assessing the evidence. *Bioelectromagnetics, 31*(2):89–101.

15. American Cancer Society. (2010). Learn about cancer: Cellular phones. Retrieved on May 11, 2011, from http://www.cancer.org/Cancer/CancerCauses/OtherCarcinogens/AtHome/cellular-phones

16. International Agency for Research on Cancer. (2011, May 31). IARC classifies radiofrequency electromagnetic fields as possibly carcinogenic to humans [Press Release No. 208]. World Health Organization. Retrieved on June 2, 2011, from http://www.iarc.fr/en/media-centre/pr/2011/pdfs/pr208_E.pdf

17. Weichenthal, S., et al. (2010). A review of pesticide exposure and cancer incidence in the Agricultural Health study cohort. *Environmental Health Perspectives, 118*(8):1117–1125.

18. Clapp, R. W., et al. (2008). Environmental and occupational causes of cancer: New evidence 2005–2007. *Reviews on Environmental Health, 23*(1):1–37.

19. Buckmaster, P. K. (2009). Sustaining acceptable indoor environmental quality. *Occupational Health and Safety, 78*(10):48, 50.

20. Norbäck, D. (2009). An update on sick building syndrome. *Current Opinion in Allergy and Immunology, 9*:55–59.

21. Centers for Disease Control and Prevention. (2011, March 3). Imported drywall and your home. Retrieved on May 12, 2011, from http://www.cdc.gov/nceh/drywall/imported_drywall_and_your_home.html

# The Mission, Vision, and Goals of Healthy People 2020

## Vision—A society in which all people live long, healthy lives.

## Mission—*Healthy People 2020* strives to:

- Identify nationwide health improvement priorities
- Increase public awareness and understanding of the determinants of health, disease, and disability, and the opportunities for progress

- Provide measurable objectives and goals that are applicable at the national, state, and local levels
- Engage multiple sectors to take actions to strengthen policies and improve practices that are driven by the best available evidence and knowledge
- Identify critical research, evaluation, and data collection needs

# Foundation Health Measures

*Healthy People 2020* includes broad, cross-cutting measures without targets that will be used to assess progress toward achieving the four overarching goals.

| Overarching Goals of *Healthy People 2020* | Foundation Measures Category | Measures of Progress |
|---|---|---|
| Attain high quality, longer lives free of preventable disease, disability, injury, and premature death | General Health Status | Life expectancy<br><br>Healthy life expectancy<br><br>Physical and mental unhealthy days<br><br>Self-assessed health status<br><br>Limitation of activity<br><br>Chronic disease prevalence<br><br>International comparisons *(where available)* |
| Achieve health equity, eliminate disparities, and improve the health of all groups | Disparities and Inequity | Disparities/inequity to be assessed by:<br>• Race/ethnicity<br>• Gender<br>• Socioeconomic status<br>• Disability status<br>• Lesbian, gay, bisexual, and transgender status<br>• Geography |
| Create social and physical environments that promote good health for all | Social Determinants of Health | Determinants can include:<br>• Social and economic factors<br>• Natural and built environments<br>• Policies and programs |
| Promote quality of life, healthy development, and healthy behaviors across all life stages | Health-Related Quality of Life and Well-Being | • Well-being/satisfaction<br>• Physical, mental, and social health-related quality of life<br>• Participation in common activities |

# Topic Areas

The Topic Areas of *Healthy People 2020* identify and group objectives of related content, highlighting specific issues and populations. Each Topic Area is assigned to one or more lead agencies within the federal government that is responsible for developing, tracking, monitoring, and periodically reporting on objectives.

1. Access to Health Services
2. Adolescent Health
3. Arthritis, Osteoporosis, and Chronic Back Conditions
4. Blood Disorders and Blood Safety
5. Cancer
6. Chronic Kidney Disease
7. Dementias, Including Alzheimer's Disease
8. Diabetes
9. Disability and Health
10. Early and Middle Childhood
11. Educational and Community-Based Programs
12. Environmental Health
13. Family Planning
14. Food Safety
15. Genomics
16. Global Health
17. Healthcare-Associated Infections
18. Health Communication and Health Information Technology
19. Health-Related Quality of Life and Well-Being
20. Hearing and Other Sensory or Communication Disorders
21. Heart Disease and Stroke

22. HIV
23. Immunization and Infectious Diseases
24. Injury and Violence Prevention
25. Lesbian, Gay, Bisexual, and Transgender Health
26. Maternal, Infant, and Child Health
27. Medical Product Safety
28. Mental Health and Mental Disorders
29. Nutrition and Weight Status
30. Occupational Safety and Health
31. Older Adults
32. Oral Health
33. Physical Activity
34. Preparedness
35. Public Health Infrastructure
36. Respiratory Diseases
37. Sexually Transmitted Diseases
38. Sleep Health
39. Social Determinants of Health
40. Substance Abuse
41. Tobacco Use
42. Vision

# Injury Prevention and Emergency Care

## Injury Prevention

During the next hour, at least 11 people will die in the United States from unintentional injuries. The causes will be diverse, including automobile crashes, drownings, poisonings (see Chapter 16), and fires. Some of those who die this hour will probably be children because unintentional, preventable injury is the number one killer of children (through young adulthood, from 1 through 21 years old) in the United States. In fact, unintentional injuries kill more children than all childhood diseases combined.

Until recently, the number of fatal unintentional injuries had been steadily declining, reaching a 68-year low of approximately 89,000 in 1994. However, that number has been rising annually since then. In 2007, almost 118,000 people died from unintentional injuries. This appendix alerts you to the most prevalent types of unintentional injuries and deaths in the United States today and discusses their causes, prevention, and emergency treatment.

## Automobile Safety

Motor vehicle crashes are the greatest cause of preventable death resulting from injuries, but the number of deaths has been dropping. In 2009, 33,808 people died on U.S. roads and highways, resulting in the lowest highway fatality rate ever recorded. Approximately 32% of the fatalities involved alcohol. In addition to deaths, motor vehicle accidents are the leading cause of unintentional injury in the United States. To keep yourself and others safe while riding in automobiles, heed the following recommendations. For general vehicle safety:

- Never drink and drive or take other drugs that impair your ability to drive.
- Always wear your seat belt; this practice reduces by half your chance of injury or death in a motor vehicle crash.
- Slow down and prepare to stop as you approach yellow lights. Many people cause automobile crashes because they try to "beat" the light.
- Yield the right of way at intersections.
- Don't tailgate; allow at least one car length for each 10 mph (e.g., stay four car lengths behind the car ahead if you are traveling at 40 mph).
- Know the traffic laws of the state in which you are driving and obey these laws.
- Read and heed traffic signs, especially railroad warning signals and gates. Always proceed cautiously across railroad tracks. Not all railroad crossings have gates or sound warnings to signal oncoming trains.
- Obey the speed limit.

**Children and Automobile Safety** To protect children while they are passengers in automobiles, follow these safety recommendations:

- Place infants and toddlers in properly secured rear-facing safety seats until they are 2 years of age or until they reach the highest weight or height allowed by their car safety seat's manufacturer.
- Always put rear-facing child safety seats in the back seat. Deploying passenger-side air bags in the front seat can injure or kill infants and toddlers in rear-facing seats.
- Children older than age 2, or those children who have outgrown the rear-facing seat before age 2, should be restrained in a forward-facing car seat with a harness *in the back seat* until they reach the highest weight and height allowed by the manufacturer.
- When children outgrow the forward-facing car seat, and until the vehicle seat belt fits properly, they should be restrained in a belt-positioning booster seat *in the back seat*. The vehicle seat belt typically fits properly when the child reaches a height of 4 feet 9 inches and they are between 8 and 12 years old.
- When adolescents reach age 13 they can ride in the front seat. Push the seat back as far as possible

to create distance between the child and the air bag.
- An infant's or child's car seat needs to be secured so tightly that it will not move more than 1 in. from side to side. Locate a certified Child Passenger Safety Seat Technician in your area to check the installation of your child's safety seat.
- Never leave a child alone in the car.

## Pedestrian Safety

Pedestrians accounted for 12% of preventable deaths involving motor vehicles in the United States and approximately 3% of motor vehicle–related injuries in 2009. Not only are drunk drivers often a cause of these injuries and deaths, but intoxicated pedestrians put themselves at increased risk. Other high-risk groups for sustaining unintentional pedestrian–automobile injuries and deaths are older adults and young children. Children are most frequently hit when they dart into traffic from between parked cars. Children younger than 10 years old do not have fully developed cognitive, developmental, behavioral, physical, and sensory abilities to be safe pedestrians on their own. To help prevent pedestrian injuries, practice these safety steps:

- Help children develop injury-prevention skills by modeling proper safety behaviors such as those listed here.
- Be sure that children younger than 10 years of age are accompanied by an older person when they cross the street.
- Cross at marked crosswalks and at corners whenever possible. Do not assume that drivers will stop because you are in a crosswalk.
- Stop, look both ways, and listen before deciding that it is safe to cross. Continue to look and listen as you cross.
- Cross only on a green light or a "walk" signal.
- Never cross between parked cars.
- Never run into the street.
- Walk on sidewalks whenever possible. If you must walk in the street, walk to the left facing traffic.
- When walking at dusk or at night, wear light colors and some type of reflective device. Walk with someone, not alone.

- Do not allow children to play in driveways, in adjacent unfenced yards, in streets, or in parking lots.

## Water Safety

In 2007, 3,443 people died from drowning, not including those involved in boat-related incidents. Drowning is the second leading cause of injury-related death for children aged 1 through 14 years, the highest rates being for children aged 1 through 4 years. (Fatalities involving automobiles are the leading cause of injury-related death for children.) Children younger than 1 year of age most often drown in bathtubs, buckets, or toilets. Children older than 1 year of age most often drown in pools, hot tubs, or spas owned by their parents, relatives, or friends, and they happen within 5 minutes of the child's being missing from sight. Children usually drown silently, so don't think that splashing or screaming will alert you to the danger.

**Safety for Small Children** To protect small children from drowning in residential pools or other accessible bodies of water, follow these safety practices:

- Provide barriers to water, such as fences and walls. If the house is part of the barrier, install door alarms so that you know when the child has gone outside, and install a power safety cover over the pool, hot tub, or spa.
- Fence gates should be self-closing and self-latching. The latch should be out of a child's reach.
- Never prop open the fence gate.
- Instruct baby-sitters about pool hazards for young children.
- If a young child is missing, check the pool first.
- Do not assume that children will not drown because they know how to swim.
- Never leave a child unsupervised near a pool, and while at the pool, watch small children continuously; do not become preoccupied with something else.
- Never leave children alone, even for a minute, when they are in or near any type of water.

**Safety for Swimmers** Even good swimmers have accidents in the water and drown. For safety in the water, follow these guidelines:

- Never swim alone.
- Don't push or jump on others.

- Check water depth before you dive or jump into the water.
- Never swim in unsupervised areas such as quarries, canals, or ponds.
- Don't swim or use a hot tub or spa while drinking alcoholic beverages or taking other drugs that could impair your judgment, impair your ability to swim, or make you drowsy. (Alcohol is involved in 25–50% of adolescent and adult deaths associated with water recreation.)

## Bicycle Safety

In 2009 in the United States, 630 people died in traffic-related bicycle crashes. Seventy-five percent of such deaths are usually caused by head injuries. Supporters of wearing bicycle helmets contend that 40–75% of head-injury deaths could be prevented if riders wore helmets. Opponents suggest that these statistics are unreliable and that most bicycle fatalities involve a crash with an automobile, a situation in which a helmet cannot protect the bicyclist. Those who take a middle stance suggest that it is prudent to wear helmets because they protect the head in many types of falls and make bicyclists more visible to automobile drivers.

As of May 2011, 21 states, the District of Columbia, and approximately 200 local governments had enacted legislation about bicycle helmets. Most of these laws pertain to children and adolescents. In 1999, the U.S. Consumer Product Safety Commission issued a new safety standard for bike helmets.

Bicycle helmets are designed to absorb much of the impact when the head hits another object like a car or the road. Often, a cyclist hits a car and then the road, so the helmet needs a strap to ensure that it stays on during multiple hits. Also, it should not be covered with any material that can catch on something during a fall and twist the cyclist's head. When purchasing a helmet, make sure that it is level on the head, covers the top of the forehead, touches all around, and is comfortably snug. Many sellers and manufacturers of helmets offer instructions about the proper fit of helmets.

Bicycle injuries are a leading cause of preventable death in children, exceeding the death rate from poisonings, falls, and firearm injuries combined. Most bicycle-related deaths occur from head trauma and are not caused by colliding with cars. Rather, children fall from their bikes or lose control of their bikes and collide with objects such as curbs and trees. Therefore, all children benefit from wearing helmets while bicycling. They should also wear helmets while being carried as passengers on adults' bikes. Have a pediatrician check a toddler's helmet, however, because the neck muscles of toddlers are weak and may be unable to properly support a helmeted head.

**Bicycle Safety Rules** For bicycling safety, follow these simple rules:

- Make yourself or your children visible with light-colored clothing and reflective tape.

- Be certain that your bicycle horn or bell is working properly.

- Drive on the right-hand side of the road in single file, obeying all traffic signs and signals. Small children should ride their bikes on the sidewalk.

- When cycling in the road, leave a distance of about 3 ft between you and parked cars. You will be more noticeable to drivers and will not be knocked off your bike by the opening doors of parked cars.

- Walk your bike at busy street corners in pedestrian crosswalks.

- Never carry a passenger on your bicycle unless you have a tandem bike or are carrying a child in a properly mounted child seat.

- When exiting a driveway into a lane of traffic, stop, look both ways, and listen to determine that it is safe to enter.

- Before turning, use hand signals and look in all directions.

- Don't ride your bike on rainy nights. Your chances of being involved in a crash are 30 times greater than on a dry night because roads are slippery, wet bicycle brakes do not work well, and automobile drivers cannot see bicyclists well in the rain.

- If you are falling off your bike, tuck and roll rather than extending an arm to break your fall.

- Children should not ride in the street until they are 10 years old, demonstrate good riding skills, and are able to observe the basic rules of the road.

# Fire Prevention

Although the number of residential fires has declined since 1980, there were 356,200 residential fires in 2009 in which 2,480 people died, not including firefighters. Most home fires are started by cooking. Lit cigarettes, cigarette lighters, or matches cause the least number of residential fires but result in the most fire-related deaths. A fewer number of fires are ignited by faulty electrical wiring or supplemental home heating devices such as wood stoves, kerosene heaters, gas-fired space heaters, and portable electric heaters than by cooking but a greater number than by cigarette-related causes.

The number of supplemental home heaters has decreased in recent years, as has the number of fires associated with them. However, supplemental heaters still cause about 13% of residential fires. Additionally, thousands of people are burned each year by coming into contact with the hot surfaces of these devices, and hundreds are poisoned by their carbon monoxide emissions (see Chapter 16).

**Home Heaters** Some safety recommendations for the use of supplemental home heaters include the following:

- Be certain that any supplemental heater is properly installed and meets building codes.

- Inspect wood stoves according to the manufacturer's directions (usually twice monthly) and have chimneys inspected and cleaned by a professional chimney sweep.

- Use a floor protector designed for use under the type of supplemental heater you have. It should extend 18 inches beyond the heater on all sides.

- Follow directions regarding how far the heater must be from combustible walls and other materials such as draperies.

- Never burn trash in a wood-burning stove because this practice could cause overheating.

- Never use gasoline to start a wood fire.

- Use only the fuel(s) the manufacturer has designated as safe in the heater.

- If using a liquid fuel, be certain that its container is well marked and is out of the reach of children.

- Place kerosene heaters out of the path of traffic and where they cannot be knocked over.

- Always fill a kerosene heater outdoors and when the heater is not operating.

- Kerosene heaters are not usually vented; therefore, keep a window ajar for ventilation.

- Use unvented gas heaters only in large, open areas that are well ventilated; do not operate vented styles unvented.

- Do not use supplemental heating devices while you are sleeping or not at home; many fires and deaths occur at these times from the unsupervised use of supplemental heaters.

- With electric heaters, follow the manufacturer's recommendations regarding the type of power cord to use. Avoid using extension cords, but if you do, be certain that it is marked with a power rating at least as high as that of the heater itself. Keep the cord stretched out and do not place anything on top of the cord.

**General Fire Prevention** Many residential fires could have been prevented with little trouble. To decrease your risk of fire, take the following precautions:

- Keep matches and cigarette lighters away from children.

- Do not store food items such as candy or other items attractive to children above the stove.

- Always check ashtrays to be certain that cigarettes are out. After a party or other gathering, check under and between the cushions of upholstered furniture to make sure that no smoldering ashes are present.

- Never place ashtrays on the arms of furniture, especially upholstered furniture that is likely to ignite from lit cigarettes or their ashes.

- Avoid placing lit candles near draperies or other flammable materials. Be certain that they do not tip easily and are not positioned where they can be easily knocked over.

- Consider purchasing clothes made out of fabrics that are difficult to ignite and tend to self-extinguish, such as 100% polyester, nylon, wool, and silk. Cotton, cotton/polyester blends, rayon, and acrylic ignite easily and burn rapidly.

- Store flammable liquids, such as gasoline and paint thinners, outside the house. They produce invisible explosive vapors.

- Install at least one smoke detector on each floor of your home and near the bedrooms. Replace the batteries annually or when they make a chirping sound.

- Plan an escape route from each room in the house. Have each family member rehearse the plan often. Designate a safe place to meet if you have to escape a fire in your home. This helps firefighters determine whether there are people in a burning building.

Source of statistics for injury prevention: American Academy of Pediatrics; Bicycle Safety Helmet Institute; Centers for Disease Control and Prevention, National Center for Injury Prevention and Control; Department of Transportation, National Highway Traffic Safety Administration; and the U.S. Fire Administration.

## Emergency Care

## When to Call for Help

Know the emergency number in your area; in most areas that number is 9-1-1. Calling for help in a medical emergency is important and may save a person's life. When a serious situation occurs, call for emergency medical help first. Do not call your doctor, the hospital, a friend, relatives, or neighbors. Calling anyone else first only wastes time.

Call for emergency help in the following situations:

- Fainting

- Chest or abdominal pain or pressure

- Sudden dizziness, weakness, or change in vision

- Difficulty breathing, shortness of breath

- Severe or persistent vomiting

- Sudden, severe pain anywhere in the body

- Suicidal or homicidal feelings

- Bleeding that does not stop after 10 to 15 minutes of pressure

- A gaping wound with edges that do not come together

- Problems with movement or sensation following an injury

- Cuts on the hand or face

- Puncture wounds

- The possibility that foreign bodies such as glass or metal may have entered a wound

- Most animal bites and all human bites

- Hallucinations and clouding of thoughts

- A stiff neck in association with a fever or a headache

- A bulging or abnormally depressed fontanel (soft spot) in infants

- Stupor or dazed behavior accompanying a high fever that is not alleviated by acetaminophen or aspirin
- Unequal pupil size, loss of consciousness, blindness, staggering, or repeated vomiting after a head injury
- Spinal injuries
- Severe burns
- Poisoning
- Drug overdose

When in doubt, CALL.

## Good Samaritan Laws

States have enacted laws to protect physicians and other medical personnel from legal actions that may arise from emergency treatment they give while not on duty. Although Good Samaritan laws cover medical personnel primarily, several states have expanded them to include laypersons who, in good faith, help others in emergency situations. Unless a person acts in a reckless or wantonly negligent manner when trying to voluntarily assist another, he or she is usually immune from conviction in a legal action. These laws vary from state to state; find out about your state's Good Samaritan laws by contacting a legal professional or checking with your local library.

## Heart Attack

For information on recognizing the signs of a possible heart attack and on how to respond, see Chapter 12.

## Poisoning

For information on preventing poisonings and how to treat a person who has been poisoned, see Chapter 16, especially the section titled "Environmental Health in and Around the Home"

## Bleeding

If a person is bleeding heavily from a wound, it is important to stop the bleeding as quickly as possible. First, take the following action, and then call for help or take the person to an emergency room.

- Protect yourself from disease by wearing medical exam gloves.
- Expose the wound by removing or cutting the clothing to see where the blood is coming from.

- Place a sterile gauze pad or a clean cloth (such as a washcloth or towel) over the entire wound and apply direct pressure with your fingers or the palm of your hand.
- If the bleeding is from an arm or leg, while still applying pressure, elevate the injured area above heart level to reduce blood flow.
- When the bleeding stops, wrap a roller gauze bandage tightly over the dressing to hold it in place and prevent further bleeding.

## Breathing Emergencies

Signs of inadequate breathing include a rate of breathing significantly less than 12 times per minute (for adults), skin that is pale or bluish and cool, and nasal flaring, especially in children. Ask someone to call for emergency care, and then if the person is not breathing:

- Tilt the head back and lift the chin to open the airway.
- Pinch the victim's nose shut, take a deep breath, and make a tight seal around the victim's mouth with your mouth.
- Slowly blow air into the victim's mouth until you see the chest rise.
- Remove your mouth to allow the air to come out, and turn your head away as you take another breath.
- Repeat one more breath.
- Check the victim for signs of circulation (breathing, coughing, or movement). If the victim is not breathing and has signs of circulation:
  - Give one breath about every 4 to 5 seconds for an adult.
  - Recheck for signs of circulation about every minute.
  - Continue this process as long as the person has signs of circulation, until help arrives.

If the first breath does not go in, retilt the victim's head and try a second breath. If the second breath does not go in, use the procedure to aid a choking victim.

## Choking

You can tell if a person is choking if he or she is unable to speak, breathe, or cough or breathes with a high-pitched wheezing. A choking victim may instinctively reach up and clutch his or her neck. To help, first tell someone to call for emergency care. Then, do the following:

- Stand behind the choking person.
- Wrap your arms around the victim's waist. (Do not allow your forearms to touch the ribs.)
- Make a fist with one hand and place the thumb side just above the victim's navel.
- Grasp your fist with your other hand.
- Press your fist into the victim's abdomen with quick inward and upward thrusts.
- Continue thrusts until the object is removed or the victim becomes unresponsive.

Each thrust should be a separate and distinct effort to dislodge the object.

## Burns

If a person is burned by fire and his or her clothing is on fire, have the victim roll on the ground using the "stop, drop, and roll" method. You can also smother the flames with a blanket or douse the victim with water. Ask someone to call for emergency help. Then, do the following:

- Remove jewelry and hot or burned clothing immediately, but do not remove clothing stuck to the skin.
- Cool the burn. Use large amounts of cool water, not ice. Immerse the burn in cool water if possible.
- Apply a thin layer of antibiotic ointment and cover the burn with dry, sterile dressings or clean cloths.
- Wait for help or transport the person to the emergency room of the local hospital.

## Heat–Related Emergencies

Everyone is susceptible to heat illness if environmental conditions overwhelm the body's temperature-regulating mechanisms. Such illnesses are progressive conditions and could become life threatening. Therefore, it is important to recognize heat-related illness early and treat it immediately.

Heat cramps are painful muscular spasms that happen suddenly, usually in the legs and abdomen. If someone has heat cramps, have him or her do the following:

- Rest in a cool place.
- Drink lightly salted cool water ($\frac{1}{4}$ tsp. salt per quart of water) or a commercial sports drink diluted to half strength.
- Lightly stretch and gently massage the cramped muscle.

Heat exhaustion is another heat-related emergency. It is characterized by heavy perspiration with normal or slightly above normal body temperatures and is caused by water or salt depletion or both. To help a person with heat exhaustion, have him or her do the following:

- Rest in a cool place.
- Drink lightly salted cool water ($\frac{1}{4}$ tsp. salt per quart of water) or a commercial sports drink diluted to half strength.
- Remove excess clothing.
- Lie down and raise the legs 8 to 12 inches, while keeping them straight.

Sponge the victim with cool water and fan him or her. If no improvement occurs within 30 minutes, seek medical attention.

In its advanced stages, heat exhaustion is called heatstroke and can cause death. It must be treated rapidly. Heatstroke is characterized by red, hot, dry skin and an altered mental state ranging from slight confusion and disorientation to coma. To treat heatstroke, send someone for emergency care and do the following:

- Have the person rest in a cool place.
- Remove clothing down to the victim's underwear.
- Keep the victim's head and shoulders slightly elevated.
- Cool the person by placing ice bags wrapped in wet towels on the wrists, ankles, groin, and neck, and in the armpits.
- Fan the person.

# APPENDIX C

## Dietary Reference Intakes for Certain Nutrients

# Food and Nutrition Board, National Academy of Sciences—National Research Council Dietary Reference Intakes for Certain Nutrients* (Abridged)

| Life Group Stage | Protein (g) | Vitamin A (µg RE) | Vitamin E (mg α-TE) | Vitamin D (µg) | Vitamin C (mg) | Thiamin (mg) | Niacin (mg) | Vitamin $B_6$ (mg) | Vitamin $B_{12}$ (µg) | Folate (µg) | Iron (mg) | Calcium (mg) | Zinc (mg) | Selenium (µg) |
|---|---|---|---|---|---|---|---|---|---|---|---|---|---|---|
| **Infants** | | | | | | | | | | | | | | |
| 0–6 mo | 9.1 | 400 | 4 | 10 | 40 | 0.2 | 2 | 0.1 | 0.4 | 65 | 0.27 | 200 | 2 | 15 |
| 7–12 mo | 11.0 | 500 | 5 | 10 | 50 | 0.3 | 4 | 0.3 | 0.5 | 80 | 11 | 260 | 3 | 20 |
| **Children** | | | | | | | | | | | | | | |
| 1–3 y | 13 | 300 | 6 | 15 | 15 | 0.5 | 6 | 0.5 | 0.9 | 150 | 7 | 700 | 3 | 20 |
| 4–8 y | 19 | 400 | 7 | 15 | 25 | 0.6 | 8 | 0.6 | 1.2 | 200 | 10 | 1,000 | 5 | 30 |
| **Males** | | | | | | | | | | | | | | |
| 9–13 y | 34 | 600 | 11 | 15 | 45 | 0.9 | 12 | 1.0 | 1.8 | 300 | 8 | 1,300 | 8 | 40 |
| 14–18 y | 52 | 900 | 15 | 15 | 75 | 1.2 | 16 | 1.3 | 2.4 | 400 | 11 | 1,300 | 11 | 55 |
| 19–30 y | 56 | 900 | 15 | 15 | 90 | 1.2 | 16 | 1.3 | 2.4 | 400 | 8 | 1,000 | 11 | 55 |
| 31–50 y | 56 | 900 | 15 | 15 | 90 | 1.2 | 16 | 1.3 | 2.4 | 400 | 8 | 1,000 | 11 | 55 |
| 51–70 y | 56 | 900 | 15 | 15 | 90 | 1.2 | 16 | 1.7 | 2.4 | 400 | 8 | 1,000 | 11 | 55 |
| >70 y | 56 | 900 | 15 | 20 | 90 | 1.2 | 16 | 1.7 | 2.4 | 400 | 8 | 1,200 | 11 | 55 |
| **Females** | | | | | | | | | | | | | | |
| 9–13 y | 34 | 600 | 11 | 15 | 45 | 0.9 | 12 | 1.0 | 1.8 | 300 | 8 | 1,300 | 8 | 40 |
| 14–18 y | 46 | 700 | 15 | 15 | 65 | 1.0 | 14 | 1.2 | 2.4 | 400 | 15 | 1,300 | 9 | 55 |
| 19–30 y | 46 | 700 | 15 | 15 | 75 | 1.1 | 14 | 1.3 | 2.4 | 400 | 18 | 1,000 | 8 | 55 |
| 31–50 y | 46 | 700 | 15 | 15 | 75 | 1.1 | 14 | 1.3 | 2.4 | 400 | 18 | 1,000 | 8 | 55 |
| 51–70 y | 46 | 700 | 15 | 15 | 75 | 1.1 | 14 | 1.5 | 2.4 | 400 | 8 | 1,200 | 8 | 55 |
| >70 y | 46 | 700 | 15 | 20 | 75 | 1.1 | 14 | 1.5 | 2.4 | 400 | 8 | 1,200 | 8 | 55 |
| **Pregnant** | | | | | | | | | | | | | | |
| 19–50 y | 71 | 770 | 15 | 15 | 85 | 1.4 | 18 | 1.9 | 2.6 | 600 | 27 | 1,000 | 11 | 60 |
| **Lactating** | | | | | | | | | | | | | | |
| 19–50 y | 71 | 1,300 | 19 | 15 | 120 | 1.4 | 17 | 2.0 | 2.8 | 500 | 9 | 1,000 | 12 | 70 |

*Daily intakes. For more information about the DRIs, go to http://ods.od.nih.gov/Health_Information/Dietary_Reference_Intakes.aspx.

*Source:* Food and Nutrition Board, Institute of Medicine, National Academies. (2010). Dietary reference intakes (DRIs): Recommended Dietary Allowances and Adequate Intakes. http://www.iom.edu/Activities/Nutrition/SummaryDRIs/

# Food Intake Patterns Based on MyPlate Recommendations

The following table indicates suggested amounts of food to consume from the basic food groups, to meet recommended nutrient intakes at 12 different calorie levels. Nutrient and energy contributions from each group are calculated according to the nutrient-dense forms of foods in each group (e.g., lean meats and fat-free milk). This appendix also includes a sample seven day menu guide for a 2000 Calorie/day food pattern.

## Daily Amount of Food from Each Group

| | 1,000 | 1,200 | 1,400 | 1,600 | 1,800 | 2,000 | 2,200 | 2,400 | 2,600 | 2,800 | 3,000 | 3,200 |
|---|---|---|---|---|---|---|---|---|---|---|---|---|
| Calorie Level[1] | | | | | | | | | | | | |
| Fruits[2] | 1 cup | 1 cup | 1.5 cups | 1.5 cups | 1.5 cups | 2 cups | 2 cups | 2 cups | 2 cups | 2.5 cups | 2.5 cups | 2.5 cups |
| Vegetables[3] | 1 cup | 1.5 cups | 1.5 cups | 2 cups | 2.5 cups | 2.5 cups | 3 cups | 3 cups | 3.5 cups | 3.5 cups | 4 cups | 4 cups |
| Grains[4] | 3 oz-eq | 4 oz-eq | 5 oz-eq | 5 oz-eq | 6 oz-eq | 6 oz-eq | 7 oz-eq | 8 oz-eq | 9 oz-eq | 10 oz-eq | 10 oz-eq | 10 oz-eq |
| Protein foods[5] | 2 oz-eq | 3 oz-eq | 4 oz-eq | 5 oz-eq | 5 oz-eq | 5.5 oz-eq | 6oz-eq | 6.5 oz-eq | 6.5 oz-eq | 7 oz-eq | 7 oz-eq | 7 oz-eq |
| Dairy[6] | 2 cups | 2 cups | 2 cups | 3 cups | 3 cups | 3 cups | 3 cups | 3 cups | 3 cups | 3 cups | 3 cups | 3 cups |

[1] **Calorie Levels** are set across a wide range to accommodate the needs of different individuals. The table "Estimated Daily Calorie Needs" can be used to help assign individuals to the food intake pattern at a particular calorie level.

[2] **Fruit Group** includes all fresh, frozen, canned, and dried fruits, and may be whole, cut-up or pureed. Any 100% fruit juice created as a form of fruit. In general, 1 cup of fruit or 100% fruit juice, or 1/2 cup of dried fruit can be considered as 1 cup from the fruit group.

[3] **Vegetable Group** includes all fresh, frozen, canned, and dried vegetables and vegetable juices. In general, 1 cup of raw or cooked vegetables or vegetable juice, or 2 cups of raw leafy greens can be considered as 1 cup from the vegetable group.

[4] **Grains Group** includes all foods made from wheat, rice, oats, cornmeal, barley, such as bread, pasta, oatmeal, breakfast cereals, tortillas, and grits. In general, 1 slice of bread, 1 cup of ready-to-eat cereal, or 1/2 cup of cooked rice, pasta, or cooked cereal can be considered as 1 ounce equivalent from the grains group. At least half of all grains consumed should be whole grains.

[5] **Protein Foods Group** in general, 1 ounce of lean meat, poultry, or fish, 1 egg, 1 Tbsp. peanut butter, 1/4 cup cooked dry beans, or 1/2 ounce of nuts or seeds can be considered as 1 ounce equivalent from the meat and beans group.

[6] **Dairy Group** includes all fluid milk products and foods made from milk that retain their calcium content, such as yogurt and cheese. Foods made from milk that have little to no calcium, such as cream cheese, cream, and butter, are not part of the group. Most dairy group choices should be fat-free or low-fat. In general, 1 cup of milk or yogurt, 1 1/2 ounces of natural cheese, or 2 ounces of processed cheese can be considered as 1 cup from the dairy group.

Although MyPlate does not include an "oils" group, some fat is essential for good health. Oils include fats from many different plants and from fish that are liquid at room temperature, such as canola, corn, olive, soybean, and sunflower oil. Some foods are naturally high in oils, like nuts, olives, some fish, and avocados. Foods that are mainly oil include mayonnaise, certain salad dressings, and soft margarine.

# Estimated Daily Calorie Needs

To determine which food intake pattern to use for an individual, the following chart gives an estimate of individual calorie needs. The calorie range for each age/sex group is based on physical activity level, from sedentary to active.

| Children | Calorie Range | | |
|---|---|---|---|
| | Sedentary* | → | Active† |
| 2–3 years | 1,000 | → | 1,400 |
| **Females** | | | |
| 4–8 years | 1,200 | → | 1,800 |
| 9–13 | 1,600 | → | 2,200 |
| 14–18 | 1,800 | → | 2,400 |
| 19–30 | 2,000 | → | 2,400 |
| 31–50 | 1,800 | → | 2,200 |
| 51+ | 1,600 | → | 2,200 |
| **Males** | | | |
| 4–8 years | 1,400 | → | 2,000 |
| 9–13 | 1,800 | → | 2,600 |
| 14–18 | 2,200 | → | 3,200 |
| 19–30 | 2,400 | → | 3,000 |
| 31–50 | 2,200 | → | 3,000 |
| 51+ | 2,000 | → | 2,800 |

* Sedentary means a lifestyle that includes only the light physical activity associated with typical day-to-day life.

† Active means a lifestyle that includes physical activity equivalent to walking more than 3 miles per day at 3 to 4 miles per hour, in addition to the light physical activity associated with typical day-to-day life.

# Sample Menus for a 2000 Calorie Food Pattern

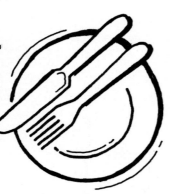

Use this 7-day menu as a motivational tool to help put a healthy eating pattern into practice, and to identify creative new ideas for healthy meals. Averaged over a week, this menu provides the recommended amounts of key nutrients and foods from each food group. The menus feature a large number of different foods to inspire ideas for adding variety to food choices. They are not intended to be followed day-by-day as a specific prescription for what to eat.

Spices and herbs can be used to taste. Try spices such as chili powder, cinnamon, cumin, curry powder, ginger, nutmeg, mustard, garlic powder, onion powder, or pepper. Try fresh or dried herbs such as basil, parsley, cilantro, chives, dill, mint, oregano, rosemary, thyme, or tarragon. Also try salt-free spice or herb blends.

While this 7-day menu provides the recommended amounts of foods and key nutrients, it does so at a moderate cost. Based on national average food costs, adjusted for inflation to March 2011 prices, the cost of this menu is less than the average amount spent for food, per person, in a 4-person family.

## DAY 1

### BREAKFAST
Creamy oatmeal (cooked in milk):
- ½ cup uncooked oatmeal
- 1 cup fat-free milk
- 2 Tbsp raisins
- 2 tsp brown sugar
- Beverage: 1 cup orange juice

### LUNCH
Taco salad:
- 2 ounces tortilla chips
- 2 ounces cooked ground turkey
- 2 tsp corn/canola oil (to cook turkey)
- ¼ cup kidney beans*
- ½ ounce low-fat cheddar cheese
- ½ cup chopped lettuce
- ½ cup avocado
- 1 tsp lime juice (on avocado)
- 2 Tbsp salsa
- Beverage: 1 cup water, coffee, or tea**

### DINNER
Spinach lasagna roll-ups:
- 1 cup lasagna noodles(2 oz dry)
- ½ cup cooked spinach
- ½ cup ricotta cheese
- 1 ounce part-skim mozzarella cheese
- ½ cup tomato sauce*
- 1 ounce whole wheat roll
- 1 tsp tub margarine
- Beverage: 1 cup fat-free milk

### SNACKS
- 2 Tbsp raisins
- 1 ounce unsalted almonds

## DAY 2

### BREAKFAST
Breakfast burrito:
- 1 flour tortilla (8" diameter)
- 1 scrambled egg
- ⅓ cup black beans*
- 2 Tbsp salsa
- ½ large grapefruit
- Beverage: 1 cup water, coffee, or tea**

### LUNCH
Roast beef sandwich:
- 1 small whole grain hoagie bun
- 2 ounces lean roast beef
- 1 slice part-skim mozzarella cheese
- 2 slices tomato
- ¼ cup mushrooms
- 1 tsp corn/canola oil (to cook mushrooms)
- 1 tsp mustard
Baked potato wedges:
- 1 cup potato wedges
- 1 tsp corn/canola oil (to cook potato)
- 1 Tbsp ketchup
- Beverage: 1 cup fat-free milk

### DINNER
Baked salmon on beet greens:
- 4 ounce salmon filet
- 1 tsp olive oil
- 2 tsp lemon juice
- ⅓ cup cooked beet greens (sauteed in 2 tsp corn/canola oil)
Quinoa with almonds:
- ½ cup quinoa
- ½ ounce slivered almonds
- Beverage: 1 cup fat-free milk

### SNACKS
- 1 cup cantaloupe balls

## DAY 3

### BREAKFAST
Cold cereal:
- 1 cup ready-to-eat oat cereal
- 1 medium banana
- ½ cup fat-free milk
- 1 slice whole wheat toast
- 1 tsp tub margarine
- Beverage: 1 cup prune juice

### LUNCH
Tuna salad sandwich:
- 2 slices rye bread
- 2 ounces tuna
- 1 Tbsp mayonnaise
- 1 Tbsp chopped celery
- ½ cup shredded lettuce
- 1 medium peach
- Beverage: 1 cup fat-free milk

### DINNER
Roasted chicken:
- 3 ounces cooked chicken breast
- 1 large sweet potato, roasted
- ½ cup succotash (limas & corn)
- 1 tsp tub margarine
- 1 ounce whole wheat roll
- 1 tsp tub margarine
- Beverage:
- 1 cup water, coffee, or tea**

### SNACKS
- ¼ cup dried apricots
- 1 cup flavored yogurt (chocolate)

# Sample Menus for a 2000 Calorie Food Pattern

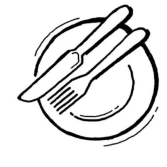

| DAY 4 | DAY 5 | DAY 6 | DAY 7 |
|-------|-------|-------|-------|

**DAY 4**

**BREAKFAST**
1 whole wheat English muffin
1 Tbsp all-fruit preserves
1 hard-cooked egg
Beverage:
1 cup water, coffee, or tea**

**LUNCH**
White bean-vegetable soup:
1 ¼ cup chunky vegetable soup with pasta
½ cup white beans*
6 saltine crackers*
½ cup celery sticks
Beverage: 1 cup fat-free milk

**DINNER**
Rigatoni with meat sauce:
1 cup rigatoni pasta (2 oz dry)
2 ounces cooked ground beef (95% lean)
2 tsp corn/canola oil (to cook beef)
½ cup tomato sauce*
3 Tbsp grated parmesan cheese
Spinach salad:
1 cup raw spinach leaves
½ cup tangerine sections
½ ounce chopped walnuts
4 tsp oil and vinegar dressing
Beverage:
1 cup water, coffee, or tea**

**SNACKS**
1 cup nonfat fruit yogurt

**DAY 5**

**BREAKFAST**
Cold cereal:
1 cup shredded wheat
½ cup sliced banana
½ cup fat-free milk
1 slice whole wheat toast
2 tsp all-fruit preserves
Beverage:
1 cup fat-free chocolate milk

**LUNCH**
Turkey sandwich
1 whole wheat pita bread (2 oz)
3 ounces roasted turkey, sliced
2 slices tomato
¼ cup shredded lettuce
1 tsp mustard
1 Tbsp mayonnaise
½ cup grapes
Beverage: 1 cup tomato juice*

**DINNER**
Steak and potatoes:
4 ounces broiled beef steak
⅔ cup mashed potatoes made with milk and 2 tsp tub margarine
½ cup cooked green beans
1 tsp tub margarine
1 tsp honey
1 ounce whole wheat roll
1 tsp tub margarine
Frozen yogurt and berries:
½ cup frozen yogurt (chocolate)
¼ cup sliced strawberries
Beverage: 1 cup fat-free milk

**SNACKS**
1 cup frozen yogurt (chocolate)

**DAY 6**

**BREAKFAST**
French toast:
2 slices whole wheat bread
3 Tbsp fat-free milk and ⅔ egg (in French toast)
2 tsp tub margarine
1 Tbsp pancake syrup
½ large grapefruit
Beverage: 1 cup fat-free milk

**LUNCH**
3-bean vegetarian chili on baked potato:
¼ cup each cooked kidney beans,* navy beans,* and black beans*
½ cup tomato sauce*
¼ cup chopped onion
2 Tbsp chopped jalapeno peppers
1 tsp corn/canola oil (to cook onion and peppers)
¼ cup cheese sauce
1 large baked potato
½ cup cantaloupe
Beverage:
1 cup water, coffee, or tea**

**DINNER**
Hawaiian pizza
2 slices cheese pizza, thin crust
1 ounce lean ham
¼ cup pineapple
¼ cup mushrooms
1 tsp safflower oil (to cook mushrooms)
Green salad:
1 cup mixed salad greens
4 tsp oil and vinegar dressing
Beverage: 1 cup fat-free milk

**SNACKS**
3 Tbsp hummus
5 whole wheat crackers*

**DAY 7**

**BREAKFAST**
Buckwheat pancakes with berries:
2 large (7") pancakes
1 Tbsp pancake syrup
¼ cup sliced strawberries
Beverage: 1 cup orange juice

**LUNCH**
New England clam chowder:
3 ounces canned clams
½ small potato
2 Tbsp chopped onion
2 Tbsp chopped celery
6 Tbsp evaporated milk
¼ cup fat-free milk
1 slice bacon
1 Tbsp white flour
10 whole wheat crackers*
1 medium orange
Beverage: 1 cup fat-free milk

**DINNER**
Tofu-vegetable stir-fry:
4 ounces firm tofu
½ cup chopped Chinese cabbage
¼ cup sliced bamboo shoots
2 Tbsp chopped sweet red peppers
2 Tbsp chopped green peppers
1 Tbsp corn/canola oil (to cook stir-fry)
1 cup cooked brown rice (2 ounces raw)
Honeydew yogurt cup:
¾ cup honeydew melon
½ cup plain fat-free yogurt
Beverage:
1 cup water, coffee, or tea**

**SNACKS**
1 large banana spread with
2 Tbsp peanut butter*
1 cup nonfat fruit yogurt

Notes:

*Foods that are reduced sodium, low sodium, or no-salt added products. These foods can also be prepared from scratch with no added salt. All other foods are regular commercial products, which contain variable levels of sodium. Average sodium level of the 7-day menu assumes that no salt is added in cooking or at the table.

**Unless indicated, all beverages are unsweetened and without added cream or whitener.

Italicized foods are part of the dish or food that precedes it.

# Sample Menus: Average Intakes

## Average amounts for weekly menu:

| Food group | Daily average over 1 week |
|---|---|
| **GRAINS** | **6.2 oz eq** |
| Whole grains | 3.8 |
| Refined grains | 2.4 |
| **VEGETABLES** | **2.6 cups** |
| Vegetable subgroups (amount per week) | |
| Dark green | 1.6 cups per week |
| Red/Orange | 5.6 |
| Starchy | 5.1 |
| Beans and Peas | 1.6 |
| Other Vegetables | 4.1 |
| **FRUITS** | **2.1 cups** |
| **DAIRY** | **3.1 cups** |
| **PROTEIN FOODS** | **5.7 oz eq** |
| Seafood | 8.8 oz per week |
| **OILS** | **29 grams** |
| **CALORIES FROM ADDED FATS AND SUGARS** | **245 calories** |

| Nutrient | Daily average over 1 week |
|---|---|
| Calories | 1975 |
| Protein | 96 g |
| Protein | 19% kcal |
| Carbohydrate | 275 g |
| Carbohydrate | 56% kcal |
| Total fat | 59 g |
| Total fat | 27% kcal |
| Saturated fat | 13.2 g |
| Saturated fat | 6.0% kcal |
| Monounsaturated fat | 25 g |
| Polyunsaturated fat | 16 g |
| Linoleic Acid | 13 g |
| Alpha-linolenic Acid | 1.8 g |
| Cholesterol | 201 mg |
| Total dietary fiber | 30 g |
| Potassium | 4701 mg |
| Sodium | 1810 mg |
| Calcium | 1436 mg |
| Magnesium | 468 mg |
| Copper | 2.0 mg |
| Iron | 18 mg |
| Phosphorus | 1885 mg |
| Zinc | 14 mg |
| Thiamin | 1.6 mg |
| Riboflavin | 2.5 mg |
| Niacin Equivalents | 24 mg |
| Vitamin B6 | 2.4 mg |
| Vitamin B12 | 12.3 mcg |
| Vitamin C | 146 mg |
| Vitamin E | 11.8 mg (AT) |
| Vitamin D | 9.1 mcg |
| Vitamin A | 1090 mcg (RAE) |
| Dietary Folate Equivalents | 530 mcg |
| Choline | 386 mg |

# Glossary

**abortion**  Removal of the embryo or fetus from the uterus before it is able to survive on its own.

**absorption**  The passage of nutrients through the walls of the intestinal tract.

**abstinence**  A method of birth control that involves refraining from vaginal intercourse.

**abuse**  Taking advantage of a relationship to mistreat a person.

**acid precipitation**  Rain, snow, or fog combined with sulfur dioxide from fossil fuel emissions.

**acquired immune deficiency syndrome (AIDS)**  A set of certain diseases and conditions that results from infection by the human immunodeficiency virus (HIV).

**acquired immunity**  Specific resistance to infection that is not inherited but develops during a person's lifetime.

**acute**  A condition or illness that tends to develop quickly and resolve within a few days or weeks.

**acute bronchitis**  A temporary inflammation of the mucous membranes.

**adipose cells**  Cells that store fat.

**aerobic**  Oxygen-requiring.

**affect**  Observable expressions of mood.

**affection**  Fondness.

**ageism**  A bias against elderly people.

**aging**  The sum of all changes that occur to an organism during its life.

**Air Quality Index (AQI)**  A guide to air quality that uses levels of various pollutants to determine its values.

**alcohol abuse**  Includes the symptoms of harmful use, but when drinking the abuser exhibits long-term social interaction problems and uses alcohol in physically dangerous situations.

**alcohol dependence (alcoholism)**  A syndrome characterized by at least three of the following symptoms: a compulsion to drink, difficulty in controlling the amount of alcohol consumed, withdrawal symptoms when alcohol is not consumed, evidence of tolerance, progressive neglect of other interests because of drinking, and continuing to use alcohol despite its physical and psychological effects on the user.

**Alzheimer's disease (AD)**  An incurable, progressive, degenerative disease that affects the functioning of the brain.

**amino acids**  The chemical units that compose proteins.

**amniocentesis**  A prenatal test performed generally between the 15th and 18th weeks of gestation, in which some of the amniotic fluid that surrounds the fetus is removed and studied to determine whether the fetus has a genetic abnormality.

**anabolic steroids**  A group of drugs that can have muscle-building effects on the body.

**analgesics**  (an-al-GEEZ-iks) Drugs that alleviate pain.

**analogs**  Drugs that are chemically similar but have different effects on the body.

**anecdotes**  Personal reports of individual experiences.

**anesthetic**  Substance that interferes with normal sensations.

**aneurysm**  (AN-you-rizm) A swollen, weakened blood vessel.

**angina pectoris**  (an-JEYE-nah PECK-tor-iss) Chest pain caused by insufficient oxygen in a portion of the heart.

**angioplasty**  (AN-jee-oh-PLAS-tee) The reconstruction of damaged blood vessels.

**anorexia nervosa**  A severe psychological disturbance in which an individual refuses to eat enough food to maintain a healthy weight.

**antibiotics**  (AN-tie-by-OT-iks) A group of chemicals that kill bacteria or inhibit their growth.

**antibodies**  Proteins that interact in a lock-and-key fashion with antigens, interfering with the normal functioning of the antigen.

**antigens**  (AN-tih-jenz) Proteins that are foreign or recognized as "nonself" by the body.

**antioxidants**  Compounds that protect cells from free-radical damage.

**appetite**  The psychological desire to eat foods that are appealing.

**arrhythmias**  (uh-RITH-me-uhs) Abnormal heartbeats.

**arteries**  Blood vessels that carry blood away from the heart.

**arthritis**  A group of diseases characterized by inflammation of the joints.

**asbestos** (as-BES-tose) A fiber-like mineral found in rocks that, when inhaled, can cause lung cancer or other lung conditions.

**asbestosis** (AS-bes-TOE-sis) A condition in which scar tissue forms in the lungs as a response to irritation by asbestos.

**assault** The intentional use of force to injure another person physically.

**asthma** (AZ-mah) A common, chronic, childhood illness characterized by sensitive airways.

**atherectomy** (ATH-er-EK-toe-me) The removal of plaque from the interior of an artery.

**atherosclerosis** (ATH-er-oh-skle-ROW-sis) Disease of large and medium-sized arteries in which the inner lining has areas that are deteriorated, thickened, and inelastic.

**atrial fibrillation** (fih-brih-LAY-shun) A type of arrhythmia in which the upper chambers of the heart contract with no set pattern.

**atrophy** A condition in which muscles lose size and strength.

**attachment** The desire to spend time with someone to give and receive emotional support.

**autoimmune diseases** Diseases in which the body perceives its own cells as foreign, attacking them and causing localized and systemic (whole-body) reactions.

**autonomy** Sense of independence and self-control.

**autopsy** Various medical examinations and tests that usually determine the cause of death.

**B cells** Specialized white blood cells (lymphocytes) that function in antibody-mediated immunity and produce antibodies.

**bacteria** Unicellular, microscopic organisms with a simple cell structure; some are pathogenic to humans and produce infections such as strep throat, bacterial pneumonia, food poisoning, and infected cuts.

**barrier methods** Types of birth control that block the path that sperm must take to reach the ovum; these forms of contraception include male condoms, female condoms, diaphragms, and cervical caps.

**basal (BAY-sl) cell carcinoma** The most common cancer of the skin, which frequently develops on portions of the skin exposed to the sun.

**benign (be-NINE) tumors** Encapsulated masses of abnormal cells that remain in one location and do not invade surrounding tissues.

**binge eating disorder** A pattern of eating excessive amounts of food in response to distress such as anxiety or depression.

**biopsy** (BI-op-see) A small piece of tissue that is taken from a growth so that the cells can be studied and a diagnosis confirmed.

**birth control (contraception)** Methods to avoid pregnancy.

**bisexual** A person who engages in sexual activity with both sexes.

**body mass index (BMI)** A standard that correlates body weight with the risk of developing chronic health conditions associated with obesity.

**Braxton-Hicks contractions** False labor; preparatory contractions that are not a part of labor.

**breech birth** A delivery in which the baby presents feet or buttocks first instead of the usual head-first position.

**bulimia nervosa** An eating disorder characterized by a craving for food that is difficult to satisfy.

**calorie** A unit of energy.

**cancer screening** An examination to detect malignancies in a person who has no symptoms.

**cancer staging** A description of the extent of the growth and metastasis of a cancer to determine appropriate therapy and prognosis.

**capillaries** (KAP-ih-LAIR-eez) Microscopic blood vessels that permeate tissues, connecting small arteries to small veins.

**carbohydrates** A class of nutrients that includes sugars and starches.

**carbon monoxide poisoning** A toxic condition that affects red blood cells' ability to carry oxygen, caused by the inhalation of the gas carbon monoxide.

**carcinogens** (kar-SIN-oh-jenz) Cancer-causing substances.

**carcinomas** (KAR-si-NO-mahz) Cancers that arise from epithelial tissues.

**cardiorespiratory fitness** The ability to perform muscular work intensely and for long periods without becoming fatigued.

**cardiovascular disease (CVD)** Disorders of the heart and blood vessels.

**caring** The expression of concern for someone's well-being.

**carpal tunnel syndrome** Numbness, pain, or pins-and-needles sensations in either of the hands that extends down the fingers, resulting from improper alignment of the wrist while engaging in repetitive-use activities.

**cataracts** A chronic condition in which the lens of the eye becomes cloudy and opaque, impairing vision.

**celiac disease** A condition characterized by hypersensitivity to gluten.

**celibacy (sexual abstinence)** Refrainment from sexual intercourse, usually by choice.

**central nervous system (CNS)** Of the two primary divisions of the nervous system, the one that consists of brain and spinal cord.

**cerebral embolism** A stroke caused by a floating blood clot that becomes lodged in a cerebral artery, blocking blood flow.

**cerebral hemorrhage** (HEM-ah-rij) A stroke caused by a burst artery that supplies the brain.

**cerebral thrombosis** A stroke caused by a stationary blood clot.

**cervix** The narrow neck of the uterus.

**chain of infection** The relationship among the factors important in the development of infectious diseases: the pathogen, transmission, and the host.

**child physical abuse** Physical violence against a child who is under 18 years of age.

**child sexual abuse** Sexual activity involving a child that takes place as a result of force or threat.

**chlamydial (klah-MID-dee-ahl) infection** An STI that results in gonorrhea-like symptoms.

**cholesterol** A type of lipid found only in animals.

**MyPlate** A practical guide for planning healthful diets.

**chorionic villus sampling (CVS)** A prenatal test performed generally between the 10th and 12th weeks of gestation, in which some of the fetal extraembryonic tissue is removed and analyzed to determine whether the fetus has a genetic abnormality.

**chronic** A condition or disease that often takes months or years to develop, progresses in severity, and can affect a person over a longer period.

**chronic bronchitis** A persistent inflammation and thickening of the lining of the bronchi.

**chronic obstructive pulmonary disease (COPD)** A syndrome that includes chronic bronchitis, asthma, and emphysema and that is characterized by extreme difficulty in breathing.

**clitoris** (KLIT-oh-ris) A female organ of sexual arousal. Located under a protective hood of tissue, the clitoris lies in front of the urethra.

**cohabitation** Unmarried persons living together.

**coitus** (KO-ih-tus) The act of a penis penetrating a vagina, often referred to as vaginal intercourse.

**coitus interruptus (withdrawal)** (KO-ih-tus in-ter-RUP-tus) A form of birth control in which the man removes his penis from his partner's vagina and genital area, interrupting intercourse before ejaculation.

**colon** Major segment of the large intestine.

**colonoscopy** (KO-lon-OS-ko-pee) A procedure in which a physician views the entire length of the colon using a flexible fiber-optic tube.

**comatose** Condition in which one is unresponsive to the environment and in a coma.

**combined oral contraceptives** "The pill" suppress ovulation through the combined actions of estrogen and progestin.

**commitment** The determination to maintain a relationship even when times are difficult.

**communicable** (ka-MYOO-ni-kah-bl) Transmissible from person to person.

**community violence** Violence between strangers or acquaintances that occurs in public settings.

**compatible** Capable of existing together in harmony.

**compulsion** The behavior that follows obsessive thoughts and reduces anxiety.

**condom** A sheath used to cover the penis during sexual intercourse to help prevent pregnancy or sexually transmitted infections.

**constipation** A condition characterized by having fewer than three bowel movements per week.

**conventional medicine** Form of medicine that relies on modern scientific principles, modern technologies, and scientifically proven methods to prevent, diagnose, and treat health conditions.

**coping strategies** Behavioral responses and thought processes that people use to deal with stressors.

**coronary arteries** Blood vessels that arise from the base of the aorta and bring freshly oxygenated blood to the heart muscle.

**coronary artery bypass graft (CABG) surgery** A surgical procedure in which healthy blood vessels are used to redirect blood flow around blocked vessels of the heart.

**coronary artery disease (CAD)** A condition in which the coronary vessels are blocked partially or completely by fatty deposits, blood clots, or both. Also commonly called coronary heart disease (CHD).

**coronary embolism** (EM-bow-lizm) A floating blood clot that lodges in an artery that brings blood to the heart muscle, blocking blood flow.

**coronary thrombosis** (throm-BOW-sis) The development of a stationary blood clot that blocks blood flow in an artery that brings blood to the heart muscle.

**corpus luteum** (KOR-pus LOO-tea-um) The ruptured follicle left behind after ovulation.

**cross-training** Incorporating a variety of aerobic activities into a fitness program.

**cunnilingus** Use of the mouth and tongue to stimulate a woman's genitals.

**cystic fibrosis (SIS-tik fie-BROH-sis) (CF)** A common, lethal, inherited disease that affects the glands that secrete mucus and sweat, resulting in multiple disorders of the lungs and pancreas.

**death** The cessation of life, which occurs soon after a person's heart or lungs stop functioning.

**defense mechanisms** Ways of thinking and behaving that reduce or eliminate anxious and guilt feelings.

**delusions** Inaccurate and unreasonable beliefs that often result in decision-making errors.

**dementia** A brain disorder that seriously affects normal cognitive abilities.

**detoxification** The process of converting harmful substances into less dangerous compounds.

**detraining** A condition characterized by atrophied and weak muscles, which occurs when skeletal muscles are not used regularly.

**diabetes mellitus ("diabetes")** A group of chronic diseases characterized by the inability to metabolize carbohydrates properly.

**diastolic (DIE-as-TOL-ik) pressure** The lower number in the blood pressure reading, which is the pressure exerted by the blood on the artery walls when the left ventricle relaxes.

**diet** One's usual pattern of food choices.

**dietary fiber** Indigestible substances produced by plants.

**Dietary Reference Intakes (DRIs)** A set of standards for evaluating the nutritional quality of diets.

**dietary supplement** A product that is consumed to add nutrients, herbs, or other plant materials to a person's diet.

**digestion** The process of breaking down large food molecules into smaller molecules that the intestinal tract can absorb.

**digital rectal exam** A test in which a physician uses a gloved finger to feel the rectum or the prostate for abnormal growths.

**disease** A process that affects the proper functioning of the body and is usually accompanied by characteristic signs and symptoms.

**distress** Events or conditions that produce unwanted or negative outcomes.

**diverticulosis** An intestinal disorder that occurs when the colon lining forms small pouches that protrude through the outer wall of the colon.

**douching** (DOOSH-ing) The use of specially prepared solutions to cleanse the vagina; not an effective birth control method.

**Down syndrome** A genetic disease usually caused by the presence of three (rather than two) number 21 chromosomes; the child is usually intellectually disabled, with a short body and a broad, flat face.

**drug abuse** The intentional improper or nonmedical use of any drug.

**drug dependence or addiction** Occurs when users develop a habitual pattern of taking drugs that produces a compulsive need, which is both physical and psychological.

**drug misuse** The temporary and improper use of a legal drug.

**drugs** Nonfood chemicals that alter the way a person thinks, feels, functions, or behaves.

**Duchenne/Becker muscular dystrophy (do-SHAYN BECK-er MUSS-ku-lar DIS-tro-fee) (DBMD)** An inherited disease in which the muscles gradually weaken and degenerate. It usually strikes boys before the age of 6 years.

**eating disorders** Persistent, abnormal eating patterns that can threaten a person's health and well-being.

**efficacy** (EF-fih-ka-see) Regarding health education, the belief that one is capable of changing his or her behavior.

**ejaculation** The emission of semen from the penis during orgasm.

**elder abuse** Use of physical or sexual violence against an elderly person.

**embolus** (EM-bow-lus) A floating blood clot.

**embryo** The 3rd through 8th weeks of gestational development.

**emergency contraception (EC)** Birth control methods that help prevent pregnancy after sexual intercourse, rather than before or during sex.

**emphysema** (EM-fih-SEE-mah) A chronic condition in which the air sacs of the lungs lose their normal elasticity, impairing respiration.

**endocrine system** A group of glands that produce hormones.

**endometrium** (EN-doe-ME-tree-um) The inner lining of the uterus.

**environmental health** The effects of environmental factors on humans and the effects of humans on their environments.

**environmental tobacco smoke (ETS)** The smoke emitted from a lit cigarette, cigar, or pipe and the smoke exhaled by smokers.

**epididymis** (EP-ih-DID-ih-mis) A coiled tube that lies on the back of each testis and in which sperm mature.

**episiotomy** (uh-pee-zee-OT-uh-me) A cut in the tissue surrounding the vaginal opening to widen it during a vaginal delivery so that the surrounding skin and tissues will be less likely to tear.

**erectile dysfunction (ED)** A sexual dysfunction in which a man is unable to develop and/or sustain an erection firm enough for penetration of the vagina. Also called impotence.

**ergogenic aids** A variety of products that supposedly enhance physical development or performance.

**estrogen** (ES-tro-jen) A hormone secreted by ovarian follicles, the groups of cells within which ova mature. With progesterone, estrogen stimulates the continued development and thickening of the uterine lining.

**euphoria** (you-FOR-ee-a) An intense feeling of well-being commonly called a "high."

**eustress** (YOU-stress) Events or conditions that create positive effects, such as making one feel happy, challenged, or successful.

**exercise** Physical activity that is usually planned and performed to improve or maintain one's physical condition.

**extrarelational sex** Sexual relationships with individuals who are not one's spouse or primary sex partner.

**fad diets**   Eating plans that are popular for a time, then quickly lose their widespread appeal.

**family (domestic) violence**   Violence or abuse between family members, people who are involved in intimate relationships, or unrelated individuals who live together.

**fecal occult (FEE-kle ok-KULT) blood test (FOBT)**   Home test that detects hidden blood in the stool.

**fellatio**   Use of the mouth and tongue to stimulate a male's genitals.

**fetal alcohol spectrum disorders (FASDs)**   A variety of incurable conditions and birth defects caused by alcohol exposure during prenatal development.

**fetal alcohol syndrome (FAS)**   The most severe FASD. Children born with FAS may suffer intellectual disability and have characteristic facial anomalies, growth deficiency, and central nervous system abnormalities.

**fetus**   The 9th through 38th weeks of gestational development.

**fight-or-flight response**   The physical responses to stressful situations that enable the body to confront or leave dangerous situations.

**flexibility**   The ability to move a muscle to any position in its normal range of motion.

**follicles**   Masses of cells in the ovaries that contain immature ova (eggs) in various stages of development. Each follicle contains one ovum.

**formaldehyde**   (form-AL-de-hide) A chemical used in the manufacture of certain building materials and furnishings; may cause health problems when released into indoor air.

**fungi**   (FUN-jeye) Cellular organisms that cannot make their own food; some are pathogenic to humans and produce infections such as athlete's foot, ringworm, and yeast infections. *Fungus* is the singular term.

**gender identity**   An individual's perception of himself or herself as male or female.

**gender role**   Patterns of behavior, attitudes, and personality attributes that are traditionally considered in a particular culture to be feminine or masculine.

**gender**   The classification of a person's sex based on many criteria, among them anatomic and chromosomal characteristics.

**general adaptation syndrome (GAS)**   The three-stage manner in which the human body responds to stress: alarm, resistance, and exhaustion.

**generalized anxiety disorder**   A condition characterized by uncontrollable chronic worrying and nervousness.

**genes**   Segments of DNA.

**genital herpes**   An STI caused by the herpes simplex virus that results in sores in the genital and anal areas.

**genital warts**   An STI caused by the human papillomavirus that results in noncancerous skin tumors of the genital area.

**genomics**   (Jee-nom-iks) The scientific study of an organism's entire set of genes.

**gerontologists**   Scientists who study aging.

**glaucoma**   (glaw-KO-mah) A chronic ailment that occurs when fluid pressure increases in the eye.

**glucose**   The most important monosaccharide in the human body.

**gonorrhea**   (GON-ah-REE-ah) An STI characterized by infection of the urethra in men and the cervix in women, usually resulting in a thick discharge from the penis or vagina.

**good health**   The ability to function adequately and independently in a constantly changing environment.

**grief**   The emotional state that nearly everyone experiences when they lose something or someone special.

**hallucinations**   False sensory perceptions that have no apparent external cause.

**harmful use**   Drinking alcoholic beverages while knowingly damaging one's physical and/or psychological health.

**hazardous waste**   Toxic chemical refuse.

**heart attack**   Myocardial infarction (MI); an area of heart muscle that dies because it does not receive enough oxygen as a result of insufficient blood supply.

**heart failure**   Ineffective pumping of the heart, which results in the overfilling of the veins that bring blood to the heart.

**heat cramps**   In a dehydrated and hot person, the signs and symptoms of heat cramps include muscular tightening and pain in the limbs or abdomen.

**heat exhaustion**   A serious form of heat illness.

**heatstroke**   A life-threatening form of heat illness.

**hemorrhoids**   Painfully swollen veins in the rectal and anal areas.

**hepatitis B virus (HBV)**   A serious infectious disease of the liver transmitted via blood or blood products.

**heredity**   The transmission of biological information, coded within genes, from parents to offspring.

**heterosexual**   A person who is sexually attracted to members of the opposite sex.

**high-density lipoproteins (HDL)**   (LIP-oh-PRO-teenz or LIE-poe-PRO-teenz) "Good" cholesterol that carries cholesterol from the cells and to the liver for removal from the body.

**holistic**   (hole-IS-tic) A characteristic involving all aspects of the person.

**homophobia**   An intense fear of or hostility toward homosexuals.

**homosexual**  A person who is sexually attracted to members of his or her own sex.

**hormones**  Chemical messengers that convey information from a gland to other cells in the body.

**hospice**  A form of health care specifically designed to give emotional support and pain relief to terminally ill people in the final stage of life.

**host**  In reference to disease, an organism that supports the growth of a pathogen; the third, and last, link in the chain of infection.

**human chorionic gonadotropin (hCG)**  In a pregnant woman, a hormone produced by embryonic tissues destined to become the placenta. Pregnancy tests rely on the detection of this hormone in the blood.

**hunger**  The physiologic drive to seek and eat food.

**hypertension**  Persistently high arterial blood pressure.

**hyperthermia**  A condition that occurs when body temperature rises above the normal range.

**hypertrophy**  A condition in which muscles become larger and stronger.

**hypnotics**  Drugs that produce trancelike effects.

**hypothermia**  Condition that occurs when the body's core temperature drops below 95°F.

**immune system**  A collection of cells and organs of the body that recognizes and combats pathogens and other foreign substances with cells and proteins that are specific for particular invaders; The specific defenses of the body that include combating infectious agents. The immune system has two branches: antibody-mediated immunity and cell-mediated immunity.

**immunity**  (im-MYOU-nih-tea) Resistance to disease.

**immunotherapy**  Manipulation of the body's immune system to rid the body of cancer.

**incest**  Sexual relations between family members who are not spouses.

**infectious (in-FEK-shus) disease**  A disease caused by bacteria, rickettsias, viruses, fungi, protozoans, or parasitic worms.

**infertility**  Inability to conceive a child after 1 year of unprotected sex.

**inherited disease**  A genetic disease transmitted solely by gene transfer from parents to offspring.

**institutional violence**  Violence that occurs mainly in institutional settings such as college campuses or workplaces.

**integrative medicine**  System of medical care that emphasizes personalized health care and disease prevention.

**interferons**  (IN-ter-FEAR-onz) Proteins produced by the body during a viral infection that protect uninfected cells from viral invasion.

**intestinal ulcer**  A sore in the lining of the esophagus, stomach, or duodenum.

**intimacy**  Disclosure of one's most personal thoughts and emotions to a trusted individual.

**intoxication**  Impairment of the functioning of the central nervous system as a result of ingesting toxic substances such as alcohol. The state of being poisoned by a drug or other toxic substance.

**intrauterine device (IUD)**  A small contraceptive device that either is covered with copper or contains a reservoir of progestin and is inserted into the uterus.

**ischemia**  (is-KI-me-ah) Insufficient blood in part of the heart.

**isometric**  A type of exercise in which the individual exerts muscular force against a fixed, immovable object.

**isotonic**  A type of exercise in which the individual exerts muscular force against a movable but constant source of resistence.

**joints**  The places where two or more bones come together.

**labia majora**  (LAY-bee-ah mah-JOR-ah) Hairy, rounded, and thick folds of skin that lie adjacent to the labia minora and extend forward to unite at the mons pubis.

**labia minora**  (LAY-bee-ah my NOR-ah) Two thin, hairless folds of skin that extend from over the clitoris to an area behind the vagina. The labia minor cover and protect the vaginal opening ad urethra.

**labor (parturition)**  (PAR-too-RISH-un) The process of childbirth.

**lead poisoning**  A toxic condition that affects the central nervous system, caused by the ingestion or inhalation of the metallic element lead.

**leukemias**  (lew-KEY-me-ahz) Cancers of the blood and related cells.

**leukocytes**  (LEWK-oh-sites) White blood cells; active in both specific and nonspecific defenses of the body.

**life expectancy**  The average number of years that an individual of a particular age can expect to live.

**life span**  The maximum number of years that members of a species can expect to live when conditions are optimal.

**lifestyle**  A way of living including behaviors that promote or impair good health and longevity.

**ligaments**  Tough bands of connective tissue that hold bones together at joints.

**lipids**  A class of nutrients that includes triglycerides and cholesterol.

**low-density lipoproteins (LDL)**  "Bad" cholesterol that carries cholesterol to the cells, including the cells that line the blood vessel walls.

**lumpectomy**  (lum-PECK-toe-me) Surgical removal of a breast tumor, including a layer of surrounding tissue.

**lymph**  (limf) Tissue fluid.

**lymphomas**  (lim-FOE-mahz) Cancers of the lymphatic system.

**macular degeneration**  A leading cause of vision loss for people age 60 years and older.

**major depressive disorder** A mood disorder characterized by persistent and profound sadness, hopelessness, helplessness, and feelings of worthlessness; lack of energy; loss of interest in usual activities; loss of the ability to concentrate; suicidal thoughts; and appetite and sleep disturbances.

**malignant melanoma** (MEL-ah-NO-mah) A deadly form of skin cancer that develops most often in persons who have been exposed to the sun in short, intense sessions, have had severe sunburn and extensive sun exposure in childhood, or have first-degree relatives who had the disease.

**malignant (mah-LIG-nant) tumors** Masses of cancer cells that invade body tissues and interfere with the normal functioning of tissues and organs.

**malnutrition** Overnutrition or undernutrition that results when diets supply improper amounts of nutrients.

**medical abortion** A method of drug-induced abortion performed within 9 weeks of the first day of the last period.

**Medicare** A federal health insurance program that provides benefits for people 65 years of age and older.

**meditation** An activity in which one relaxes by mentally focusing on a single word, object, or thought.

**menarche** (meh-NAR-key) The first menstruation.

**menses** (MEN-seez) The menstrual period; the sloughing of the endometrium.

**menstrual (MEN-strool-al) cycle** The monthly changes in the levels of the female sex hormones that orchestrate physiologic changes in the ovaries and uterus.

**metabolic rate** The amount of energy the body requires to fuel cellular activities during a specified time.

**metabolism** All chemical reactions that take place in the body.

**metastasize** (meh-TAS-tah-size) The ability of cancer cells to spread from where they develop to another part of the body.

**minerals** A class of inorganic nutrients that includes several elements, such as iron, calcium, and zinc.

**mons pubis** A mound of fatty tissue that lies over the pubic bone, cushioning it.

**motivation** The force or drive that leads people to take action.

**mourning** The culturally defined way in which survivors observe bereavement.

**municipal solid waste** Nonhazardous refuse generally collected from homes and offices.

**muscular endurance** A muscle's ability to contract repeatedly without becoming fatigued.

**muscular strength** The ability to apply maximum force against an object that is resisting this force.

**mutation** (mew-TAY-shun) In reference to human biology, a change in a gene or a chromosome; damaged genes.

**myotonia** An increase in muscle tension throughout the body during sexual arousal.

**narcotics** Drugs that induce euphoria and sleep as well as alter the perception of pain.

**natural family planning (fertility awareness)** Formerly called the rhythm method; a group of birth control techniques in which a couple abstains from sexual intercourse during the time of the month when a woman is most likely to conceive.

**neurotransmitters** Chemicals produced and released by nerves that convey information between most nerve cells.

**nicotine** An addictive psychoactive drug found in tobacco.

**noncommunicable** Not transmissible from person to person.

**noninfectious (NON-in-FEK-shus) disease** Illness caused by genetic abnormalities, by interactions between hereditary and environmental factors, or solely by environmental factors.

**nonspecific immunity** A variety of defense mechanisms that combat any type of damage to the body, including the invasion of infectious agents.

**nutrient requirement** The minimum amount of a nutrient that prevents that nutrient's deficiency disease.

**nutrients** Substances in food that are necessary for growth, repair, maintenance of tissues.

**obesity** A condition in which the body has an excessive and unhealthy amount of fat. Obese people have BMIs of 30 or more.

**obsession** A repetitive thought that produces anxious feelings.

**oncogenes** (ONG-ko-geenz) Tumor genes that manufacture altered proteins that speed cell growth and decrease the level of cell differentiation.

**optimal wellness** A sense that one is functioning at his or her best level.

**orgasm** The peak of sexual excitement.

**osteoporosis** An age-related condition in which bones lose density, becoming weak and breaking easily.

**ovaries** Internal organs of female sexual reproduction within which eggs (ova) develop.

**overweight** A condition in which the body has more fat, muscle, bone, and/or water than a person whose weight is normal. Overweight people have BMIs of between 25 and 30.

**ovulation** The maturation and release of an egg from an ovary, usually each month from puberty to menopause.

**ozone holes** Depleted areas of the ozone ($O_3$) layer in the upper atmosphere.

**panic disorder** Psychological condition that features panic attacks, unpredictable episodes of extreme anxiety, and loss of emotional control.

**Papanicolaou (PAP-eh-nik-eh-LOUW) test (Pap test)** A screening procedure for cervical cancer in which cells from the cervical canal are removed and then smeared on a glass slide for microscopic examination.

**passive smoking** The inhalation, by nonsmokers, of tobacco smoke in the air.

**pathogen** (PATH-oh-jen) A disease-causing agent of infection; the first link in the chain of infection.

**pedophile** (PE-doe-file) An individual who is sexually attracted to children.

**penis** A cylindrical external organ of sexual reproduction in males, which hangs in front of the scrotum.

**periodontal (PER-ee-oh-DON-tal) disease** A disorder of the tissues that support the teeth.

**peripheral nervous system (PNS)** Of the two primary divisions of the nervous system, the one that consists of nerves, which relay information to and from the CNS.

**peripheral vascular disease** Any blockage of vessels other than those to the heart.

**persistent vegetative state** Condition in which a person has a nonfunctioning cerebral cortex and is in an irreversible coma.

**personality** A set of distinct thoughts and behaviors that characterizes a person's response to situations.

**pesticides** Chemicals that kill plant and animal pests and that can cause poisoning when ingested.

**phagocytosis** (FAG-oh-sigh-TOE-sis) The process of white blood cells ingesting foreign cells and debris, such as the dirt or dead cells in a cut.

**phobia** An intense and irrational fear of an object or a situation.

**physical activity** Movement that occurs when skeletal muscles contract.

**physiology** The study of bodily functions.

**phytochemicals** A group of nonnutrients that are produced by plants and may have beneficial effects on the body.

**placebo** A sham treatment that has no known physical effects; an inactive substance.

**placenta** (plah-SEN-tah) A structure that develops after implantation of a fertilized ovum in the uterine wall and consists of maternal and fetal tissues that secrete hormones that help maintain the pregnancy.

**plaques** (plaks) Fatty deposits in artery walls.

**polyabuse** Abusing more than one drug at a time.

**portal of entry** Site on or in the body where pathogens enter.

**pre-embryo** The first 2 weeks of gestational development.

**pregnancy** The gestational process; the process of development of a new individual from fertilization until birth.

**premature (rapid) ejaculation** A common male sexual dysfunction in which a man consistently attains orgasm either before or shortly after intercourse and before he wishes it to occur.

**premenstrual syndrome (PMS)** Symptoms such as anxiety, mood swings, aches, and cramps that occur prior to the menses and that significantly interfere with daily life.

**probiotics** Live bacteria that may benefit health.

**progesterone** (pro-JES-te-rone) A hormone secreted by the corpus luteum. With estrogen, progesterone stimulates the continued development and thickening of the uterine lining.

**prostate gland** A single, walnut-sized gland that lies just below the bladder, surrounding the urethra. The prostate produces a milky alkaline fluid that is added to the ejaculate.

**proteins** A class of nutrients that are needed to build, maintain, and repair cells.

**psychoactive** Having mind-altering or mood-altering effects.

**psychological adjustment** Changing one's thoughts, attitudes, and behaviors to cope effectively with the demands of the environment.

**psychological growth** The process of learning from one's experiences.

**psychology** The study of the mental processes that influence human behavior.

**psychoneuroimmunology** (SIGH-ko-NEW-ro-im-mu-NOL-lo-gee) The study of the relationships between the nervous and immune systems.

**puberty** (PEW-ber-tea) A stage of sexual development during which the endocrine (hormone) and reproductive systems mature.

**pubic louse** A close relative of fleas that causes sexually transmitted infestation; also called crabs.

**quackery** The practice of medicine without having the proper training and credentials.

**radical mastectomy** Surgical removal of a breast, underlying muscle, and underarm fat and lymph nodes as a treatment for breast cancer.

**radon gas** A colorless, odorless, radioactive gas present in the rocks and soils in many areas in the United States that, when inhaled, can cause mutations in cells.

**rape** Sexual intercourse by force or with a person who is incapable of legal consent.

**rectum** The lower part of the large intestine.

**respect** The feeling that another has value and deserves attention.

**risk factor** A characteristic that increases an individual's chances of developing a health problem.

**sarcomas** (sar-KO-mahz) Cancers that arise from connective or muscle tissue.

**satiety** The feeling that enough food has been eaten to relieve hunger and turn off appetite.

**scabies** (SKAY-beez) An infestation of the pubic area in which a spider-like organism burrows into the skin and lays eggs there.

**schizophrenia** A form of psychosis.

**scrotum** (SKRO-tum) The sac of skin in which the testes are enclosed and hang outside the body.

**sedatives** Drugs that produce calming effects.

**self-esteem** The extent to which a person feels worthy and useful.

**semen** The ejaculate; the secretions of the accessory sex glands (called seminal fluid) and sperm.

**seminal vesicles** (SEM-ih-nal VES-ih-klz) Paired male sex organs located near the junction of the two vasa deferentia, which produce thick fructose-containing secretions that are added to the ejaculate.

**senescence** (seh-NES-ens) The stage of life that begins at age 65 years and ends with death.

**set point** A theoretical level of body fat that resists weight loss efforts.

**sexism** Discrimination and bias against one sex.

**sexologists** Scientists who study human sexuality.

**sexual harassment** Intentional use of annoying sexually related comments or behaviors to intimidate or coerce people into unwanted sexual activity.

**sexual intercourse** Penetration of the vagina by a penis.

**sexual orientation** The direction of a person's romantic thoughts, feelings, and attractions toward people of the same or different sex.

**sexual reproduction** The fertilization of an egg (*ovum*; plural, *ova*) by a sperm.

**sexual stereotype** The widespread association of certain perceptions with one gender.

**sexual violence** Gaining sexual activity through force or threat of force.

**sexuality** The aspect of personality that encompasses a person's sexual thoughts, feelings, attitudes, and actions.

**sexually transmitted infection (STI)** Infection spread from person to person by intimate sexual contact, primarily anal or vaginal intercourse and oral sex.

**sick building syndrome** A variety of vague health-related problems reported by many occupants of large buildings.

**sigmoidoscopy** (SIG-moid-OS-ko-pee) A procedure in which a physician views the lower portion of the colon via a flexible fiber-optic tube.

**signs** Observable and measurable features of an illness.

**smog** (smoke and fog) A haze in the atmosphere formed by various pollutants.

**specific immunity** Defense mechanism carried out by the immune system.

**spermicides** Chemicals that kill sperm.

**sprain** Generally refers to an injured ligament.

**squamous (SKWAY-muss) cell carcinoma** A common form of skin cancer that develops from exposure to noxious chemicals and high levels of x-rays, as well as from trauma.

**stent** A springlike mesh device that is implanted within an artery to cover compressed plaque, support the artery, and smooth the artery wall.

**sterilization** A permanent form of birth control that requires a surgical procedure.

**strain** Generally refers to an injured muscle or tendon.

**stress** A complex series of psychological and physical reactions that occur as one responds to a situation.

**stressors** Events that produce physical or psychological demands on an individual.

**stroke** A brain injury that occurs when arteries that supply the brain become blocked and prevent blood flow or become damaged and leak blood onto or into the brain.

**sudden cardiac arrest** Cessation of the heartbeat.

**surgical abortion** Includes various methods of induced abortion in which the contents of the uterus are physically removed.

**symptoms** Subjective complaints of illness.

**synergism** (SIH-ner-jism) The multiplied effects produced by taking combinations of certain drugs.

**syphilis** (SIF-ih-lis) An STI that can progress from skin sores to more generalized symptoms (e.g., weight loss and muscle pain) to life-threatening, tissue-destroying skin abnormalities.

**systolic (sis-TOL-ik) pressure** The higher number in the blood pressure reading, which is the pressure exerted by the blood on the artery walls when the left ventricle contracts.

**T cells** specialized white blood cells (lymphocytes) that function in cell-mediated immunity; there are four types of T cells.

**T. vaginalis infection** An STI caused by a protozoan, resulting in infection of the urethra in men and of the urethra and walls of the vagina in women.

**targeted therapies** Drugs or other substances that block the growth and spread of cancer by interfering with specific molecules involved in tumor growth and progression.

**temperament** The predictable way an individual responds to situations and others, such as being pleasant, outgoing, or shy.

**temporomandibular (TEM-pe-row-man-DIB-you-ler) joint** The place where the lower jaw bone (mandible) attaches to the temporal bone of the skull.

**tendons**   Tough bands of tissue that connect many skeletal muscles to bones.

**teratogens**   Various environmental influences such as drugs, alcohol, viruses, and dietary deficiencies that can damage the embryo or fetus early in pregnancy.

**testes**   (TES-tease) The male reproductive organs that produce sperm (the male sex cells) and testosterone (a male sex hormone).

**testicular (tes-TIK-you-lar) self-examination (TSE)**   A self-screening test that males can perform to detect cancer of the testicles.

**testimonials**   Individual claims about the value of a product.

**testosterone**   A male sex hormone (androgen) that plays a role in the development of functionally mature sperm and is responsible for the development and maintenance of male secondary sexual characteristics such as the deepening of the voice and the growth of facial hair.

**thermic effect of food (TEF)**   The small amount of energy that the body uses to digest, absorb, and process the nutrients from foods.

**thrombus**   (THROM-bus) A stationary blood clot.

**tolerance**   A physiologic response in chronic users of drugs in which increased amounts of the drug are required to achieve effects previously produced by lower amounts.

**total mastectomy**   (mas-TEK-toe-me) Surgical removal of a breast and involved lymph nodes for the treatment of breast cancer.

**toxic chemicals**   Poisonous substances present in the home, workplace, or outdoor environments that affect human health.

**toxicity**   (tok-SIH-si-tea) Poisonous quality.

**transgender**   An umbrella term for various groups of people who do not conform to traditional gender roles.

**transient ischemic (is-KI-mik) attacks (TIAs)**   Minor strokes that usually cause no permanent damage and have signs that last for only a short time.

**transmission**   In reference to disease, the means by which a pathogen gets to a host; the second link in the chain of infection.

**triglycerides**   The most prevalent form of lipids in foods; often called fat.

**tubal ligation**   Female sterilization that is performed by cutting and tying off the uterine tubes so that the sperm and egg cannot unite.

**tumor-suppressor genes**   Pieces of hereditary material that slow cell growth; anti-oncogenes.

**urinary incontinence**   The inability to control the flow of urine from the bladder.

**uterine tubes**   Passageways that extend from each ovary to the uterus.

**uterus**   A hollow, muscular, pear-shaped organ that protects and nourishes the embryo/fetus during development.

**vaccine**   A preparation of a killed or weakened pathogen or its antigenic parts to be administered to a person to induce immunity and thereby prevent infectious disease.

**vagina**   A tube about 10 cm (approximately 4 in.) long that receives the penis during intercourse, allows the passage of the menstrual flow, and is a birth canal.

**vaginismus**   A sexual dysfunction of women in which the lower portion of the vagina contracts involuntarily at the anticipation of penetration, preventing it.

**value**   The belief that an idea, object, or action has worth.

**vas deferens**   (VAS DEF-er-enz) A tube that links the epididymis and the urethra, the passageway through which sperm exit the body.

**vasectomy**   Male sterilization that is performed by cutting and tying off the vas deferens to prevent sperm from becoming part of the ejaculate.

**vasocongestion**   A condition in which the spongy tissue of the penis and clitoris expands with blood during sexual arousal.

**veins**   Blood vessels that return blood to the heart.

**violence**   Interpersonal uses of force that are not socially sanctioned.

**virus**   Hereditary material surrounded by a coat of protein; some viruses are pathogenic to humans and produce infections such as the common cold, influenza, mumps, measles, chicken pox, hepatitis, and AIDS.

**vitamins**   A class of organic nutrients that help regulate growth; release energy from carbohydrates, fats, and proteins; and maintain tissues.

**vulva**   The collective term for the external female genitals. The vulva surrounds the vaginal opening.

**withdrawal**   A temporary physical and psychological state that occurs when certain drugs are discontinued.

**yeast infection**   A condition in which the fungus *Candida albicans* grows in the vagina or on the penis; also known as candidiasis or moniliasis.

## CHAPTER 1

**SELF-ASSESSMENT 1**

# Healthstyle

T his self-test, which is a modified version of one developed by the U.S. Public Health Service, assesses several health-related behaviors. Although these behaviors apply to most individuals, pregnant women, and people with chronic health concerns should follow the advice of their physicians. Answer each of the following questions by circling the number of the response that applies best to you. Add the number of points under each health-related behavior category to obtain a score for that category. Use the scoring guide at the end of the test to determine the level of risk you are incurring by your health-related behavior.

## Tobacco, Alcohol, and Other Drugs

If you have never used tobacco products, enter a score of 10 for this section, and skip questions 1 and 2.

| | Almost Always | Sometimes | Almost Never |
|---|---|---|---|
| 1. I avoid using tobacco products. | 2 | 1 | 0 |
| 2. I smoke only low-tar cigarettes. | 2 | 1 | 0 |
| | | Smoking Score: _____ | |
| 3. I avoid drinking alcoholic beverages, or I drink no more than one or two drinks a day. | 2 | 1 | 0 |
| 4. I avoid using alcohol or other drugs (especially illegal drugs) as a way of handling stressful situations or problems in my life. | 2 | 1 | 0 |
| 5. I avoid driving while under the influence of alcohol and other drugs. | 2 | 1 | 0 |
| 6. I am careful not to drink alcohol when taking certain pain medications or when pregnant. | 2 | 1 | 0 |
| 7. I read and follow the label directions when using prescribed and over-the-counter drugs. | 2 | 1 | 0 |
| | | Alcohol and Other Drugs Score: _____ | |

# Eating Habits

| | Almost Always | Sometimes | Almost Never |
|---|---|---|---|
| 8. I eat a variety of foods each day, including fruits and vegetables, whole-grain products, lean meats, low-fat dairy products, seeds, nuts, and dry beans. | 3 | 1 | 0 |
| 9. I limit the amount of animal fat in my food, which includes cream, butter, cheese, and fatty meats. | 3 | 1 | 0 |
| 10. I limit the amount of salt that I eat, by avoiding salty foods and not using salt at the table. | 2 | 1 | 0 |
| 11. I avoid eating too much sugar, by eating few sweet snacks and sugary soft drinks. | 2 | 1 | 0 |

Eating Habits Score: _____

# Exercise/Fitness

| | Almost Always | Sometimes | Almost Never |
|---|---|---|---|
| 12. I maintain a body weight that is reasonable for my height. | 3 | 1 | 0 |
| 13. I do vigorous exercise (for example, running, swimming, or brisk walking) for at least 30 minutes at least three times a week. | 3 | 1 | 0 |
| 14. I do exercises to enhance my muscle tone and flexibility (for example, yoga or calisthenics) for 15 to 30 minutes at least three times a week. | 2 | 1 | 0 |
| 15. I use part of my leisure time participating in individual, family, or team activities that increase my level of physical fitness (for example, gardening, bowling, or golf). | 2 | 1 | 0 |

Exercise/Fitness Score: _____

# Stress Management

| | Almost Always | Sometimes | Almost Never |
|---|---|---|---|
| 16. I take time every day to relax. | 2 | 1 | 0 |
| 17. I find it easy to express my feelings without harming others. | 2 | 1 | 0 |
| 18. I recognize and prepare for events or situations that are likely to be stressful. | 2 | 1 | 0 |
| 19. I have close friends, relatives, or others to whom I can talk about personal matters and contact for help when needed. | 2 | 1 | 0 |
| 20. I participate in hobbies that I enjoy or group activities such as religious or community organizations. | 2 | 1 | 0 |

Stress Management Score: _____

and cons carefully, however, before making your final decision. You may decide to change even if your reasons not to change outrank your reasons to change.

## Implementing the Change

1. **Set a target date to begin the new behavior or reach the goal.** Depending on the type of decision, a behavior change could involve setting a beginning date and a goal date. For example, you could decide to lose 10 pounds by May 31st, then begin changing your eating and physical activity patterns tomorrow.

2. **Identify and list the factors that will help you reach your goal and those that will stand in the way of reaching your goal.**

   *Factors that help*

   My roommate has also decided to lose weight.

   I just got a check for my birthday to buy a new outfit when I lose 10 pounds.

   My student fees include the use of the health facility.

   *Factors that hinder*

   My mother insists that I eat a lot of food when I visit.

   My roommate keeps lots of high-calorie snacks in the house.

   I'm so busy that finding a time to exercise is difficult.

3. **Prepare an action plan for making the change.** An action plan specifies how you will change your behavior to meet your goal.

   a. **Identify alternative methods for reaching your goal.**

      **Example**

      **Alternative 1:** Consume a 1,200-calorie diet that consists of eating only one meal a day and drinking a diet supplement for breakfast and lunch.

      **Alternative 2:** Consume a 1,200-calorie diet that permits three nutritious meals daily.

      **Alternative 3:** Consume a 1,200-calorie diet and increase exercise by 30 minutes a day.

      **Alternative 4:** Go to a weight loss clinic for help.

   b. **Gather information about each method.** Seek information that supports and criticizes each method. (People tend to gather data that only support what they think they want to do.) Ask yourself questions to guide your information gathering.

      **Example:** How long do people who reduce their caloric intake without exercising keep the weight off? By which method am I more likely to lose weight fastest? Is it better for my health to lose weight as quickly as possible, or does the length of time not matter? What changes will I have to make in my life if I decide to eat more nutritious foods and exercise? Are diet supplement drinks safe? Where can I find information about the caloric content of foods?

   c. **Choose the method that fits your situation best.**

      **Example:** After researching alternative methods, you decide to follow a 1,200-calorie-per-day, diet and increase the amount of exercise you engage in each day.

   d. **Consider the factors that can help or hinder your effort to change (see step 2).** What can you do that will take advantage of the helps and minimize the hindrances? For example, keep plenty of low-calorie snacks on hand to avoid being tempted by your roommate's supply of high-calorie munchies. Also, discuss the situation with your roommate to enlist his or her support in your effort.

4. **Change the lifestyle behavior that you have decided to improve by implementing the action plan you developed in step 3.**

5. **Chart your daily progress toward your goal.** Track your progress on a regular basis. Recording your weight once a week, for example, may be helpful. Are you losing weight?

6. **Evaluate how effective you were in reaching your goal.** Did your plan work? What can you learn from the experience?

   **Example:** You lost 5 pounds instead of 10 pounds. What seemed to keep you from reaching your goal? What can you do differently that might help you succeed? Do you need more time to lose weight, or do you need to reevaluate your decision?

*Factors that help:* _____

*Factors that hinder:* _____

3. Prepare an action plan for making the change.
   a. Identify alternative methods for reaching your goal.
   b. Gather information about each method.
   c. Choose the method that fits your situation best.
   d. Consider the factors that can help or hinder your effort to change (see step 2).

4. Change the lifestyle behavior that you have decided to improve by implementing the action plan that you developed in step 3.

5. Chart your daily progress toward your goal.

6. Evaluate how effective you were in reaching your goal.

*SELF-ASSESSMENT 2*

# K6 Serious Psychological Distress Assessment

Answer the following questions by checking the statement that best applies.

| During the past 30 days, how often did you feel? | All of the time 4 | Most of the time 3 | Some of the time 2 | A little of the time 1 | None of the time 0 |
|---|---|---|---|---|---|
| So sad that nothing could cheer you up? | | | | | |
| Nervous? | | | | | |
| Restless or fidgety? | | | | | |
| Hopeless? | | | | | |
| That everything was an effort? | | | | | |
| Worthless? | | | | | |
| **Total** | | | | | |

**Scoring:** To score the K6, add the points for each of the questions together. Scores can range from 0 to 24. A threshold of 13 or more points indicates a high degree of distress and possibility of serious mental illness.

*Source:* National Center for Health Statistics (reviewed 2007). Serious psychological distress. Retrieved June 15, 2007, from http://www.cdc.gov/nchs/datawh/nchdefs/seriouspsydistress.htm.

# Taking Steps to Reduce Your Stress

**F**ollow the steps of the decision-making and implementation model to identify and change a health-related habit that contributes to your level of stress. For example, do you work too many hours per week? Are you in a relationship that causes you continual stress? Are you trying to take care of your home and family with no help while going to school and working part-time?

## Deciding to Change

1. Identify the problem, goal, or question.
2. List the reasons you should make this change and the reasons you should not.

## Choices

Reasons to change behaviors (pros):

| *Points* | *Reasons* |
|---|---|
| ____ | _____ |
| ____ | _____ |
| ____ | _____ |
| ____ Total | |

Reasons not to change behaviors (cons):

| *Points* | *Reasons* |
|---|---|
| ____ | _____ |
| ____ | _____ |
| ____ | _____ |
| ____ Total | |

3. Draw a conclusion by adding the points in the pros section and then in the cons section. If the point total of the pros section is greater than the total of the cons section, you are probably ready to make a change in your life that reduces stress. If your cons outweigh your pros, you may not be motivated to make the change now. Study your list of pros and cons carefully, however, before making your final decision. You may decide to change even if your reasons not to change outrank your reasons to change.

## Implementing the Change

1. Set a target date to begin the new behavior or reach the goal.
2. Identify and list the factors that will help you reach your goal and those that will stand in the way of reaching your goal.

   *Factors that help:* _____

   *Factors that hinder:* _____

3. Prepare an action plan for making the change.

    **a.** Identify alternative methods for reaching your goal.

       *Alternative 1:* _____

       *Alternative 2:* _____

       *Alternative 3:* _____

       *Alternative 4:* _____

    **b.** Gather information about each method.

    **c.** Choose the method that fits your particular situation best.

    **d.** Consider the factors that can help or hinder your effort to change (see step 2).

4. Change the lifestyle behavior that you have decided to improve by implementing the action plan you developed in step 3.

5. Chart your daily progress toward your goal.

6. Evaluate how effective you were in reaching your goal.

# Am I in an Abusive Intimate Relationship?

Read the following statements and indicate whether you agree or disagree with them. Draw a circle around your answer. Your responses can help you assess whether you are in an abusive intimate relationship.

| | | |
|---|---|---|
| 1. My partner often embarrasses me in front of others. | Yes | No |
| 2. My partner often criticizes my appearance, belittles my accomplishments, or makes fun of my ideas. | Yes | No |
| 3. My partner frequently uses threats to make me to do what he/she wants. | Yes | No |
| 4. My partner has told me that I'm worthless without him/her. | Yes | No |
| 5. When my partner physically hurts me, he/she apologizes or says, "It was an accident," or "I didn't mean to hurt you." | Yes | No |
| 6. My partner frequently has trouble controlling his/her anger. | Yes | No |
| 7. My partner often makes me feel guilty when I want to spend time away from him/her. | Yes | No |
| 8. My partner mistreats me when he/she gets drunk or high on drugs. | Yes | No |
| 9. My partner usually blames me for his/her problems. | Yes | No |
| 10. My partner pressures me for sex when I don't want it. | Yes | No |
| 11. I often think about breaking up with my partner, but I don't because I'm afraid of what he/she might do to me or to himself/herself. | Yes | No |
| 12. My friends and family members have told me that my partner is abusing me. | Yes | No |
| 13. When I'm with others, I usually make excuses for my partner's abusive behavior. | Yes | No |
| 14. I often sacrifice what I would like to do because I'm afraid of how my partner will respond if I don't follow his/her plans. | Yes | No |
| 15. I often avoid saying or doing things that might anger my partner because I'm afraid that he/she will hurt me. | Yes | No |

If you agreed with any of these statements, you may be in an abusive relationship. If you're not sure that your partner is abusive, seek counseling from a licensed professional therapist. If you are afraid of your partner, get help immediately. Contact your campus counseling center or a local domestic violence intervention center listed in your "Yellow Pages" phone book. The phone number for the National Domestic Violence Hotline is 1-800-799-7233.

# Can You Reduce Your Risk of Violence?

**F**ollow the steps of the decision-making and implementation model to identify and change a health-related habit that contributes to your risk of violence. For example, do you ignore basic security measures? Are you involved in an abusive relationship that you feel hopeless about improving or terminating? Does your work, family, and college schedule force you to be exposed to risky situations and places?

## Deciding to Change

1. Identify the problem, goal, or question.
2. List the reasons you should make this change and the reasons you should not.

## Choices

Reasons to change behaviors (pros):

| Points | Reasons |
| --- | --- |
| ____ | _____ |
| ____ | _____ |
| ____ | _____ |
| ____ | Total |

Reasons not to change behaviors (cons):

| Points | Reasons |
| --- | --- |
| ____ | _____ |
| ____ | _____ |
| ____ | _____ |
| ____ | Total |

3. Draw a conclusion by adding the points in the pros section and then in the cons section. If the point total of the pros section is greater than the total of the cons section, you are probably ready to make a change in your life that reduces your risk of violence. If your cons outweigh your pros, you may not be motivated to make the change now. Study your list of pros and cons carefully, however, before making your final decision. You may decide to change even if your reasons not to change outrank your reasons to change.

## Implementing the Change

1. Set a target date to begin the new behavior or reach the goal.
2. Identify and list the factors that will help you reach your goal and those that will stand in the way of reaching your goal.

*Factors that help:* _____

*Factors that hinder:* _____

3.  Prepare an action plan for making the change.

    **a.**  Identify alternative methods for reaching your goal.

        *Alternative 1:* _____

        *Alternative 2:* _____

        *Alternative 3:* _____

        *Alternative 4:* _____

    **b.**  Gather information about each method.

    **c.**  Choose the method that fits your particular situation best.

    **d.**  Consider the factors that can help or hinder your effort to change (see step 2).

4.  Change the lifestyle behavior that you have decided to improve by implementing the action plan you developed in step 3.

5.  Chart your daily progress toward your goal.

6.  Evaluate how effective you were in reaching your goal.

Changing Health Habits   **607**

Student Workbook

# Contraceptive Comfort and Confidence Scale

The following series of questions, which are adapted from the Contraceptive Comfort and Confidence Scale, is designed to help you assess whether the method of contraception that you are using or may be considering for future use is or will be effective for you.

With regard to the method of birth control you are currently using or are considering using, answer YES or NO to the following questions:

1. Have you had problems using this method before?

2. Are you afraid of using this method?

3. Would you really rather not use this method?

4. Will you have trouble remembering to use this method?

5. Have you ever become pregnant using this method? (Or, has your partner ever become pregnant using this method?)

6. Will you have trouble using this method correctly?

7. Do you still have unanswered questions about this method?

8. Does this method make menstrual periods longer or more painful?

9. Does this method cost more than you can afford?

10. Could this method cause you or your partner to have serious complications?

11. Are you opposed to this method because of religious beliefs?

12. Is your partner opposed to this method?

13. Are you using this method without your partner's knowledge?

14. Will using this method embarrass your partner?

15. Will using this method embarrass you?

16. Will you enjoy intercourse less because of this method?

17. Will your partner enjoy intercourse less because of this method?

18. If this method interrupts lovemaking, will you avoid using it?

19. Has a nurse or doctor ever told you (or your partner) not to use this method?

20. Is there anything about your personality that could lead you to use this method incorrectly?

**21.** Does this method leave you at risk of being exposed to HIV or other sexually transmissible infections?

Total number of YES answers: _____

## Interpreting Your Score

Most individuals will have a few "yes" answers. Yes answers predict potential problems. If you have more than a few yes responses, you may want to talk to your physician, counselor, partner, or a friend. Talking it over can help you decide whether to use this method or how to use it so it will be effective. In general, the more yes answers you have, the less likely you are to use this method consistently and correctly.

In choosing a method of contraception, keep in mind that if you want a highly effective method of contraception and a method that is highly effective in preventing transmission of STIs, you may have to use two methods. Hence, any method of contraception (except abstinence, of course) should be combined with condom use for maximum protection against STIs.

*Source:* Adapted from Hatcher, R. A., Stewart, F., Trussell, J., Kowal, D., Guest, F., Stewart, G. K., & Cates, W. (1990). *Contraceptive technology: 1990–1992* (15th ed., rev.) (p. 150). New York: Irvington.

CHAPTER 5

SELF-ASSESSMENT 2

# Attitudes Toward Timing of Parenthood Scale (ATOP)

## Directions

Circle the response that most closely represents your feelings. The options are strongly agree (SA), agree (A), undecided (U), disagree (D), and strongly disagree (SD).

| | SD | D | U | A | SA |
|---|---|---|---|---|---|
| 1. The best time to begin having children is usually within the first two years of marriage. | 1 | 2 | 3 | 4 | 5 |
| 2. It is important for a young couple to enjoy their social life first and to have children later in the marriage. | 1 | 2 | 3 | 4 | 5 |
| 3. A marriage relationship is strengthened if children are born in the early years of marriage. | 1 | 2 | 3 | 4 | 5 |
| 4. Women are generally happier if they have children early in the marriage. | 1 | 2 | 3 | 4 | 5 |
| 5. Men are generally tied closer to the marriage when there are children in the home. | 1 | 2 | 3 | 4 | 5 |
| 6. Most young married women lack self-fulfillment until they have a child. | 1 | 2 | 3 | 4 | 5 |
| 7. Young couples who do not have children are usually unable to do so. | 1 | 2 | 3 | 4 | 5 |
| 8. Married couples who have mature love for each other will be eager to have a child as soon as possible. | 1 | 2 | 3 | 4 | 5 |
| 9. Couples who do not have children cannot share in the major interests of their friends who are parents, and are therefore left out of most social circles. | 1 | 2 | 3 | 4 | 5 |
| 10. Children enjoy their parents more when the parents are nearer their own age; therefore, parents should have children while they are still young. | 1 | 2 | 3 | 4 | 5 |
| 11. In general, research indicates that the majority of couples approaching parenthood for the first time have had little or no previous child care experience beyond sporadic baby-sitting, a course in child psychology, or occasional care of younger siblings. Considering your background preparation for parenthood, would you judge that you are well prepared for the parenting experience? | 1 | 2 | 3 | 4 | 5 |

Items 1 through 10 are from the Attitudes Toward Timing of Parenthood Scale (Maxwell & Montgomery, 1969). Item 11 was an additional item constructed to determine perceived degree of preparation for parenthood.

**Scoring:** Response options that favor early parenthood receive the highest score (5 points), and those that favor delayed parenthood receive the lowest score (1 point). The range of possible scores is from 10 to 50. Item number 2 is reverse scored, so if you choose option 4, change it to 2 (or vice versa); if you chose option 5, change it to 1 (or vice versa). Then sum the value of the options you selected for all items to compute your total score.

**Reliability and validity:** No reliability information was provided. The scale's developers, Maxwell and Montgomery (1969), reported that in an item analysis, each of the original 10-scale items discriminated significantly between upper- and lower-quartile groups. In their study of 96 married women, consistent attitudes and behavior were found; those who waited longer before having their first child scored lower on the ATOP.

**Interpreting your score:** Maxwell and Montgomery (1969) found that the following factors related to lower scores (favoring delay of parenting): higher age of respondent, higher education level and socioeconomic status, and having fewer children. Studies in the decade following publication of this measure reveal that women in the late 1970s and early 1980s were more likely than Maxwell and Montgomery's original sample to favor delayed parenthood (Knaub, Eversol, & Voss, 1981, 1983). In the 1983 study of 213 female students at a large midwestern university (Knaub, Eversoll, & Voss, 1983), the mean total score (on items 1 through 10) on the ATOP was 21.

Researchers using this measure typically present the percentage of respondents who agree and disagree with each item. Following is a table that summarizes the responses of 213 female students at a large midwestern university (Knaub, Eversoll, & Voss, 1983) and 76 male students from colleges in four states (Eversoll, Voss, & Knaub, 1983). Percentages for the response options "strongly agree" and "agree" are combined, as are the percentages for "disagree" and "strongly disagree."

## ATOP Items by Percent of Respondents Agreeing and Disagreeing (Refer to questions at the beginning of this assessment)

| | Women | | | Men | | |
| --- | --- | --- | --- | --- | --- | --- |
| | Agree | Disagree | Undecided | Agree | Disagree | Undecided |
| Question 1 | 7.5 | 86.8 | 5.7 | 6.6 | 84.1 | 9.2 |
| Question 2 | 78.8 | 10.8 | 11.3 | 76.0 | 11.8 | 13.2 |
| Question 3 | 6.6 | 76.9 | 16.5 | 10.5 | 68.5 | 21.0 |
| Question 4 | 5.2 | 72.7 | 22.1 | 5.3 | 58.0 | 36.5 |
| Question 5 | 34.9 | 44.8 | 20.8 | 21.1 | 56.6 | 22.4 |
| Question 6 | 8.9 | 81.7 | 9.4 | 7.9 | 72.4 | 19.7 |
| Question 7 | 2.8 | 93.9 | 2.8 | 2.6 | 88.2 | 9.2 |
| Question 8 | 4.3 | 84.4 | 11.3 | 9.2 | 81.6 | 9.2 |
| Question 9 | 14.6 | 77.8 | 7.5 | 15.8 | 78.9 | 5.3 |
| Question 10 | 15.6 | 71.2 | 13.2 | 19.8 | 64.5 | 15.8 |
| Question 11 | 34.7 | 53.1 | 12.2 | | | |

*Sources:* Data from Eversoll, D. B., Voss, J. H., & Knaub, P. K. (1983). Attitudes of college females toward parenthood timing. *Journal of Home Economics*, 75:25–29.

Knaub, P. K., Eversoll, D. B., & Voss, J. H. (1981). Student attitudes toward parenthood: Implications for curricula in the 1980s. *Journal of Home Economics*, 73:34–37.

Knaub, P. K., Eversoll, D. B., & Voss, J. H. (1983). Is parenthood a desirable adult role? An assessment of attitudes held by contemporary women. *Sex Roles*, 9:355–362. Reprinted with kind permission from Springer Science and Business Media and Patricia K. Knaub.

Maxwell, J. W., & Montgomery, J. E. (1969). Societal pressure toward early parenthood. *Family Coordinator*, 18:340–344.

**CHANGING HEALTH HABITS**

# Do You Want to Improve Your Reproductive Health?

Do you need to change a behavior that relates to or affects your reproductive health? For example, if you are sexually active, are you using contraception irregularly, risking pregnancy? Are you using a method that does not provide the level of protection you desire? The "Deciding to Change" section of the Changing Health Habits worksheet can help you determine whether you are ready to alter your behaviors to improve your reproductive health. Use the "Implementing the Change" section of the worksheet if you decide to make the necessary changes.

## Deciding to Change

1. Identify the problem, goal, or question.
2. List the reasons you should make this change and the reasons you should not.

## Choices

Reasons to change behaviors (pros):

| *Points* | *Reasons* |
| --- | --- |
| ____ | _____ |
| ____ | _____ |
| ____ | _____ |
| ____ | Total |

Reasons not to change behaviors (cons):

| *Points* | *Reasons* |
| --- | --- |
| ____ | _____ |
| ____ | _____ |
| ____ | _____ |
| ____ | Total |

3. Draw a conclusion by adding the points in the pros section and then in the cons section. If the point total of the pros section is greater than the total of the cons section, you are probably ready to make a change in your life that improves your reproductive health. If your cons outweigh your pros, you may not be motivated to make the change now. Study your list of pros and cons carefully, however, before making your final decision. You may decide to change even if your reasons not to change outrank your reasons to change.

## Implementing the Change

1. Set a target date to begin the new behavior or reach the goal.
2. Identify and list the factors that will help you reach your goal and those that will stand in the way of reaching your goal.

   *Factors that help:* _____

   *Factors that hinder:* _____

3. Prepare an action plan for making the change.

   a. Identify alternative methods for reaching your goal.

      *Alternative 1:* _____

      *Alternative 2:* _____

      *Alternative 3:* _____

      *Alternative 4:* _____

   b. Gather information about each method.

   c. Choose the method that fits your particular situation best.

   d. Consider the factors that can help or hinder your effort to change (see step 2).

4. Change the lifestyle behavior that you have decided to improve by implementing the action plan you developed in step 3.
5. Chart your daily progress toward your goal.
6. Evaluate how effective you were in reaching your goal.

**SELF-ASSESSMENT 1**

# Male Sexual Quotient Self-Assessment Questionnaire

This self-assessment addresses sexual function and satisfaction in men. It is designed to help men determine whether there are aspects of their sexual experience that could benefit from talking with their partner, consulting their physicians, and seeking treatment.

Answer this questionnaire honestly based on the last 6 months of your sex life, rating your answer as follows.

1 = Infrequently or rarely
2 = Sometimes
3 = Nearly 50% of the time
4 = Most of the time
5 = Always

1. Is your desire high enough to encourage you to initiate sexual intercourse? _____

2. Do you feel confident in your ability of seduction? _____

3. Do you feel that foreplay is enjoyable and satisfying for both you and your partner? _____

4. Is your own sexual performance affected by your partner's sexual satisfaction? _____

5. Can you maintain an erection sufficiently in order to complete sexual activity in a satisfactory way? _____

6. After sexual stimulation, is your erection hard enough to ensure satisfying intercourse? _____

7. Are you able to consistently obtain and maintain an erection whenever you have sexual activity? _____

8. Are you able to control ejaculation so that sexual activity lasts as long as you want? _____

9. Are you able to reach orgasm during sex? _____

10. Does your sexual performance encourage you to enjoy sex more frequently? _____

# Male Sexual Quotient (MSQ) Scoring

Total maximum score: 50

The MSQ equals total score multiplied by 2. Higher scores indicate greater sexual function and satisfaction with such function.

| | |
|---|---|
| 82–100 | Highly satisfied: I am very sexually satisfied and enjoy my sex life to the maximum. |
| 62–80 | Partially satisfied: I enjoy sex, but there is some room for improvement. |
| 42–60 | Average: I am concerned that my sexual enjoyment really could be better. |
| 22–40 | Dissatisfied: I feel that my sex life does not give me enough satisfaction. |
| 0–20 | Highly dissatisfied: I am very concerned that I don't get any satisfaction from my sex life. |

*Source:* Abdo, C. H. N. (2007). The Male Sexual Quotient: A brief, self-administered questionnaire to assess male sexual satisfaction. *Journal of Sexual Medicine, 4:*382–389. Reprinted with permission of Wiley-Blackwell.

# The Love Attitudes Scale

Listed below are several statements that reflect different attitudes about love. For each statement, fill in the response that indicates how much you agree or disagree with the statement. The items refer to a specific love relationship. Whenever possible, answer the questions with your current partner in mind. If you are not currently in a love relationship, answer the questions with your most recent partner in mind. If you have never been in love, answer in terms of what you think your responses would most likely be.

## For Each Statement

1 = strongly agree with the statement
2 = moderately agree with the statement
3 = neutral—neither agree nor disagree
4 = moderately disagree with the statement
5 = strongly disagree with the statement

1. My partner and I have the right physical "chemistry" between us. _____

2. I feel that my partner and I were meant for each other. _____

3. My partner and I really understand each other. _____

4. My partner fits my ideal standards of physical beauty/handsomeness. _____

5. I believe that what my partner doesn't know about me won't hurt him/her. _____

6. I have sometimes had to keep my partner from finding out about other lovers. _____

7. My partner would get upset if he/she knew of some of the things I've done with other people. _____

8. I enjoy playing the "game of love" with my partner and a number of other partners. _____

9. Our love is the best kind because it grew out of a long friendship. _____

10. Our friendship merged gradually into love over time. _____

11. Our love is really a deep friendship, not a mysterious, mystical emotion. _____

12. Our love relationship is the most satisfying because it developed from a good friendship. _____

13. A main consideration in choosing my partner was how he/she would reflect on my family. _____

14. An important factor in choosing my partner was whether or not he/she would be a good parent. _____

15. One consideration in choosing my partner was how he/she would reflect on my career. _____

16. Before getting very involved with my partner, I tried to figure out how compatible his/her hereditary background would be with mine in case we ever had children. _____

17. When my partner doesn't pay attention to me, I feel sick all over. _____

18. Since I've been in love with my partner I've had trouble concentrating on anything else. _____

19. I cannot relax if I suspect that my partner is with someone else. _____

20. If my partner ignores me for a while, I sometimes do stupid things to try to get his/her attention back. _____

21. I would rather suffer myself than let my partner suffer. _____

22. I cannot be happy unless I place my partner's happiness before my own. _____

23. I am usually willing to sacrifice my own wishes to let my partner achieve his/hers. _____

24. I would endure all things for the sake of my partner. _____

## Scoring

Add your scores for the following groups of questions: 1–4, 5–8, 9–12, 13–16, 17–20, and 21–24. Each of these six groupings of questions corresponds to one of Lee's six styles of loving. Your lowest group score means that you most closely align yourself with that style of loving. Table 6-1 in *Essential Concepts for Healthy Living*, Sixth Edition, lists meanings and characteristics for each of Lee's six styles of loving.

1–4 = Eros
5–8 = Ludus
9–12 = Storge
13–16 = Pragma
17–20 = Mania
21–24 = Agape

*Source:* Hendrick, C., Hendrick, S. S., & Dicke, A. (1998). The love attitudes scale: Short form. *Journal of Social and Personal Relationships, 15*:147–159.

## CHANGING HEALTH HABITS

# Would a Behavior Change Improve Your Relationship?

**D**o you need to change a behavior that relates to or affects your relationships? For example, are your communication patterns ineffective with those close to you, such as your lover, spouse, or parents? Are you having trouble communicating effectively with other persons, such as a friend or your boss? Do you want to change those patterns so that you will be more effective in maintaining successful relationships? The "Deciding to Change" section of the Changing Health Habits worksheet can help you determine whether you are ready to alter your behaviors to improve your communication skills. Use the "Implementing the Change" section of the worksheet if you decide to make the necessary changes.

## Deciding to Change

1. Identify the problem, goal, or question.
2. List the reasons you should make this change and the reasons you should not.

## Choices

Reasons to change behaviors (pros):

| Points | Reasons |
| --- | --- |
| ____ | _____ |
| ____ | _____ |
| ____ | _____ |
| ____ | Total |

Reasons not to change behaviors (cons):

| Points | Reasons |
| --- | --- |
| ____ | _____ |
| ____ | _____ |
| ____ | _____ |
| ____ | Total |

3. Draw a conclusion by adding the points in the pros section and then in the cons section. If the point total of the pros section is greater than the total of the cons section, you are probably ready to make a change in your life that improves your communications skills. If your cons outweigh your pros, you may not be motivated to make the change now. Study your list of pros and cons carefully, however, before making your final decision. You may decide to change even if your reasons not to change outrank your reasons to change.

## Implementing the Change

1. Set a target date to begin the new behavior or reach the goal.
2. Identify and list the factors that will help you reach your goal and those that will stand in the way of reaching your goal.

   *Factors that help:* _____

   *Factors that hinder:* _____

3. Prepare an action plan for making the change.

   a. Identify alternative methods to reach your goal.

   *Alternative 1:* _____

   *Alternative 2:* _____

   *Alternative 3:* _____

   *Alternative 4:* _____

   b. Gather information about each method.

   c. Choose the method that fits your particular situation best.

   d. Consider the factors that can help or hinder your effort to change (see step 2).

4. Change the lifestyle behavior that you have decided to improve by implementing the action plan you developed in step 3.
5. Chart your daily progress toward your goal.
6. Evaluate how effective you were in reaching your goal.

## CHAPTER 7

**CHANGING HEALTH HABITS**

# Are You Using Drugs Inappropriately?

**A**re you taking any drugs now, such as caffeine or much stronger drugs, that may be habit forming, may have negative health effects, and that were not prescribed by your healthcare practitioner? If you are using drugs inappropriately, follow the steps of the decision-making and implementation model to identify and change a drug-related habit.

## Deciding to Change

1. Identify the problem, goal, or question.
2. List the reasons you should make this change and the reasons you should not.

## Choices

Reasons to change behaviors (pros):

| *Points* | *Reasons* |
| --- | --- |
| _____ | _____ |
| _____ | _____ |
| _____ | _____ |
| _____ | Total |

Reasons not to change behaviors (cons):

| *Points* | *Reasons* |
| --- | --- |
| _____ | _____ |
| _____ | _____ |
| _____ | _____ |
| _____ | Total |

3. Draw a conclusion by adding the points in the pros section and then in the cons section. If the point total of the pros section is greater than the total of the cons section, you are probably ready to make a change in your life regarding a drug-related habit. If your cons outweigh your pros, you may not be motivated to make the change now. Study your list of pros and cons carefully, however, before making your final decision. You may decide to change even if your reasons not to change outrank your reasons to change.

## Implementing the Change

1. Set a target date to begin the new behavior or reach the goal.
2. Identify and list the factors that will help you reach your goal and those that will stand in the way of reaching your goal.

   *Factors that help:* _____

   *Factors that hinder:* _____

3. Prepare an action plan for making the change.

  a. Identify alternative methods for reaching your goal.

  *Alternative 1:* _____

  *Alternative 2:* _____

  *Alternative 3:* _____

  *Alternative 4:* _____

  b. Gather information about each method.

  c. Choose the method that fits your particular situation best.

  d. Consider the factors that can help or hinder your effort to change (see step 2).

4. Change the lifestyle behavior that you have decided to improve by implementing the action plan you developed in step 3.

5. Chart your daily progress toward your goal.

6. Evaluate how effective you were in reaching your goal.

**CHANGING HEALTH HABITS**

# Do You Want to Change a Smoking or Drinking Habit?

Follow the steps of the decision-making and implementation model to identify and change a health-related habit that concerns your drinking of alcoholic beverages or your use of tobacco. For example, are you a heavy smoker who would like to smoke less or stop smoking cigarettes completely? Do you have drinking habits that you would like to change, such as drinking a six-pack in front of the TV every night, drinking on an empty stomach, or drinking too much at parties and sporting events?

## Deciding to Change

1. Identify the problem, goal, or question.
2. List the reasons you should make this change and the reasons you should not.

## Choices

Reasons to change behaviors (pros):

| **Points** | **Reasons** |
| --- | --- |
| ____ | _____ |
| ____ | _____ |
| ____ | _____ |
| ____ | Total |

Reasons not to change behaviors (cons):

| **Points** | **Reasons** |
| --- | --- |
| ____ | _____ |
| ____ | _____ |
| ____ | _____ |
| ____ | Total |

3. Draw a conclusion by adding the points in the pros section and then in the cons section. If the point total of the pros section is greater than the total of the cons section, you are probably ready to make a change in your life regarding a smoking or drinking habit. If your cons outweigh your pros, you may not be motivated to make the change now. Study your list of pros and cons carefully, however, before making your final decision. You may decide to change even if your reasons not to change outrank your reasons to change.

## Implementing the Change

1. Set a target date to begin the new behavior or reach the goal.
2. Identify and list the factors that will help you reach your goal and those that will stand in the way of reaching your goal.

*Factors that help:* _____

*Factors that hinder:* _____

3. Prepare an action plan for making the change.

    **a.** Identify alternative methods for reaching your goal.

        *Alternative 1:* _____

        *Alternative 2:* _____

        *Alternative 3:* _____

        *Alternative 4:* _____

    **b.** Gather information about each method.

    **c.** Choose the method that fits your particular situation best.

    **d.** Consider the factors that can help or hinder your effort to change (see step 2).

4. Change the lifestyle behavior that you have decided to improve by implementing the action plan you developed in step 3.

5. Chart your daily progress toward your goal.

6. Evaluate how effective you were in reaching your goal.

**SELF-ASSESSMENT 1**

# Assessing the Nutritional Quality of Your Diet

Measure or estimate the amounts of everything you eat and drink for 3 days. For each day, record this information on a daily food record-keeping form (see the next page). To determine the nutritional value of your food items, you can use the "SuperTracker" tools at https://www.choosemyplate.gov/SuperTracker/default.aspx. The textbook's Web site (go.jblearning.com/alters6e) includes a content link in Chapter 9 for a Web site with a dietary analysis tool that you can use to determine the nutritional value of foods.

At the end of each day, add the amounts in each column and write the totals at the bottom of the form. Determine your average intake of calories and nutrients for that period. (Add the three daily totals for calories, then divide by 3. Do the same for each nutrient listed in the record-keeping form.) You can evaluate the nutritional quality of your diet by comparing your average intakes with the DRIs for those nutrients, which are shown in Appendix C.

1.  Write a one-page description of the nutritional quality of your diet; in your summary, provide answers to the following questions:
    a.  Did your average intake of calories and nutrients meet at least 75% of the DRIs for your age and gender?
    b.  If your average intake of one or more nutrients did not meet 75% of the DRIs, which foods could you add to your diet to boost the amounts of the nutrient(s) you are lacking?
    c.  For each of the 3 days, what percentage of your calories were from protein, fat, and alcohol?
    d.  If the percentage of calories from fat exceeded 35%, which foods contributed to your high fat intake?

2.  Do you need to make any changes to improve the nutritional quality of your diet? Would you like to eat more fruits or vegetables? Should you replace whole or reduced-fat (2%) milk with nonfat milk? Do you need more calcium or iron in your diet? Do you think you eat too much sugar, salt, or fat?

3.  Use your responses to number 2 to complete the Changing Health Habits activity for this chapter.

Daily Food Record

Name _____

Date _____

| Food Item | Amount Eaten | Calories | Prot. (g) | Fat* (g) | Vit. D (μg) | Vit. C (mg) | Vit. E (mg) | Folate (μg) | Calcium (mg) | Iron (mg) |
|---|---|---|---|---|---|---|---|---|---|---|
| | | | | | | | | | | |
| | | | | | | | | | | |
| | | | | | | | | | | |
| | | | | | | | | | | |
| | | | | | | | | | | |
| | | | | | | | | | | |
| | | | | | | | | | | |
| | | | | | | | | | | |
| | | | | | | | | | | |
| | | | | | | | | | | |
| | | | | | | | | | | |
| | | | | | | | | | | |
| | | | | | | | | | | |
| | | | | | | | | | | |
| | | | | | | | | | | |
| | | | | | | | | | | |
| | | | | | | | | | | |
| | | | | | | | | | | |
| | | | | | | | | | | |
| **Totals** | | | | | | | | | | |

*No DRI

Total calories from alcohol _____

# Diabetes Risk Test

**▲. American Diabetes Association.**

# ALERT!DAY

# ARE YOU AT RISK?

# DIABETES RISK TEST

Calculate Your Chances for Type 2 or Pre-Diabetes

The American Diabetes Association has revised its Diabetes Risk Test according to a new, more accurate statistical model. The updated test includes some new risk factors, and projects risk for pre-diabetes as well as diabetes.

This simple tool can help you determine your risk for having pre-diabetes or diabetes. Using the flow chart, answer the questions until you reach a colored shape. Match that with a risk message shown below.

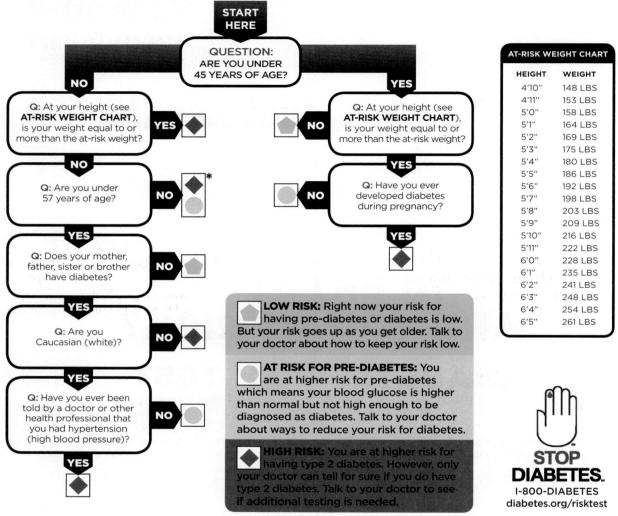

**START HERE**

**QUESTION:** ARE YOU UNDER 45 YEARS OF AGE?

**NO**

**Q:** At your height (see **AT-RISK WEIGHT CHART**), is your weight equal to or more than the at-risk weight?
YES ◆

NO

**Q:** Are you under 57 years of age?
NO ◆ ● *

YES

**Q:** Does your mother, father, sister or brother have diabetes?
NO ⬠

YES

**Q:** Are you Caucasian (white)?
NO ◆

YES

**Q:** Have you ever been told by a doctor or other health professional that you had hypertension (high blood pressure)?
NO ●

YES
◆

**YES**

**Q:** At your height (see **AT-RISK WEIGHT CHART**), is your weight equal to or more than the at-risk weight?
⬠ NO

YES

**Q:** Have you ever developed diabetes during pregnancy?
● NO

YES
◆

**LOW RISK:** Right now your risk for having pre-diabetes or diabetes is low. But your risk goes up as you get older. Talk to your doctor about how to keep your risk low.

**AT RISK FOR PRE-DIABETES:** You are at higher risk for pre-diabetes which means your blood glucose is higher than normal but not high enough to be diagnosed as diabetes. Talk to your doctor about ways to reduce your risk for diabetes.

**HIGH RISK:** You are at higher risk for having type 2 diabetes. However, only your doctor can tell for sure if you do have type 2 diabetes. Talk to your doctor to see if additional testing is needed.

| AT-RISK WEIGHT CHART | |
|---|---|
| **HEIGHT** | **WEIGHT** |
| 4'10" | 148 LBS |
| 4'11" | 153 LBS |
| 5'0" | 158 LBS |
| 5'1" | 164 LBS |
| 5'2" | 169 LBS |
| 5'3" | 175 LBS |
| 5'4" | 180 LBS |
| 5'5" | 186 LBS |
| 5'6" | 192 LBS |
| 5'7" | 198 LBS |
| 5'8" | 203 LBS |
| 5'9" | 209 LBS |
| 5'10" | 216 LBS |
| 5'11" | 222 LBS |
| 6'0" | 228 LBS |
| 6'1" | 235 LBS |
| 6'2" | 241 LBS |
| 6'3" | 248 LBS |
| 6'4" | 254 LBS |
| 6'5" | 261 LBS |

**STOP DIABETES.**
1-800-DIABETES
diabetes.org/risktest

*Your risk for diabetes or pre-diabetes depends on additional risk factors including weight, physical activity and blood pressure.

Source: 2011 American Diabetes Association. From www.diabetes.org. Reprinted with permission from "The American Diabetes Association".

*Factors that help:* _____

*Factors that hinder:* _____

3. Prepare an action plan for making the change.

   a. Identify alternative methods for reaching your goal.

      *Alternative 1:* _____

      *Alternative 2:* _____

      *Alternative 3:* _____

      *Alternative 4:* _____

   b. Gather information about each method.

   c. Choose the method that fits your particular situation best.

   d. Consider the factors that can help or hinder your effort to change (see step 2).

4. Change the lifestyle behavior that you have decided to improve by implementing the action plan you developed in step 3.

5. Chart your daily progress toward your goal.

6. Evaluate how effective you were in reaching your goal.

## CHAPTER 10

SELF-ASSESSMENT

**Student Workbook**

# How Much Energy Do You Use Daily?

**U**se the following activity to estimate your daily caloric needs.

### A. Estimating energy needs for basal metabolism:

**1.** Convert your body weight to kilograms. Since each pound equals about 2.2 kilograms, divide your weight in pounds by 2.2 to obtain your weight in kilograms.

_____ weight in pounds ÷ 2.2 = _____ kilograms (kg)

**2.** To sustain its basal metabolic needs, the body needs about 1.0 calorie per kg of body weight per hour (men) or 0.9 calorie per kg of body weight per hour (women). To estimate the amount of calories you need for basal metabolism in an hour, multiply your body weight (kg) by 1.0 if you are male or 0.9 if you are female.

_____ body weight (kg) × 1.0 or 0.9 = _____ calories per hour

**3.** To estimate the amount of calories you need for basal metabolism in a day, multiply the amount of calories you obtained in step 2 by 24 (hours in a day).

_____ calories per hour × 24 hours = _____ calories per day (basal metabolism)

## B. Estimating energy needs for physical activity:

**4.** To determine your energy needs for physical activity, you can keep records of every activity you perform during the day, and the time spent engaging in each activity. An easier, but less precise way to estimate your energy expenditures for physical activity is to use the following rule of thumb. To use this method, choose the category of physical activity in the table on the next page that best describes your usual physical activity level. For example, if you spend most of your day sitting while taking classes, studying, and watching TV, you probably have a very light level of activity. If you sit some of the time, but move around while working, you might rate your level of physical activity as light. If you are on your feet most of the time and engage in strenuous work such as lifting heavy objects, you are probably expending energy at the heavy level of intensity.

My activity level is _____

5. Note the Activity Factor in the table below for your level of intensity and gender. For example, if you are male, and you consider your overall physical activity pattern to be in the moderate range, your Activity Factor is 1.7.

The Activity Factor for my gender and level of physical activity intensity is _____

6. Multiply your basal metabolic energy needs (the number of calories per day estimated in step 3) by the Activity Factor (step 5).

___ calories for basal metabolism × __ Activity Factor = ____ calories for physical activity

7. To estimate the number of calories you expend each day for the thermic effect of food (TEF), multiply the number of calories determined in step 6 by 0.10.

_____ calories × 0.10 = ___ calories for TEF

8. To estimate your total energy needs for a day, add the number of calories determined in steps 6 and 7.

_____ calories for basal metabolism and physical activity

+ _____ calories for TEF

= _____ total calories

This is an estimation of the total number of calories you use each day. If you take in more calories than needed, they may be converted to body fat.

9. If you completed the assessment in Chapter 9, you were able to determine an average number of calories that you consumed during the three-day record-keeping period. Is your average caloric intake about the same, greater than, or less than the total number of calories that you need for a day?

_____ about the same _____ greater than _____ less than

10. If you continue to consume this average amount of calories, explain what may happen to your body weight.

| | | Activity Factor | |
|---|---|---|---|
| Intensity | Physical Activity | Men | Women |
| Very light | Standing, sitting, driving, typing, sewing, cooking, playing cards or a musical instrument | 1.3 | 1.3 |
| Light | Walking on a level surface at 2.5 to 3.0 mph, carpentry, child care, golf, sailing, table tennis | 1.6 | 1.5 |
| Moderate | Walking 3.5 to 4.0 mph, gardening, carrying a load, cycling, skiing, tennis, dancing | 1.7 | 1.6 |
| Heavy | Walking uphill carrying a load; digging by hand; playing basketball, football, or soccer; climbing | 2.1 | 1.9 |
| Exceptionally heavy | Athletic training or participation in professional or world-class events | 2.4 | 2.2 |

Source: Reprinted with permission from *Recommended dietary allowances* (10th Ed.). Copyright © 1989 by the National Academy of Sciences. Courtesy of the National Academies Press, Washington, D.C.

### CHANGING HEALTH HABITS

# Altering Caloric Intake and Physical Activity

D o you need to lose or gain weight? The "Deciding to Change" section of the Changing Health Habits worksheet can help you determine whether you are ready to alter your caloric intake and physical activity level to gain or lose weight. If you decide to change some of your eating and physical activity habits, use the "Implementing the Change" section of the worksheet to help you make the necessary lifestyle changes.

## Deciding to Change

1. Identify the problem, goal, or question.
2. List the reasons you should make this change and the reasons you should not.

## Choices

Reasons to change behaviors (pros):

| Points | Reasons |
|--------|---------|
| ____ | _____ |
| ____ | _____ |
| ____ | _____ |
| ____ | Total |

Reasons not to change behaviors (cons):

| Points | Reasons |
|--------|---------|
| ____ | _____ |
| ____ | _____ |
| ____ | _____ |
| ____ | Total |

3. Draw a conclusion by adding the points in the pros section and then in the cons section. If the point total of the pros section is greater than the total of the cons section, you are probably ready to make the lifestyle changes necessary to lose or gain weight. If your cons outweigh your pros, you may not be motivated to make the change now. Study your list of pros and cons carefully, however, before making your final decision. You may decide to change even if your reasons not to change outrank your reasons to change.

## Implementing the Change

1. Set a target date to begin the new behavior or reach the goal.
2. Identify and list the factors that will help you reach your goal and those that will stand in the way of reaching your goal.

   *Factors that help:* _____

   *Factors that hinder:* _____
3. Prepare an action plan for making the change.

   a. Identify alternative methods for reaching your goal.

   *Alternative 1:* _____

   *Alternative 2:* _____

   *Alternative 3:* _____

   *Alternative 4:* _____

   b. Gather information about each method.

   c. Choose the method that fits your particular situation best.

   d. Consider the factors that can help or hinder your effort to change (see step 2).
4. Change the lifestyle behavior that you have decided to improve by implementing the action plan you developed in step 3.
5. Chart your daily progress toward your goal.
6. Evaluate how effective you were in reaching your goal.

# Cardiorespiratory Fitness: The Rockport Fitness Walking Test™

This activity assesses cardiorespiratory (aerobic) fitness. To perform the test, you need a watch with a second hand to record your time, and you need to wear good walking shoes and loose clothes. You should have your physician's consent before undertaking this exercise test.

## Instructions

1. Find a measured track or measure 1 mile using your car's odometer on a level uninterrupted road.
2. Warm up by walking slowly for 5 minutes.
3. Walk 1 mile as fast as you can, maintaining a steady pace. Note the time that you began walking.
4. When you complete the mile walk, record your time to the nearest second and keep walking at a slower pace. Count your pulse for 15 seconds and multiply by 4, then record this number. This gives you your heart rate per minute after your test walk.

   Heart rate at the end of a mile walk: _____ beats per minute

   Time to walk the mile: _____ minutes

5. Remember to stretch once you have cooled down.
6. To find your cardiorespiratory fitness level, refer to the appropriate Rockport Fitness Walking Test™ charts according to your age and sex. These show established fitness norms from the American Heart Association.

   Using your fitness level chart, find your time in minutes and your heart rate per minute. Follow these lines until they meet, and mark this point on your chart. This tells you how fit you are compared to other individuals of your sex and age category. Level 5 represents the highest fitness level.

   These charts are based on weights of 170 lb for men and 125 lb for women. If you weigh substantially less, your cardiovascular fitness will be slightly underestimated. Conversely, if you weigh substantially more, your cardiovascular fitness will be slightly overestimated.

**MEN'S FITNESS LEVEL CHART**   **WOMEN'S FITNESS LEVEL CHART**

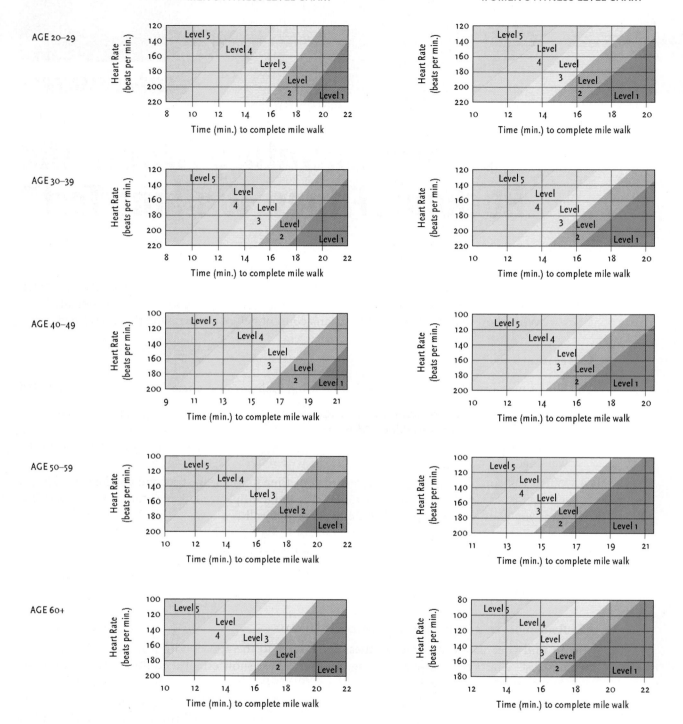

*Source:* Courtesy of the Rockport Company, Inc.

# Push-Up Test for Muscular Endurance

**T**he push-up test can help assess your muscular endurance. To take the test, follow these instructions.

## Procedure

### Men

- Assume the standard position for a push-up, with the body rigid and straight, toes tucked under, and hands about shoulder-width apart and straight under the shoulders.
- Lower the body until the elbows reach 90 degrees. Some prefer to place an object such as a paper cup beneath to touch.
- Return to the starting position with the arms fully extended.
- The most common error is not keeping the back straight and rigid throughout the entire push-up.
- Count the number of push-ups you can perform in one minute.
- See the accompanying table for your fitness level.

### Women

Women tend to have less upper body strength and therefore should use the modified push-up position to assess their upper body endurance. The test is performed as follows:

- Directions are the same for women as for men, except that women should perform the test from the bent-knee position. Make sure that your hands are slightly ahead of your shoulders in the up position so that when you are in the down position, your hands are directly under the shoulders.
- Keep the back straight and rigid throughout the entire push-up.
- Count the number of push-ups you can perform in one minute.
- See the accompanying table to rate your muscular endurance.

*Note:* Women who wish to do full-body push-ups can rate their performances by using the table on the next page.

## Muscular Endurance Ratings
## 1 Minute Push-Up

| Males | | | | | |
|---|---|---|---|---|---|
| | | | Age | | |
| % | 20–29 | 30–39 | 40–49 | 50–59 | |
| 99 | 100 | 86 | 64 | 51 | |
| 95 | 62 | 52 | 40 | 39 | Superior |
| 90 | 57 | 46 | 36 | 30 | |
| 85 | 51 | 41 | 34 | 28 | |
| 80 | 47 | 39 | 30 | 25 | Excellent |
| 75 | 44 | 36 | 29 | 24 | |
| 70 | 41 | 34 | 26 | 21 | |
| 65 | 39 | 31 | 25 | 20 | |
| 60 | 37 | 30 | 24 | 19 | Good |
| 55 | 35 | 29 | 22 | 17 | |
| 50 | 33 | 27 | 21 | 15 | |
| 45 | 31 | 25 | 19 | 14 | |
| 40 | 29 | 24 | 18 | 13 | Fair |
| 35 | 27 | 21 | 16 | 11 | |
| 30 | 26 | 20 | 15 | 10 | |
| 25 | 24 | 19 | 13 | 9.5 | |
| 20 | 22 | 17 | 11 | 9 | Poor |
| 15 | 19 | 15 | 10 | 7 | |
| 10 | 18 | 13 | 9 | 6 | |
| 5 | 13 | 9 | 5 | 3 | Very Poor |
| n | 1,045 | 790 | 364 | 172 | |

Total n = 2,371

*Note:* Norms are based on worksite wellness program participants.

## Muscular Endurance Ratings
## 1 Minute Modified Push-Up

| Females | | | | | |
|---|---|---|---|---|---|
| | **Age** | | | | |
| **%** | **20–29** | **30–39** | **40–49** | **50–59** | |
| 99 | 70 | 56 | 60 | 31 | |
| 95 | 45 | 39 | 33 | 28 | Superior |
| 90 | 42 | 36 | 28 | 25 | |
| 85 | 39 | 33 | 26 | 23 | |
| 80 | 36 | 31 | 24 | 21 | Excellent |
| 75 | 34 | 29 | 21 | 20 | |
| 70 | 32 | 28 | 20 | 19 | |
| 65 | 31 | 26 | 19 | 18 | |
| 60 | 30 | 24 | 18 | 17 | Good |
| 55 | 29 | 23 | 17 | 15 | |
| 50 | 26 | 21 | 15 | 13 | |
| 45 | 25 | 20 | 14 | 13 | |
| 40 | 23 | 19 | 13 | 12 | Fair |
| 35 | 22 | 17 | 11 | 10 | |
| 30 | 20 | 15 | 10 | 9 | |
| 25 | 19 | 14 | 9 | 8 | |
| 20 | 17 | 11 | 6 | 6 | Poor |
| 15 | 15 | 9 | 4 | 4 | |
| 10 | 12 | 8 | 2 | 1 | |
| 5 | 9 | 4 | 1 | 0 | Very Poor |
| *n* | 579 | 411 | 246 | 105 | |

Total n = 1,341

*Note:* Norms are based on worksite wellness program participants.

## Muscular Endurance Ratings
## 1 Minute Full-Body Push-Up*

| Females | Age | | | |
|---|---|---|---|---|
| % | 20–29 | 30–39 | 40–49 | Endurance Level |
| 99 | 53 | 48 | 23 | |
| 95 | 42 | 39.5 | 20 | Superior |
| 90 | 37 | 33 | 18 | |
| 85 | 33 | 26 | 17 | |
| 80 | 28 | 23 | 15 | Excellent |
| 75 | 27 | 19 | 15 | |
| 70 | 24 | 18 | 14 | |
| 65 | 23 | 16 | 13 | |
| 60 | 21 | 15 | 13 | Good |
| 55 | 19 | 14 | 11 | |
| 50 | 18 | 14 | 11 | |
| 45 | 17 | 13 | 10 | |
| 40 | 15 | 11 | 9 | Fair |
| 35 | 14 | 10 | 8 | |
| 30 | 13 | 9 | 7 | |
| 25 | 11 | 9 | 7 | |
| 20 | 10 | 8 | 6 | Poor |
| 15 | 9 | 6.5 | 5 | |
| 10 | 8 | 6 | 4 | |
| 5 | 6 | 4 | 1 | |
| 1 | 3 | 1 | 0 | Very Poor |

* Full-body push-ups are generally used by law enforcement and public safety organizations. These norms are based on >1000 female U.S. Army soldiers who were tested in the 1990s by the U.S. Army.

Reprinted with permission from The Cooper Institute, Dallas, Texas, from *Physical Fitness Assessments and Norms for Adults and Law Enforcement*. Available online at http://www.cooperinstitute.org.

# Sit-and-Reach Test for Flexibility Assessment

The sit-and-reach test can help assess your flexibility. Read the following precautions, and if they do not apply, take the test.

## Precautions

If any of the following apply, seek medical advice before performing the test.

- You are presently suffering from acute back pain.
- You are currently receiving treatment for back pain.
- You have ever had a surgical operation on your back.
- A healthcare professional told you to never exercise your back.

## Procedure

Warm up. Stop the test if pain occurs. Do not perform fast, jerky movements.

### Step 1:

Sit on the floor with your legs straight and knees together. Your toes should point upward toward the ceiling and rest against the side of a box.

### Step 2:

Place one hand over the other. The tips of your two middle fingers should be on top of each other.

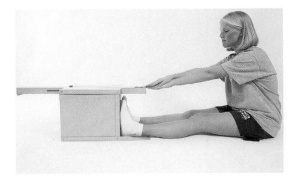

## Step 3:

Slowly stretch forward without bouncing or jerking. Stop when tightness or discomfort occurs in the back or legs. Measure how far your hands reached on the top of the box.

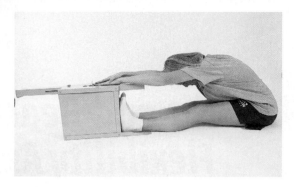

## Step 4:

Repeat this test two more times and record scores.

First attempt           _____ points

Second attempt       _____ points

Third attempt         _____ points

| How to score (average of 3 attempts) | |
| --- | --- |
| Reached well past toes and side of box | 1 point; excellent |
| Reached just to toes | 2 points; good |
| Up to 4 inches from toes (did not reach side of box) | 3 points; fair |
| More than 4 inches from toes (did not reach side of box) | 4 points; poor |

*Source:* David Imrie. (1998). *Back power.* Toronto, Canada: Stoddart. Reprinted with permission of the author.

Total points = _____ divided by 3 = _____ points, which is rated as _____.

**SELF-ASSESSMENT 4**

# Check Your Physical Activity and Heart Disease IQ

est your knowledge about the effects that physical activity can have on your heart. Mark each statement true or false. Answers are on the following page.

| | | |
|---|---|---|
| 1. Regular physical activity can reduce your chances of getting heart disease. | T | F |
| 2. Most people get enough physical activity from their normal daily routines. | T | F |
| 3. You don't have to train like a marathon runner to become more physically fit. | T | F |
| 4. Exercise programs do not require a lot of time to be very effective. | T | F |
| 5. People who need to lose some weight are the only ones who will benefit from regular physical activity. | T | F |
| 6. All exercises give you the same benefits. | T | F |
| 7. The older you are, the less active you need to be. | T | F |
| 8. It doesn't take a lot of money or expensive equipment to become physically fit. | T | F |
| 9. There are many risks and injuries that can occur with exercise. | T | F |
| 10. You should consult a doctor before starting a physical activity program. | T | F |
| 11. People who have had a heart attack should not start any physical activity program. | T | F |
| 12. To help stay physically active, include a variety of activities. | T | F |

**How well did you do?**

# Answers to the Check Your Physical Activity and Heart Disease IQ Quiz

1. *True*. Heart disease is almost twice as likely to develop in inactive people. Being physically inactive is a risk factor for heart disease, along with cigarette smoking, high blood pressure, high blood cholesterol, and being overweight. The more risk factors you have, the greater your chance for heart disease. Regular physical activity (even mild to moderate exercise) can reduce this risk.

2. *False*. Most Americans are very busy but not very active. Every American adult should make a habit of getting at least 30 minutes of low to moderate levels of physical activity daily. This includes walking, gardening, and walking up stairs. If you are inactive now, begin by doing a few minutes of activity each day. If you only do some activity every once in a while, try to work something into your routine everyday.

3. *True*. Low- to moderate-intensity activities, such as pleasure walking, stair climbing, yard work, housework, dancing, and home exercises can have both short- and long-term benefits. If you are inactive, the key is to get started. One great way is to take a walk for 10 to 15 minutes during your lunch break, or take your dog for a walk every day. At least 30 minutes of physical activity every day can help improve your heart health.

4. *True*. It takes only a few minutes a day to become more physically active. If you don't have 30 minutes in your schedule for an exercise break, try to find two 15-minute periods or even three 10-minute periods. These exercise breaks will soon become a habit you can't live without.

5. *False*. People who are physically active experience many positive benefits. Regular physical activity gives you more energy, reduces stress, and helps you to sleep better. It helps to lower high blood pressure and improves blood cholesterol levels. Physical activity helps to tone your muscles, burns off calories to help you lose extra pounds or stay at your desirable weight, and helps control your appetite. It can also increase muscle strength, help your heart and lungs work more efficiently, and let you enjoy your life more fully.

6. *False*. Low-intensity activities—if performed daily—can have some long-term health benefits and can lower your risk of heart disease. Regular, brisk, and sustained exercise for at least 30 minutes, three to four times a week, such as brisk walking, jogging, or swimming, is necessary to improve the efficiency of your heart and lungs and burn off extra calories. These activities are called aerobic—meaning the body uses oxygen to produce the energy needed for the activity. Other activities, depending on the type, may give you other benefits such as increased flexibility or muscle strength.

7. *False*. Although we tend to become less active with age, physical activity is still important. In fact, regular physical activity in older persons increases their capacity to do everyday activities. In general, middle-aged and older people benefit from regular physical activity just as young people do. What is important, at any age, is tailoring the activity program to your own fitness level.

8. *True*. Many activities require little or no equipment. For example, brisk walking only requires a comfortable pair of walking shoes. Many communities offer free or inexpensive recreation facilities and physical activity classes. Check your shopping malls, as many of them are open early and late for people who do not wish to walk alone, in the dark, or in bad weather.

9. *False*. Under normal conditions, exercise does not involve many risks and injuries. However, the most common risk in exercising is injury to the muscles and joints. Such injuries are usually caused by exercising too hard for too long, particularly if a person has been inactive. To avoid injuries, try to build up your level of activity gradually, listen to your body for warning pains, be aware of possible signs of heart problems (such as pain or pressure in the left or mid-chest

area, left neck, shoulder, or arm during or just after exercising, or sudden light-headedness, cold sweat, pallor, or fainting), and be prepared for special weather conditions.

10. *True.* You should ask your doctor before you start (or greatly increase) your physical activity **if** you have a medical condition such as high blood pressure, have pains or pressure in the chest and shoulder, feel dizzy or faint, get breathless after mild exertion, are middle-aged or older and have not been physically active, or plan a vigorous activity program. If none of these apply, start slow and get moving.

11. *False.* Regular physical activity can help reduce your risk of having another heart attack. People who include regular physical activity in their lives after a heart attack improve their chances of survival and can improve how they feel and look. If you have had a heart attack, consult your doctor to be sure you are following a safe and effective exercise program that will help prevent heart pain and further damage from overexertion.

12. *True.* Pick several different activities that you like doing. You will be more likely to stay with it. Plan short-term and long-term goals. Keep a record of your progress, and check it regularly to see the progress you have made. Get your family and friends to join in. They can help keep you going.

*Source:* U.S. Department of Health and Human Services, National Institutes of Health, National Heart, Lung, and Blood Institute. Retrieved May 27, 2011, from http://www.nhlbi.nih.gov/actintime/rhar/bpa_quiz.htm.

# Do You Want to Be More Physically Active?

After completing the cardiorespiratory fitness assessment in the workbook, do you think you need to increase your physical activity level to become more fit? The "Deciding to Change" section of the Changing Health Habits worksheet can help you identify the health benefits of adding physical activity to your schedule and decide whether you are ready to do so. If you choose to increase your present level of physical activity, use the "Implementing the Change" section of the worksheet to help you.

## Deciding to Change

1. Identify the problem, goal, or question.
2. List the reasons you should make this change and the reasons you should not.

## Choices

Reasons to change behaviors (pros):

| Points | Reasons |
|--------|---------|
| _____ | _____ |
| _____ | _____ |
| _____ | _____ |
| _____ | Total |

Reasons not to change behaviors (cons):

| Points | Reasons |
|--------|---------|
| _____ | _____ |
| _____ | _____ |
| _____ | _____ |
| _____ | Total |

3. Draw a conclusion by adding the points in the pros section and then in the cons section. If the point total of the pros section is greater than the total of the cons section, you are probably ready to make a change that increases your level of physical activity. If your cons outweigh your pros, you may not be motivated to make the change now. Study your list of pros and cons carefully, however, before making your final decision. You may decide to change even if your reasons not to change outrank your reasons to change.

## Implementing the Change

1. Set a target date to begin the new behavior or reach the goal.
2. Identify and list the factors that will help you reach your goal and those that will stand in the way of reaching your goal.

   *Factors that help:* _____

   *Factors that hinder:* _____

3. Prepare an action plan for making the change.

   a. Identify alternative methods for reaching your goal.

      *Alternative 1:* _____

      *Alternative 2:* _____

      *Alternative 3:* _____

      *Alternative 4:* _____

   b. Gather information about each method.

   c. Choose the method that fits your situation best.

   d. Consider the factors that can help or hinder your effort to change (see step 2).

4. Change the exercise-related behavior that you have decided to improve by implementing the action plan you developed in step 3.
5. Chart your daily progress toward your goal.
6. Evaluate how effective you were in reaching your goal.

**SELF-ASSESSMENT**

# What is Your Risk of Developing Heart Disease or Having a Heart Attack?

I n general, the higher your LDL level and the more risk factors you have (other than LDL), the greater your chances of developing heart disease or having a heart attack. Some people are at high risk for a heart attack because they already have heart disease. Other people are at high risk for developing heart disease because they have diabetes (which is a strong risk factor) or a combination of risk factors for heart disease. Follow these steps to find out your risk for developing heart disease.

**Step 1:** Check the following table to see how many of the listed risk factors you have; these are the risk factors that affect your LDL goal.

## Major Risk Factors That Affect Your LDL Goal

- Cigarette smoking
- High blood pressure (140/90 mmHg or higher or on blood pressure medication)
- Low HDL cholesterol (less than 40 mg/dl)*
- Family history of early heart disease (heart disease in father or brother before age 55; heart disease in mother or sister before age 65)
- Age (men 45 years or older; women 55 years or older)

* If your HDL cholesterol is 60 mg/dl or higher, subtract 1 from your total count.

Even though obesity and physical inactivity are not counted in this list, they are conditions that need to be corrected.

**Step 2:** How many major risk factors do you have? If you have two or more risk factors in the bulleted list above, use the risk scoring tables at the end of this assessment (which include your cholesterol levels) to find your risk score. Risk score refers to the chance of having a heart attack in the next 10 years, given as a percentage. My risk score is _____%.

**Step 3:** Use your medical history, number of risk factors, and risk score to find your risk of developing heart disease or having a heart attack in the following table.

| If You Have | You Are in Category |
|---|---|
| Heart disease, diabetes, or risk score more than 20%* | I. High Risk |
| 2 or more risk factors and risk score 10–20% | II. Next Highest Risk |
| 2 or more risk factors and risk score less than 10% | III. Moderate Risk |
| 0 or 1 risk factor | IV. Low-to-Moderate Risk |

* Means that more than 20 of 100 people in this category will have a heart attack within 10 years.

My risk category is _____.

## Treating High Cholesterol

The main goal of cholesterol-lowering treatment is to lower your LDL level enough to reduce your risk of developing heart disease or having a heart attack. The higher your risk, the lower your LDL goal will be. To find your LDL goal, see the bulleted list that follows for your risk category. There are two main ways to lower your cholesterol:

1. Therapeutic lifestyle changes (TLC): Includes a cholesterol-lowering diet (called the TLC diet), physical activity, and weight management. TLC is for anyone whose LDL is above goal.

2. Drug treatment: If cholesterol-lowering drugs are needed, they are used together with TLC treatment to help lower your LDL.

If you are in . . .

- **Category I, Highest Risk**, your LDL goal is less than 100 mg/dl. You will need to begin the TLC diet to reduce your high risk even if your LDL is below 100 mg/dl. If your LDL is 100 or above, you will need to start drug treatment at the same time as the TLC diet. If your LDL is below 100 mg/dl, you may also need to start drug treatment together with the TLC diet if your doctor finds your risk is very high—for example, if you had a recent heart attack or have both heart disease and diabetes.

- **Category II, Next Highest Risk**, your LDL goal is less than 130 mg/dl. If your LDL is 130 mg/dl or above, you will need to begin treatment with the TLC diet. If your LDL is 130 mg/dl or more after 3 months on the TLC diet, you may need drug treatment along with the TLC diet. If your LDL is less than 130 mg/dl, you will need to follow the heart-healthy diet for all Americans, which allows a little more saturated fat and cholesterol than the TLC diet.

- **Category III, Moderate Risk**, your LDL goal is less than 130 mg/dl. If your LDL is 130 mg/dl or above, you will need to begin the TLC diet. If your LDL is 160 mg/dl or more after you have tried the TLC diet for 3 months, you may need drug treatment along with the TLC diet. If your LDL is less than 130 mg/dl, you will need to follow the heart-healthy diet for all Americans.

- **Category IV, Low-to-Moderate Risk**, your LDL goal is less than 160 mg/dl. If your LDL is 160 mg/dl or above, you will need to begin the TLC diet. If your LDL is still 160 mg/dl or more after 3 months on the TLC diet, you may need drug treatment along with the TLC diet to lower your LDL, especially if your LDL is 190 mg/dl or more. If your LDL is less than 160 mg/dl, you will need to follow the heart-healthy diet for all Americans.

To reduce your risk for heart disease or keep it low, it is very important to control any other risk factors you may have, such as high blood pressure and smoking.

## Lowering Cholesterol with Therapeutic Lifestyle Changes

TLC is a set of things you can do to help lower your LDL cholesterol. The main parts of TLC are:

- *The TLC diet.* This is a low-saturated-fat, low-cholesterol eating plan that calls for less than 7% of calories from saturated fat and less than 200 mg of dietary cholesterol per day. The TLC diet recommends only enough calories to maintain a desirable weight and avoid weight gain. If your LDL is not lowered enough by reducing your saturated fat and cholesterol intakes, the amount of soluble fiber in your diet can be increased. Certain food products that contain plant stanols or plant sterols (for example, cholesterol-lowering margarines) can also be added to the TLC diet to boost its LDL-lowering power.

- *Weight management.* Losing weight if you are overweight can help lower LDL and is especially important for those with a cluster of risk factors that includes high triglyceride and/or low HDL levels and being overweight with a large waist measurement (more than 40 inches for men and more than 35 inches for women).

- *Physical activity.* Regular physical activity (30 minutes on most, if not all, days) is recommended for everyone. It can help raise HDL and lower LDL and is especially important for those with high triglyceride and/or low HDL levels who are overweight with a large waist measurement.

---

Foods low in saturated fat include fat-free or 1% dairy products, lean meats, fish, skinless poultry, whole-grain foods, and fruits and vegetables. Look for soft margarines (liquid or tub varieties) that are low in saturated fat and contain little or no trans fat (another type of dietary fat that can raise your cholesterol level). Limit foods high in cholesterol, such as liver and other organ meats, egg yolks, and full-fat dairy products.

Good sources of soluble fiber include oats, certain fruits (such as oranges and pears) and vegetables (such as brussels sprouts and carrots), and dried peas and beans.

---

## Drug Treatment

Even if you begin drug treatment to lower your cholesterol, you will need to continue your treatment with lifestyle changes. This will keep the dose of medicine as low as possible, and lower your risk in other ways as well. There are several types of drugs available for cholesterol lowering, including statins, bile acid sequestrants, nicotinic acid, fibric acids, and cholesterol absorption inhibitors. Your doctor can help decide which type of drug is best for you. The statin drugs are very effective in lowering LDL levels and are safe for most people. Bile acid sequestrants also lower LDL and can be used alone or in combination with statin drugs. Nicotinic acid lowers LDL and triglycerides and raises HDL. Fibric acids lower LDL somewhat but are used mainly to treat high triglyceride and low HDL levels. Cholesterol absorption inhibitors lower LDL and can be used alone or in combination with statin drugs.

---

*Note:* Before beginning any diet and exercise regimen, you should speak with your physician to be sure it is right for you. Your physician will also advise you whether you should begin drug treatment to lower your cholesterol level.

---

Once your LDL goal has been reached, your doctor may prescribe treatment for high triglycerides and/or a low HDL level, if present. The treatment includes losing weight if needed, increasing physical activity, quitting smoking, and possibly taking a drug.

### Resources

For more information about lowering cholesterol and lowering your risk for heart disease, write to the NHLBI Health Information Center, P.O. Box 30105, Bethesda, MD, 20824-0105 or call 301-592-8573.

*Source:* National Heart, Lung, and Blood Institute. (2005). *High blood cholesterol: What you need to know.* Retrieved from http://www.nhlbi.nih.gov/health/public/heart/chol/hbc_what.htm.

# Risk Scoring Tables: Estimate of Ten-Year Risk for Coronary Heart Disease

## Men

(Framingham Point Scores)*

| Age | Points |
|-----|--------|
| 20–34 | −9 |
| 35–39 | −4 |
| 40–44 | 0 |
| 45–49 | 3 |
| 50–54 | 6 |
| 55–59 | 8 |
| 60–64 | 10 |
| 65–69 | 11 |
| 70–74 | 12 |
| 75–79 | 13 |

| Total Cholesterol | Points | | | | |
|-------------------|--------------|--------------|--------------|--------------|--------------|
| | Age 20–39 | Age 40–49 | Age 50–59 | Age 60–69 | Age 70–79 |
| <160 | 0 | 0 | 0 | 0 | 0 |
| 160–199 | 4 | 3 | 2 | 1 | 0 |
| 200–239 | 7 | 5 | 3 | 1 | 0 |
| 240–279 | 9 | 6 | 4 | 2 | 1 |
| ≥280 | 11 | 8 | 5 | 3 | 1 |

| | Points | | | | |
|-----------|--------------|--------------|--------------|--------------|--------------|
| | Age 20–39 | Age 40–49 | Age 50–59 | Age 60–69 | Age 70–79 |
| Nonsmoker | 0 | 0 | 0 | 0 | 0 |
| Smoker | 8 | 5 | 3 | 1 | 1 |

## Women

(Framingham Point Scores)*

| Age | Points |
|-----|--------|
| 20–34 | −7 |
| 35–39 | −3 |
| 40–44 | 0 |
| 45–49 | 3 |
| 50–54 | 6 |
| 55–59 | 8 |
| 60–64 | 10 |
| 65–69 | 12 |
| 70–74 | 14 |
| 75–79 | 16 |

| Total Cholesterol | Points | | | | |
|-------------------|--------------|--------------|--------------|--------------|--------------|
| | Age 20–39 | Age 40–49 | Age 50–59 | Age 60–69 | Age 70–79 |
| <160 | 0 | 0 | 0 | 0 | 0 |
| 160–199 | 4 | 3 | 2 | 1 | 1 |
| 200–239 | 8 | 6 | 4 | 2 | 1 |
| 240–279 | 11 | 8 | 5 | 3 | 2 |
| ≥280 | 13 | 10 | 7 | 4 | 2 |

| | Points | | | | |
|-----------|--------------|--------------|--------------|--------------|--------------|
| | Age 20–39 | Age 40–49 | Age 50–59 | Age 60–69 | Age 70–79 |
| Nonsmoker | 0 | 0 | 0 | 0 | 0 |
| Smoker | 9 | 7 | 4 | 2 | 1 |

| HDL (mg/dl) | Points |
|---|---|
| ≥60 | −1 |
| 50–59 | 0 |
| 40–49 | 1 |
| <40 | 2 |

| HDL (mg/dl) | Points |
|---|---|
| ≥60 | −1 |
| 50–59 | 0 |
| 40–49 | 1 |
| <40 | 2 |

| Systolic BP (mmHg) | If Untreated | If Treated |
|---|---|---|
| <120 | 0 | 0 |
| 120–129 | 0 | 1 |
| 130–139 | 1 | 2 |
| 140–159 | 1 | 2 |
| ≥160 | 2 | 5 |

| Systolic BP (mmHg) | If Untreated | If Treated |
|---|---|---|
| <120 | 0 | 0 |
| 120–129 | 1 | 3 |
| 130–139 | 2 | 4 |
| 140–159 | 3 | 5 |
| ≥160 | 4 | 6 |

| Point Total | 10-Year Risk (%) |
|---|---|
| <0 | <1 |
| 0 | 1 |
| 1 | 1 |
| 2 | 1 |
| 3 | 1 |
| 4 | 1 |
| 5 | 2 |
| 6 | 2 |
| 7 | 3 |
| 8 | 4 |
| 9 | 5 |
| 10 | 6 |
| 11 | 8 |
| 12 | 10 |
| 13 | 12 |
| 14 | 16 |
| 15 | 20 |
| 16 | 25 |
| ≥17 | ≥30 |

10-year risk _____%

| Point Total | 10-Year Risk (%) |
|---|---|
| <9 | <1 |
| 9 | 1 |
| 10 | 1 |
| 11 | 1 |
| 12 | 1 |
| 13 | 2 |
| 14 | 2 |
| 15 | 3 |
| 16 | 4 |
| 17 | 5 |
| 18 | 6 |
| 19 | 8 |
| 20 | 11 |
| 21 | 14 |
| 22 | 17 |
| 23 | 22 |
| 24 | 27 |
| ≥25 | ≥30 |

10-year risk _____%

* The Framingham Heart Study is a long-term ongoing medical study conducted by the National Heart, Lung, and Blood Institute.

### CHANGING HEALTH HABITS

# Reducing Your Risk of Cardiovascular Disease

In completing the "Applying What You Have Learned" questions for this chapter in the textbook, you analyzed your lifestyle to determine which modifiable risk factors are raising your probability of developing cardiovascular disease. Then you described how you could modify your behavior to lower your risk of developing cardiovascular disease. Pick one of these behaviors and take the following steps to facilitate change.

## Deciding to Change

1. Identify the problem, goal, or question.
2. List the reasons you should make this change and the reasons you should not.

## Choices

Reasons to change behaviors (pros):

| Points | Reasons |
|---|---|
| ____ | _____ |
| ____ | _____ |
| ____ | _____ |
| ____ | Total |

Reasons not to change behaviors (cons):

| Points | Reasons |
|---|---|
| ____ | _____ |
| ____ | _____ |
| ____ | _____ |
| ____ | Total |

3. Draw a conclusion by adding the points in the pros section and then in the cons section. If the point total of the pros section is greater than the total of the cons section, you are probably ready to make a change in your life that reduces your risk of cardiovascular disease. If your cons outweigh your pros, you may not be motivated to make the change now. Study your list of pros and cons carefully, however, before making your final decision. You may decide to change even if your reasons not to change outrank your reasons to change.

## Implementing the Change

1. Set a target date to begin the new behavior or reach the goal.
2. Identify and list the factors that will help you reach your goal and those that will stand in the way of reaching your goal.

   *Factors that help:* _____

   *Factors that hinder:* _____

3. Prepare an action plan for making the change.

   a. Identify alternative methods to reach your goal.

   *Alternative 1:* _____

   *Alternative 2:* _____

   *Alternative 3:* _____

   *Alternative 4:* _____

   b. Gather information about each method.

   c. Choose the method that fits your situation best.

   d. Consider the factors that can help or hinder your effort to change (see step 2).

4. Change the lifestyle behavior that you have decided to improve by implementing the action plan you developed in step 3.
5. Chart your daily progress toward your goal.
6. Evaluate how effective you were in reaching your goal.

### CHANGING HEALTH HABITS

# Modifying Behavior to Reduce Cancer Risk

**I**n completing the "Applying What You Have Learned" questions for this chapter in the textbook, you analyzed your lifestyle to determine which modifiable risk factors are raising your probability of developing cancer. Then you described how you could modify your behavior to lower your risk of developing cancer. Pick one of these behavior changes and follow the following steps to facilitate change.

## Deciding to Change

1. Identify the problem, goal, or question.
2. List the reasons you should make this change and the reasons you should not.

## Choices

Reasons to change behaviors (pros):

| *Points* | *Reasons* |
|---|---|
| ____ | _____ |
| ____ | _____ |
| ____ | _____ |
| ____ | Total |

Reasons not to change behaviors (cons):

| *Points* | *Reasons* |
|---|---|
| ____ | _____ |
| ____ | _____ |
| ____ | _____ |
| ____ | Total |

3. Draw a conclusion by adding the points in the pros section and then in the cons section. If the point total of the pros section is greater than the total of the cons section, you are probably ready to make a change that reduces your risk of cancer. If your cons outweigh your pros, you may not be motivated to make the change now. Study your list of pros and cons carefully, however, before making your final decision. You may decide to change even if your reasons not to change outrank your reasons to change.

## Implementing the Change

1. Set a target date to begin the new behavior or reach the goal.
2. Identify and list the factors that will help you reach your goal and those that will stand in the way of reaching your goal.

   *Factors that help:* _____

   *Factors that hinder:* _____

3. Prepare an action plan for making the change.
   a. Identify alternative methods for reaching your goal.

      *Alternative 1:* _____

      *Alternative 2:* _____

      *Alternative 3:* _____

      *Alternative 4:* _____

   b. Gather information about each method.
   c. Choose the method that fits your particular situation best.
   d. Consider the factors that can help or hinder your effort to change (see step 2).
4. Change the lifestyle behavior that you have decided to improve by implementing the action plan you developed in step 3.
5. Chart your daily progress toward your goal.
6. Evaluate how effective you were in reaching your goal.

## CHAPTER 14

**SELF-ASSESSMENT**

# STI Attitude Scale

## Directions

Please read each statement carefully: STIs are sexually transmitted infections, once called venereal diseases. Record your first reaction by circling the letter that best describes how much you agree or disagree with the idea.

**Use this key:**

SA = Strongly agree; A = Agree; U = Undecided;

D = Disagree; SD = Strongly disagree.

*Remember:* STIs means sexually transmitted infections, such as gonorrhea, syphilis, genital herpes, chlamydia, HPV, and AIDS.

1. How one uses his or her sexuality has nothing to do with STIs.

   SA        A        U        D        SD

2. It is easy to use the prevention methods that reduce one's chances of getting an STI.

   SA        A        U        D        SD

3. Responsible sex is one of the best ways of reducing the risk of STIs.

   SA        A        U        D        SD

4. Getting early medical care is the main key to preventing harmful effects of STIs.

   SA        A        U        D        SD

5. Choosing the right sex partner is important in reducing the risk of getting an STI.

   SA        A        U        D        SD

6. A high rate of STIs should be a concern for all people.

   SA        A        U        D        SD

7. People with an STI have a duty to get their sex partners to seek medical care.

   SA        A        U        D        SD

8. The best way to get a sex partner to STI treatment is to take him or her to the doctor with you.

   SA        A        U        D        SD

9. Changing one's sex habits is necessary once the presence of an STI is known.

    SA　　A　　U　　D　　SD

10. I would dislike having to follow the medical steps for treating an STI.

    SA　　A　　U　　D　　SD

11. If I were sexually active, I would feel uneasy doing things before and after sex to prevent getting an STI.

    SA　　A　　U　　D　　SD

12. If I were sexually active, it would be insulting if a sex partner suggested we use a condom to avoid STIs.

    SA　　A　　U　　D　　SD

13. I dislike talking about STIs with my peers.

    SA　　A　　U　　D　　SD

14. I would be uncertain about going to the doctor unless I was sure I really had an STI.

    SA　　A　　U　　D　　SD

15. I would feel that I should take my sex partner with me to a clinic if I thought I had an STI.

    SA　　A　　U　　D　　SD

16. It would be embarrassing to discuss STIs with one's partner if one were sexually active.

    SA　　A　　U　　D　　SD

17. If I were to have sex, the chance of getting an STI makes me uneasy about having sex with more than one person.

    SA　　A　　U　　D　　SD

18. I like the idea of sexual abstinence (not having sex) as the best way of avoiding STIs.

    SA　　A　　U　　D　　SD

19. If I had an STI, I would cooperate with public health persons to find the sources of the STI.

    SA　　A　　U　　D　　SD

20. If I had an STI, I would avoid exposing others while I was being treated.

    SA　　A　　U　　D　　SD

21. I would have regular STI checkups if I were having sex with more than one partner.

    SA　　A　　U　　D　　SD

22. I intend to look for STI signs before deciding to have sex with anyone.

    SA　　A　　U　　D　　SD

23. I will limit my sexual activity to just one partner because of the chances I might get an STI.

    SA　　A　　U　　D　　SD

24. I will avoid sexual contact anytime I think there is even a slight chance of getting an STI.

    SA　　A　　U　　D　　SD

25. The chance of getting an STI would not stop me from having sex.

    SA　　A　　U　　D　　SD

26. If I had a chance, I would support community efforts toward controlling STIs.

    SA　　A　　U　　D　　SD

27. I would be willing to work with others to make people aware of STI problems in my town.

    SA　　A　　U　　D　　SD

**Scoring**   Calculate total points for each subscale and total scale, using the point values below.
For items 1, 10–14, 16, 25: Strongly agree = 5 points; Agree = 4 points; Undecided = 3 points; Disagree = 2 points; and Strongly disagree = 1 point.
For items 2–9, 15, 17–24, 26, 27: Strongly agree = 1 point; Agree = 2 points; Undecided = 3 points; Disagree = 4 points; and Strongly disagree = 5 points.

Total scale: items 1–27

Belief subscale: items 1–9

Feeling subscale: items 10–18

Intention to act subscale: items 19–27

## Interpretation

High score predisposes one toward high-risk STI behavior. Low score predisposes one toward low-risk STI behavior.

Yarber, Torabi, and Veenker (1989) developed the STI Attitudes Scale by administering three experimental forms of 45 items each. Respondents were 2,980 students in six secondary school districts in the Midwest and East. Based on statistical analysis, the scale was reduced to the final 27 items. Reliability coefficients for the entire scale and the three subscales ranged from 0.48 to 0.73. The developers reported evidence of construct validity in that the scale was sensitive to positive attitude changes resulting from STI education.

From "Development of a three-component STD attitude scale" from *Journal of Sex Education and Therapy* by W.L. Yarber, 15:36–39. Copyright © 1989 by American Association of Sex Educators Couns. & Ther. in the format Textbook via Copyright Clearance Center. Reprinted with permission of American Association of Sex Educators Couns. & Ther.

# Reducing Your Risk of Contracting an STI

I n completing the "Applying What You Have Learned" questions for this chapter in the textbook, you analyzed your risk for contracting STIs. Then you determined what you could do to lower your risk of contracting a sexually transmitted infection. Pick one of these behavior changes and take the following steps to facilitate change.

## Deciding to Change

1. Identify the problem, goal, or question.
2. List the reasons you should make this change and the reasons you should not.

## Choices

Reasons to change behaviors (pros):

| *Points* | *Reasons* |
|---|---|
| ____ | _____ |
| ____ | _____ |
| ____ | _____ |
| ____ Total | |

Reasons not to change behaviors (cons):

| *Points* | *Reasons* |
|---|---|
| ____ | _____ |
| ____ | _____ |
| ____ | _____ |
| ____ Total | |

3. Draw a conclusion by adding the points in the pros section and then in the cons section. If the point total of the pros section is greater than the total of the cons section, you are probably ready to make a change that reduces your risk of contracting an STI. If your cons outweigh your pros, you may not be motivated to make the change now. Study your list of pros and cons carefully, however, before making your final decision. You may decide to change even if your reasons not to change outrank your reasons to change.

## Implementing the Change

1. Set a target date to begin the new behavior or reach the goal.
2. Identify and list the factors that will help you reach your goal and those that will stand in the way of reaching your goal.

   *Factors that help:* _____

   *Factors that hinder:* _____

3. Prepare an action plan for making the change.

   a. Identify alternative methods to reach your goal.

      *Alternative 1:* _____

      *Alternative 2:* _____

      *Alternative 3:* _____

      *Alternative 4:* _____

   b. Gather information about each method.

   c. Choose the method that fits your particular situation best.

   d. Consider the factors that can help or hinder your effort to change (see step 2).

4. Change the lifestyle behavior that you have decided to improve by implementing the action plan you developed in step 3.
5. Chart your daily progress toward your goal.
6. Evaluate how effective you were in reaching your goal.

# Preparing for Aging and Death

**A**nswer the following questions. Depending on your situation, some of the questions may not apply.

| | | | |
|---|---|---|---|
| 1. | Are you doing anything to increase your chances of living a long and healthy life? | ___ Yes | ___ No |
| | If you answered yes, discuss the steps you are taking to live a long and healthy life. | | |
| 2. | How do you want to spend your retirement years? Are you doing anything to prepare for retirement? | ___ Yes | ___ No |
| | If you answered yes, what actions are you taking to prepare for retirement? | | |
| 3. | How do you feel about elderly people? Do you think they are "over the hill" and should be "put out to pasture?" | ___ Yes | ___ No |
| | Why do you feel this way about older adults? | | |
| 4. | Do you worry about growing old? | ___ Yes | ___ No |
| | If you do, what worries you about aging? | | |
| 5. | Have you prepared a will and a living will or durable power of attorney? | ___ Yes | ___ No |
| | If yes, have you informed your family about these documents? | ___ Yes | ___ No |
| | Have you selected a guardian for your children? | ___ Yes | ___ No |
| | Have you discussed guardianship with this individual? | ___ Yes | ___ No |
| 6. | Have you thought about your funeral? | ___ Yes | ___ No |
| | If you have thought about your funeral, what kind of funeral would you want? | | |
| | Do you want to be buried or cremated? | | |
| | Have you discussed your wishes with your family? | ___ Yes | ___ No |
| | Have you made funeral prearrangements? | ___ Yes | ___ No |
| 7. | Have you considered donating your body or your tissues or organs after your death? | ___ Yes | ___ No |
| | If you want to donate your body, tissues, or organs, have you made any preparations and informed relatives? Do you carry a card in your wallet that identifies you as a donor? | ___ Yes | ___ No |
| 8. | If you were told that you have a terminal disease and have only 6 months to live, how would you spend these last months of your life? | | |
| 9. | Have you written your obituary? | ___ Yes | ___ No |
| | What would you like people to remember most about you? | | |

Examine your responses to these questions; there are no correct answers.

## CHANGING HEALTH HABITS

# Can Changing a Health Habit Extend Your Life?

D o you have a habit, such as cigarette smoking, that increases your chances of dying prematurely? Which habit? The "Deciding to Change" section of the Changing Health Habits worksheet can help you determine whether you are ready to change this habit. If you decide to change, use the "Implementing the Change" section of the worksheet to help you make the necessary lifestyle changes.

## Deciding to Change

1. Identify the problem, goal, or question.
2. List the reasons you should make this change and the reasons you should not.

## Choices

Reasons to change behaviors (pros):

| *Points* | *Reasons* |
|---|---|
| ____ | _____ |
| ____ | _____ |
| ____ | _____ |
| ____ Total | |

Reasons not to change behaviors (cons):

| *Points* | *Reasons* |
|---|---|
| ____ | _____ |
| ____ | _____ |
| ____ | _____ |
| ____ Total | |

3. Draw a conclusion by adding the points in the pros section and then in the cons section. If the point total of the pros section is greater than the total of the cons section, you are probably ready to make the lifestyle changes necessary to change the unhealthy habit. If your cons outweigh your pros, you may not be motivated to make the change now. Study your list of pros and cons carefully, however, before making your final decision. You may decide to change even if your reasons not to change outrank your reasons to change.

## Implementing the Change

1. Set a target date to begin the new behavior or reach the goal.

2. Identify and list the factors that will help you reach your goal and those that will stand in the way of reaching your goal.

   *Factors that help:* _____

   *Factors that hinder:* _____

3. Prepare an action plan for making the change.

   a. Identify alternative methods to reach your goal.

   *Alternative 1:* _____

   *Alternative 2:* _____

   *Alternative 3:* _____

   *Alternative 4:* _____

   b. Gather information about each method.

   c. Choose the method that fits your particular situation best.

   d. Consider the factors that can help or hinder your effort to change (see step 2).

4. Change the lifestyle behavior that you have decided to improve by implementing the action plan you developed in step 3.

5. Chart your daily progress toward your goal.

6. Evaluate how effective you were in reaching your goal.

**SELF-ASSESSMENT 1**

# Poison Lookout Checklist

The home areas listed below are the most common sites of accidental poisonings. Follow this checklist to learn how to correct situations that may lead to poisonings. If you answer no to any questions, fix the situation quickly. Your goal is to have all your answers be yes.

## The Kitchen

|   |   | Yes | No |
|---|---|---|---|
| 1. | Do all harmful products in the cabinets have child-resistant caps? Products like furniture polishes, drain cleaners, and some oven cleaners should have safety packaging to keep little children from accidentally opening the packages. | ____ | ____ |
| 2. | Are all potentially harmful products in their original containers? There are two dangers if products aren't stored in their original containers. Labels on the original containers often give first aid information if someone should swallow the product. And if products are stored in containers like drinking glasses or soda bottles, someone may think it is food and swallow it. | ____ | ____ |
| 3. | Are harmful products stored away from food? If harmful products are placed next to food, someone may accidentally get a food and a poison mixed up and swallow the poison. | ____ | ____ |
| 4. | Have all potentially harmful products been put up high and out of reach of children? The best way to prevent poisoning is making sure that it's impossible to find and get at the poisons. Locking all cabinets that hold dangerous products is the best poison prevention. | ____ | ____ |

## The Bathroom

|   |   | Yes | No |
|---|---|---|---|
| 1. | Did you ever stop to think that medicines could poison if used improperly? Many children are poisoned each year by overdoses of aspirin. If aspirin can poison, just think of how many other poisons might be in your medicine cabinet. | ____ | ____ |
| 2. | Do your aspirins and other potentially harmful products have child-resistant closures? Aspirins and most prescription drugs come with child-resistant caps. Check to see that yours have them, and that they are properly secured. Check your prescriptions before leaving the pharmacy to make sure the medicines are in child-resistant packaging. These caps have been shown to save the lives of children. | ____ | ____ |

| | Yes | No |
|---|---|---|
| 3. Have you thrown out all out-of-date prescriptions? As medicines get older, the chemicals inside them can change. So what was once a good medicine may now be a dangerous poison. Flush all old drugs down the toilet. Rinse the container well, then discard it. | _____ | _____ |
| 4. Are all medicines in their original containers with the original labels? Prescription medicines may or may not list ingredients. The prescription number on the label will, however, allow rapid identification by the pharmacist of the ingredients should they not be listed. Without the original label and container, you can't be sure of what you're taking. After all, aspirin looks a lot like poisonous roach tablets. | _____ | _____ |
| 5. If your vitamins or vitamin/mineral supplements contain iron, are they in child-resistant packaging? Most people think of vitamins and minerals as foods and, therefore, nontoxic, but a few iron pills can kill a child. | _____ | _____ |

## The Garage or Storage Area

Did you know that many things in your garage or storage area that can be swallowed are terrible poisons? Death may occur when people swallow such everyday substances as charcoal lighter, paint thinner and remover, antifreeze, and turpentine.

| | Yes | No |
|---|---|---|
| 1. Do all these poisons have child-resistant caps? | _____ | _____ |
| 2. Are they stored in the original containers? | _____ | _____ |
| 3. Are the original labels on the containers? | _____ | _____ |
| 4. Have you made sure that no poisons are stored in drinking glasses or soda bottles? | _____ | _____ |
| 5. Are all these harmful products locked up and out of sight and reach? | _____ | _____ |

When all your answers are yes, then continue this level of poison protection by making sure that whenever you buy potentially harmful products, they have child-resistant closures and are kept out of sight and reach. Post the number of the Poison Control Center near your telephone.

*Source:* Consumer Product Safety Commission. CPSC Document 4383.

CHAPTER **16**

# Checklist for the Prevention of Carbon Monoxide Poisoning

**C**arbon monoxide is often referred to as CO, which is its chemical symbol. Unlike many gases, CO is odorless, colorless, tasteless, and nonirritating. Red blood cells absorb CO over 200 times more readily than oxygen. As levels of CO in the air rise, this gas replaces oxygen in the bloodstream. As a result, body tissues are damaged and may die of a lack of oxygen. Knowing the major causes of carbon monoxide poisoning and using measures to eliminate them will prevent many needless tragedies.

The following questions relating to various areas in your environment will help you in dealing properly with the unseen, deadly hazard of carbon monoxide. The questions have been divided into sections that may directly apply to your particular situation. You can compare your answers with the correct explanation provided at the end of the list of questions.

## Questions

Draw a circle around your answer.

## The Home, Cabin, and Camper

Most questions will apply equally to homeowners, campers, and to those who rent. Renters, however, should refer any questions regarding maintenance to the management.

| | | | |
|---|---|---|---|
| 1. | Have you had the fireplace draft and the drafts of other fuel-burning appliances checked by an expert within the past year? | Yes | No |
| 2. | Have all gas appliances been checked annually for proper operation? | Yes | No |
| 3. | Are all combustion appliances properly vented? | Yes | No |
| 4. | Has your chimney vent been checked for defects within the past year? | Yes | No |
| 5. | Have you patched any vent pipe with tape, gum, or other substances? | Yes | No |
| 6. | Are all horizontal vent pipes to fuel appliances perfectly level? | Yes | No |
| 7. | Do you use your gas range or oven for heating? | Yes | No |
| 8. | Does the cooling unit of your gas refrigerator give off an odor? | Yes | No |
| 9. | Have you ever used a charcoal grill such as a barbecue grill for cooking within your home, cabin, or camper other than in a vented fireplace? | Yes | No |
| 10. | Have you ever brought burning charcoal into your home, cabin, or camper for heating purposes? | Yes | No |

| | | | |
|---|---|---|---|
| 11. | Do you consider portable flameless chemical heaters (catalytic) safe for use in your cabin, camper, or home? | Yes | No |
| 12. | Have you ever used a portable gas camp stove in your home, cabin, or camper for heating purposes? | Yes | No |

## The Auto

| | | | |
|---|---|---|---|
| 13. | Have you had a reliable mechanic check the exhaust system of your car within the past year? | Yes | No |
| 14. | Do you ever run your auto engine in the garage while the garage door is shut? | Yes | No |
| 15. | Do you leave the door closed between your attached garage and your house when you run your car engine? | Yes | No |
| 16. | Do you keep your windows slightly open while driving in heavy traffic, although you have an air conditioner? | Yes | No |
| 17. | While driving your station wagon, do you lower the tailgate to get a greater flow of air in the car? | Yes | No |

## Other

| | | | |
|---|---|---|---|
| 18. | When you are selecting gas equipment, do you buy only those items that carry the seal of a national testing agency, such as the American Gas Association or the Underwriters' Laboratory? | Yes | No |
| 19. | Have you ever converted, or are you about to convert, a fuel burner from one fuel to another without having it done by an expert? | Yes | No |
| 20. | As an overnight guest at motels or hotels that have heating units located in the room, do you read operating instructions or ask how such appliances operate? | Yes | No |

## *Correct Answers*

### The Home, Cabin, and Camper

1. *Yes.* A yearly checkup of all fuel-burning venting systems in the home is desirable.

2. *Yes.* A yearly checkup of all combustion appliances is suggested. In many areas, upon request, the gas company will provide this service.

3. *Yes.* All gas appliances must have adequate ventilation so that CO will not accumulate.

4. *Yes.* Chimney vents often become blocked by debris, causing a buildup of CO. They should be checked annually.

5. *No.* Often a makeshift patch can lead to an accumulation of CO, and therefore should be avoided.

6. *No.* In-room vent pipes should be on a slight incline as they go toward the exterior. This will reduce leaking of toxic gases in case the joints or pipes are improperly fitted.

7. *No.* Using a gas range for heating can result in the accumulation of CO.

8. *No.* An unusual odor from a gas refrigerator often is the result of defects within the cooling unit. Odorless CO also may be given off.

9. *No.* The use of barbecue grills indoors will quickly result in dangerous levels of CO.

10. *No.* Burning charcoal—whether black, red, gray, or white—gives off CO.

11. *No.* Although catalytic heaters produce heat without flame, combustion is occurring that can cause the production of CO.

12. *No.* Using a gas camp stove for heating the home, cabin, or camper can result in the accumulation of CO.

## The Auto

13. *Yes.* Small leaks in the exhaust system of a car can lead to an accumulation of CO in the interior.

14. *No.* CO can rapidly build up while your auto engine is operated in a closed garage. Never run your car in a garage unless the outside door is open to provide ventilation.

15. *Yes.* CO can easily escape from a garage through a connecting door that opens into the house, although the garage door is open. Doors connecting a garage and house should be kept closed when the auto is running.

16. *Yes.* Even with an air conditioner, CO can be drawn into a car while it is being driven slowly in heavy traffic. Therefore, windows should be slightly opened.

17. *No.* If the tailgate is open, be sure to open vents or windows to increase the flow of air in the car. If the tailgate window is open and the other windows or the vents are closed, CO from the exhaust will be drawn into the car.

## Other

18. *Yes.* Buy only equipment carrying the seal of a national testing agency; otherwise, one may get poorly designed equipment, which may soon result in the production of CO.

19. *No.* An expert is needed to make proper modifications and to evaluate the venting capabilities of your appliance.

20. *Yes.* Even with adequately designed and properly installed heating equipment, the improper operation of this equipment can result in its malfunctioning and lead to the production of CO. Therefore, be sure you understand the correct way to operate any fuel-burning appliance before using it.

*Source:* Centers for Disease Control and Prevention. HEW Pub. No.(CDC) 77 8335.

**CHANGING HEALTH HABITS**

# Can You Reduce Environmental Threats to Your Health?

In completing the "Applying What You Have Learned" questions for this chapter, you analyzed your interactions with the environment to develop a list of environmental threats to your health. Determine ways in which you could change your behavior to remove or reduce these environmental threats. Pick one of these behaviors and use the following steps to facilitate change.

## Deciding to Change

1. Identify the problem, goal, or question.
2. List the reasons you should make this change and the reasons you should not.

## Choices

Reasons to change behaviors (pros):

| *Points* | *Reasons* |
| --- | --- |
| ____ | _____ |
| ____ | _____ |
| ____ | _____ |
| ____ | Total |

Reasons not to change behaviors (cons):

| *Points* | *Reasons* |
| --- | --- |
| ____ | _____ |
| ____ | _____ |
| ____ | _____ |
| ____ | Total |

3. Draw a conclusion by adding the points in the pros section and then in the cons section. If the point total of the pros section is greater than the total of the cons section, you are probably ready to make a change in your life that reduces environmental risks to your health. If your cons outweigh your pros, you may not be motivated to make the change now. Study your list of pros and cons carefully, however, before making your final decision. You may decide to change even if your reasons not to change outrank your reasons to change.

## Implementing the Change

1. Set a target date to begin the new behavior.
2. Identify and list the factors that will help you change this behavior and those that will stand in your way.

    *Factors that help:* _____

    *Factors that hinder:* _____

3. Prepare an action plan for making the change.

    a. Identify alternative methods for reaching your goal.

       *Alternative 1:* _____

       *Alternative 2:* _____

       *Alternative 3:* _____

       *Alternative 4:* _____

    b. Gather information about each method.

    c. Choose the method that fits your particular situation best.

    d. Consider the factors that can help or hinder your effort to change (see step 2).

4. Change the lifestyle behavior that you have decided to improve by implementing the action plan you developed in step 3.

5. Chart your daily progress toward your goal.

6. Evaluate how effective you were in reaching your goal.

Student Workbook

# Index

strokes and, 388
suicide and, 56, 62
venous disease and, 379
violence and, 102, 109, 113
General adaptation syndrome (GAS), 74–76
Generalized anxiety disorder, 52
Generativity, 44
Genes, 11
Gene therapy, 482, 494
Genetics
*See also* Heredity
aging and, 505–506
counseling, 131–132, 494
diseases, 454–459, 494
health status and, 11–14
life expectancy and, 504
metabolic rate and, 315
obesity and, 322, 324–325
Genital herpes, 482–483
Genital warts, 483–486
Genomics, 11–14, 458
German measles, 130, 132, 461, 462
Gerontologists, 502
Gestational diabetes mellitus (GDM), 130, 138, 314
GHB (gamma hydroxybutyrate), 207, 211
Ginkgo biloba, 27, 28, 220, 511, 514
Ginseng, 27, 28, 170
Glaucoma, 508
Globesity, 313–314
Glucosamine sulfate, 301
Glucose, 277
Gluten, 288–289
Glycemic index (GI), 280
Gonorrhea, 487–489
Good health, 5
Good Samaritan laws, 564
Gout, 314
Green tea, 419
Grief (grieving), 525–527
Growth, psychological, 45
Guarana, 28

Hallucinations, 48, 49, 214
Hallucinogens, 214–215, 224
Hamer, Dean, 179
Hangovers, 243
Harmful use, 233
Hashish, 213
Hate crimes, 98
Hazardous waste, 549
Headaches, 81–82
Health
components of, 6–7
continuum, 6
defined, 5
good, 5
promotion, 9–10, 17–18
status of Americans, 2–3, 7–11
wellness and, 5–6
Health care practitioner-patient relationship, 30–31

healthfinder, 22
Health food, 274
Health information, analyzing
addiction, 223
Alzheimer's disease, 512–513
cell phones and cancer, 542–543
college drinking, strategies to reduce, 240
exercises, alternatives for outdated, 352–353
folic acid, 159
garlic, 305
herbal tea to reduce anger, 114
Internet, 22–23
model for, 19–22
mood and anxiety, 65
sample analysis of an ad, 24
sleeplessness, 85
tanning beds, 440–441
tips for, 19–23
trans fats, 400–403
websites, 190
weight-loss products, 331
Health insurance, 8
Health on the Net Foundation, 22
Health-related behavior
changing, 14–15
making positive decisions about, 15–17
*Healthy People 2000*, 9
*Healthy People 2010*, 10, 313
*Healthy People 2020*, 9–10, 109, 440–441
goals of, 556–558
Heart
attacks, 381, 384–387, 564
chambers of, 378
failure, 384
rates, target, 346–347
Heat
cramps, 363
emergency care, 565–566
exhaustion, 363–364
stroke, 363–364
Height tables, 313, 314
Helper T cells, 470–471
Hemochromatosis, 295
Hemoglobin, 254, 294
Hemorrhoids, 281, 282
Hepatitis, alcoholic, 241
Hepatitis B virus (HBV), 437, 476
Hepatitis C, 460
Herbs, use of, 26–28, 474–475
cancer and, 418–419
for depression, 56
to reduce anger, 114
sex and use of, 170
for stress, 82, 83
Herceptin, 436
Heredity
*See also* Genetics
alcoholism and, 234
breast cancer and, 432
cardiovascular disease and, 389
defined, 41

hypertension and, 392
mental illnesses and, 50
metabolic rate and, 315
obesity and, 322, 324–325
personality development and, 41
Heroin, 212
Herpes simplex virus, 482–483
Heterosexual, 177
Hierarchy of Human Needs, 44–45
High blood pressure. *See* Hypertension
High-density lipoproteins (HDL), 389–391
High-fructose corn syrup (HFCS), 278
Hispanics (Latinos)
depression in, 56
diabetes in, 280
health status of, 12
hypertension in, 392
prostate cancer in, 441
testicular cancer in, 442
Histamine, 468
HIV (human immunodeficiency virus), 460
people at risk for, 480
progression of, 477–479
protection against, 480–481
statistics, 476–477, 478
transmission of, 479–480
treatment of, 481–482
Hives, 287
Hochbaum, Godfrey, 5
Holistic, 5–6
Holmes, Thomas, 76–78
Home security measures, 109–110
Homeopathy, 26, 473
Homophobia, 179
Homosexuality, 177–179
Honey, 279, 463
Hormone replacement therapy (HRT), 157, 398, 432, 434
Hormones
cancer and, 432–436
defined, 73
reproductive/sex, 128, 157, 166–167
stress, 73–74
Hospice, 519–520
Host, 460, 461, 465–466
Huang ch'i, 419
Human chorionic gonadotropin (hCG), 134, 135
Human Genome Project, 458
Human immunodeficiency virus. *See* HIV
Human papilloma virus (HPV), 427, 437, 476, 483–484
Human T-cell leukemia virus (HTLV), 437
Humor, use of, 87
Hunger, 324, 553
Huntington's disease, 494
Hydrogenation, 284
Hydrostatic weighting, 319

Hypertension, 256, 380, 392–393, 396–397
Hyperthermia, 363
Hypertrophy, 349
Hyperventilation, 88
Hypnotics, 211
Hypoactive sexual desire disorder (HSDD), 172
Hypomania, 57
Hypnotic, 210, 211
Hypothalamus, 324
Hypothermia, 364–365

Identity, 44
Illegal drugs, defined, 201
Illicit drugs, defined, 202
Imagery, 89–90
Immune system
alcohol consumption and suppression of, 242
defined, 78, 467
effects of aging on, 507
role of, 466–471
stress and, 78
Immunity
acquired, 471–472
defined, 466, 467
nonspecific, 466–469
specific, 466, 467, 469–471
Immunizations, 472
Immunotherapy, 415, 421
Implanon, 151
Implantation bleeding, 134
Implants, contraceptive, 151
Impotence, 171
Impulse control disorders, 53–54
Inborn immunity, 471
Incest, 113, 115
Induced abortion, 154, 155
Induction, 155
Infants (infancy)
age for, 31
AIDS, 480
birth defects, 130, 131, 133, 263, 303–304, 399, 493–494
cardiovascular health, 399
chlamydial infections, 489
drug abuse and, 130, 133, 206, 222
genetic disorders, 494
gonorrhea and, 488
health concerns, 31
herpes virus and, 483
honey, given to, 279, 463
infectious diseases, 494–495
life expectancy of, 3
maternal alcohol consumption and affects on, 263–264
maternal smoking and affects on, 264
metabolic rate and, 316
nutritional needs, 304
obesity and, 313
psychological health, 39–40
psychosocial stages of personality development, 44
weight management, 335

# Photo Credits

## Special Features
Diversity in Health © Mike Flippo/ShutterStock, Inc.; Managing Your Health © Kzenon/ShutterStock, Inc.; Consumer Health © sevenke/ShutterStock, Inc.; Healthy Living Practices © djgis /ShutterStock, Inc.; Across the Life Span © Galina Barskaya /ShutterStock, Inc.

## Chapter 1
Opener © aricvyhmeister/ShutterStock, Inc.; 1.1 © Marek Slusarczyk/ShutterStock, Inc.; 1.3 © Hung Chung Chih /ShutterStock, Inc.; page 9 Courtesy of Judy Schmidt/CDC; 1.5 © digitalskillet/ShutterStock, Inc.; page 11 © Hemera /Thinkstock; page 13 © allen russell/Alamy Images; page 16 © AbleStock; page 17 © iofoto/ShutterStock, Inc.; page 22 © Courtesy of Health On the Net Foundation www. HealthOnNet.org; 1.8 © Stuart Pearce/Pixtal/age fotostock; page 27 © iStockphoto/Thinkstock; page 29 © Zina Seletskaya /ShutterStock, Inc.; 1.9 © iStockphoto/Thinkstock

## Chapter 2
Opener © Blaine Harrington III/Alamy Images; page 42 © Jim Wark/Lonely Planet Images/Alamy Images; page 44 © ClickPop /ShutterStock, Inc.; page 47 © Ilike/ShutterStock, Inc.; page 48 © auremar/ShutterStock, Inc.; 2.3 © dundanim/ShutterStock, Inc.; 2.4 © Dustie/ShutterStock, Inc.; page 54 © neal and molly jansen/Alamy Images; page 55 © Bubbles Photolibrary /Alamy Images; page 58 © Bubbles Photolibrary/Alamy Images; 2.6 © Mercier Serge/Maxppp/Landov; page 61 © Anetta /ShutterStock, Inc.; 2.7 © Photodisc; page 64 © Noam Armonn /ShutterStock, Inc.; page 65 © Jack Hollingsworth/Photodisc

## Chapter 3
Opener © PhotoCreate/Shutterstock, Inc.; page 72 © Digital Vision/Thinkstock; page 75 © Serget Skleznev/ShutterStock, Inc.; page 79 © iStockphoto/Thinkstock; page 80 © Martin Novak/Dreamstime.com; 3.3 © CLIFF LIPSON/CBS/Landov; page 82 © Paul Maguire/ShutterStock, Inc.; page 85 © l i g h t p o e t/ShutterStock, Inc.; page 86 © Thomas Barwick /Getty Images; 3.4 © Photos.com; page 90 © Aspen Photo /ShutterStock, Inc.; 3.6, 3.7 © Photodisc

## Chapter 4
Opener © Monalyn Gracia/age fotostock; 4.1 © Jonathan Nourok/PhotoEdit, Inc.; page 99 © Digital Media Pro /ShutterStock, Inc.; page 100 © Jupiterimages/Comstock /Thinkstock; 4.2 © Tatiana Belova/ShutterStock, Inc.; page 106 © Galina Barskaya/ShutterStock, Inc.; 4.3 © Kevin Lamarque /Reuters/Landov; 4.4 © kentannenbaum/Fotolia.com; page 108 © GARY C. CASKEY/UPI/Landov; 4.5 © Hemera Technologies

/AbleStock.com/Thinkstock; page 113 © Margot Petrowski /ShutterStock, Inc.; page 114 © Janis Christie/Photodisc

## Chapter 5
Opener © Phototake/Alamy Images; 5.4 © Professor P.M. Motta, G. Macciarelli, S.A Nottola/SPL/Photo Researchers, Inc.; 5.A © Chris Ryan/OJO Images/Getty Images; 5.8 © Ralph Hutchings /Visuals Unlimited; 5.9 © Custom Medical Stock Photo; 5.10 © Neil Bromhall/Science Photo Library/Photo Researchers, Inc.; 5.11 © Petite Format/Nestle/Science Source/Photo Researchers, Inc.; 5.14A © Custom Medical Stock Photo; 5.17D, F, G Courtesy of the Cervical Barrier Advancement Society and Ibis Reproductive Health; page 159 Courtesy of CDC

## Chapter 6
Opener © dpaint/ShutterStock, Inc.; 6.4 © Dewayne Flowers /ShutterStock, Inc.; 6.A © Blue Jean Images/Digital Vision /Thinkstock; 6.B © Lizette Potgieter/ShutterStock, Inc.; 6.C © Per-Anders Pettersson/Getty Images; 6.6A © Susan Sterner/AP Photos; 6.6B © Helga Esteb/ShutterStock, Inc.; page 181 © Mike Wintroath/AP Photos; 6.10 © Bassittart/ShutterStock, Inc.; 6.13 © Pixland/Thinkstock; page 191 Courtesy of Google, Inc.

## Chapter 7
Opener © CREATISTA/ShutterStock, Inc.; 7.1 © Evan Agostini /AP Photos; 7.2 © Rick Wilking/Reuters/Landov; 7.4 © Chicago /PA Photos/Landov; 7.A © Peter Smolka/dpa/Landov; 7.5 Courtesy of Paul Thompson, Kiralee Hayashi, Arthur Toga, Edythe London/UCLA; 7.6 © Images from the Faces of Meth V 1, 2005 CD©, Multnomah County Sheriff's Office; 7.7 © Medical-on-Line/Alamy Images; 7.8 © Nigel Cattlin/Holt Studios International/Photo Researchers, Inc.; 7.10 © Bob Cheung/ShutterStock, Inc.; page 216 (amyl nitrate) © Martyn Vickery/Alamy Images; 7.11 Courtesy of DEA; 7.12 © Krzysztof Slusarczyk/Shutterstock, Inc.

## Chapter 8
Opener Courtesy of U.S. Food and Drug Administration; 8.1 © MCT/Landov; page 240 © Corbis; 8.2A © SIU /Visuals Unlimited; 8.2B © PhotoEdit, Inc.; 8.A © PhotoEdit /Alamy Images; 8.10A, B © Matt Meadows/Getty Images; 8.11 © Ellis Neel, Alamogordo Daily News/AP Photos; 8.12 Courtesy of J.S. Greenspan, B.D.S., University of California, San Francisco; Sol Silverman, Jr., D.D.S./CDC; 8.14 © iStockphoto/Thinkstock; 8.16 © Richard Pipes/Albuquerque Journal/AP Photos

## Chapter 9
Opener © Photodisc/Thinkstock; 9.2 © ÊDenis Pepin /ShutterStock, Inc.; page 275 © Jupiterimages/Polka Dot

/Thinkstock; page 277 © Valentyn Volkov/ShutterStock, Inc.; page 279 © Thomas Northcut/Digital Vision/Thinkstock; page 280 © Steve Cukrov/ShutterStock, Inc.; page 281 © iStockphoto/Thinkstock; page 284 © Hemera/Thinkstock; page 285 © tkemot/Shutterstock Inc.; page 286 © Dan Peretz/Shutterstock Inc.; 9.6 © Photodisc; page 287 © Noam Armonn/Shutterstock Inc.; 9.8 © Andy Lidstone/ShutterStock, Inc.; page 291 © Stephen Bonk/ShutterStock, Inc.; 9.9 © Bill Aron/PhotoEdit, Inc.; 9.10 © Mitch Hrdlicka/Photodisc; page 297 © Picsfive/Shutterstock Inc.; page 298 © AbleStock; 9.11 Courtesy of the USDA; page 304 © iStockphoto/Thinkstock; page 305 (scientist and garlic) © Photodisc; 9.13 © De Visu/Shutterstock Inc.

## Chapter 10

Opener Courtesy of CDC; page 312 © Dr. Dennis Kunkel/Visuals Unlimited; page 315 © Brian Chase/ShutterStock, Inc.; 10.5 © David Young-Wolff/PhotoEdit, Inc.; 10.6 © Photodisc; 10.7 Courtesy of COSMED USA, Inc.; page 323 (photo of woman) Courtesy of Library of Congress, Prints & Photographs Division, Curtis (Edward S.) Collection [Reproduction Number LC-USZ62-112212]; page 324 © Sander Crombeen/ShutterStock, Inc.; page 325 © karamysh/ShutterStock, Inc.; page 326 Courtesy of Bill Branson/National Cancer Institute; page 328 © Konstantin Sutyagin/ShutterStock, Inc.; 10.13 © Girish Menon/ShutterStock, Inc.; 10.14 © Goga/ShutterStock, Inc.

## Chapter 11

Opener © Vereshchagin Dmitry/ShutterStock, Inc.; page 344 © Wendy Hope/Stockbyte/Thinkstock; 11.3 © LiquidLibrary; 11.4 © Kristy-Anne Glubish/Design Pics Inc./Alamy Images; 11.5B © Photos.com; 11.9 © Jason DeCrow/AP Photos; 11.11 (top) © Andrew Haddon/ShutterStock Inc.; (bottom) © Coprid/ShutterStock Inc.; page 364 © Courtesy of Neil Malcom Winkelmann; 11.C © Thomas Barrat/ShutterStock, Inc.; 11.14 © Photodisc; 11.15 © Don Tremain/Photodisc/Getty Images

## Chapter 12

Opener © Image Source/age fotostock; 12.2 © Audie/ShutterStock, Inc.; 12.5 © Simon Fraser/Science Photo Library/Photo Researchers, Inc.; 12.9 © Linda Stelter/Birmingham News/Landov; 12.10 © Joe Skipper/Reuters/Landov; 12.11 © W. Ober/Visuals Unlimited; 12.12 © Mehau Kulyk/Science Photo Library/Photo Researchers, Inc.; 12.13 (photo) © Brand X Pictures/Thinkstock

## Chapter 13

Opener © Michel Spingler/AP Photos; 13.1 © Carolina Biological Supply Co./Visuals Unlimited, Inc.;

13.4A Courtesy of Dr. Giovanni Di Chiro, Neuroimaging Section, National Institute of Neurologic/National Cancer Institute; 13.4B © National Cancer Institute/Photodisc/Getty Images; 13.A (astragalus) Courtesy of John Martin; (Camellia) © Tracing Tea/ShutterStock Inc.; 13.5 Courtesy of the James M. Slater, M.D. Proton Treatment and Research Center, Loma Linda University Medical Center; 13.7A Courtesy of Robert Fingland; 13.8 © John Radcliffe Hospital/Photo Researchers, Inc.; 13.10 © Photodisc; 13.11 Courtesy of National Cancer Institute; page 441 © Stockbyte/Thinkstock

## Chapter 14

Opener © Mike Blake/Reuters/Landov; 14.A © Dr. Stanley Flegler/Visuals Unlimited; 14.1A © PhotoCreate/ShutterStock, Inc.; 14.6 Courtesy of CDC; 14.7 © Science Photo Library/Photo Researchers, Inc.; 14.8 Courtesy of James Gathany/CDC; 14.9 (top) © iStockphoto/Thinkstock; (bottom) Courtesy of Jim Gathany/CDC; 14.11 © Prof. S.H.E. Kaufman & Dr. J.R. Golecki/SPL/Photo Researchers, Inc.; 14.C © motorolka/ShutterStock, Inc.; 14.18 © BioPhoto Associates/Photo Researchers, Inc.; 14.19 Courtesy of National Cancer Institute; 14.21 © Courtesy Dr. Wiesner/CDC; 14.24 Courtesy of Dr. Gavin Hart and Dr. N. J. Fiumara/CDC; 14.26 © Visuals Unlimited; 14.28 © Oliver Meckes, Science Source/Photo Researchers, Inc.

## Chapter 15

Opener © Larry Beckner/Great Falls Tribune/AP Photos; 15.1 © Launette/AP Photos; page 503 © Martin Puddy/age fotostock; page 507 © STILLFX/ShutterStock, Inc.; 15.4 © Dr. Ken Greet/Visuals Unlimited; page 511 © Hamera Technologies/PhotoObjects.net/Thinkstock; page 512 © Mel Curtis/Photodisc/Getty Images; page 514 © LiquidLibrary; 15.6 © mauritius images/age fotostock; 15.7 Courtesy of Library of Congress, Prints and Photographs Division. [Reproduction number LC-DIG-ppmsca-11042]; page 519 © Monkey Business Images/Dreamstime.com; 15.8 © Schindler Family Photo/AP Photos; page 526 © David Kay/ShutterStock Inc.; 15.11 © Cheryl Casey/ShutterStock, Inc.

## Chapter 16

Opener © Aurora Photos/Alamy Images; 16.3 © Chitose Suzuki/AP Photos; 16.4 Courtesy of Tim McCabe/USDA NRCS; 16.5 © Imagechina/AP Photos; 16.6 © Peter Clark/ShutterStock, Inc.; 16.7A © Jupiterimages/Photos.com/Thinkstock; 16.7B © Chad Littlejohn/ShutterStock, Inc.

Unless otherwise indicated, all photographs and illustrations are under copyright of Jones & Bartlett Learning or have been provided by the authors.